LEGAL ASPECTS OF MIDWIFERY

THIRD EDITION

Bridgit Dimond

MA LLB DSA AHSM ACIA Barrister-at-law
Emeritus Professor of the University of Glamorgan, UK

Foreword by
Dr Robyn Phillips

Professional Adviser (Midwifery), Health Professions Wales

BfM **Books *for* Midwives**

Edinburgh   London   New York   Oxford   Philadelphia   St Louis   Sydney   Toronto   2006

BOOKS FOR MIDWIVES
An imprint of Elsevier Limited

First published 1994
Second Edition 2002
Reprinted 2003 (twice)
Third Edition 2006

ISBN 0 7506 8817 3

British Library Cataloguing in Publication Data
A catalogue record for this book is available from the British Library

Library of Congress Cataloging in Publication Data
A catalog record for this book is available from the Library of Congress

Knowledge and best practice in this field are constantly changing. As new research and experience broaden our knowledge, changes in practice, treatment and drug therapy may become necessary or appropriate. Readers are advised to check the most current information provided (i) on procedures featured or (ii) by the manufacturer of each product to be administered, to verify the recommended dose or formula, the method and duration of administration and contraindications. It is the responsibility of the practitioner, relying on their own experience and knowledge of the patient, to make diagnoses, to determine dosages and the best treatment for each individual patient, and to take all appropriate safety precautions.

To the fullest extent of the law, neither the publisher nor the editors assume any liability for any injury and/or damage.

The Publisher

Printed in Europe

Legal Aspects of Midwifery

For Elsevier:

Commissioning Editor: Mary Seager
Development Editor: Rebecca Nelemans
Project Manager: Emma Riley
Designer: Andy Chapman

for Bette

Contents

Foreword

I was delighted and honoured when Bridgit asked me to write the foreword to this third edition of her excellent book, *Legal Aspects of Midwifery*.

Professor Bridgit Dimond is a renowned expert on the legislation relating to healthcare. She has published extensively on the law and its application to many of the healthcare professions and also to specific aspects of care, for example, confidentiality and consent. Those who have had the good fortune to attend Professor Dimond's lectures, study days or workshops will appreciate the depth and vastness of her knowledge and her particular skills in relating this to clinical practice for a variety of professions. Professor Dimond has always been able to gain spontaneous interaction with participants; the law comes alive through her unique ability and commensurate skill in using discussion and questions to apply 'legal aspects' to practical clinical situations relevant to an individual or specific audience.

Similarly with this book, Professor Dimond engages the reader and makes the law and legal frameworks interesting and relevant through her comprehensive and practical coverage of the subject and sound use of case study examples. As in the previous edition, the arrangement of the book is in six discrete but connected areas, each with a clear introduction and outline. An updated explanation of the law and legislation in Chapter 1 places midwifery practice firmly in context and sets the scene for the chapters which follow. However, the book is also designed for the reader to be able to easily access individual sections and topic areas. In this third edition there are a number of new and updated areas which Professor Dimond outlines in her preface. All are fundamental to the scope of a midwife's practice, which is what makes this book such an essential reference. Underpinning 'every day' midwifery practice, however, are the chapters on the new Midwives Rules and Fitness to Practise Rules, together with new Nursing and Midwifery Council (NMC) standards for Local Supervising Authorities (LSA).

The role of midwives as independent, autonomous practitioners is strengthened by a clear understanding of how to practise within a legislative framework, as well as a professional regulatory one. Practising autonomously, whether self employed or employed within the National Health Service, requires the midwife to understand and use this knowledge to enhance, not inhibit, the delivery of safe care. Professor Dimond's clear and logical explanations, supported by helpful case study examples, facilitate all midwives, wherever they practise, to do so with confidence and competence. As Professor Dimond herself advocates, the aim of the book is not to frighten but to empower midwives to practise with confidence, knowing that the law is there to protect them as well as their clients.

This third edition of *Legal Aspects of Midwifery* continues to make an important contribution to midwifery education and practice and to maternity care in general. It enables midwives to understand the legal framework of their practice and to take into consideration the legal and ethical issues inherent within it. The book is a key source of information for midwives, students, other health professionals and also the lay reader. Midwives are indeed fortunate to have recourse to such a valuable and updated text on the law and its application to midwifery with which to underpin and support their practice.

Dr Robyn Phillips
Professional Adviser (Midwifery)
Health Professions Wales

Preface to the Third Edition

Some 5 years have elapsed since the Second Edition of this book was written and significant changes in the NHS and the laws relating to Midwifery Practice have occurred. The impact of the incorporation of the European Convention into the laws of the UK as a result of the Human Rights Act 1998, which came into force in England in October 2000, is now becoming clear. Other additions to the book include the New Midwives Rules, standards for Local Supervising Authorities (LSAs) and guidance by the Nursing and Midwifery Council (NMC) and new Fitness to Practise Rules, which came into force in August 2004. Chapter 12 is a new chapter on the laws relating to teenage pregnancy, since this presents many concerns to the midwife. Other inclusions are the Human Tissue Act 2004, the Mental Incapacity Act 2005, new Complaint Regulations 2004, which came into force in July 2004, the Female Genital Mutilation Act 2003, the Domestic Violence, Crime and Victims Act 2004, Health and Social Care (Community Health and Standards) Act 2003 and the Gender Recognition Act 2004.

Other developments include a revised and re-named NMC Code of Professional Conduct: standards for conduct, performance and ethics which includes a new clause on professional indemnity insurance cover. There are many recommendations from the National Institute for Health and Clinical Excellence (NICE) relevant to mid-wifery practice and their legal significance is considered in Chapter 13. Foundation NHS trusts are a new phenomenon and the Healthcare Commission replaces the Commission for Health Improvement. The significance of these and other Department of Health initiatives is explored.

ARRANGEMENT OF THE BOOK

The structure of the Second Edition has been retained. The book is divided into six discrete areas:

- Professional Issues: registration, education and the role of the statutory bodies, supervision, professional conduct proceedings and the Rules, Codes and the Scope of Professional Practice

- Client Rights: looking at issues from the client's perspective

- Litigation and Accountability: the personal and professional accountability of the midwife in the civil and criminal courts, and issues relating to health and safety laws

- Management Issues: the organisation of the NHS, employment law, the position of the independent midwife and the regulations relating to private maternity hospitals

– Statutory Provisions: relating to births, deaths, human fertilisation and embryology, abortion and other statutes

– Specific Situations: different aspects of the midwife's role including the midwife as teacher, researcher, and in relation to children and the mentally disordered.

My aim, as always, is not to frighten the reader, but to provide information which a midwife can use with confidence, knowing that the law is there to protect her and her clients.

Acknowledgements

I would like to thank all those hundreds of midwives who, by raising their concerns with me, have provided the situations and problems which this book aims to resolve. My special thanks go to Dorothy Walters, for using her contacts with colleagues and fellow Supervisors to direct me toward some of the issues they wanted to see covered in this book, and for being such a generous source of information and help. Also to Ruth Gammon for her helpful comments and Helene Shaw of the Department of Health. I would like to thank officers at the Royal College of Midwives and Royal College of Nursing, particularly Angela Perrett. I would also like to acknowledge the support and assistance of Robyn Phillips (who has provided a further Foreword), and that of her predecessor as Professional Officer for Midwives at the Welsh National Board, the late Ruth Davies, who was much loved and respected. I also wish to thank my family for their constant encouragement and Bette for her great support. It is to her that this book is dedicated.

The copyright of the Stationery Office for Statute and Statutory Instruments and of the various publishers for law reports and of the Clinical Negligence Scheme for Trusts and National Health Service Litigation Authority for their reports are acknowledged. The author wishes to thank them all for being able to quote from their works.

Abbreviations

ACAS	Advisory, Conciliation and Arbitration Service
ACMD	Advisory Council on the Misuse of Drugs
ACPC	Area Child Protection Committee
AID	Artificial Insemination by Donor
AIDS	Acquired Immune Deficiency Syndrome
AIH	Artificial Insemination by Husband
ARC	AIDS Related Condition
CCC	Conduct and Competence Committee
CHAI	Commission for Healthcare Audit and Inspection (Formerly CHI)
CHC	Community Health Council
CHI	Commission for Health Improvement (Replaced by CHAI)
CHRE	Council for Healthcare Regulatory Excellence (Formerly CRHP)
CPS	Crown Prosecution Service
CRHP	Council for the Regulation of Healthcare Professionals (now the CHRE)
DGH	District General Hospital
DH	Department of Health
DHA	District Health Authority
DHSS	Department of Health and Social Security (Divided in 1989 into DH and DSS)
DNA	Deoxyribonucleic Acid
DSS	Department of Social Security
EC	European Community
ECHR	European Court of Human Rights
ECR	Extra-Contractual Referral
EEC	European Economic Area
EWC	Expected Week of Confinement
EWTD	European Working Time Directive
FGM	Female Genital Mutilation
FHSA	Family Health Service Authority
GP	General Practitioner
HFEA	Human Fertilisation and Embryology Authority
ITP	Intention to Practise
IV	Intravenous(ly) or Intravenous infusion

IVF	*In vitro* Fertilisation
JP	Justice of the Peace
LREC	Local Research Ethics Committee
LSA	Local Supervising Authority
LSAMO	Local Supervising Authority Midwifery Officer
MCA	Maternity Care Assistant
MHAC	Mental Health Act Commission
MHRT	Mental Health Review Tribunal
MPP	Maternity Pay Period
NHS	National Health Service
NICE	National Institute for Clinical Excellence
NICE	(from 1 April 2005) National Institute for Health and Clinical Excellence
NMC	Nursing and Midwifery Council
NPfIT	National Programme for Information Technology
NSF	National Service Framework
PALS	Patient Advocacy and Liaison Services
PBC	Prudential Borrowing Code
PPC	Preliminary Proceedings Committee
PPI	Patient and Public Involvement
PREP	Post-Registration Education and Practice
RCM	Royal College of Midwives
RCOG	Royal College of Obstetricians and Gynaecologists
RHA	Regional Health Authority
RSCPHN	Registered Specialist Community Public Health Nurses
SCIG	Social Care Information Governance
SI	Statutory Instrument
SMS	Security Management Service
SOAD	Second Opinion Appointed Doctor
SoM	Supervisor of Midwives
TCM	Traditional Chinese Medicine
UKCC	United Kingdom Central Council for Nursing, Midwifery and Health Visiting
WHO	World Health Organization

Table of Cases

Table of Statutes

Statutory Instruments

European Directives

INTRODUCTION

In this Section, we explore how laws are formed and the structure of the legal system in the UK.

Chapter 1
THE LEGAL SYSTEM

WHAT IS THE LAW?

'It is against the law' is a powerful statement, and anyone making it should be able to declare the source of the law to which reference is being made. If the statement is accurate, then either an Act of Parliament/Statutory Instrument (known as a statute or 'legislation') or a decided case would be cited. (See the Glossary for further explanations of legal terms.)

LEGISLATION

Legislation consists both of Acts of Parliament (with approval by the Houses of Commons and Lords, and the Queen's signature) and directives and regulations emanating from the European Community, which we as a member state are required to implement and obey.

Legislation can be primary or secondary. Primary legislation consists of Acts of Parliament, known as statutes, which come into force at a date set either in the initial Act of Parliament or subsequently fixed by order of a Minister (i.e. by Statutory Instrument). The date of enforcement is often later than the date the Act is passed by the two Houses of Parliament and signed by the Crown.

The statute sometimes gives power to a Minister to enact more detailed laws, and this is known as secondary legislation. Regulations have to be laid before the Houses of Parliament and in certain circumstances have to receive express approval. Statutory Instruments which are quoted in the text are an example of this secondary legislation.

Section 60 of the Health Act 1999 gives power to Her Majesty to make by Order in Council provisions for the regulation of various health professions. The Order[1] relating to the establishment of the Nursing and Midwifery Council (NMC) in turn gives power to the NMC to make rules regulating the practice of midwifery (Article 40(1)). Under Article 45, the approval of the Privy Council shall be required for any exercise by the Council of a power to make rules under this Order.

DECIDED CASES

The other main source of law is 'the decisions of the courts'. This source is known as case law, or judge-made law, or the common law. The courts form a hierarchy and the highest court in this country is the House of Lords (different in composition from the House of Lords in Parliament, since only the law lords hear cases, not the bishops, hereditary peers and life peers who all sit in Parliament). If the House of Lords sets out a specific rule, then this is binding on all courts in the country, except itself, i.e. the House of Lords does not have to follow its own principles. A principle set out by a senior court is known as a precedent. Judges decide cases which may involve interpretation of Acts of Parliament, or situations where there does not appear to have been any enacted law or relevant case. Recent decisions of the House of Lords have included the Pinochet case[2] where it was held that a ruler of another state was subject to law and could be lawfully arrested while a request for extradition to another state was considered. Another decision[3] was the ruling that an adult who lacked mental competence to give consent to admission, could be admitted to a psychiatric hospital without being placed under the Mental Health Act 1983,[4] a decision which was subsequently overturned by the European Court of Human Rights in Strasbourg.[5]

Following the Hillsborough football disaster, the House of Lords had to rule on whether it was lawful to withdraw artificial feeding from a patient in a persistent vegetative state.[6] It held that artificial feeding for Tony Bland could cease, on the basis that that was in his best interests. (This case is considered in Ch. 9.)

Each decision of the courts is reported, so that lawyers and judges can refer to the case, and the principles it established (known as the *ratio decidendi*) can be applied to any matters in dispute. If there is a dispute between a case and a statute, the latter would take priority: judges have to follow an Act of Parliament. Parliament can enact legislation which would overrule a principle established in the courts.

Appeals can be made to the European Court of Justice in Luxembourg, which gives interpretations of European laws. Their decisions are binding on the courts of member states.

THE HUMAN RIGHTS ACT 1998

This country was a signatory of the European Convention in 1951 and accepted the articles on human rights. However, the Convention was not incorporated into our law at that time. If a person considered his or her rights had been infringed, then he or she had to take the case to Strasbourg, to the European Court of Human Rights, to argue the case there. Parliament has now passed the Human Rights Act 1998. This came into force on 2 October 2000 for England and Wales (in Scotland the Act came into force earlier, on devolution). It is discussed in detail in Chapter 6, and the

Articles of the European Convention on Human Rights, set out in Schedule 1 to the Human Rights Act 1998, can be found in Appendix One to this book.

The main features of the Human Rights Act 1998 are that it:
- requires all public authorities to implement the articles of the European Convention on Human Rights

- gives a right to anyone who alleges that a public authority has failed to respect those rights to bring an action in the courts of this country and

- enables judges who consider that legislation is incompatible with the Articles of the Convention to refer that legislation back to Parliament.

CHANGES TO THE LAW

Law is dynamic. As conflicts and disputes arise and are brought before the courts, the judges have to decide in the light of existing statutes and decided cases which are binding upon them, the principles which apply. In that sense there is always a law, the judges simply declare it. New legislation is enacted which may overrule existing case law, change existing statutes and statutory instruments or fill gaps created by technological developments. (See for example Ch. 27 and laws relating to embryology and genetic developments.)

EFFECT OF THE EUROPEAN COMMUNITY

Since the UK signed the Treaty of Rome in 1972, the UK has become one of the member states of the European Community. The effect of this is that the UK is now subject to the laws made by the Council of Ministers and the European Commission. In addition, secondary legislation of the European Community in the form of regulations is binding on the member states. Directives of the Community must be incorporated by Act of Parliament into the law of each member state. (See for example the European Directive 80/155/EEC, Article 4, which sets out the definition of the activities of a midwife and is considered in Ch. 2.)

CRIMINAL LAWS AND CIVIL LAWS

A major distinction in the law of the UK is that between criminal laws and civil laws.

CRIMINAL LAWS

These laws, mostly derived from statutes, create offences which can be followed by criminal proceedings in the form of a prosecution. An example of a statutory provi-

sion giving rise to criminal proceedings is Article 45 of the Nurses, Midwives
Health Visitors Order[7] which makes it a criminal offence for a person other th
registered midwife or doctor, or student of either, to attend a woman in childb
except in an emergency (see Ch. 25).

An example of case law which gives rise to criminal proceedings is the definition of
murder, which was set out in a case in the seventeenth century. Most of our criminal
laws are enforced by prosecutions brought by the Crown Prosecution Service, which
was created in 1985. Other bodies also have powers to prosecute in specific cases,
e.g. the Health and Safety Inspectorate, the National Society for the Prevention of
Cruelty to Children and Environmental Health Officers.

There are other criminal laws such as those created by Local Authority powers known
as by-laws, which create local offences. There is also a right of an individual to bring
a private prosecution, but this can be costly and of uncertain benefit.

CIVIL LAWS

These are laws (both statutory and case law) which enable citizens to claim remedies
against other citizens or organisations as a result of a civil wrong. A large group of
civil wrongs are known as torts, of which negligence is the main one, but the group
also includes action for breach of statutory duty, nuisance and defamation. Actions
for breach of contract are not included in the definition of tort.

An example of a statute which can give rise to civil action is the Congenital Disabilities
(Civil Liability) Act 1976, which gives a child who is born alive the right to sue in
respect of negligence which led to him or her suffering from a congenital defect.
(This is considered in Ch. 17.)

An example of a case which applies to civil proceedings is that of Whitehouse v.
Jordan[8] in which an obstetrician was sued for negligence on the grounds that he had
allegedly pulled too long and too hard in a trial of forceps. The House of Lords held
that an error of clinical judgement may or may not be evidence of negligence, and
that it had not been established that Dr Jordan failed to follow the reasonable standard of care required in the circumstances, based on the approved standard of practice at the time. (The case is considered in detail in Ch. 14.)

Some acts may be actionable as both a criminal offence and a civil wrong.
(For example, in Ch. 7, the action for trespass to the person is discussed.) This
action can be brought where treatment is given without the consent of the individual and in the absence of other factors which would be a defence to the action
(e.g. acting out of necessity). A trespass may however also be a criminal act of
assault, and there could be a prosecution in the criminal courts. It can be seen
from this that there is not necessarily a moral difference between a crime and a civil
wrong.

WHAT ABOUT ETHICS?

Some civil and criminal wrongs may also be ethically wrong. Some may not be considered as ethical issues. For example, failure to register the birth of a baby may not give rise to ethical issues if it has occurred simply from absent-mindedness. It would however be a criminal offence. In this book, we are concerned with the law and therefore there can be little discussion of ethical issues. However, the reader is referred to the Further Reading list at the end of this book, for sources on ethics in midwifery. Codes of Practice and conduct are not in themselves 'laws'. They do however provide guidance for professional practice, and could be used in evidence in civil or professional conduct proceedings to demonstrate that reasonable practice has not been followed. (This is further discussed in Ch. 5.)

LEGAL PERSONNEL

Lawyers in this country are trained as solicitors or barristers. The former, in the past, have had direct dealings with clients and arranged with barristers (known as Counsel) for the paperwork to be drafted and for representation of the client in court. Now, increasingly, solicitors are being trained for advocacy and have rights of presenting a case in court. Eventually this may lead to a single legal profession.

Solicitors and barristers share a common foundation training: either a law degree or success in the Common Professional Examination. Then would-be solicitors undertake practical training with a firm of solicitors, and take the Law Society's Part 2 examination, called the Legal Practice Course, while would-be barristers study for the Bar with an approved institution (such as the Council for Legal Education) and are then 'called' to the bar by the Inn of Court to which they belong. A barrister who wishes to practise must then undertake pupillage for a year where they are attached to a practising barrister. Senior barristers are eligible to 'take silk', i.e. they become Queen's Counsel (QC) appointed by the Queen on the basis of recommendations made by the Lord Chancellor.

LEGAL AID AND CONDITIONAL FEES

Major changes have been made to the legal aid system under the Access to Justice Act 1999.

Part I of the Act provides for two new schemes, replacing the existing legal aid scheme, to secure the provision of publicly-funded legal services for people who need them. It establishes a Legal Services Commission to run the two schemes, and enables the Lord Chancellor to give the Commission orders, directions and guidance about how it should exercise its functions. It requires the Commission to establish, maintain and develop a Community Legal Service. The Community Legal Service fund replaces the legal aid fund in civil and family cases. The Commission is also responsible for a Criminal Defence Service, which replaced the legal aid scheme in criminal cases. The scheme is intended to ensure that people suspected or accused of a crime are properly represented, while securing better value for money than is possible under the legal aid scheme. The Legal Services Commission is empowered to secure these services through contracts with lawyers in private practice, or by providing them through salaried defenders (employed directly by the Commission or by non-profit-making organisations established for the purpose).

Part II of the Access to Justice Act 1999 makes changes to facilitate the private funding of litigation. A scheme known as 'no win, no fee' or conditional fee system has been introduced. By this system, potential litigants can agree with lawyers terms on which they will be represented. Insurance cover is taken out to meet the expenses of witnesses and other costs arising, in case the action is lost. The 1999 Act amends the law on conditional fee agreements between lawyers and their clients; in particular it allows the additional fees payable to a solicitor in a successful case in a 'no win, no fee' agreement to be recovered from the other side. The Court of Appeal has agreed that the cost of taking out insurance at a reasonable premium could be recovered from the losing party.[9]

It is impossible in a work of this size to deal adequately with the complexities of the legal system and the procedures which are followed. The interested reader is therefore referred to the works in the list of Further Reading at the end of this book.

QUESTIONS AND EXERCISES

1. Look at the Glossary at the beginning of this book and identify the words and terms with which you are not familiar.

2. Try and arrange a visit to a court of law, and make notes of the procedure which is followed, the language used, the level of formality followed (e.g. in clothes which are worn) and the purpose of the proceedings. What preparations would you need to make if you were required to give evidence?

3. Look at Appendix 1 to this book which sets out Schedule 1 to the Human Rights Act 1999. Consider those Articles which would appear to be relevant to the practice of midwifery and the rights of the woman and discuss with colleagues what action needs to be taken to implement them. (Refer to Ch. 6 for further discussion on human rights.)

References

1 The Nursing and Midwifery Order 2001 Statutory Instrument 2002, No. 253.

2 R v. Evans and others *ex parte* Pinochet Ugarte. Times Law Report, 26 November 1998 HL.

3 R v. Bournewood Community and Mental Health NHS Trust *ex parte* L [1998] 1 All ER 634 HL.

4 R. v. Bournewood Community and Mental Health NHS Trust *ex parte* L The Times 30 June 1998; [1999] AC 458.

5 L. v United Kingdom (Application No 45508/99) Times Law Report, 19 October 2004.

6 Airedale NHS Trust v. Bland [1993] 1 All ER 821.

7 The Nurses, Midwives and Health Visitors Order 2001. Statutory Instrument 2002, No 253.

8 Whitehouse v. Jordan [1981] 1 All ER 267.

9 Callery v. Gray; Russell v. Pal Pak Corrugated Ltd. Times Law Report, 18 July 2001.

SECTION A

PROFESSIONAL ISSUES

In this Section, professional issues relating to midwifery practice are considered. The first chapter looks at the role of the NMC in the registration and education of midwives. The next chapter considers those aspects which relate to the Supervisor of Midwives and the Local Supervising Authority. The last two chapters consider the regulations which relate to fitness to practise proceedings and the nature of the Midwives Rules and Standards, the Code of professional conduct, standards for conduct, performance and ethics and other NMC (formerly UKCC) guidance.

Chapter 2
MIDWIFERY
PROFESSIONAL REGULATION

This chapter considers the following topics:

- What is a midwife?

- Role constitution and function of the statutory bodies

- The Midwifery Committee of the NMC

- Registration and false claims to registration

- Pre-registration education and training

- Post-registration education and practice (PREP)

WHAT IS A MIDWIFE?

The origin of the term in Middle and Old English means 'with a woman' (Middle and Old English mid = with; Middle English wif = a woman). Churchill's medical directory gives a present day meaning as 'a healthcare worker who may or may not be formally trained and is not a physician, that delivers babies and provides associated maternal care'.

The same directory defines midwifery as 'the practice of obstetrics by a midwife', a definition which may not be universally accepted in view of the present debate concerning the separate role of obstetricians and midwives in childbirth.

The definition adopted by the World Health Organization from the International Conference of Midwives (1972) and the International Federation of Gynaecologists and Obstetricians (1973), as adapted in 1991 and 1992 is set out at the end of the Midwives Rules and Standards.[1]

The definition includes the following:

She must be able to give the necessary supervision, care and advice to women during pregnancy, labour and the postpartum period; to conduct deliveries on her own responsibility and to care for the newborn and the infant.

Care includes:

- preventative measures

- the detection of abnormal conditions in mother and child

- the procurement of medical assistance

- the execution of emergency measures in the absence of medical help

- health counselling and education, not only for the women, but also within the family and community

- antenatal education and preparation for parenthood, certain areas of gynaecology, family planning and child care.

She may practise in hospitals, clinics, health units, domiciliary conditions or in any other service.

The definition adopted by the EU Second Midwifery Directive[2] 80/155/EEC/ Article 4 on activities of a midwife is also set out at the end of the NMC Midwives Rules and Standards and is shown in Box 2.1.

Box 2.1 Activities of a midwife laid down by the EC in the Second Midwifery Directive

Member states shall ensure that midwives are at least entitled to take up and pursue the following activities:

- to provide sound family planning information and advice

- to diagnose pregnancies and monitor normal pregnancies; to carry out examinations necessary for the monitoring of the development of normal pregnancies

- to prescribe or advise on the examinations necessary for the earliest possible diagnosis of pregnancies at risk

- to provide a programme of parenthood preparation and a complete preparation for childbirth including advice on hygiene and nutrition

- to care for and assist the mother during labour and to monitor the condition of the fetus in utero by the appropriate clinical and technical means

- to conduct spontaneous deliveries including where required an episiotomy and in urgent cases a breech delivery

- to recognise the warning signs of abnormality in the mother or infant which necessitate referral to a doctor and to assist the latter where appropriate; to take the necessary emergency measures in the doctor's absence, in particular the

▶

manual removal of the placenta, possibly followed by manual examination of the uterus

– to examine and care for the newborn infant; to take all initiatives which are necessary in case of need and to carry out where necessary immediate resuscitation

– to care for and monitor the progress of the mother in the postnatal period and to give all the necessary advice to the mother on infant care to enable her to ensure the optimum progress of the newborn infant

– to carry out the treatment prescribed by a doctor

– to maintain all necessary records.

And as amended by the European Union Directive 89/594/EEC:

– advising of pregnant women, involving at least 100 prenatal examinations

– supervision and care of at least 40 women in labour

– the student should personally carry out at least 40 deliveries; where this number cannot be reached owing to the lack of available women in labour, it may be reduced to minimum of 30, provided that the student participates actively in 20 further deliveries

– active participation with breech deliveries. Where this is not possible because of lack of breech deliveries, practice may be in a simulated situation

– performance of episiotomy and initiation into suturing. Initiation shall include theoretical instruction and clinical practice. The practice of suturing includes suturing the wound following an episiotomy and a simple perineal laceration. This may be in a simulated situation if absolutely necessary

– supervision and care of 40 women at risk in pregnancy, or labour or postnatal period

– supervision and care (including examination) of at least 100 postnatal women and healthy newborn infants

– observation and care of the newborn requiring special care including those born pre-term, post-term, underweight or ill

– care of women with pathological conditions in the fields of gynaecology and obstetrics

– initiation into care in the field of medicine and surgery. Initiation shall include theoretical instruction and clinical practice.

The NMC has updated the standards for proficiency for pre-registration midwifery education.[3]

The essential competencies required in midwifery practice were considered at an International Confederation of Midwives in 2003.[4]

New rules relating to education, registration and registration appeals came into force in August 2004.[5] This Order in Council sets out the educational requirements for registration and re-registration as follows:

(1) Where an approved programme of education leads to the award of a qualification listed in the Annex to the Nursing Directive or Midwifery Directive, it shall comply with the training requirements in Articles 1 and 2 of the Second Nursing Directive or Articles 1 and 3 of the Second Midwifery Directive (the requirements of which are reproduced in paras 1, 2(b), 3, 4, A and B of Schedule 1 and paras 1, 2, 3, 4, A and B of Schedule 2).

(2) The requirements for entry to an approved programme of education shall include the requirements of Article 1.2(a) of the Second Nursing Directive or Article 1.2 of the second Midwifery Directive (the requirements of which are reproduced in para 2(a) of Schedule 1 and para 2 of Schedule 2).

(3) A registrant must undertake such continuing professional development as the Council shall specify in standards in accordance with Article 19(1) of the Order.

(4) A person applying for registration, renewal or re-admission

(a) who first applies for registration more than 5 years after being awarded an approved qualification;

(b) whose registration has lapsed and who applies for readmission to the register, unless in the 5 years before the date of her application for readmission to the register she has practised for at least 750 hours; or

(c) who, subject to para (5) has practised for less than 450 hours in the 3 years preceding the date of an application for renewal of registration,

shall undertake such education and training or gain such experience as the Council specifies in standards in accordance with Article 19(3) of the Order.

(5) Until 2 years after the coming into force of these rules, a person may satisfy para (4)(c) if she has practised for 750 hours or more in the 5 years preceding the date of her application.

Under the European Nursing and Midwifery Qualifications Designation Order of Council 2004,[6] the recognised qualifications for nurses and midwives in other EU states are set out. Part 2 sets out the recognised Midwifery Diplomas under the EC Nursing[7] and Midwifery Directive.[8]

There is no doubt that in relation to normal births, the duties set out above are extremely comprehensive. Although midwives in this country have not enjoyed a smooth path historically, as 'The Art and Science of Midwifery' by Louise Silverton[9] shows, they do at present enjoy a higher status and protection in law than their colleagues in America.[10] Their present situation in law contrasts greatly with the limited recognition of the scope of midwifery in certain American states quoted by Louise Silverton.[11] She cites the situation in California, where the state law which governs the practice of nurse-midwives prohibits them from using any instrument to assist the birth of the child (with the exception of those used to clamp and cut the umbilical cord) or from prescribing or administering, either before or during birth, drugs or medications other than laxatives or disinfectants. Reference could also be made to the gripping thriller by Chris Bohjalian, 'Midwives',[12] a novel about a midwife in Vermont and her prosecution following a home delivery, as a contrast between the legal position of midwives in that state of the USA and in the UK.

MIDWIVES IN THE UK

The Nursing and Midwifery Council statistical analysis of the register for 1 April 2003 to 31 March 2004[13] shows that there were 43 636 midwives qualified to practise on the Register. The numbers of midwives with an effective registration were:

Women	33 578
Men	108
Not recorded	1

The NMC tentatively suggested that the downward trend of numbers of practising midwives may have been reversed, though one cannot discern too much from one year's figures.

The age breakdown for practising midwives showed that:

Below 25	1.61%
25–29	5.85%
30–39	26.88%
40–49	33.94%
50–54	11.62%
over 55	15.6%

The NMC makes the comment that these figures show that a greater proportion of midwives are under 50 (76%) than is the case for the Register as a whole (73%). However, it also shows a smaller proportion under 30 (7.5%) than for the Register as a whole (10.5%).

The NMC also notes that the long-term trend has seen a shift away from full-time working in midwifery towards part-time working. It is not known how many midwives have several part-time posts.

The vast majority of practising midwives work in an NHS trust (including community): only 44 are identified as working in private practice; 511 work for an agency; 105 for a family practitioner; 1529 work in a midwifery bank; 694 are identified as midwifery teachers/lecturers and 468 work for a private institution. (Many midwives may of course operate in more than one of these fields.)

ROLE CONSTITUTION AND FUNCTION OF THE STATUTORY BODIES

In April 2002, the Nursing and Midwifery Council began its work, taking over from the UKCC as the registration body for nurses, midwives and health visitors. It had existed in shadow form since May 2001 when the Department of Health announced the appointment of the President, members and alternates. Existing guidance from the UKCC will remain effective until such time as the NMC replaces it.

The events leading up to the establishment of the NMC were as follows:

The Government commissioned an independent review of the Nurses, Midwives and Health Visitors Act 1997 from JM Consulting Ltd. Its report was published in February 1999. The Government accepted its main recommendations, that the UKCC and the four National Boards should be replaced by a smaller, more strategic Nursing and Midwifery Council with stronger lay input and ultimate ownership of the setting and monitoring of standards of training and conduct. Following publication of the Department of Health's Modernising Regulation consultation document, draft orders were published in April 2001 and, after a further consultation period, came into force in April 2002.[14]

The constitution of the NMC is shown in Box 2.2.

**Box 2.2 Constitution of the NMC
(Schedule 1 Part 1 to the Orders in Council)**

The Council shall consist of:

– 12 members who are appointed by the Council on being elected under the electoral scheme ('Registered members')

– 11 members who are appointed by the Privy Council ('lay members')

Alternate members

▶

In addition the Council shall appoint 12 members of the Council (referred to as 'alternate members') who have been elected under the election scheme, who may not attend or vote at a Council meeting unless their corresponding registrant member is unable to do so.

THE ELECTION SCHEME

The details for this are set out in Para. 2 of Schedule 1. The Council has the power to provide rules for the scheme but the scheme must provide for:

(a) A person seeking election as a registrant member or alternate member:

    i.   is registered in the part of the register for which he seeks election but no person may be elected for more than one part of the register at a time

    ii. in respect of a national constituency, lives or works wholly or mainly in that national constituency

    iii. is not the subject of any allegation, investigation or proceedings concerning his fitness to practise; and

    iv. is wholly or mainly engaged in the practice, teaching or management of the profession in respect of which he is registered and seeks election or in research in those fields.

(b) at least one registrant member and one alternate member shall be appointed from each part of the register and the number of members from each part shall be equal

(c) at least one member shall be elected from each of the national constituencies for each part of the register

(d) a person may only vote:

    i.   in respect of one part of the register

    ii. for candidates who represent a part of the register in which he is registered at the time of the election and

    iii. for a candidate seeking election for the constituency in which he wholly or mainly lives or works or, if he does not wholly or mainly live or work in any constituency, the constituency he has selected or to which he has been assigned in accordance with prescribed criteria

(e) a person may vote even if he is residing or works outside the UK

(f) where someone ceases to be a member or alternate member a replacement may be appointed by the Council.

LAY MEMBERS

The Privy Council, after consulting such persons as it considers appropriate, shall appoint lay members from among persons who are not and never have been on the Register, and who have such qualifications, interests and experience as, in the opinion of the Privy Council, will be of value to the Council in the performance of its functions. At least one of the PC appointed members shall be appointed from each country of the UK and that member shall live or work (wholly or mainly) in the country concerned.

TENURE OF MEMBERS

Each member's term of office will be for a period of 4 years.

PRESIDENT

The first president was appointed after open competition. In future, members of the Council shall elect the president from among themselves for a term of 4 years.

STANDING ORDERS

The Council may make standing orders in respect of the Council, its committees and sub-committees, but not in respect of any of the Practice Committees.

The functions of the NMC, which under Schedule 3 Para. 8(2) of the Health Act 1999 cannot be delegated to any other body, are shown in Box 2.3.

Box 2.3 Functions of the NMC which cannot be delegated

- Keeping the register of members admitted to practise

- Determining the standards of education and training for admission to practise

- Giving advice about standards of conduct and performance

- Administering procedures (including making rules) relating to misconduct, unfitness to practise and similar matters.

PERFORMANCE OF FUNCTIONS

Under Article 3(4) and (5) of the Order, the Council is required to follow several stipulations in performing its functions. These are shown in Box 2.4.

Box 2.4 NMC performance of functions

The main objective of the Council in exercising its functions shall be to safeguard the health and wellbeing of persons using or needing the services of registrants.

(a) In exercising its functions, the Council shall: (a) Have proper regard to the interests of all registrants and prospective registrants and persons referred to in para. (4) in each of the countries of the UK and to any differing considerations applying to the professions to which this Order applies and to groups within them and cooperate wherever reasonably practicable with:

    i.   employers and prospective employers of registrants

    ii. persons who provide, assess or fund education or training for registrants or prospective registrants, or who propose to do so

    iii. persons who are responsible for regulating or coordinating the regulation of other health and social care professionals, or of those who carry out activities in connection with services provided by those professions or the professions regulated under this Order.

The NMC is also required to inform and educate registrants and the public about its work (Article 3(13) of the Order).

Before establishing any standards or giving guidance, the Council shall consult representatives of any group of persons it considers appropriate, including, as it sees fit, representatives of:

– registrants or classes of registrants

– employers of registrants

– users of the services of registrants

– persons providing, assessing or funding education or training for registrants and prospective registrants.

The Council shall publish any standards it establishes and any guidance it gives (Article 3(15)).

POWERS OF THE COUNCIL

The powers of the Council are set out in Paragraph 15 of Schedule 1 Part 1 of the NMC Order 2001.[15] They include power to borrow, to appoint such staff as it may determine necessary, to pay salaries, pensions, fees and allowances for members and to set up or abolish any of its committees except statutory committees. Where it appears to the Council that any statutory committee is failing to perform its functions adequately, the Council may give a direction as to the proper performance of those functions. Where it has given directions but is satisfied that the committee has failed to comply with the direction, the Council may exercise any power of that committee or do any act or other thing authorised to be done by that committee.

STATUTORY COMMITTEES

These are the following:

- Investigating Committee

- Conduct and Competence Committee

- Health Committee

- Midwifery Committee.

The Investigating Committee, the Conduct and Competence Committee and the Health Committee are also referred to as the 'Practice Committees'. Their constitution and functions are explained below.

THE MIDWIFERY COMMITTEE OF THE NMC

Part VIII of the Order for the NMC sets out the statutory provisions relating to midwifery. Article 41 states that the role of the Midwifery Committee shall be to advise the Council, at the Council's request or otherwise, on any matter affecting midwifery. The Council is required to 'consult the Midwifery Committee on the exercise of its functions in so far as it affects midwifery including any proposal to make rules under Article 42'. Article 42 is shown in Box 2.5.

Box 2.5 Article 42

1. In addition to its functions under other provisions in this Order, the Council shall by rules regulate the practice of midwifery and the rules may in particular:

▶

(a) Determine the circumstances in which and the procedure by means of which a midwife may be suspended from practice

(b) require midwives to give notice of their intention to practise to the Local Supervising Authority (LSA) for the area in which they intend to practise

(c) require midwives to attend courses of instruction in accordance with the rules.

2. If rules are made requiring midwives to give the notice referred to in 1(b) above, the LSA shall inform the Council of any notices given to it under those rules.

Rules were created under these provisions in 2004[16] and together with the role of the Local Supervising Authority under Article 43 are discussed in Chapter 3.

The NMC has the power to make provision by standing orders for the composition, members, quorum, procedure, standards for the attendance and performance of members and the performance of the functions of the Midwifery Committee. The Chairman is required to be a member of Council and the majority of members must be practising midwives. The Council must have regard to the guidance issued by the Commissioner for Public Appointments when selecting non-Council members for the Committee. No person who is a member of the Council or the Midwifery Committee by virtue of his membership of any profession may take part in any proceedings of the Committee in any period during which he is the subject of any investigations, proceedings or a determination against him concerning his fitness to practise his profession. The powers of the Midwifery Committee may be exercised even though there is a vacancy among its members. No proceedings of the Midwifery Committee shall be invalidated by any defect in the appointment of a member.

REGISTRATION

Under Article 4, the NMC is required to appoint a Registrar to hold office for such period and on such terms as the Council may determine and who shall have such functions as the Council may direct. Article 5 requires the Council to establish and maintain a register of qualified nurses and midwives. The Council shall from time to time establish the standards of proficiency necessary to be admitted to the different parts of the Register, being standards it considers necessary for safe and effective practice under that part of the Register.

The Register shall show, in relation to each registrant, such address and other details as the Council may prescribe.

The Register may be divided into such parts as the Privy Council may by order determine, on a proposal by the Council or otherwise (Article 6(1)). Each part shall have a designated title indicative of different qualifications and different kinds of education or training, and a registered professional is entitled to use the title corresponding to the part of the Register in which he is registered. Rules can be made under Article 7 for the keeping of the Register.

A new Register came into being on 1 August 2004. The new register replaces the earlier 15 parts with three: nurses, midwives and a new category of registered specialist community public health nurses (RSCPHN). Other changes introduced in August 2004 include:

- The nurses' part of the register has two sub-parts: one for current first level registered nurses, and one for current second level registered nurses
- Specialisms such as adult nursing and mental health no longer have separate parts but are recorded on a nurse's register entry
- The midwives' part is open to all those who hold a midwifery qualification
- All health visitors are automatically recorded as RSCPHNs
- The addition of other categories such as school nurses and occupational health nurses is being phased in
- New entrants and those renewing their registration will have to provide declarations of good health and good character. (This is considered in Ch. 4.)

ACCESS TO THE REGISTER

The Council shall make the Register available for inspection by members of the public at all reasonable times and shall publish the Register in such a manner and at such times as it considers appropriate (Article 8).

REGISTRATION

Under Article 9, a person seeking admission to a part of the Register shall be entitled to be registered in that part if the application is made in the prescribed form and manner and the applicant:

(a) satisfies the Registrar that he/she holds an approved qualification awarded:

  i. within such period not exceeding 5 years, ending with the date of the application, as may be prescribed; or

  ii. before the prescribed period mentioned above and he has met such requirements as to additional education, training, and experience as the Council may specify under Article 19(3)

(b) satisfies the Registrar in accordance with the Council's requirements mentioned in Article 5 that he is capable of safe and effective practice as nurse or midwife and

(c) has paid the prescribed fee.

RENEWAL OF REGISTRATION

Under Article 10, provisions for renewal of registration and readmission require the applicant to satisfy the Registrar, in addition to other requirements, that he has met any prescribed requirements for continuing professional development within the prescribed time.

Under Article 11, visiting EEA (European Economic Area) nurses and midwives are deemed to be registered.

PRE-REGISTRATION EDUCATION AND TRAINING

Article 13 defines what is meant by an approved qualification. The definition is shown in Box 2.6.

Box 2.6 Approved qualification (Article 13)

For the purpose of this Order, a person is to be regarded as having an approved qualification if:

(a) he has a qualification awarded in the UK which has been approved by the Council as attesting to the standard of proficiency it requires for admission to the part of the Register in respect of which he is applying

(b) he is an EEA national and has a qualification of the kind mentioned in Article 14; or

(c) he has, elsewhere than in the UK, undergone training in nursing or midwifery and either:

    i. holds a qualification which the Council is satisfied attests to a standard of proficiency comparable to that attested by a qualification referred to in sub-paragraph (a); or

    ii. the Council is not so satisfied, but the applicant has undergone in the UK or elsewhere such additional training and experience as satisfies the Council,

---

following any test of competence as it may require him to take, that he has the requisite standard of proficiency for admission to the part of the register in respect of which he is applying; and in either case

iii. he is not an EEA national or exempt person and he satisfies prescribed requirements as to knowledge of English.

The NMC shall determine procedures to assess whether qualifications granted by institutions outside the UK and experience of practice outside the UK are of a comparable standard to those approved inside the UK and shall, where it sees fit, keep a list of comparable qualifications which it shall keep under review.

EDUCATION AND TRAINING

Article 15 gives the responsibility to the Council from time to time to establish:

(a) the standards of education and training necessary to achieve the standards of proficiency it has established under Article 5(2)

(b) the requirements to be satisfied for admission to, and continued participation in, such education and training which may include requirements as to good health and good character.

These standards shall be set out in rules made by the Council and shall include such matters as the outcomes to be achieved by that education and training. The Council is required to ensure that universities and other bodies concerned with such education and training are notified of the NMC's standards and requirements and take appropriate steps to ensure that these standards and requirements are met. The information which the Council must give to any institution providing the education, training or test of competence is set out in Article 17.

Article 18 covers the refusal or withdrawal of approval of courses, qualifications and institutions.

Under Article 19, the Council may make rules requiring registered nurses and midwives to undertake such continuing professional development as it shall specify in standards. The rules may, in particular, make provision with respect to registrants who fail to comply with any requirements of the rules including provision for their registration to cease to have effect.

Under Article 20, the National Assembly for Wales may create or designate a body with which the Council may enter into any such arrangements as are referred to in

Article 15(6) of the Order in order to perform its functions under Article 15(5)(b) in respect of the standards established under Article 15(1) or 19(4) or (6).

VISITORS

The Council may appoint persons (Visitors) to visit any place at which any relevant education and training, examinations or test of competence is given or to be given (Article 16).

REQUIREMENTS FOR PRE-REGISTRATION MIDWIFERY PROGRAMMES NMC CIRCULAR[17]

Standards are set by the NMC covering the following topics:

Standards for the proficiency for pre-registration midwifery programmes of education

Standards for the Lead Midwife for Education
1. Appointment of the Lead Midwife for Education
2. Development, delivery and management of midwifery programmes of education
3. Signing the supporting declaration for good health and good character

Standards for admission to, and continued participation in, pre-registration midwifery programmes
4. Age of entry
5. General entry requirements
6. Interruption in pre-registration midwifery programmes of education
7. Admission with advanced standing
8. Transfer between approved educational institutions

Standards for the structure and nature of pre-registration midwifery programmes
9. Academic standards of programme
10. Length of programme
11. Student support
12. Balance between clinical practice and theory
13. Supernumerary status
14. Assessment strategy

Standards of education to achieve the NMC standards of proficiency
This sets out guiding principles and the international definition of a midwife and the Second Midwifery Directive (see Box 2.1 above).

15. Standards of education to achieve the NMC standards of proficiency.

The standards reflect the requirements of the EC Midwifery Directives.[18]

POST-REGISTRATION EDUCATION AND PRACTICE (PREP)

The United Kingdom Central Council had published, in March 1994, the standards it had set in relation to post-registration education and practice for registered practitioners. A handbook was published in 2001 which was revised by the NMC in 2002 and again in August 2004[19] to bring it in line with the Nursing and Midwifery Order 2001. The two PREP standards set by the NMC are shown in Box 2.7.

Box 2.7 PREP standards

The PREP (practice) standard: you must have worked in some capacity by virtue of your nursing and midwifery qualification during the previous 5 years for a minimum of 100 days (750 h), or have successfully undertaken an approved return to practice course.

The PREP (continuing professional development) standard: you must have undertaken and recorded your continuing professional development (CPD) over the 3 years prior to the renewal of your registration. All registered nurses, midwives have been required to comply with this standard since April 1995. Since April 2000, registrants need to have declared on their Notification of Practice (NOP) form that they have met this requirement when they renew their registration. The PREP CPD standard requires:

- At least 5 days or 35 h of learning activity relevant to your practice during the 3 years prior to your renewal of registration

- Maintain a personal professional profile (PPP) of your learning activity

- Comply with any request from the NMC to audit how you have met these requirements.

IMPLICATIONS OF PREP FOR MIDWIVES

Midwives were originally the only group of practitioners registered by the UKCC who had statutorily to comply with minimum standards of post-registration training and education. This has now been extended to all registrants. The requirement of a personal professional profile underlines the emphasis on the practitioner being responsible for her own development and competence. It is part of the philosophy set out in the Code of Professional Conduct, standards for conduct, performance and ethics to be updated by the NMC in 2005 (see Ch. 5) which requires the practitioner to be accountable and responsible for the development of her own professional practice. Examples given in the PREP handbook of PREP (CPD) learning for midwives include direct client care using structured/formal learning and direct client care using unstructured/informal learning.

Many different schemes for the structure of the personal professional profile have been marketed.

ADVANCED MIDWIFERY AND NURSING PRACTICE

The UKCC had recognised that many practitioners would undertake additional studies in pursuit of advanced midwifery and nursing practice and such studies were likely to be at Masters level. The Council did not, however, at that stage, propose a formal preparation and qualification with explicit links with the Council's register for advanced midwifery practice. Initially, it was not the intention of the UKCC to include advanced midwifery practice in its standards for specialist practice as part of the post-registration education and practice proposals. The UKCC in 1997 stated:

'The Council recognises that many practitioners will undertake additional studies in pursuit of advanced midwifery practice and such studies are likely to be at Masters level. The Council does not, however, at this stage, propose a formal preparation and qualification with explicit links with the Council's Register. Many midwives hope that this is only for the immediate short term and that eventually there will be formal recognition for the skills to be acquired through advanced midwifery practice by Council itself'.[20]

The UKCC considered that advanced practice was not about specific tasks but involved a broader concept of nursing, midwifery and health visiting, an important part of which is advancing the practice of others. In 1998 and 1999 the UKCC carried out a series of consultations about higher level practice and launched pilot studies. There was a general feeling amongst many midwives, reflected in RCM reports, that midwives already practised at a 'higher level'.[21] In 2000, the UKCC received a report on the possibility of measuring higher level practice,[22] which the Midwifery Committee of the UKCC felt was not entirely appropriate to midwifery practice. The UKCC found a survey of maternity service users supported the idea of higher level practice for midwives.[23]

The concept of advanced midwifery practice is analysed by Sookhoo and Butler (1999).[24] The authors emphasise that advanced practice in midwifery is not synonymous with extending the role of the midwife, but about developing midwifery practice in order to enhance quality of care. They suggest from their study that advanced midwifery practice requires an expertise associated with skills and knowledge to enable the provision of holistic client-orientated care, and any programmes leading to advanced midwifery practitioner status should be client-centred as opposed to organisation-centred. Following their definition, it would appear that it should be part of the professional development of every midwife to secure advanced practice. Undoubtedly, the new status of Consultant midwife is linked to the concept of advanced practice.

In April 2001, the UKCC published a document bringing together all its guidance relating to specialist practice, preparatory to providing further clarification of the UKCC standards for specialist practice.[25] This covers the areas shown in Box 2.8.

Box 2.8 UKCC standards for specialist practice

– PREP

– Recording the qualification of specialist practice

– Transitional arrangements 1.11.95–31.10.98

– Preparation for specialist practice

Standards for specialist community nursing education and practice

– General practice nursing

– Community mental health nursing

– Community learning disabilities nursing

– Public health nursing/health visiting

– Occupational health nursing

– Community nursing in the home/district nursing

– School nursing

Annexe 1 Health visitor training rules

Annexe 2 Parts of the UKCC Register

There has been no statement by the NMC on advanced midwifery practice but it is understood that at the time of writing its Midwifery Committee is considering the issue.

PUBLIC INVOLVEMENT AND THE NMC

The UKCC published its strategy for public involvement in 2000,[26] which emphasised that the main function of the Council was to protect the public through professional standards and therefore it was only right that the public should be involved in all aspects of its work. The NMC has embraced this policy,[27] stating the importance of involving the public in its work. It has established a Public Involvement Working Group (PIWG) to review and update the strategy set out by the UKCC, working with other health and social care regulators to promote public involvement. The public are involved in the following areas of the NMC work: 11 out of 23 voting members of Council are lay people; lay people are involved in fitness to practise hearings; an independent reference (which acts as a sounding board when policy work and ideas are at an early stage) which includes lay members from a wide variety of backgrounds. The NMC is also considering how patients might be involved in its work.

THE FUTURE

August 2004 marked a watershed in the history of the midwifery profession with the introduction of a new Registrar, the publication of the new Midwives Rules and Standards, and new Fitness to Practise Procedures introduced. The NMC is now well established and has begun to stamp its own character on registered practitioners within its statutory framework and is taking further the work of regulation and protecting the public.

QUESTIONS AND EXERCISES

1. If you were to stand for election to the NMC, what duties would you expect to undertake?

2. To what extent do you consider the Midwifery Committee is able to protect the educational and practice standards of registered midwives?

3. The National Boards were abolished at the end of March 2002. Who now undertakes the functions which they formerly carried out?

4. You are now required to provide declarations of good health and good character when re-registering as an NMC registered practitioner. How would you define those terms?

References

1 NMC Midwives Rules and Standards. August 2004 incorporating Nursing and Midwifery Council (Midwives) Rules Order of Council 2004 Statutory Instrument 2004/1764.

2 Second EC Midwifery Directive 80/155/ECC as amended by Directive 89/594/EEC.

3 Nursing and Midwifery Council. Standards for proficiency for pre-registration midwifery education August 2004 (replacing the UKCC. 2000. Requirements for pre-registration midwifery programmes. Registrar's Letter 25/2000).

4 Fullerton J, Severino R, Brogan K., et al. The International Confederation of Midwives' study of essential competencies of midwifery practice. Midwifery 2003; 19(3):174–190.

5 The Nursing and Midwifery Council. (Education, Registration and Registration Appeals) Rules Order of Council 2004 SI 2004 No. 1767.

6 European Nursing and Midwifery Qualifications Designation Order of Council 2004 S I 2004 No. 1766.

7 EC Directive 77/452 (the Nursing Directive).

8 EC Directive 80/154 (the Midwifery Directive).

9 Silverton L. The Art and Science of Midwifery. Hemel Hempstead: Prentice Hall; 1993.

10 Bryce R. Five women in Lost Angeles were facing up to six years in prison for operating an independent birthing centre. The US has no national qualification standards for lay midwives (as distinct from certified nurse-midwives) so their work is regulated by individual states. The Guardian, 26 July 1993; 31.

11 Silverton L. The enhanced role of the midwife. In: Hunt G, Wainwright P, eds. Expanding the role of the nurse. Oxford: Blackwell Scientific Publications; 1994:151–161.

12 Bohjalian C. Midwives: a novel. New York: Vintage Contemporaries; 1998.

13 The Nursing and Midwifery Council. Statistical Analysis of the Register, 1 April 2003–31 March 2004. NMC; December 2004.

14 The Nursing and Midwifery Order 2001, Statutory Instrument 2002 No 253.

15 The Nursing and Midwifery Order 2001, Para. 15 of Schedule 1, Part 1.

16 Nursing and Midwifery Council (Midwives) Rules Order of Council 2004, Statutory Instrument 2004/1764.

17 Nursing and Midwifery Council Standards for proficiency for pre-registration midwifery education August 2004 (replacing the UKCC. 2000. Requirements for pre-registration midwifery programmes. Registrar's Letter 25/2000).

18 EC Midwifery Directives 80/154/ECC; 80/155/ECC as amended by Directive 89/594/EEC.

19 Nursing and Midwifery Council. PREP Handbook, revised edition. NMC; August 2004.

20 UKCC 1997. Registrar's Letter: The Council's decision on PREP and advanced practice. London: UKCC; 1997.

21 Anderson T. Midwives already practise at a higher level. Comment on Royal College of Midwives Report: Higher Level Midwives – who needs them? Practising Midwife 1999; 2(3):4–5.

22 UKCC. Future work on a higher level of practice to be part of the wider post-registration framework: UKCC Council Report. London: UKCC; 2001.

23 UKCC. Users of midwifery services support the idea of higher level practice for midwives. London: UKCC; 2000.

24 Sookhoo ML and Butler MS. An analysis of the concept of advanced midwifery practice. Br J Midwifery 1999; 7(11):690–693.

25 UKCC. Standards for specialist education and practice. London: UKCC; 2001.

26 UKCC. Strategy for public involvement. London: UKCC; 2000.

27 Nursing and Midwifery Council News, October 2004.

Chapter 3
MIDWIFERY SUPERVISION

Midwives are unique among health professionals in having a system of supervision prescribed by statute. It was initiated under the Midwives' Act 1902 which set up medical and non-medical Supervisors of Midwives. No specific qualifications were required for the latter and this defect was addressed under the Midwives' Act 1936, which required that Supervisors of Midwives had adequate experience of midwifery. The present arrangements for midwifery supervision are set up under the Health Act 1999 and the Orders in Council made under that Act which amend the Nurses, Midwives and Health Visitors Act 1997. Further modifications result from the new Midwives Rules which came into force in August 2004.[1] The NMC has provided guidance on the Rules.[2] Reference should be made to Developments in the Supervision of Midwives edited by Mavis Kirkham for an overview of supervision.[3] The English National Board issued guidelines for midwives on the statutory supervision of midwives which clarified the role of the Supervisor.[4] This has now been updated by the NMC.[5]

Some acknowledge supervision to be such a useful system that they advocate its extension to other health professionals. Others, particularly independent midwives, whose clients may come from a variety of districts and who therefore may find that they are reporting to more than 20 Supervisors of Midwives, wish to see radical changes in the supervisory system, if not its abolition. The aim of this chapter will be to collate the statutory and guidance provisions relating to the appointment and role of the Supervisor of Midwives, and discuss these in relation to the legal issues which arise and the present debate as to the future role of supervision. Of particular value as reference material is the English National Board pack, Preparation of Supervisors of Midwives.[6]

This chapter looks at:

- The statutory framework for supervision

- The definition and functions of the Local Supervising Authority

- The appointment and role of the Supervisor of Midwives

- The duty of the midwife in relation to the LSA and Supervisor of Midwives

- Legal aspects of the supervision of midwifery

- The future.

THE STATUTORY FRAMEWORK FOR SUPERVISION

There is a statutory requirement for the establishment of Local Supervising Authorities (LSAs) and for the appointment of Supervisors of Midwives. This is laid down in the Order in Council set up under the Health Act 1999. Provision is given in the Articles of the Order in Council for rules relating to supervision to be made which have binding force. The principal Rules were enacted in 1983, amended in 1998 and the new Rules date from August 2004. The Rules are in turn amplified by the guidance given in the NMC booklet.[7] The new Midwives Rules and Standards and the guidance in the NMC booklet replace the earlier Midwives Code of Practice. The midwife is also subject to the NMC Code of Professional Conduct: standards for conduct, performance and ethics. The Code does not have statutory force, but clearly failure to follow the Code will be taken into account in any investigation and/or hearing of fitness to practise. Discussion of the Midwives Rules and Standards can be found in Chapter 5.

THE PRINCIPAL LEGISLATION

The following provisions are made under Part VIII of the Orders in Council.[8]

Article 42

1. The Council shall by rules regulate the practice of midwifery and the rules may in particular:

   (a) determine the circumstances in which and the procedure by means of which a midwife may be suspended from practice

   (b) require midwives to give notice of their intention to practise to the Local Supervising Authority (referred to in this part as 'the LSA') for the area in which they intend to practise

   (c) require midwives to attend courses of instruction in accordance with the rules.

2. If rules are made requiring midwives to give the notice referred to in 1(b) above, the LSA shall inform the Council of any notices given to it under those rules.

DEFINITION AND FUNCTIONS OF THE LOCAL SUPERVISING AUTHORITIES

The definition of the LSA is given in Schedule 4 of the Nursing and Midwifery Order 2001[8] and is shown below:

LSA means:

– in England and Wales, Health Authorities

– in Scotland, Health Boards, and

– in Northern Ireland, Health and Social Services Boards.

Provisions relating to the local supervision of midwives are made under Part VIII of the Nursing and Midwifery Order 2001, made under the Health Act 1999 and shown in Box 3.1.

Box 3.1 Duties of Local Supervising Authorities

Article 43

1. Each Local Supervising Authority shall:

   (a) exercise general supervision, in accordance with rules under Article 42, over all midwives practising in its area

   (b) where it appears to it that the fitness to practise of a midwife in its area is impaired, report it to the Council, and

   (c) have power in accordance with the Council's rules to suspend a midwife from practice.

2. The Council may prescribe the qualifications of persons who may be appointed by the LSA to exercise supervision over midwives within its area, and no person shall be so appointed who is not qualified.

3. The Council may by rules from time to time establish standards for the exercise by LSAs of their functions and may give guidance to LSAs on these matters.

NEW RULES ON SUPERVISION IN MIDWIFERY

New rules in relation to the supervision of midwifery and the role of the LSA came into force on 1 August 2004 and the NMC has provided standards and guidance on the new rules.[7] The new rules cover the following aspects of the role of the LSA and midwifery supervision:

Rule 3	Notification of intention to practise
Rule 4	Notifications by local supervising authority

Rule 5   Suspension from practice by a local supervising authority

Rule 10   Inspection of premises and equipment

Rule 11   The eligibility for appointment as a Supervisor of Midwives

Rule 12   The supervision of midwives

Rule 13   The local supervising authority midwifery officer

Rule 14   The exercise by a local supervising authority of its functions

Rule 15   Publication of local supervising authority procedures and

Rule 16   Annual Report of the LSA.

Notification of intention to practise (ITP)

It is the statutory duty of a midwife who intends to practise to notify her intention to do so, to the Local Supervising Authority. Rule 3 sets out the provisions in relation to this duty. The NMC guidance makes it clear that notification in accordance with the procedures is the responsibility of the midwife. The LSA has a duty to inform the Council, in such form and at such frequency as requested by the Council, of any notice given to it under Rule 3. There is provision in Rule 3(3) for the notice to be given, in an emergency, after the time when she commences to practise, provided that it is given within 48 hours of that time. Under Rule 4, which covers the notifications by the Local Supervising Authority, each Local Supervising Authority shall publish:

a. the name and address of its midwifery officer for the submission of a notice under Rule 3(1)

b. the date by which a midwife must give notice under Rule 3(1) in accordance with Rule 3(2b).

Under the NMC standards set for Rule 4 the LSA must:

– publish annually the name and address of the person to whom the notice must be sent

– publish annually the date by which it must receive intention to practise forms from midwives in its area

– ensure accurate completion and timely delivery of intention to practise data to the NMC by the 20th of each month.

The NMC issued guidance to Supervisors of Midwives (SoMs), local supervising authority midwifery officers (LSAMOs) and local supervising authorities (LSAs) about changes to the Intention to Practise Rules (ITP)[9] which came into force in April 2005. This supplements the guidance given in Rules 3 and 4 of the Midwives Rules and Standards. A new requirement is that there must be a countersignature by a named Supervisor of Midwives. Only a midwife with effective registration can give notice of intention to practise. If she has not met her PREP requirements, then her registration has lapsed. Midwives are now sent a personalised ITP form. The requirement that the supervisor must countersign it gives the supervisor the opportunity to confirm the midwife's continued eligibility to practise. The ITP data is sent by the LSA to the NMC electronically.

Suspension from practice
It must be clarified that there are various forms of suspension.

– There is suspension from practice by the LSA, which is the subject of this discussion. Suspension from practice must, however, be distinguished from two other forms of suspension:

 - The right of an employer to suspend from the workplace an employee who is alleged to be in breach of the terms of the contract of employment, or incapable by reason of physical or mental disability to perform her functions adequately. This is considered in Chapter 22 and can apply to all employees.

 - The NMC has the power to suspend from the Register or make an interim suspension.

NMC suspension or interim suspension
Rule 5 of the Midwives Rules requires the LSA to notify Council of any suspension of a midwife and also places obligations upon the Practice Committee once it is informed by Council of such a suspension. It must consider whether or not to make an interim suspension order or interim conditions of practice order in respect of the midwife concerned. If the Practice Committee does not make an interim suspension order, the LSA must revoke the suspension; if the Practice Committee does make an interim suspension order, but this is subsequently revoked, the LSA must revoke their suspension. The effect of an interim suspension from the Register is that the practitioner is no longer able to work as a registered practitioner, and this may mean that she would be suspended or dismissed from her employment. In its guidance on Rule 5 the NMC states:

> There is a difference between suspension from practice and suspension from duty. If the midwife is employed within the NHS or private sector, the employer may suspend them from duty whilst management investigations take place. These are separate from any investigation the local supervising authority may undertake. Suspension from duty will only affect the midwife's employment with an organisation and they can continue to work for another employer.

Rule 5 of the Midwives Rules is set out in Box 3.2.

The power of suspension set out in Box 3.2 covers both employed midwives within the NHS and independent midwives who practise in the district of the LSA.

Box 3.2 Suspension from practice by LSA (Rule 5 of Midwives Rules)

1. Subject to the provisions of this rule a local supervising authority may, following an appropriate investigation (which is to include, where appropriate, seeking the views of the midwife concerned) suspend from practice

    (a) a midwife against whom it has reported a case for investigation to the Council, pending the outcome of the Council's investigation; or

    (b) a midwife who has been referred to a Practice Committee of the Council, pending the outcome of that referral

2. Where it exercises its powers to suspend a midwife from practice, a local supervising authority shall

    (a) immediately notify the midwife concerned in writing of the decision to suspend her and the reason for the suspension, and supply her with a copy of the documentation which it intends to submit to the Council in accordance with sub-paragraph (b); and thereafter

    (b) immediately report to the Council in writing any such suspension and details of the investigation carried out by the local supervising authority that led to that suspension.

The Rules have been amended so that there is no longer any obligation upon the LSA to suspend a midwife from practice when necessary for the purpose of preventing the spread of infection. However, the definition of fitness to practise includes physical health and condition and therefore if a midwife has been reported to Council for investigation, this could include midwives who present a danger to their patients.

Another change to the rules is that Rule 39, which required a midwife to be medically examined, has not been replaced.

There are at any one time only a tiny number of midwives who are suspended from practice. The NMC annual report on Fitness to Practise does not divide those registrants who were subject to professional conduct proceedings into their specialisms.[10]

Inspection of premises and equipment
Rule 10 is set out in Box 3.3.

There are no additional powers of enforcement given by either the Act or the Rules in relation to the inspection of premises, and it is assumed that the midwife will

Box 3.3 Inspection of premises and equipment (Rule 10)

1. A practising midwife shall give to a Supervisor of Midwives, a local supervising authority and the Council every reasonable facility to monitor her standards and methods of practice and to inspect her records, her equipment and any premises that she is entitled to permit them to enter, which may include such part of the midwife's residence as may be used for professional purposes.

2. A practising midwife shall use her best endeavours to permit inspection from time to time of all places of work in which she practises, other than the private residence of a woman and baby she is attending, by persons nominated by the Council for this purpose, one of whom shall be a practising midwife.

The duty of the midwife to give reasonable facility to the monitoring of her standards and her methods of practice is new and in its guidance on this rule the NMC makes it clear that it is the midwife's responsibility to let the LSA and the NMC monitor her standards and methods of practice.

obey the obligations placed upon her under the rules, since she can be removed from the Register for professional misconduct (see Ch. 4). No offences are created under the Act other than those in relation to registration and to attendance at childbirth (see Ch. 25). The aim of the legislation is not to create criminal offences in relation to enforcement but to secure self-regulation of the profession through the powers given to the NMC and its committees.

Local Supervising Authority: Information

Rule 15 requires the LSA to publish the information shown in Box 3.4.

Box 3.4 Discharge of functions by a LSA (Rule 15)

Each local supervising authority shall publish

(a) the name and address of its midwifery officer, together with the procedure for reporting all adverse incidents relating to midwifery practice or allegations of impaired fitness to practise of practising midwives within its area and the procedure by which it will investigate any such reports;

(b) the procedure by which it will deal with complaints or allegations against its midwifery officer or Supervisor of Midwives within its area.

The NMC has supplemented this rule with standards relating to the procedures for ensuring the LSA midwifery officer is notified of all incidents that cause serious concern and also relating to procedures about allegations against the LSA midwifery officer or Supervisor of Midwives.

APPOINTMENT AND ROLE OF THE SUPERVISOR OF MIDWIVES

The NMC has issued guidance on the selection and appointment of local supervising authority midwifery officers.[11] The circular emphasises the importance of excellent communication and dialogue between the LSAs and the NMC on all matters affecting the regulation of midwifery practice, including the function of the LSA in statutory supervision. The LSAMO must be able to have direct access to the NMC in relation to these matters and the NMC will, in future, provide advice and support to the LSA during the recruitment of LSAMOs. The NMC emphasises that it is concerned with protecting the public, not with managing and developing services, but recognises the need for a consistent standard across the UK in the selection and appointment of LSAMOs. It also recognises that it is for employers to determine the final job description and role specification, to ensure these reflect local NHS structures.

If an LSAMO's employer requires her to undertake any other role or work, this is entirely separate from the statutory supervision of midwives in the LSA area.

The NMC circular sets out the statutory functions of the LSAMO and cites Articles 42 and 43 on the Rules of midwifery practice and the local supervision of midwives.

The NMC does not specify any maximum number of midwives that an individual Supervisor of Midwives should supervise.

The eligibility for appointment as a Supervisor of Midwives is set out in Rule 11 and can be found in Box 3.5.

Box 3.5 Eligibility for appointment as a Supervisor of Midwives (Rule 11)

1. A local supervising authority shall appoint an adequate number of Supervisors of Midwives to exercise supervision over practising midwives in its area.

2. To be appointed for the first time as a Supervisor of Midwives, in accordance with Article 43 of the Order, a person shall

▶

▶

(a) be a practising midwife;

(b) have three years' experience as a practising midwife of which at least one shall have been in the 2-year period immediately preceding the appointment; and

(c) have successfully completed a programme of a type mentioned in para. (5) within the 3-year period prior to her first appointment as a Supervisor of Midwives.

3. For any subsequent appointment as a Supervisor of Midwives, a person must have practised in such a role for 3 years within the 5-year period prior to the new appointment.

4. In the case of a national of an EEA state (or other person entitled to be treated for the purpose of appointment as a Supervisor of Midwives, no less favourably than a national of such a state by virtue of an enforceable community law right or any enactment giving effect to a community obligation) the conditions in para. (2) or (3) shall be satisfied if, in the opinion of the Council, a person has had comparable training or experience within or outside the EEA.

5. The provider, content and duration of a programme referred to in para. (2c) shall be such as the Council shall from time to time specify for the purposes of this rule.

6. Following her appointment, a Supervisor of Midwives shall complete such periods of study relating to the supervision of midwives as the Council shall from time to time require.

The NMC has set standards for LSAs to follow in ensuring that Supervisors of Midwives meet the requirements shown in Box 3.5. NMC guidance emphasises the supportive role which the supervisor should be fulfilling and states that:

The success of supervision reflects the ability of those who do it and it is, therefore, important to get the right person into the role. To become a Supervisor of Midwives, a midwife will need to go through a selection process set by the local supervising authority, which meets the standards set by the NMC.

Regulations relating to the Supervision of Midwives are set out in Rule 12, which is shown in Box 3.6.

Box 3.6 The supervision of midwives (Rule 12)

1. Each practising midwife shall have a named Supervisor of Midwives from among the Supervisors of Midwives appointed by the local supervising authority covering her main area of practice.

2. A local supervising authority shall ensure that:

   (a) each practising midwife within its area has a named Supervisor of Midwives

   (b) at least once a year, each Supervisor of Midwives meets each midwife for whom she is the named Supervisor of Midwives to review the midwife's practice and to identify her training needs;

   (c) all Supervisors of Midwives within its area maintain records of their supervisory activities, including any meeting with a midwife; and

   (d) all practising midwives within its area have 24-hour access to a Supervisor of Midwives.

THE DUTIES OF THE SUPERVISOR OF MIDWIVES

Rule 12 (see Box 3.6) sets out the basic duties of the supervisor. They are amplified in the guidance provided by the NMC. This sees the role as including:

– Offering continuity of support to the midwife

– Liaising with other supervisors if the midwife practises outside the area

– Advice and guidance being available at all times in each LSA (not necessarily from the named supervisor)

– Statutory supervision at least once per year, to discuss personal and professional development with an agreed record of any meeting

The NMC requires LSAs to ensure that there is support for the Supervisor of Midwives and the standards require the LSA to:

– Monitor the provision of protected time and administrative support for Supervisors of Midwives

– Promote woman-centred, evidence-based midwifery practice

– Ensure that Supervisors of Midwives maintain accurate data and records of all their supervisory activities and meetings with the midwives they supervise

The NCM also requires the LSA to set standards for Supervisors of Midwives that incorporate the following broad principles:

– Supervisors of Midwives are available to offer guidance and support to women accessing maternity services

– Supervisors of Midwives give advice and guidance regarding woman-centred care and promote evidence-based midwifery practice

– Supervisors of Midwives are directly accountable to the local supervising authority for all matters relating to the statutory supervision of midwives

– Supervisors of Midwives provide professional leadership

– Supervisors of Midwives are approachable and accessible to midwives to support them in their practice.

The NMC guidance on these standards emphasises the importance of resources being made available to maximise the effectiveness of supervision of midwives. The LSA is required to monitor to ensure that the number of Supervisors of Midwives and the resources available to them are sufficient. It suggests that regular meetings take place between the supervisors and the LSA midwifery officer to ensure up-to-date information is exchanged, thereby giving opportunity for discussion to provide advice and support.

LOCAL SUPERVISING AUTHORITY MIDWIFERY OFFICER (RULE 13)

The requirement that each LSA appoints a midwifery officer is a new provision in the Rules and is set out in Box 3.7.

Box 3.7 Local supervising authority midwifery officer (Rule 13)

1. Each local supervising authority shall appoint a local supervising authority midwifery officer who shall be responsible for exercising its functions in relation to the supervision of midwives including in relation to the appointment of Supervisors of Midwives under Rule 11(1)

2. A local supervising authority shall not appoint a person to the post of local supervising authority midwifery officer unless

   (a) she is a practising midwife; and

   (b) she meets the standards of experience and education set by the Council from time to time.

Standards set by the NMC for LSAs to fulfil in implementing Rule 13 require the LSA to act as follows:

– observe the NMC core criteria and person specification

– involve an NMC nominated and appropriately experienced midwife in the selection and appointment process

– manage the performance of the appointed LSA midwifery officer

– provide designated time and administrative support for a local supervising authority midwifery officer to discharge the statutory supervisory function

– arrange for the local supervising authority midwifery officer to complete an annual audit of the practice and supervision of midwives within its area to ensure the requirements of the NMC are being met.

The NMC guidance recognises that the LSA sits within a NHS authority and the LSA midwifery officer is subject to the terms and conditions of that employment. It refers to NMC circulars which cover core standards for appointments to these posts. It recommends good communication between the LSA and the Council to enhance the protection of the public and suggests that women should have access to the LSA midwifery officer if they wish to discuss any aspect of their care that they do not feel has been addressed through other channels. The NMC guidance also highlights the pivotal role in clinical governance played by the LSA midwifery officer by ensuring that the standard of supervision of midwives and midwifery practice meets that required by the NMC. She is expected to promote openness and transparency in exercising supervision over midwives and the role is impartial in that it does not represent the interests of any health service provider.

EXERCISE BY A LSA OF ITS FUNCTIONS (RULE 14)

Rule 14 is set out in Box 3.8.

Box 3.8 Exercise by a LSA of its functions (Rule 14)

Where a local supervising authority (in relation to the exercise of its functions as to the supervision of midwives) has concerns about whether a local supervising authority midwifery officer or a Supervisor of Midwives meets the Council's standards, it shall discuss those concerns with the Council.

NMC guidance suggests that the LSA is able to use the NMC as a resource in helping them to manage a variety of situations related to professional concerns.

The NMC has a duty to provide the LSA with advice and guidance in respect of the exercise of their functions.

ANNUAL REPORT OF THE LSA

Rule 16 requires every local supervising authority each year to submit a written report to the NMC by such date and containing such information as the NMC may specify. In its standards on Rule 16, the NMC has specified 1 June as the required date and set the following minimum contents:

- numbers of Supervisor of Midwives appointments, resignations and removals

- details of how midwives are provided with continuous access to a Supervisor of Midwives

- details of how the practice of midwifery is supervised

- evidence that service users have been involved in monitoring supervision of midwives and assisting the local supervising authority midwifery officer with the annual audits

- evidence of engagement with higher education institutions in relation to supervisory input into midwifery education

- details of any new policies relating to the supervision of midwives

- evidence of developing trends affecting midwifery practice in the local supervision authority

- details of the number of complaints regarding the discharge of the supervisory function

- reports on all local supervising authority investigations undertaken during the year.

The NMC monitors the performance of the LSAs by the annual report and by regular visits to the LSA.

PERSONAL CONTACT BETWEEN SUPERVISOR AND MIDWIFE

The guidance provided on Rule 12, the supervision of midwives (see above), states that having a named Supervisor of Midwives means that the supervisor will be able to offer continuity of support. The midwife can also expect a supervisor (not necessarily her named supervisor) to be available to her at all times for advice and guidance. It is for the LSA to determine how 24-hour access to a Supervisor of Midwives for advice and support is organised. The guidance also suggests that if the relationship is not beneficial to both midwife and supervisor, either of them can request a change. It recommends that the midwife should arrange to meet with her supervisor at least once a year for the purpose of statutory supervision. The NMC guidance states:

This provides you with the opportunity to discuss your personal and professional development.

It also notes that an agreed record of any meeting will assist in continuity of support and although the records are confidential between the midwife and supervisor, they may be disclosed in certain circumstances in an LSA or NMC investigation into fitness to practise or by order of the court.

DUTY OF MIDWIFE IN RELATION TO THE LSA AND SUPERVISOR OF MIDWIVES

To assist the reader, a compilation of the duties of the midwife (taken both from the Rules, the Standards and the guidance), in relation to supervision and midwifery practice is set out in Box 3.9. Further discussion can be found in the chapters relating to records (Ch. 15), drugs (Ch. 20) and professional practice (Ch. 5).

Box 3.9 Duties of midwife in relation to her Supervisor of Midwives and her practice

(a) Give notice of her intention to practise to the Supervisor of Midwives in the district (i.e. the geographical jurisdiction of the Supervisor of Midwives) in which she intends to work (Rule 3). Notice must be given in the prescribed form. Where the midwife works in more than one district or LSA, she must notify her intention to practise to the Supervisor of Midwives in each different district or LSA (Rule 3.2).

(b) Notify change of name and address to the NMC (Rule 3 Guidance).

(c) Maintain her professional knowledge and competence (Code Para. 6 and see standard on Rule 6, below).

(d) Should consult her Supervisor of Midwives (Guidance on Rule 12). (The changes brought about by PREP are considered in Ch. 2.)

(e) Must provide midwifery care in accordance with such standards as the NMC may specify from time to time, to a woman and baby during the antenatal, intranatal and postnatal periods (Rule 6.1).

(f) In an emergency, or where a deviation from the norm which is outside her current sphere of practice becomes apparent in the mother or baby during the antenatal, intranatal or postnatal periods, a practising midwife shall call such qualified health professional as may reasonably be expected to have the necessary skills and experience to assist her in the provision of care (Rule 6.3).

(g) Cannot arrange for anyone to act as a substitute, other than another practising midwife or a registered medical practitioner (Standards on Rule 6).

(h) Must make sure the needs of the woman or baby are the primary focus of her practice (Standards on Rule 6).

(i) Should work in partnership with the woman and her family (Standards on Rule 6).

(j) Should enable the woman to make decisions about her care based on her individual needs, by discussing matters fully with her (Standards on Rule 6).

(k) Should respect the woman's right to refuse any advice given (Standards on Rule 6).

(l) Is responsible for maintaining and developing her own competence (Standards on Rule 6).

(m) Must ensure she becomes competent in any new skills required for her practice (Standards on Rule 6).

(n) Is responsible for familiarising herself with her employer's policies (Standards on Rule 6).

(o) Must keep, as contemporaneously as is reasonable, continuous and detailed records of observations made, care given and medicine and any form of pain relief administered by her to a woman or baby (Rule 9.1).

(p) Records cannot be destroyed (Rule 9.3).

(q) Immediately before ceasing to practise or if she finds it impossible or inconvenient to preserve her records safely, a midwife must transfer them to her employer or the LSA (Rule 9.4).

(r) The transfer of records must be recorded (Rule 9.5).

(s) Provide every reasonable facility to the supervisor, LSA and NMC to monitor her standards and methods of practice and to inspect her records, her equipment and any premises she is entitled to permit them to enter (Rule 10.1).

SUPERVISION RECORDS

The NMC in its guidance[12] on Rule 9 of the Midwives Rules relating to records states that:

The majority of supervisors' records relate to information such as continuing professional development and support. They could be regarded as personnel files and should be kept for seven years. A copy of these records could also be given to the midwife. Any supervisory records relating to investigation of a clinical incident, alleged misconduct or incompetence relating to a midwife must be kept for 25 years.

Under Rule 10, the midwife is obliged to give every facility for her records to be inspected. The NMC says in its guidance on this Rule:

It is your responsibility to let the local supervising authority and the NMC monitor your standards and methods of practice. This may include allowing access to your records, equipment and place of work.

LEGAL ASPECTS OF THE SUPERVISION OF MIDWIFERY

The Supervisor of Midwives is not vicariously liable for the negligence of the midwife. The midwife must accept personal responsibility and accountability for her actions. If she is at fault she cannot lay the blame upon the Supervisor of Midwives and argue that the supervisor should have told her otherwise or warned her of certain dangers.

On the other hand, the Supervisor of Midwives may be the manager of the midwife. In this situation, there may be matters relating to resources which are properly the responsibility of the manager. The midwife would have to show that she drew any dangers relating to the health and safety of mother and child to the attention of the manager and did all that she reasonably could to ensure that the clients were safe.

NEGLIGENCE BY THE SUPERVISOR OF MIDWIVES

If the Supervisor of Midwives is negligent in carrying out her duties as set out in the Rules, the Standards, the guidance and NMC publication 'The Code of professional conduct: standards for conduct, performance and ethics', then she may face fitness to practise proceedings before the Conduct and Competence Committee of the NMC (see Ch. 4) as being guilty of professional misconduct. Unless harm has been caused as a reasonably foreseeable result of her negligence, she is not likely to face civil proceedings for compensation for the harm arising from her negligence.

If she has misinformed the midwife, who as a result of reliance upon the supervisor's information has caused harm to the mother or baby, then the midwife, if sued for negligence, would have to show that reliance upon the supervisor's information was reasonable and would have been the practice followed by any responsible midwife. This might be difficult to establish.

LSA MIDWIFERY OFFICER

Any midwife appointed as the LSA midwifery officer will have a contract of employment with the health authority which acts as the LSA. The core standards issued by the NMC for such appointments should be followed.

MIDWIVES APPOINTED BY THE LSA

Is there a legal relationship between Supervisor of Midwives and midwife? The conclusion from the Rules and the Standards is that it is not the intention of the NMC to create a legal relationship between them so that either one could sue the other. The Supervisor of Midwives is not professionally accountable for the professional standards of practice of the midwife she supervises, but she is answerable in her own right for failings in her role as Supervisor of Midwives to the NMC and to the LSA. She is also answerable to her employer as a practising midwife.

EMPLOYMENT SITUATION OF SUPERVISORS OF MIDWIVES

While the supervisors are appointed by the LSA, they rarely receive any payment from the LSA but are usually employed by the NHS Trust. It is helpful if their work as Supervisor of Midwives is recognised by their employer and included in their contract of employment with the trust, so that the trust would be seen to be vicariously liable both for their work as a midwife within the trust and also for their activities as a supervisor. In addition, the contract would clearly have to give them time to undertake their work of midwifery supervision.

SUPERVISORS OF MIDWIVES AND LINE MANAGEMENT SUPERVISION

Supervisors of midwives might, in addition to being the midwifery supervisor for an individual midwife, also be her line manager. Where there is this dual role, it is important if possible to keep them separate, so that the midwife is aware when the other midwife is acting as her line manager rather than as her Supervisor of Midwives. The distinction between the two roles is not always clear to midwives, as research carried out by Barbara Burden and Tricia Jones shows.[13]

In 2001, the UKCC issued a position statement[14] providing advice for the Local Supervising Authorities and Supervisors of Midwives and setting out the recurring issues and themes of the reports considered by the Midwifery Committee. It identifies major issues relating to clinical practice, women's experience of care, organisational issues, and lists those issues particularly relevant to midwifery practice, Supervisors of Midwives, midwifery managers and midwifery educationalists. A similar position paper is provided for NHS employers,[15] which is considered in Chapter 21. To some extent the NMC Standards and guidance on the new Rules published in 2004 overtake the UKCC position statement, but some of the guidance is still relevant.

THE FUTURE

The debate over the role of the Supervisor of Midwives is ongoing. In 1998 the ENB supported research into the evaluation of the impact of the supervision of midwives on professional practice and the quality of midwifery care, which considered a range of different models of supervision of midwives.[16] Further research of the kind carried out by Elizabeth Gaffney,[17] where midwives are asked what they want from their supervisors, is essential to ensure that supervision of midwives in the future is designed to meet the clinical needs of midwives and to support their professional practice. The ENB has also investigated the extent to which statutory supervision of midwives enables midwives to contribute to the work of primary care groups and health improvement programmes[18] (see Ch. 21).

The clinical supervision as reflective practice recommended by the UKCC for non-midwife practitioners is very different from the system of midwifery supervision,[19] and there may be continuing debate over the preferred form of supervision. As clinical supervision is increasingly introduced for nurses and health visitors, the pressure grows to redefine the role of the Supervisor of Midwives.[20] The NMC has clarified the role of the supervisor and set national standards for practice and for the LSAs and its Midwifery Officer. Margaret Rodger argues strongly for the role of the Supervisor of Midwives in protecting the public health.[21]

QUESTIONS AND EXERCISES

1. How do you see the future of midwifery supervision? Do you consider that all practitioners registered with the NMC should be subject to statutory supervision?

2. You are considering becoming a Supervisor of Midwives. Prepare a protocol for the role of the Supervisor of Midwives.

3. Identify the issues which you, as a practising midwife, would wish to take to a Supervisor of Midwives.

4. Identify the advantages and disadvantages of the system of midwifery supervision and consider ways, if any, of overcoming the disadvantages.

References

1 Nursing and Midwifery Council (Midwives) Rules Order of Council 2004, Statutory Instrument 2004/1764.

2 NMC. Midwives Rules and Standards. NMC; August 2004.

3 Kirkham M. Developments in the supervision of midwives. Oxford: Books for Midwives Press; 2000.

4 English National Board. Supervision of midwives. London: ENB; 1996.

5 Nursing and Midwifery Council. Preparation and supervision of midwives. New NMC edition; August 2002.

6 English National Board. Preparation of Supervisors of Midwives: an open learning programme. The four modules cover the statutory basis to the role of the supervisor; the role in supporting good midwifery practice; the role and responsibility in dealing with alleged professional misconduct; and the role in professional development. London: ENB; 1992.

7 NMC. Midwives Rules and Standards, August 2004, incorporating Nursing and Midwifery Council (Midwives) Rules Order of Council 2004, Statutory Instrument 2004/1764.

8 The Nursing and Midwifery Order 2001. SI 2002 No 253.

9 Nursing and Midwifery Council. Guidance on the revised Intention to Practise process. Circular 2/2005; January 2005.

10 Nursing and Midwifery Council. Fitness to Practise. Annual Report 2003–4.

11 Nursing and Midwifery Council. Guidance on selection and appointment of Local Supervising Authority Midwifery Officers. Circular 23/2004; July 2004.

12 Nursing and Midwifery Council. Midwives Rules and Standards, August 2004.

13 Burden B, Jones T. Midwives' perceptions of supervisors and managers. Br J Midwifery 1999; 7:547–552.

14 UKCC. Strengthening and supporting the midwifery contribution to maternity care for women and their families. Registrar's Letter 23/2001; 2001.

15 UKCC. Strengthening and supporting the midwifery contribution to maternity care for women and their families. Registrar's Letter 22/2001; 2001.

16 Stapleton H, Duerden J, Kirkham M. Evaluation of the impact of the supervision of midwives on professional practice and the quality of midwifery care. London: ENB; 1998. Online. Available: enb. resources@easynet.co.uk

17 Gaffney E. What do midwives want from their supervision? The Practising Midwife 1998; 1:24–26.

18 English National Board. Midwives and Public Health: an identification of the extent to which statutory supervision of midwives enables midwives to contribute to the work of primary care groups and health improvement programmes. London: ENB; 2000.

19 Derbyshire F. Clinical supervision within midwifery. In: Kirkham M, ed. Developments in the supervision of midwives. Oxford: Books for Midwives Press; 2000:169–176.

20 Deery R. Improving relationships through clinical supervision: Parts 1, 2. Br J Midwifery 1999; 7:160–163; 251–254.

21 Rodger M. The Supervisor of Midwives' role in protecting the public. MIDIRS Midwifery Digest 2004; 14:541–544.

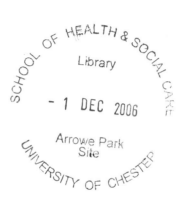

Chapter 4

PROFESSIONAL ACCOUNTABILITY AND THE NMC

The midwife, as a registered practitioner, is accountable to the NMC for her conduct. This chapter looks at the principles and procedures relating to misconduct in the light of the changes brought about by the Health Act 1999, the Nursing and Midwifery Order 2001.[1]

The topics covered in this chapter are:

– The function of the NMC in maintaining standards

– The Investigating Committee

– The Conduct and Competence Committee

– The Health Committee

– Procedural rules for the investigation of allegations

– A case of alleged misconduct.

THE FUNCTION OF THE NMC IN MAINTAINING STANDARDS

The NMC has the duty of giving advice about standards of conduct and performance and administering procedures (including making rules) relating to misconduct, unfitness to practise and similar matters (Schedule 3, Para. 8 of the Health Act 1999). Its update of the Code of Professional Conduct against fitness to practise will be assessed.[2]

Under Article 21 of the Nursing and Midwifery Order 2001 SI 2002 No 253:

1. The Council shall

    (a) establish and keep under review the standards of conduct, performance and ethics expected of registrants and prospective registrants and give them such guidance on these matters as it sees fit; and

    (b) establish and keep under review effective arrangements to protect the public from persons whose fitness to practise is impaired.

2. The Council may also from time to time give guidance to registrants, employers and such other persons as it thinks appropriate in respect of standards for the education and training, supervision and performance of persons who provide services in connection with those provided by registrants.

3. Before establishing any standards or arrangements mentioned in Para. (1), the Council shall consult the Conduct and Competence Committee in addition to the persons mentioned in Article 3(14).

ALLEGATIONS

The provisions of Article 22 apply where any allegation is made against a registered person to the effect that:

(a) his fitness to practise is impaired by reason of:

    i. misconduct

    ii. lack of competence

    iii. a conviction or caution in the UK for a criminal offence; or a conviction elsewhere for an offence, which if committed in England and Wales, would constitute a criminal offence

    iv. his physical or mental health, or

    v. a determination by a body in the UK responsible under any enactment for the regulation of a health or social care profession to the effect that his fitness to practise is impaired, or a determination by a licensing body elsewhere to the same effect;

(b) an entry in the register relating to him has been fraudulently procured or incorrectly made.

Article 22 also applies even if the allegation is based on a matter alleged to have occurred outside the UK or at a time when the person against whom the allegation is made was not registered.

Under Article 22(4) rules may provide that where a Practice Committee finds that a person has failed to comply with the standards mentioned in Article 21(1) such failure shall not be taken of itself to establish that his fitness to practise is impaired, but may be taken into account in any proceedings under this Order.

PROCEDURE FOLLOWING ALLEGATION

If the allegation relates to a fraudulent entry in the Register, then it is referred to the Investigating Committee.

In other cases, the allegation is referred to:

i. persons appointed by the Council in accordance with any rules made under Article 23 or

ii. a Practice Committee.

HEARINGS ARE TO BE HELD

(a) in the UK country in which the registered address of the person concerned is situated; or

(b) if he is not registered and resides in the UK, in the country in which he resides; or

(c) in any other case, in England.

PUBLICATION OF DECISIONS

Under Article 22(9) the Council is required to publish without delay particulars of any Orders and decisions made by a Practice Committee and of its reasons for them.

The Council may also disclose to any person any information relating to a person's fitness to practise which it considers it to be in the public interest to disclose.

SCREENERS

The NMC may by rules provide for the appointment of Screeners to whom allegations may be referred. A Screener may be a member of Council, and of any of its committees except a Practice Committee. Employees of Council are prohibited from being screeners.

There must be a panel of at least two Screeners considering an allegation; one of the panel must be a lay person and one must be a registrant from the same field as the person concerned. The number of registrants on the panel cannot exceed the number of lay persons.

The functions of the screeners

The functions of the Screeners include the following:

– considering the allegation and establishing whether, in their opinion, power is given by the Order to deal with it if it proves to be well founded

- if the power is given, of referring the matter together with a report of the results of their consideration to such Practice Committee as they see fit

- if the power is not given, of closing the case

  - where there are two Screeners, the lay person agrees, or

  - where there are more than two Screeners, it is the decision of the majority

- if either of these conditions is not satisfied, the Screeners may refer the matter to the Practice Committee

- where requested to do so by a Practice Committee, of mediating in any case with the aim of dealing with the allegation without it being necessary for the Health Committee or the Conduct and Competence Committee, as the case may be, to reach the stage at which it would arrange a hearing in accordance with Article 32(2f)

- in the event that mediation fails, of referring the matter back to the Practice Committee which referred it to the Screeners.

No person may act as a Screener or sit on a Practice Committee in respect of a particular case if he has been involved in that case in any other capacity.

THE INVESTIGATING COMMITTEE

The Investigating Committee is required to investigate any allegation appropriately referred to it (Article 26). Following the referral it shall:

- Notify without delay the person against whom the allegation is made and invite him to submit written representations within a prescribed period

- Where it sees fit, notify the person making the allegations of these representations and invite him to deal within a specified period with any points raised by the Committee in respect of these representations

- Take such other steps as are reasonably practicable to obtain as much information as possible about the case

- Consider in the light of the information which it has been able to obtain and any representations or other observations, whether in its opinion there is a case to answer or an entry has been fraudulently procured or incorrectly made.

The NMC has the power to draw up rules to make provision for the procedure to be followed by the Investigating Committee (see below procedures for Fitness to Practise hearings). Article 25 gives the Council power to require disclosure of documents by any person who is believed to be able to supply information or produce any document which appears relevant to the discharge of any functions of the Practice Committee. No person can be required to disclose information which is prohibited by or under any other enactment.

CASE TO ANSWER

Where the Investigating Committee reaches a decision that there is a case to answer, it shall notify in writing both the registered professional concerned and the person making the allegation of the decision, giving its reasons.

The Investigating Committee must then undertake mediation or refer the case to:

– Screeners, for them to undertake mediation

– the Health Committee

– the Conduct and Competence Committee.

Alternatively, it may make an interim order under Article 31 (see below).

This does not apply in the case of a fraudulent entry on the Register, where if the Investigating Committee are satisfied that this has occurred, it can make an order that the Registrar remove or amend the entry. In this case, the registered practitioner concerned has the right of appealing to the court under Article 38 within 28 days of the notice of the order.

NEW EVIDENCE

If new evidence becomes available, the Investigating Committee can review or revoke any order it has made.

CONDUCT AND COMPETENCE COMMITTEE (CCC)

The duties of the CCC are:

– Having consulted the other Practice Committees as it thinks appropriate, advise the Council on

  - the performance of the Council's functions in relation to standards of conduct, performance and ethics expected of registrants and prospective registrants

  - requirements as to good character and good health to be met by registrants and prospective registrants, and

  - the protection of the public from persons who are unfit to practise, and

– consider

  - any allegation referred to it by the Council, Screeners, the Investigating Committee or the Health Committee, and

  - any application for restoration referred to it by the Registrar.

THE HEALTH COMMITTEE

The functions of the Health Committee (Article 28) are to consider:

– any allegations referred to it by the Council, Screeners, the Investigating Committee or the Conduct and Competence Committee, and

– any application for restoration referred to it by the Registrar.

Under Article 29, the Health Committee and the Conduct and Competence Committee may:

– refer the matter to Screeners for mediation or itself undertake mediation

– decide that it is not appropriate to take further action

– issue a striking off order

– issue a suspension order (lasting up to 1 year)

– issue a conditions of practice order (lasting up to 3 years)

– issue a caution order (lasting up to 5 years).

If the person concerned appeals, or where new evidence becomes available, then there are powers, depending upon the order and the Committee concerned, to confirm the order, extend the period for which the order has effect (subject to the maximums indicated above), reduce the period, revoke the order, vary any condition, or replace the order with another.

INTERIM ORDERS BY A PRACTICE COMMITTEE

Article 31 enables an interim suspension order to be made:

if the Committee is satisfied that it is necessary for the protection of members of the public or is otherwise in the public interest, or is in the interests of the registered professional concerned, for the registration of that person to be suspended or to be made subject to conditions.

PROCEDURAL RULES FOR THE INVESTIGATION OF ALLEGATIONS

Article 32 requires the Council to make rules as to the procedure to be followed by the Health Committee and the Conduct and Competence Committee in considering any allegation. The required content of these rules is set out in Article 32(2) and is shown in Box 4.1.

Box 4.1 Article 32(2) requirements for contents of Rules

(2) The rules shall, in particular, make provision:

(a) empowering each Committee to refer to the other any allegation which it considers would be better dealt with by that other Committee;

(b) empowering each Committee, before it holds any hearing to which sub-paragraph (f) applies, where it considers that it would assist it in performing its functions, to hold a preliminary meeting in private attended by the parties and their representatives and any other person it thinks appropriate;

(c) requiring the person concerned to be given notice of the allegation without delay;

(d) giving the person concerned an opportunity to submit written representations within a prescribed period;

(e) for the Committee, where it sees fit, to notify the person making the allegation of the representations provided under sub-paragraph (d) and to invite him to deal within a prescribed period with any points raised by the Committee in respect of those representations;

(f) giving the person concerned an opportunity to put his case at a hearing if:

(i) before the end of the prescribed period, he asks for a hearing; or

(ii) the Committee considers that a hearing is desirable;

(g) entitling the person concerned to be represented whether by a legally qualified person or otherwise at any such hearing;

(h) where an allegation is referred by the Council, Screeners or the Investigating Committee to the Health Committee or the Conduct and Competence Committee, for the Council to give notice of that referral to specified persons who shall include the Secretary of State, the Scottish Ministers, the National Assembly for Wales and the Department of Health, Social Services and Public Safety in Northern Ireland and, where they are known, to any person referred to in Article 25 para. (2a) or (b);

(i) giving any person, other than the person concerned, who, in the opinion of the relevant Committee, taking account of any criteria included in the rules, has an interest in proceedings before it, the opportunity to submit written representations;

(j) requiring a hearing before a Committee to be held in public except in so far as may be provided by the rules;

(k) requiring the Committee to notify the person concerned of its decision, its reasons for reaching that decision and of his right of appeal;

(l) requiring the person by whom the allegation was made to be notified by the Committee of its decision and of its reasons for reaching that decision;

(m) empowering the Committee to require persons (other than the person concerned) to attend and give evidence or to produce documents;

(n) about the admissibility of evidence;

(o) enabling the Committee to administer oaths;

(p) where the person concerned has been convicted of a criminal offence, for the conviction to be proved by the production of a certified copy of the certificate of conviction, or, in Scotland, an extract conviction, relating to the offence and for the findings of fact upon which the conviction is based to be admissible as proof of those facts.

(3) Each stage in proceedings under Part V and Article 37 shall be dealt with expeditiously and the Committee concerned may give directions as to the conduct of the case and for the consequences of failure to comply with such directions (which may include the making of an order or refusal of an application if the failure to comply was without reasonable excuse).

(4) The Council may provide in the rules for the Chairman of the Committee to hold the meeting referred to in para. (2b) or to give the directions mentioned in para. (3) and, subject to the agreement of the parties to his acting on behalf of the Committee, to take such action as the Committee would be competent to take at such a meeting.

(5) In this Article 'parties' means the Council and the person requirements as to good character and good health concerned.

REQUIREMENTS AS TO GOOD CHARACTER AND GOOD HEALTH

Guidance has been provided by the NMC on how the declarations that a prospective registrant is of good character and good health should be made.[3] It covers the situation pre-entry to the training school, pre-first registration and for continuing registration. The NMC recognises that 'good health' is a relative concept and states:

In other words, a registrant may have a disability, such as impaired hearing, or a health condition, such as depression, epilepsy, diabetes or heart disease, and yet be perfectly capable of safe and effective practice. However, there are some conditions which would be likely to affect a practitioner's ability to practise safely and effectively. These include alcoholism or drug abuse.

As far as good character is concerned the NMC states:

Good character is not easy to define. An important determinant of good character is the individual's commitment to compliance with the Code. The absence of convictions or formal cautions issued by the police is not sufficient evidence of good character and there are some convictions which the Council would not regard as being incompatible with fitness to practise and, therefore, registration. It depends on the seriousness of the conviction and the circumstances in which the offence was committed. The absence of relevant convictions, as determined by the Council, is integral to the meaning of good character. Another factor that might throw into question a registrant's good character is if they are currently suspended by another regulatory body or have been found guilty of misconduct or lack of fitness to practise by such a body. Likewise if they are subject to a determination by a licensing body elsewhere to the same effect.

The declaration is made by the registrant who will have to declare that she is of sufficiently good health and good character to be capable of safe and effective practice. A supporting declaration must be provided by those applying for entry to the register, whether for the first time or after a break in registration. It can be made by persons listed in the Education, Registration and Registration Appeals Rules.[4] In all cases the person making the supporting declaration must not be a relative or employee of the applicant.

FITNESS TO PRACTISE RULES

Rules came into force on 1 August 2004 on Fitness to Practise procedures[5] which were drawn up by the Nursing and Midwifery Council and approved by the Privy Council and the Department of Health. These cover the areas shown in Box 4.2.

The areas covered in Box 4.2 provide the detailed regulations which flesh out the basic requirements of fitness to practise procedures set out in the articles of the Nurses and Midwives Order and discussed above. The full details can be obtained from the

Box 4.2 Fitness to Practise Rules

Investigating Committee

3. Notice provisions

4. Procedure of the Investigating Committee where the allegation relates to impairment of fitness to practise

5. Procedure of the Investigating Committee where the allegation relates to a fraudulent or incorrect entry in the register

6. Notice of decision

7. Reconsideration of allegation after a finding of no case to answer

Interim Orders

8. Notice and procedure

Conduct and Competence Committee and Health Committee

9. Action upon referral of an allegation

10. Meetings and hearings

11. Notice of hearing

12. Procedure of the Conduct and Competence Committee and the Health Committee

13. Notice of decision

14. Referral of allegation from the Conduct and Competence Committee to the Health Committee

15. Referral of allegation from the Health Committee to the Conduct and Competence Committee

Procedure at hearings

16. Application of Part 5

17. Interpretation

▶

18. Preliminary meetings

19. Public and private hearings

20. Representation and entitlement to be heard

21. Absence of the practitioner

22. Witnesses

23. Vulnerable witnesses

24. Order of proceedings at initial hearing

25. Order of proceedings at a review or restoration hearing

26. Order of proceedings at an interim orders hearing

27. Notes and transcript of proceedings

General

28. Amendment of the charge

29. Joinder

30. Burden of proof

31. Evidence

32. Postponements and adjournments

33. Cancellation of hearing

34. Service of documents

Stationery Office website[6] and the NMC has provided a summary of the main changes.[7] The main changes are:

– Changes in terminology: allegations are now made about a practitioner's fitness to practise compared with allegations of professional misconduct or ill health
– Lack of competence: allegations of this can be made for the first time

– New sanctions: *Where fitness to practise is found to be impaired*: caution (of between 1 and 5 years); a Conditions of Practice Order; suspension of up to 1 year; or striking off the register.

– *In cases of lack of competence or health:* striking off can occur only if suspension or conditions of practice have been in place continuously for the preceding 2 years.

– Restorations: Those struck off may not apply to be restored until 5 years have elapsed.

RESTORATION TO THE REGISTER

Provision for restoration to the Register is made in Article 33. No application for restoration can be made before the end of the period of 5 years beginning with the date on which the striking off order was made.

LEGAL ASSESSORS

The Council is required to appoint legal assessors to advise the Screeners, the Practice Committees or the Registrar on questions of law, and to perform other functions which the Council confers on them by its rules. There are stipulations relating to who is eligible to be a legal assessor (Article 34).

MEDICAL ASSESSORS

Medical assessors are to be appointed by the Council to give advice to the same persons as the legal assessors, and there are similar provisions relating to eligibility or non-eligibility (Article 35).

REGISTRANT ASSESSORS

The Council may appoint these under Article 36. They have the general function of giving advice to the Council, the committees of the Council, Screeners or the Registrar on matters of professional practice arising in connection with any matter which the Registrar or any of the bodies is considering. They may also have other functions conferred on them by rules of Council. Conditions of eligibility for appointment as professional assessors are set.

APPEALS

Part VI of the Order lays down the rules which apply to the holding of appeals.

These cover appeals to the Council against a decision made by the Registrar and also appeals to court. The establishment of a Nursing and Midwifery Independent Tribunal which had been envisaged in the draft Order was deleted from the final Order.

A CASE OF ALLEGED MISCONDUCT

The following is an example of a case of alleged misconduct by a midwife appearing before the Professional Conduct Committee.

A 48-year-old woman appeared before the Professional Conduct Committee following an incident during the course of her professional work as a Registered Midwife some months earlier. She had come to midwifery at a mature age as a direct entrant (i.e. with no previous nursing qualification), but at the time of the incident had 9 years' experience as a midwife.

She was employed as a Community Midwife in a large city, and had a student midwife attached (her first after 3 years without).

The charges she faced arose from allegations that she failed to urgently summon medical aid when there was evidence of likely distress, and failed to adequately supervise a student midwife (approximately 2 months into training).

The circumstances were as follows:

The Community Midwives used a Community/General Practitioner Unit for the deliveries for which they had a responsibility. It was located at a hospital, immediately next to and only divided by an unlocked door from the Consultant Obstetrics Unit. One night, at about 12.15 a.m., the midwife had a call from the hospital to say that an 18-year-old woman had arrived at the Community Midwifery Unit, and that she was one of that midwife's patients. The midwife immediately telephoned her new student (whom she had not met) and asked her to travel to the Unit. The midwife arrived at approximately 12.50 a.m., 5 min before her student. She found that the patient was one who had made several local house moves in a short time, had never been found at home by the midwife when visiting, and had received no antenatal care. During the 5 min before the student arrived, the midwife, with a little difficulty, located a fetal heart beat, which she did not record but subsequently described as 'soft but regular'. (The hospital midwife who had called her to this unexpected patient had checked when the patient arrived, and she had recorded the fetal heart as 'strong'.)

When the student arrived, the midwife asked her to go through the required admission and examination procedures. One of her first actions was to take the patient's blood pressure, which she found to be significantly raised, especially the diastolic pressure. The student expressed concern at the finding which she recorded, but it was not checked, and she was told to continue with her examination. She could not find a fetal heart beat but was told that the midwife had done so, with difficulty. The student was asked if she had attached fetal scalp electrodes before, and replied that she had only watched the procedure being done. She was told to apply electrodes after completing a vaginal examination.

She tried her best to comply with the instruction, and eventually succeeded after some difficulty, the patient being in some distress and preferring to lie on her side. Some 9 min after the scalp electrodes had been attached, the student observed the recording was not being properly made, not least because the paper was 'burning' but her concern seemed not to be shared or understood. The midwife seemed content with the figures flashing on the visual recording. After a further slight delay, the student took it upon herself to go to seek aid at the Consultant Unit, whence she returned with a Midwifery Sister. The Sister immediately saw that the equipment was not properly set up, in that the paper roll was not aligned or mounted on the sprocket holes. She corrected this, and checked and corrected the attachment of the electrodes. Then, having observed the recording then showing, she said to the midwife: 'I would call for medical assistance urgently if I were you'. It was then approximately 1.25 a.m.

The Sister departed, and the midwife told the student to continue and complete her admission procedures. These were eventually completed just before 1.45 a.m., at which time the fetal heart recording was showing cause for real concern, and the blood pressure taken by the student indicated a further increase. Only then, with the admission/examination procedures complete in her view, did the midwife go to call the patient's General Practitioner by telephone. She found that his calls were redirected to a deputising service, to whom she then spoke. They said that the only doctor on duty with obstetric experience was engaged in another part of the city, and would not be free to leave there until about 2.10 a.m. and would arrive at approximately 2.30 a.m.

On her return to the ward where the patient was in the care of the student, the midwife found the situation deteriorating further. She telephoned the deputising service again, and they told her they would arrange a police escort to get the doctor there as quickly as possible.

Several minutes later (by now it was approximately 2.05 a.m.) there was a sudden prolapse of the cord. The student's immediate reaction was to apply pressure to the fetal head to prevent it constricting the cord. The midwife said that she left the student with the patient, went through the door to the Consultant Unit, and shouted 'prolapsed cord' very loudly, several times. The Sister who had visited earlier and her senior colleague rushed to the patient. They quickly assessed the situation, summoned 'hospital medical aid' (which was on call in the Unit) and moved the patient. Within minutes a caesarean had been performed. Unfortunately, the patient was delivered of a fresh male stillbirth.

The evidence to prove that the sequence of events had been as described came from the student, the Sister, a nursing officer and from the midwife herself. She denied the charges, though agreeing to the sequence of events. She insisted that they had done the right things in the right order, and that she had summoned medical aid as soon as the admission procedures were completed. The Committee found the facts proved, and considered them to constitute misconduct.

At the mitigation stage, it emerged that there was considerable antipathy between the midwifery staff of the Consultant Unit and the community midwives who used the other Unit. The midwife's manager said that the midwife only rarely took the in-service training opportunities provided, and that she had required counselling on the subject of student supervision on a number of occasions, culminating in the removal of students for a significant period.

The Committee decided that the midwife should be removed from the Register.

Clearly, the Committee was not convinced that the public were safe if the midwife remained on the Register. Their concern was her total obsession with procedures and her indifference as to what was actually happening to the woman.

This case was heard before the Professional Conduct Committee, but it is also an example of a case which could result in several different hearings (it is not known whether in fact any of these other proceedings took place):

- An action in the civil courts could be commenced by the parents seeking to claim compensation for the death of the child.
- The events could also lead to criminal proceedings if the Crown Prosecution Service took the view that the actions of the midwife amounted to gross negligence of criminal proportions.
- The midwife would also face disciplinary proceedings before the employer. Even if the employer were to allow her to keep her post, once she was removed from the Register she would be unable to practise as a midwife.

In the Annual Report of the UKCC for 1999/2002 it was reported that there was one appeal to the High Court following removal from the Register. A midwife was removed from the Register by the Professional Conduct Committee after having been found guilty on one charge of misconduct. The midwife had been employed on a night shift and the charge was that she failed to summon medical assistance when it was appropriate to do so. She challenged the decision on two grounds. The first was that there was insufficient evidence to support the charge. The High Court rejected this argument and maintained that although the Committee had heard conflicting evidence, it comprised professional people and experts in the field of midwifery who were able to assess the evidence. The second ground for appeal was that, in finding one charge not proven, the Committee had acted inconsistently in finding a second charge proven. The Court also rejected this argument, and stated that the particular charge required an intent to deceive and that the Committee was entitled to reject this charge if it considered that there was no such intent.

CASE STUDY: ANNUAL REPORT 2003-2004

In its Annual Report for 2003-2004[8] the NMC published a case study of a midwife working on a labour ward who was alleged to have failed to take action when the CTG recording showed decelerations; failed to monitor the progress of labour in an appropriate way; failed to seek medical assistance in the second stage of labour when there were fetal heart abnormalities; failed to check the dilations of the cervix by vaginal examination, failed to replace the CTG paper and failed to keep proper and adequate records. The midwife admitted that the proven facts amounted to misconduct and she was found guilty of misconduct and following details of mitigation her name was removed from the register.

COUNCIL FOR THE REGULATION OF HEALTHCARE PROFESSIONALS (CRHP) (SUBSEQUENTLY KNOWN AS THE COUNCIL FOR HEALTHCARE REGULATORY EXCELLENCE) (CHRE)

Section 25 of the National Health Service Reform and Health Care Professions Act 2002 provided for the establishment of a body corporate known as the Council for the Regulation of Healthcare Professionals (CRHP). Set up in the wake of the Kennedy Report into children's heart surgery at Bristol Royal Infirmary,[9] its remit covers nine regulatory bodies including the NMC. It is an independent body, which reports annually to Parliament. Its functions are set out under s. 25(2) of the Act and shown below:

– To promote the interests of patients and other members of the public in relation to the performance of their functions by the GMC, GDC, NMC, HPC and other health professional registration bodies and by their committees and officers

– To promote best practice in the performance of those functions

– To formulate principles relating to good professional self-regulation, and to encourage regulatory bodies to conform to them and

– To promote cooperation between regulatory bodies; and between them, or any of them, and other bodies performing corresponding functions.

Under Section 29 of the NHS Reform and Health Care Professions Act 2002, if the Council considers that a decision by one of the healthcare professions' regulatory bodies under its jurisdiction (e.g. the NMC, GMC, etc.) is unduly lenient, and it would be desirable for the protection of members of the public for the Council to take action, it can refer the case to the relevant court (i.e. High Court in England and Wales). The court then has the power to dismiss the appeal, allow the appeal and quash the relevant decision; substitute for the relevant decision any other decision which could have been made by the committee or person concerned, or, remit the case to the committee or other person concerned to dispose of the case in accordance with the directions of the court. The referral must be within 4 weeks beginning with the last date on which the practitioner concerned has the right to appeal against the decision. The High Court held in March 2004 that the Council for the Regulation of Healthcare Professionals had the right to refer cases to court even after an acquittal by the appropriate regulatory body. The GMC had challenged the CRHP's right to refer the case of Dr Ruscillo to the court. In another case, the High Court held that where a decision of the GMC was referred by the Council for the Regulation of Healthcare Professionals to the High Court, the question for the court was whether the GMC had been unduly lenient and not whether the decision was wrong.[10] These judgements were confirmed on appeal.[11]

In July 2004, the CRHP changed its name to the Council for Healthcare Regulatory Excellence (CHRE) and announced that the Council's corporate identity would be officially launched with publication of its first annual report to Parliament in the Autumn of 2004. This Annual Report for 2003/2004[12] outlines the actions which it has undertaken since being set up in April 2003 including:

– undertaking a performance review of the work of the regulators;

– considering the disciplinary decisions of the regulators: of 213 cases considered the CHRE closed 176 without further action; referred 15 to a case meeting and sent seven to the High Court (one of which it later withdrew);

– promoting good practice by enhancing communication between the regulators, considering future consultation on its power under s. 27 to change regulators' rules and developing principles of good practice;

– publishing a landmark study of the nine regulators' work; and

– identifying some of the future challenges including increased mobility of healthcare professionals, adapting to the demands of new workforce trends such as team working and building on good practice in relation to public involvement, complaints, fitness to practise procedures, diversity standards and education.

FIFTH SHIPMAN REPORT

The fifth report of this Inquiry was published in December 2004.[13] It considers the handling of complaints against GPs, the raising of concerns about GPs, the procedures of the General Medical Council and the revalidation of doctors and makes significant recommendations for the more effective regulation of GPs. In March 2005, the Chief Medical Officer announced that, in the light of the Fifth Shipman Report, a review of medical revalidation was being carried out, starting with a call for ideas.[14]

This has led to the postponement of the GMC's revalidation scheme. The review aims to give advice on further measures necessary to strengthen procedures for assuring the safety of patients in situations where a doctor's performance or conduct pose a risk to patients, ensure the operation of an effective system of revalidation and modify the role, structure and functions of the GMC. Many of the detailed changes for GMC procedures recommended in the Fifth Shipman Report could also apply, where appropriate, to the NMC, as could the results from the CMO's review.

CONCLUSIONS

Major changes have taken place in the accountability of health professionals to their registration body. The Government's intention in the NHS Plan was to raise the standards of registered practitioners and ensure that the public were protected from those who were unworthy to be placed on, or remain on, the Register. The constitution and procedures for dealing with fitness to practise of the Health Professions Council are similar to the NMC, and significant changes have taken place in the powers and procedures of the General Medical Council. There are however still considerable differences between the ways in which these registration bodies function, and there is every likelihood that as the new Councils establish themselves, they will lead to greater similarities in the state regulation of the conduct of all health professionals. This uniformity will be accelerated as a result of the establishment of the Council for the Regulation of Healthcare Professionals (now called the Council for Healthcare Regulatory Excellence) acting as a central regulator for the health registration bodies[15] and also as a result of the recommendations of the Fifth Shipman Report. The DoH consultation document on a new statutory compensation scheme for clinical negligence, Making Amends,[16] recommends that there should be an enforceable duty of candour on health professionals. (This is discussed in Ch. 14.) It remains to be seen the extent to which the new machinery and workings of fitness to practise, competence and health committees of the NMC raise standards of professional practice and the protection of the general public in comparison with the work of its predecessor the UKCC. It is highly likely that within the next 2 years, there will be significant changes to our current system of professional conduct hearings and registration and re-registration provisions. Possibly the CHRE could take over the role currently played by the NMC, GMC and other health profession registration bodies.

QUESTIONS AND EXERCISES

1. How would you define fitness to practise?

2. You are asked by a colleague who is facing fitness to practise proceedings to accompany her as a friend. Outline the stages which you would expect the

hearing to follow and consider the types of evidence she would require to defend herself.

3. Evaluate the role of the Health Committee of the NMC. Do you think that there could be an overlap between the functions of the Health Committee and that of the Conduct and Competence Committee?

4. You have been fined for parking on double yellow lines while visiting a client in the course of your employment. To your horror, you discover that someone has reported this to the NMC. Outline the stages which will follow and the procedures which exist for each stage.

References

1 The Nursing and Midwifery Order 2001, Statutory Instrument 2002 No 253.

2 Nursing and Midwifery Council. Code of professional conduct: standards for conduct, performance and ethics. NMC; 2004.

3 Nursing and Midwifery Council Guidance 06/04. Requirements for evidence of good health and good character. NMC; 2004

4 Nursing and Midwifery Council. (Education, Registration and Registration Appeals) Rules 2004 (SI 2004/1767). Norwich: The Stationery Office; 2004. Online. Available: www.hmso.gov.uk

5 The Nursing and Midwifery Council. (Fitness to Practise) Rules Order of Council 2004, SI No 1761.

6 HMSO. Online. Available: www.hmso.legislation.uk

7 NMC Circular 16/2004 20 July 2004.

8 Nursing and Midwifery Council. Fitness to Practise Annual Report 2003–4.

9 Bristol Royal Infirmary Learning from Bristol: the report of the public inquiry into children's heart surgery at the Bristol Royal Infirmary 1984–1995 (Chaired by Professor Ian Kennedy). Command Paper CM 5207 July 2001. Online. Available: http://www.bristol-inquiry.org.uk

10 Council for the Regulation of Healthcare Professionals v. General Medical Council and Another. The Times Law Report, 1 September 2004.

11 Council for the Regulation of Health Care Professionals v. General Medical Council (Sub nom Ruscillo); Council for the Regulation of Health Care Professionals v. Nursing and Midwifery Council (Sub nom Truscott) [2004] EWCA Civ 1356, [2005] 1 WLR 717.

12 Council for Healthcare Regulatory Excellence. Online. Available: www.chre.org.uk

13 The Shipman Inquiry Fifth Report Safeguarding Patients: Lessons from the Past – Proposals for the Future. Command Paper CM 6394 December 2004; Stationery Office. Online. Available: www. the-shipman-inquiry.org.uk/reports.asp

14 Chief Medical Officer. DoH Review of Medical Revalidation: A call for ideas. London: DoH; 2005: 3 March.

15 Dimond B. Law for midwives step by step: Part 39 Health Professions Regulation. Br J Midwifery 2002; 10(3):180.

16 Department of Health Making Amends. A consultation paper setting out proposals for reforming the approach to clinical negligence in the NHS. CMO; June 2003.

Chapter 5

THE MIDWIVES RULES AND CODE OF PRACTICE, THE CODE OF PROFESSIONAL CONDUCT AND THE SCOPE OF PROFESSIONAL PRACTICE

The midwife is the only professional (other than registered nurses who are fever nurses) of those registered by the NMC to be subject to rules made specifically for her profession. The Midwives Rules have legal force and are binding upon the practitioner. In contrast, the NMC Standards and guidance and the Code of Professional Conduct: standards for conduct, performance and ethics, like the other NMC advisory papers, do not have the force of law, but failure to follow the codes could be used in evidence in proceedings on fitness to practise, conduct and competence proceedings.

THE MIDWIVES RULES

The Midwives Rules which came into force on 1 August 2004[1] replace the Rules which were revised in 1998.[2] They replace the Midwives Rules and Code of Practice and in the publication by the NMC[3] each of the new rules is accompanied by NMC standards and guidance. The new Rules cover the topics shown in Box 5.1.

Box 5.1 Midwives Rules 2004

Rule 1 Citation and commencement

Rule 2 Interpretation

Rule 3 Notification of intention to practise (see Ch. 3)

Rule 4 Notification by local supervising authority (see Ch. 3)

Rule 5 Suspension from practice by a local supervising authority

Rule 6 Responsibility and sphere of practice

Rule 7 Administration of medicines

Rule 8 Clinical trials

Rule 9 Records

Rule 10 Inspection of premises and equipment

Rule 11 Eligibility for appointment as a Supervisor of Midwives

Rule 12 The supervision of midwives

Rule 13 The local supervising authority midwifery officer

Rule 14 Exercise by a local supervising authority of its functions

Rule 15 Publication of local supervising authority procedures

Rule 16 Annual Report

RULE 6 RESPONSIBILITY AND SPHERE OF PRACTICE

Rule 6 sets out the midwife's responsibility and sphere of practice and is shown in Box 5.2.

Box 5.2 Rule 6: Responsibility and sphere of practice

1. A practising midwife is responsible for providing midwifery care, **in accordance with such standards as the Council may specify from time to time**, to a woman and baby during the antenatal, intranatal and postnatal periods.

2. Except in an emergency, a practising midwife shall not provide any care, or undertake any treatment, which she has not been trained to give.

3. In an emergency, or where a deviation from the norm which is outside her current sphere of practice becomes apparent in a woman or baby during the antenatal, intranatal or postnatal periods, a practising midwife shall call such qualified health professional who may reasonably be expected to have the requisite skills and experience to assist her in the provision of care.

The words in bold were added in the new Rule as an amendment to the old Rule 40. Other changes include the omission of the words 'midwifery' and 'either before or after registration as a midwife' from sub-para. 1 and the omission of registered medical practitioner from the emergency provisions of sub-para. 3.

The NMC has set standards and provided guidance for the implementation of Rule 6. The Standards are shown in Box 5.3.

Box 5.3 NMC Standards for Rule 6: Responsibility and sphere of practice

A midwife:

– cannot arrange for anyone to act as a substitute, other than another practising midwife or a registered medical practitioner

– must make sure the needs of the woman or baby are the primary focus of her practice

– should work in partnership with the woman and her family

– should enable the woman to make decisions about her care based on her individual needs, by discussing matters fully with her

– should respect the woman's right to refuse any advice given

– is responsible for maintaining and developing her own competence

– must ensure she becomes competent in any new skills required for her practice

– is responsible for familiarising herself with her employer's policies.

In addition, the NMC has provided guidance noting the definition of the activities of a midwife as set by the Federation of International Gynaecologists and Obstetricians and the World Health Organization, which are given on p. 36 of the NMC Midwives Rules and Standards booklet (see Ch. 2 of this book)

The NMC guidance covers the accountability of the midwife which cannot be taken by or given to another registered practitioner; her professional accountability for students; the necessity for good team working; fully informing the woman about significant risks and giving her full information; action to be taken if the woman rejects the midwife's advice (which is recognised as the woman's right); the need for the midwife to keep clinically up to date to ensure that she can carry out effectively emergency procedures such as resuscitation, for the woman or baby. The NMC also advises that where new skills are learnt which do not necessarily become part of the role of all midwives, each employing authority should have a locally agreed guideline, which meets the NMC standards. The NMC also advises the midwife to determine her professional indemnity insurance status and take appropriate action (see Ch. 13 and also Ch. 23, on the independent midwife).

THE CODE OF PROFESSIONAL CONDUCT: STANDARDS FOR CONDUCT, PERFORMANCE AND ETHICS AND OTHER NMC GUIDANCE AND ADVISORY PAPERS

Like all other registered practitioners, the midwife has also a duty to observe the Code of Professional Conduct: standards for conduct, performance and ethics[4] and the other guidance issued by the NMC. While these do not have the force of law (i.e. breach of the Paragraphs does not automatically constitute an offence), a practitioner's failure to observe the guidance can be used in fitness to practise hearings.

The midwife should however be aware of certain problems which she may confront in developing her practice. Those discussed here include:

- Definition of competence

- Protecting the employee who asserts her incompetence

- Resisting pressures of work

- Definition of job description.

DEFINITION OF COMPETENCE

Since the midwife is personally responsible for her own professional development she needs to have some benchmark to determine whether she has the appropriate competence to practise in a new field. Attendance of an approved course with assessment procedures may still be an important criterion for competence but it will be more difficult to assess competence in the workplace as new procedures, equipment and methods of work are introduced. The introduction of water births is one example where initially there were no clear standards or criteria for competence. The same problem confronts the employer who has the responsibility to ensure that his employees are competent, and the employer will be looking for criteria to determine the competence of new and existing employees to work in new fields of practice. The NMC in its guidance on Rule 6 (see above) states that where the midwife is required to learn new skills, which do not necessarily become part of the role of all midwives, each employing authority should have a locally agreed guideline, which meets the NMC standards.

PROTECTION OF THE EMPLOYEE WHO ASSERTS HER INCOMPETENCE

If the midwife knows that she is being asked to work outside her field of competence she has a clear duty under the Midwives Rules, Standards and Guidance and the Code of Professional Conduct: standards for conduct, performance and ethics, to make that known to her employers and to practise only within her sphere of competence. However, employees who are under pressure from other professionals or managers to work outside their sphere of competence must be protected. The midwife should make known both to her Supervisor of Midwives and also to her line manager, any unacceptable pressures upon her and potential dangers for the client. Unfortunately at present, while there is a legal requirement for the midwife to undertake a specific number of days of professional development to remain on the register, there is no statutory requirement for an employer to fund the cost of such professional development for a midwife, and there is inconsistency across the country over whether midwives obtain paid time off work and/or obtain the costs of any study days. Ultimately, it is the midwife's personal responsibility to ensure that she is competent and that she obtains the necessary training and supervised practice before moving into new areas.

RESISTING PRESSURES OF WORK

The employee whose scope of practice is enlarged must be protected from the dangers of lowering standards. Since the skill mix is changing and more non-registered employees are being employed in ratio to registered practitioners, new techniques and work methods will have to be devised to protect standards of practice and the patients from harm. However, the law makes illegal any delegation of the activity of attendance at childbirth to a non-midwife or non-doctor (see Ch. 25).

There are pressures on the midwife to work outside her competence, as the situation in Box 5.4 illustrates.

Box 5.4 Considerable pressure

When new laws were introduced making it illegal for the junior doctors to exceed 56 hours working per week, midwives found that they were expected to act as first assistants for an emergency caesarean section. They asked the obstetricians if they could receive training for this role, but were told that midwives could not take on a surgical activity. What is the law?

There are clear dangers to patient safety in allowing the situation identified above to continue. Either acting as first assistant is recognised as an expanded role activity for midwives, who then receive the appropriate training, or sufficient doctors are employed to ensure that midwives would not have to take on that activity. A midwife would be entitled to refuse to act in a situation where she is not competent, unless in an emergency the risks of not acting outweighed the risks of acting. There are of course many examples of hospitals providing the training for midwives to act as first assistants in theatres. For example, the developments at the Gloucester Royal Hospital[5] enabled midwives to expand their roles to include suturing, episiotomies and perineal lacerations, assisting in theatre with caesarean sections, and carrying out cardiotocographic interpretations, venesection and intravenous cannulation.

PROTECTION OF THE EMPLOYEE

The government has recognised the need to protect staff from being victimised if they bring attention to the hazards at work. Following a consultation exercise on the Secretary of State's guidance on relations with the public and media, the NHS Management Executive issued guidance EL(93)51, published 8 June 1993. This guidance made it clear that:

Under no circumstances are employees who express their views about health service issues in accordance with this guidance to be penalised in any way for doing so. (Para. 6)

This guidance was followed by a circular bringing the Public Interest Disclosure Act 1998 to the attention of staff and requiring all NHS trusts to implement the Act.[6] All NHS employers have the responsibility for establishing a local procedure for staff to raise concerns with the management including the highest level of local management and ultimately with the Chairman of the authority or trust. Any member of staff who raises concerns is protected from victimisation (see Ch. 22 and whistle-blowing).

Many trusts now incorporate within their contracts of employment terms that registered practitioners should follow the professional guidance of their registration bodies as part of the contract of employment. Such terms should prevent a conflict between the duties required of a practitioner by their employer and by their professional registration body. This was a recommendation of the Report of the Inquiry into the Bristol Royal Infirmary children's heart surgery,[7] but was rejected by the Department of Health in respect of the contracts of medical practitioners.

DEFINITION OF JOB DESCRIPTION

The midwife must ensure that as her expected duties enlarge she has a clear agreement with the employer over what she is expected to undertake in relation to other staff, particularly medical staff. This is of particular importance in the development of midwife-managed units where there may not be 24-hour medical cover and where the midwife should identify the skills she requires in order to be able to care for the mother and baby appropriately. (This is further considered in Ch. 24, which also considers the expanded role of the midwife.)

All employers have the right in law to define the job description of the employee. The employee has an implied duty to obey the reasonable orders of the employer and to undertake all duties with all reasonable care and skill. What is 'reasonable' may lead to discussion. For example, is it 'reasonable' to ask a midwife to work on the gynaecology wards when the midwifery unit is not busy? What is reasonable would depend upon the duration of that work, and the capacity in which the midwife is required to work. It would, for example, be unreasonable to ask a direct entry midwife to be a staff nurse, if she does not have the competence; it may be reasonable to ask the midwife to help out for an afternoon, in the appropriate capacity, but unreasonable to ask her to work there for 3 months which would de-skill her as a midwife. 'Reasonableness' must therefore be defined in the context of what is lawful, what would be the recommendations of the professional registration body, and what would be within the job description of the midwife. Where instructions of the employer are unreasonable, then it would be lawful for the midwife to refuse to obey them.

Where the midwife is aware that a policy of the trust appears to conflict with the rights of clients/mothers, or with the regulations and guidance of the NMC, and with her own right to use her professional judgement, she should ensure that this is brought to the attention of her Supervisor of Midwives and the senior managers so that the dispute can be resolved before it gives rise to problems in practice. If necessary, the internal procedure set up under the Public Interest Disclosure Act 1998 could be used to ensure that she is not victimised as a result of bringing the concern to the attention of managers.

WATER BIRTHS

The development of skills in handling births in water can be used as an example of the application of the principles of professional development.

Much publicity was given in 1993 to the tragic deaths of two babies delivered in water, one in Sweden, the other in Bristol. The baby in Sweden died after being delivered with the help of two midwives, but not in a hospital.[8] In Bristol, a baby died after the mother spent part of the labour in a birthing pool at St Michael's Hospital. A second baby was born, with brain damage, 18 months later. Professor Stirrat said that in both cases the children appear to have been deprived of oxygen: 'We think that something happened during the first stage of labour. We speculate that it might have been the temperature of the water. We think that the fetal temperature might have gone up, and that stressed the baby'.[9] As a result of the publicity given to these events, several trusts decided to inform their midwives that they should not participate in water births either in the community or in trust hospitals.

In Hertfordshire, two midwives were disciplined when they assisted in a home confinement when the mother refused to get out of the bath. The trust had a policy of allowing women to labour in water, but not to give birth in water.[10] One midwife received a final written warning, which meant that she would be dismissed if she committed another transgression in the next 2 years, the other received a final written warning and was required to undergo 3 months' updating. The Chief Executive of the trust made it clear that:

- the technique of delivering in water is still not fully evaluated

- the contract between purchaser and provider does not include the provision of water births

- no staff are trained in water births

- the trust would have no defence if a medical catastrophe were to occur

- any patient wishing to have a water birth may book at other hospitals

- if evidence becomes available to confirm the safe and effective nature of the technique then the trust will revise its policies.

Research has now been conducted by the National Perinatal Epidemiology Unit in Oxford, commissioned by the Department of Health, into the safety of water births. The survey was initiated in response to a recommendation of the Commons Select Committee that all hospitals should provide the pools where practicable.[11] In September 2000, a set of evidence-based practical guidelines for midwives on using water in labour and birth was prepared by Ethel Burns and Sheila Kitzinger (2000)[12] with the intention that they will be regularly updated. The guidelines are based upon advice from midwives experienced in using birth pools and upon a wide range of published studies and can be used in any care setting. Ethel Burns has also published an analysis of the data on the use of water births taken from 1300 women and shows that water immersion can be a safe and satisfying choice for women in childbirth who have experienced an uncomplicated pregnancy.[13] Garland and Jones (2000)[14] showed, using a five-centre audit, how audit data was able to make a useful contribution to evidence-based practice. A brief outline of the essential issues to consider in a water birth is given in the latest edition of Mayes' Midwifery.[15]

Where there is a simple direction from the employer forbidding certain activities within the course of employment, several issues emerge:

- How is the standard of care determined in a water birth case?

- How is competence on the part of the midwife determined?

- To what extent is the midwife bound to obey the policies of the trust?

HOW IS THE STANDARD OF CARE DETERMINED?

In Chapter 13, the Bolam Test is discussed. This is the test used by judges to determine the standard of care which can be expected of the defendant in a case.

The standard of care expected is the standard of the ordinary skilled man exercising and professing to have that special skill.[16]

Evidence would be given in court by experts as to the practice which they would have expected to see followed in the case of such a method of delivery and birth. Yet this is difficult in an area which is still the subject of research and innovation. Initially it may have been difficult to define a set standard. However, over recent years, many centres have developed the use of birthing pools, and skills and standards have developed as seen above. Any midwife who wishes to take part in water births must ensure that she has kept up-to-date with recent developments and constantly improved her practice. In any dispute over the standard of care which should have been followed in a water birth, expert evidence would be given to the court by specialists over what standard the client could have expected according to the Bolam Test.

The Royal College of Midwives has published guidelines on water births[17] and is currently mounting a campaign for normal birth.[18]

Increasingly, guidance and recommended practice from the National Institute for Health and Clinical Excellence (NICE) will be referred to in defining standards of practice across most clinical areas. Their guidance will create a presumption that that advice should be followed, and the clinical practitioner will have to show reasonable grounds why the guidance did not apply for that particular patient (see Ch. 21 on NICE).

HOW IS COMPETENCE DETERMINED?

In a field which is constantly developing, it is very difficult for the midwife to pinpoint the moment at which she is competent to assist in a water birth delivery. Attendance at a recognised centre, with assessment, is obviously desirable. However, this is a field which shows clearly the value of the principles laid down by the NMC in the Code of Professional Conduct: standards for conduct, performance and ethics and in the guidance in the Midwives Rules and Standards. The midwife has to check out her own competence by assisting at water births under the control of more experienced midwives, learning as much as she can from what has been written, and delivering her first water birth baby under supervision. As with all other skills it will need constant updating in the light of research findings.

OBEDIENCE TO THE POLICIES OF THE TRUST

It is hoped that policies of trusts relating to midwifery services and practice will comply with the NMC guidance and with the policies established by the Local Supervising Authority (see Ch. 3) in conjunction with the Supervisor of Midwives. Where there is a clash, then clearly the midwife must take the advice of her senior manager and supervisor. The midwife has a contractual duty to obey the reasonable instructions of her employer. It is not possible to say that there will never be a clash between the instructions of her employer and the Midwives Rules and the NMC guidance. However, it is extremely unlikely. The midwife is bound by the Rules: the trust must accept that and many trusts now incorporate the NMC Code of Professional Conduct: standards for conduct, performance and ethics, within the contracts of employment of their registered practitioners. The NHS Trust as the provider of services must ensure through its risk management policies that precautions are taken to prevent any possibility of claims through litigation. One way of safeguarding this is through ensuring that staff are trained and competent.

If, however, a trust is to attempt to define in detail what a midwife can and cannot do, it raises questions as to the midwife's professional clinical judgement and the role it plays in her contract of employment. Rule 6, on the definition of the responsibility and sphere of practice of the practising midwife, would appear to leave little scope for trusts to define what is or is not in the competence of the midwife. In Chapter 6, a case where a midwife refused to accept the Trust's instructions not to assist in a home birth is considered.

CONCLUSIONS

The midwife is perhaps more fortunate than other practitioners registered with the NMC in that she has clear rules of conduct which are legally binding upon her. The new rules in force since August 2004 and the standards and guidance provided by the NMC provide a clear statutory framework for her practice. Ultimately however, like all other registered practitioners it is her personal and professional responsibility to ensure that she is competent, up to date and her professional development is maintained.

QUESTIONS AND EXERCISES

1. Identify activities which you do not at present undertake as part of your role as a midwife and consider how you could develop the expertise to undertake those activities within the principles laid down by the NMC.

2. What limits do you consider should be placed by Act of Parliament on the functions and role of the midwife?

3. Consider whether there are any potential conflicts between your job description and the policies relating to midwifery laid down by your employer (see Ch. 24).

4. Obtain a copy of the procedure set up by your employer as a result of the Public Interest Disclosure Act 1998 and analyse how it would apply in the event of your being aware of a major health and safety concern.

5. What role do you consider that the Consultant midwife plays, and what is its likely impact upon advanced midwifery practice (see Ch. 24)?

References

1 Nursing and Midwifery Council (Midwives) Rules Order of Council 2004, Statutory Instrument 2004/1764.

2 Nurses, Midwives and Health Visitors. (Midwives Amendment) Rules Approval Order, SI 1998 No 2649.

3 Nursing and Midwifery Council Midwives Rules and Standards, August 2004.

4 Nursing and Midwifery Council Code of professional conduct: standards for conduct, performance and ethics. NMC; 2004.

5 Ramsay B. Senior house officer training. When midwives perform obstetric tasks at night, trainees can spend more supervised time in clinics. BMJ 1997; 314:1830.

6 Department of Health Public Interest Disclosure Act. Health Service Circular 1999; 198.

7 Bristol Royal Infirmary. Learning from Bristol: the report of the public inquiry into children's heart surgery at the Bristol Royal Infirmary 1984–1995. Command Paper CM 5207; 2001. Online. Available: www.bristol-inquiry.org.uk

8 George N. The Times, 16 October 1993.

9 Laurance J, Berrington L. The Times, 16 October 1993.

10 Lewison H. Br J Midwifery 1994; 2:146–147.

11 Royal College of Obstetricians and Gynaecologists. Guidelines: birth in water. January 2001. Online. Available: www.rcog.org.uk/guidelines/birthwater.html

12 Burns E, Kitzinger S. Midwifery guidelines for use of water in labour. Oxford: Oxford Centres for Health Care Research and Development, Oxford Brookes University; 2000. Online. Available: www.sheilakitzinger.com/WaterBirth.htm

13 Burns E. Waterbirth. MIDIRS Midwifery Digest 2001; 11(s2):s10–13.

14 Garland D, Jones K. Waterbirths – supporting practice with clinical audit. MIDIRS Midwifery Digest 2000; 10:333–336.

15 Henderson C and Macdonald S, eds. Mayes' Midwifery, 13th edn. London: Baillière Tindall; 2004:500–501.

16 Bolam v. Friern Hospital Management Committee QBD [1957] 2 All ER 118.

17 Royal College of Midwives. The use of water in labour and birth: Position Paper 1a. RCM Midwives J 2000; 3:374–375.

18 Royal College of Midwives Campaign for Normal Birth 2005. Online. Available: www.rcmnormalbirth.net

SECTION B

CLIENT RIGHTS

This Section considers the legal issues relating to a woman and her legal rights in childbirth. It begins by considering the implications of the Human Rights Act 1998 and then looks at the changing background to the provision of maternity services and the legal implications of this. Specific topics such as the right to give consent, confidentiality, access and the rights of the fetus are considered in subsequent chapters in this section. A further chapter is concerned with the issues arising from teenage pregnancies.

Chapter 6
WOMAN-CENTRED CARE
The Human Rights Act 1998

Following the Second World War, the UK, together with many other European countries, was a signatory to the European Convention on Human Rights. People who considered that their rights had been infringed could take a case to the European Court of Human Rights which was based in Strasbourg. (This is entirely separate from the European Economic Community which has its European Court of Justice in Luxembourg.) In 1998 the Human Rights Act was passed. This was brought into force for England, Wales and Northern Ireland on 2 October 2000 and for Scotland on devolution. Its main effect was to place a duty upon public authorities and those organisations exercising functions of a public nature to implement the articles of the Convention. In addition, those people who considered that their rights as set out in the European Convention on Human Rights had been infringed could take public authorities to court in this country, instead of going to Strasbourg. These Articles are set out in Schedule 1 to the Act and can be found in Appendix 1 of this book. Articles 2, 3, 5, 6, 8, 9, 10 and 14 are likely to be of particular concern to midwifery practice.

ARTICLE 2

Everyone's right to life shall be protected by law. No one shall be deprived of his life intentionally save in the execution of a sentence of a court following his conviction of a crime for which this penalty is provided by law.

Recent decisions of the courts show how this right is interpreted. For example in a recent case,[1] parents lost their attempt to ensure that a severely handicapped baby born prematurely was resuscitated if necessary. The judge ruled that the hospital should provide him with palliative care to ease his suffering, but should not try to revive him as that would cause unnecessary pain (the case is considered in Ch. 9).

In another case, the President of the Family Division, Dame Elizabeth Butler-Sloss, held that withdrawal of life-sustaining medical treatment was not contrary to Article 2 of the Human Rights Convention and the right to life, where the patient was in a persistent vegetative state. The ruling was made on 25 October 2000 in cases involving Mrs M, 49, who suffered brain damage during an operation abroad in 1997 and was diagnosed as being in a persistent vegetative state (PVS) in October 1998 and Mrs H, 36, who fell ill in America as a result of pancreatitis at Christmas 1999.[2]

Article 2 was also invoked in the case involving the separation of Siamese twins, in which the Court of Appeal decided on 22 September 2000 that they could be separated even though this would undoubtedly lead to the death of the one who depended upon the heart and the lungs of the other. The Court of Appeal defended its decision on the grounds that the baby who had a chance of survival was having its lifeblood drained away by the other who had no chance of survival if she were to be separated, and therefore doctors were acting on behalf of that one in self-defence. Acting in self-defence can be a justification for depriving another of the right to life. The parents, who had refused to give consent to the operation of separation, decided against appealing to the House of Lords. At the inquest, a unique finding of death was made, the coroner resorting to a 'narrative verdict':

Mary died after surgery to separate her from her conjoined twin, and that the surgery was permitted by order of the High Court, confirmed by the Court of Appeal.[3]

There could be more cases heard where patients and relatives urge the courts to accept that there has been an infringement of Article 2 of the European Convention on Human Rights. For example, it may be used if a person is marked down as Not for Resuscitation (NFR) and the relatives disagree with the clinicians. In addition, the Article may also be relied upon where a patient alleges that failure to provide health services is infringing her right to life. However, it has to be established that there is an intention to take life and this has proved the stumbling block to those who have argued that letting die in the case of persistent vegetative state patients or severely disabled babies is a breach of Article 2[4] (see Ch. 9).

In the case where a woman suffering the terminal stages of motor neurone disease applied to the High Court for a declaration that it would be lawful for her husband to assist her in ending her life,[5] the High Court held that Articles 2 and 3 of the European Convention on Human Rights did not protect the right to procure one's own death or confer a right to die. The right to the dignity of life was not a right to die with dignity but the right to live with as much dignity as could possibly be afforded until that life reached its natural end (see also Ch. 9). The High Court held that the Director of Public Prosecutions had no power under the Suicide Act to give an undertaking not to consent to the prosecution of a person for aiding and abetting, counselling or procuring of a suicide of another, where the acts which might constitute such an offence had not yet occurred or been investigated. The House of Lords dismissed Diane Pretty's appeal, holding that there was no conflict between the Articles of the European Convention on Human Rights and Section 2(1) of the Suicide Act 1961 which made it a criminal offence to aid and abet a suicide.[6] She also lost her application to the European Court of Human Rights, the court holding that there was no incompatibility between the Suicide Act 1961 and the articles of the European Convention.[7] In the case of Osman v. United Kingdom,[8] the ECHR held that the obligation to preserve life was not absolute especially in the context of operational choices, priorities and resources.

ARTICLE 3

No one shall be subjected to torture or to inhuman or degrading treatment or punishment.

While it is hoped that torture does not take place in healthcare, there are evident examples of degrading and inhuman treatment. Most midwives would probably agree that a recent case where a pregnant prisoner was handcuffed to the bed during her labour would appear to be a *prima facie* breach of this right (see below). The European Court of Human Rights has ruled that corporal punishment by parents to discipline their children was a breach of Article 3 of the European Convention on Human Rights.[9] A step-father had on several occasions beaten a 9-year-old boy with a garden cane. The step-father had been prosecuted for assault occasioning actual bodily harm, but had been acquitted by the jury who accepted his defence that the caning had been necessary and reasonable to discipline the boy. The European Court of Human Rights held that ill-treatment must attain a minimum level of severity if it is to fall within the scope of Article 3. It depended on all the circumstances of the case, such as the nature and context of the treatment, its duration, its physical and mental effects and in some instances, the sex, age and state of health of the victim. In finding that there had been a breach of Article 3, the court awarded the boy £10 000 against the UK government, and costs. The UK government acknowledged that UK law failed to provide adequate protection to children and should be amended. Subsequently, guidance was issued by the government on the use of corporal punishment against children (see Ch. 32 and Child protection).

In the case of Z. v. UK 1999[10] the Commission found a violation of Article 3 arising from the failure of the local authority to take action in respect of serious ill-treatment and neglect caused to four siblings by their parents over a period of more than four and a half years.

Midwives should analyse their practice and the way in which the mothers are treated right through antenatal, intrapartum and postnatal care and decide if there are grounds for believing that this Article is not respected. Action should then be taken to remedy the situation in order to prevent possible litigation.

Article 3 and women prisoners

It was reported in 1994 that a prisoner who was transferred to Wythenshawe hospital for the delivery of her child was handcuffed during the confinement.[11] It appeared that she had absconded three times before and therefore staff kept her handcuffed at all times, including during the birth.

A prison service spokesman stated that guidelines had been issued to cover such a situation and the Director General of the Prison Service at that time issued an official apology to the mother. The RCM welcomed the apology given by the Director General of the Prison Service to the prisoner, who had been moved from Styal prison to Wythenshawe Hospital for the delivery.[12] Hansard reported that a letter from the Director General read out in Parliament confirmed that:

Handcuffs must be removed in any case if the doctor treating the patient so requests.[13]

It might have been thought that with these promises of new guidelines and apologies, a situation of handcuffing a woman during labour would not recur. Yet, in 1996 it was reported that Annette Walker was taken from Holloway prison to the Whittington Hospital in handcuffs, where she spent 10 hours in labour chained to a bed, in the presence of a male and a female officer.[14] Ann Widdecombe, the Home Office Minister, defended the action initially, saying that Whittington Hospital had not been concerned about the handcuffing of women prisoners while in labour at their hospital. However, she subsequently apologised for this inaccurate statement.[15] It was later reported that the Home Office, following discussions with the RCM, was dropping the policy of keeping pregnant women in handcuffs during labour and delivery.[16] Subsequently, supported by AIMS, Annette Walker sued the prison service and accepted £19 000 compensation.[17]

In 2003, the European Court of Human Rights held that inadequate medical care by prison authorities towards a prisoner which caused distress and discomfort but which did not amount to physical or psychological injury could amount to a breach of Article 3.[18]

For further information on mothers in prison see Cading-Paull (1994).[19] Price and Ridge (2001) also consider the implications for pregnant women in prison.[20] Yet, shackling of pregnant women continued: Theresa McDonagh, a pregnant woman, was shackled to a radiator for 5 hours when she appeared in court on a £27 theft charge.[21] Many individuals and organisations have fought valiantly to ensure that the rules are changed: Sheila Kitzinger and the National Childbirth Trust, Beverley Beech and AIMS, the Maternity Alliance, the Royal College of Midwives, and the Howard League for Penal Reform to name only a few. Their campaigning has ensured that such gross breaches of human rights are brought to public attention and promises secured over improvements. Sheila Kitzinger reviews the current challenges facing those concerned about pregnant women in prison.[22] See also Sally Price's articles[23] and a case study illustrating the work of the Howard League for Penal Reform by Finola Farrant.[24]

ARTICLE 5

Everyone has the right to liberty and security of person. No one shall be deprived of his liberty save in the following cases and in accordance with a procedure prescribed by law.

Many exceptions are then given, including:

(f) the lawful detention of persons for the prevention of the spreading of infectious diseases, or persons of unsound mind, alcoholics or drug addicts or vagrants.

The House of Lords decided in the Bournewood case[25] that a person who lacked the mental capacity to consent to admission to psychiatric hospital could be detained there in his best interests without being detained under the Mental Health Act 1983. However, the European Court of Human Rights subsequently held that the NHS Trust was in breach of Article 5.[26] As a consequence of this decision, the Department of Health is consulting on how the 'Bournewood gap' should be filled[27] (see Ch. 7). A new Mental Capacity Act is to be brought into force in April 2007 making provision for decision-making on behalf of mentally incapacitated adults (see Ch. 7) and a second draft Mental Health Bill is being considered (see Ch. 33). The Court of Appeal has held that in the absence of statutory provision for mentally incapacitated adults, the court did have an inherent power to hear issues involved in the day-to-day care of such persons and to grant declarations in the best interests of mentally incapable persons.[28]

ARTICLE 6: THE RIGHT TO A FAIR TRIAL

This right will have significant implications since it applies not just to criminal charges but also to the determination of civil rights and obligations. It would there-fore apply to disciplinary actions and other such forums, where at present employees may not have representation and they may be in a very weak situation compared with the employer. A challenge that the proceedings of the UKCC failed to comply with Article 6[29] led to the UKCC reviewing its procedures.[30] Originally, the arrange-ments for the new Nursing and Midwifery Council took into account the provisions of the Human Rights Act 1998 by establishing an appeal process to a Nursing and Midwifery Independent Appeals Tribunal (Articles 35–37). However, this was subse-quently removed from the draft statutory provisions on the grounds that the existing system of appeals satisfied the provisions of the Human Rights Articles. (This is con-sidered in Ch. 4.)

ARTICLE 8

1. *Everyone has the right to respect for private and family life, his home and his correspondence.*

2. *There shall be no interference by a public authority with the exercise of the right except such as is in accordance with the law and is necessary in a democratic society in the interests of national security, public safety or the economic wellbeing of the country, for the prevention of disorder or crime, for the protection of health or morals, or for the pro-tection of the rights and freedoms of others.*

This right requires greater sensitivity about patient privacy than has been shown in the past within healthcare. The traditional ward round, where a curtain is seen as a sound-proof barrier but in fact all those on the ward can hear the intimate details of a patient's diagnosis, prognosis and treatment, will have to be reviewed. Many other actions may have to be taken in order to ensure that this right of the patient is recognised and protected. The Caldicott Guardians, whose role is considered in Chapter 10, will have to take on the responsibility for ensuring that there is no breach of Article 8.

The respect for family life did not enable a prisoner to obtain artificial insemination[31] and it was held that high security restrictions on child visits were valid and not a breach of Article 8.[32] In contrast, a woman in Holloway prison won her appeal against the decision that her baby would be taken away from her at birth.[33] This was held to be a breach of Article 8 of the Human Rights Convention and the United Nations Convention on the Rights of the Child. Article 8 of the European Convention could be interpreted as giving a baby a right to be breast-fed if the mother so wished, and of continuing contact with the mother, irrespective of her being in custody. In contrast, the High Court has ruled in two cases (brought by P and by Q) that the policy of the prison service that children should cease to live·with their mothers in prison at 18 months old was lawful and not contrary to Article 8.[34] Article 8 gave a right to respect for family life and the qualifications contained in Article 8.2 were in play by reason of the legality, recognised by Article 5, of the prisoner's imprisonment. The Court of Appeal held[34] that the prison service was entitled to have a policy that children aged 18 months should cease to stay with their mothers in prison, but such a policy should not be operated rigidly. The reasons for the need for flexibility were first, the aim of promoting the welfare of the child (which had to be related to the circumstances of the prison) and second, the interference with the child's family life had to be justified under Article 8.2 of the Human Rights Convention. The Court dismissed the appeal of P but allowed the appeal of Q.

A patient at Ashworth High Security Hospital lost his application for judicial review on the grounds that the provisions relating to the discretionary power of the Special Hospitals to record and listen to a random 10% of telephone calls infringed his right to respect for privacy under Article 8. The court held that the recording was a justified infringement of Article 8 since it was a proportionate measure and necessary to achieve security for high-risk patients.[35] In contrast, the interception of private phone calls by an employer were held to be a violation of Article 8.[36] Alison Halford won her case claiming violation by the Merseyside Police, her employer, since the Interception of Communications Act 1985 only applied to a public telecommunications system.

The concept of private life includes the right to have information such as official records, photographs, letters and diaries and medical information kept private and confidential. In the case of Gunn-Russo v. Nugent Care Society and the Secretary of State for Health[37] it was held that the Secretary of State had no power to compel a voluntary adoption agency to disclose adoption records to an adopted person, but the disclosure of adoption records by such an agency required a balancing exercise to be conducted between disclosure and confidentiality.

Article 8 has to be interpreted in relation to Article 10 which recognises a right to freedom of expression. Both Articles 8 and 10 are qualified by specified circumstances in which the right is limited, and the courts will balance one against the other in determining whether there has been a breach of either Article. For example when the Beckhams sought an injunction to prevent publication of their nanny's account of their home life, arguing that their right to a private life should be supported, they lost because they had promoted their image of a harmonious family.[38]

OTHER SIGNIFICANT ARTICLES

While these Articles have been looked at in detail, there are others which have considerable significance for healthcare. Article 14, for example, prohibits discrimination and this is considered in Chapter 22 on employment. Article 2 of the First Protocol recognises a right to education, which may be significant for staff who are caring for children with long-term illnesses. Parents also have the right to ensure that such education and teaching is in conformity with their own religious and philosophical convictions.

HUMAN RIGHTS AND THE NHS

An Audit Commission report[39] on Human Rights in the public sector in September 2003 showed that 73% of NHS trusts are not taking action to adopt a strategy for human rights. Health bodies consistently lag behind other public services in recognising human rights issues and are vulnerable to the risk of challenge because they are failing to protect themselves and will not secure service improvement. The Audit Commission emphasised the importance of developing a human rights culture in each public organisation. It suggested the following steps:

– learning lessons from case law

– raising awareness

– developing strategy, policies and procedures to promote human rights

– managing complaints effectively using human rights

– ensuring contractors comply with human rights legislation.

THE DATA PROTECTION ACT 1998 AND THE FREEDOM OF INFORMATION ACT 2000

This legislation also recognises many rights of the patient in the protection of confidential information and in the right of access to information held by public authorities. The Data Protection Act is considered in Chapter 10 and the Freedom of Information Act is considered in Chapter 7.

STATUTORY DUTY TO PROVIDE MATERNITY SERVICES

In Chapter 21, the statutory authorities within the NHS are considered, along with the duty placed upon the Secretary of State to provide services for expectant and nursing mothers and young children 'as he considers are appropriate as part of the health service'. While this is not an absolute duty, it is impossible to have a waiting list in maternity care: nature does not wait. Therefore minimum standards for ante-natal, intrapartum and postnatal care must be provided. In other fields of healthcare, court actions against the Secretary of State for the provision of services have usually failed. Thus patients who had been waiting several years for hip replacement opera-tions in the West Midlands failed in their action against the Secretary of State[40] and a mother who was concerned at the delay in providing her child with heart surgery lost her case.[41] The court held that it was not for the court to substitute its own judgement for that of those responsible for the allocation of resources. It would only interfere if there had been a failure to allocate funds in a way which was reasonable or where there had been breaches of public duties. The same principle was followed in the much-publicised case of Jamie Bowen, a 10-year-old girl who suffered from leukaemia. She needed another course of chemotherapy and a bone marrow trans-plant, after the first one failed. The Health Authority took medical advice that there was a very low chance of success and therefore would not allocate the funds for this additional treatment. Her father brought a court action and the High Court judge suggested that the Health Authority should review its decision. The Court of Appeal upheld the decision of the Health Authority.[42] The Court of Appeal were unable to fault the process of reasoning of the Health Authority and allowed its appeal. The Master of the Rolls (Sir Thomas Bingham) stated:

while I have every sympathy with B, I feel bound to regard this as an attempt – wholly understandable, but nevertheless misguided – to involve the court in a field of activity where it is not fitted to make any decision favourable to the patient.

An anonymous donor then came forward and paid for further treatment for the child, but she died 1 year later.

There have, however, been some recent cases which suggest that the court may be taking a more interventionalist role. Thus, where a Health Authority had a blanket policy not to fund trans-sexual operations, the court held that any policy of funding by a health authority must have genuine regard for the clinical needs of the indi-vidual and recognise the possibility of exceptional circumstances.[43] The court did not, however, consider that there had been a breach of Articles 3 or 8 of the European Convention. In a second case, the court held that failure by a Health Authority to permit the prescribing of Beta Interferon for multiple sclerosis patients in its area, was not in accordance with guidance issued by the Department of Health.[44] A decla-ration was granted that the policy adopted by the Health Authority was unlawful and an 'order of mandamus' was made, requiring the defendants to formulate and implement a policy which took full and proper account of national policy as stated in the circular.

Failure by an NHS trust or Health Authority to provide reasonable services for the care of pregnant women, mothers and babies could therefore lead to action against the Authority and the Secretary of State for breach of a statutory duty. Such a case may be supported by an allegation of failure to comply with the Articles of Human Rights (especially Articles 2 and 3, see above). It does not follow, however, that a woman would be successful in suing for failure to provide a specific form of care, such as a water birth. There is built into the statutory provisions a discretion over the services to be provided. Now that the National Service Framework in child and maternity services has been published, women will be able to bring a complaint if their local services fall below the minimum outlined in these standards (see Ch. 21).

MATERNITY SERVICES DEVELOPMENTS AND STANDARDS

The Health Committee of the House of Commons reported on Maternity Services in February 1992.[45] Its main recommendations are shown in Box 6.1. These are culled from nine pages of recommendations and it is difficult to give credit to the wide-ranging and comprehensive scope of the report in this short account.

Box 6.1 Main recommendations of the House of Commons (Winterton) report

- The relationship between the woman and the care-givers is recognised as being of fundamental importance.

- Schemes should be set up enabling women to get to know one or two health professionals during pregnancy who will be with them during labour and delivery whether at home or in hospital, and who will continue the care of the mother and baby after birth.

- The majority of maternity care should be community based and near to the woman's home, and obstetric and other specialist care should be readily available by referral from midwives or GPs.

- Those GPs who wish to provide a continuum of care throughout pregnancy, labour and the puerperium should be able to do so; and their training should equip them to do so.

- Women needing intensive obstetric care within the NHS should also be able to enjoy continuity of care and carer, so far as is possible.

- Within a hospital, women should be able to exercise choice as to the personnel who will be responsible for their care.

▶

– The woman having a baby should be seen as the focus of care; and professionals providing that care should identify their needs and develop arrangements to meet them which are based on full and equal cooperation between all those charged with her care.

– Proper attention should be paid to the needs of the baby, with particular regard to skilled resuscitation at birth, examination for abnormalities, and the encouragement of breastfeeding.

The Secretary of State responded by setting up an expert panel under the chairmanship of Baroness Cumberlege to consider the recommendations and make proposals for implementation.[46] A consensus conference was held in March 1993, arranged by the King's Fund Centre for the Department of Health. Following the consensus conference a statement drawn up by an independent panel was submitted as evidence to the Expert Committee on Maternity Services.[47]

Changing Childbirth, the report of the expert committee, was published in August 1993.[48] The recommendations are given under four main headings:

1. Woman-centred care

2. Professional support

3. Accessible maternity services

4. Effective and efficient services.

Box 6.2 shows the indicators of success as set out in Chapter 5 of the Cumberlege recommendations.

Box 6.2 Indicators of success

Within 5 years:

1. All women should be entitled to carry their own notes.

2. Every woman should know one midwife who ensures continuity of her midwifery care – the named midwife.

3. At least 30% of women should have the midwife as the lead professional.

4. Every woman should know the lead professional who has a key role in the planning and provision of her care.

▶

5. At least 75% of women should know the person who cares for them during their delivery.

6. Midwives should have direct access to some beds in all maternity units.

7. At least 30% of women delivered in a maternity unit should be admitted under the management of the midwife.

8. The total number of antenatal visits for women with uncomplicated pregnancies should have been reviewed in the light of the available evidence and the RCOG guidelines.

9. All front-line ambulances should have a paramedic able to support the midwife who needs to transfer a woman to hospital in an emergency.

10. All women should have access to information about the services available in their locality.

The government responded warmly to the report of the expert advisory committee and NHS authorities were required to review maternity services in the light of the report's recommendations and develop a strategy for implementing these within the resources available.

The NHS Management Executive (EL(94)9) instructed NHS authorities to reflect the Expert Maternity Group's recommendations in NHS contracts for 1995–1996. The guidance required purchasers to draw up implementation plans for Changing Childbirth and ensure that its recommendations were reflected in both their 3–5 year purchasing strategy and their 1995/6 purchasing plans. Purchasers were also requested to set a date by which they expected to be able to offer a Changing Childbirth service, as defined in Annex A of the circular. Regional strategies were also to be prepared. An advisory group was established to support the NHS in implementing Changing Childbirth. A Patient's Charter leaflet was to be issued to set out what the current Patient's Charter rights and standards mean for pregnant women.

RECENT INITIATIVES

The NHS Plan[49] envisages major changes and initiatives in the NHS including maternity services. Following the NHS Plan, the strategic document 'Delivering the Best' was published to identify midwives' contribution to the NHS Plan.[50] This document identified five challenges for midwives:

1. Excellence in midwifery practice

2. Dynamic leadership

3. Partnerships with women

4. Improving Public Health

5. Working with others

and outlined how they could be achieved.

Following the NHS White Paper[51] and the Health Act 1999, several institutions were established: the National Institute for Clinical Excellence and the Commission for Healthcare Audit and Inspection (now known as the Healthcare Commission and replacing the Commission for Health Improvement). These organisations and their significance are considered in Chapter 21. An All-Party Parliamentary Group on Maternity was set up, chaired by Julia Brown MP,[52] which is discussed in Chapter 21. A Maternity and Neonatal Workforce Group (MNWG) was set up under the Chairmanship of Dr Sheila Adam, the Deputy Chief Medical Officer of Health. It reported to the Department of Health in January 2003[53] and made strong recommendations on the models of care required to meet specified standards of maternity care (see Ch. 24), and gave guidance to NHS trusts on changes in service provision and to primary care trusts on commissioning maternity care services in the future.

Increasingly therefore over future years, there will be greater emphasis on nationally set standards for maternity provision based on researched evidence. In addition, the NHS Plan places greater emphasis on the involvement and representation of the patient in healthcare. This may eventually have a major impact upon the running of midwifery and obstetric departments.

NATIONAL SERVICE FRAMEWORK FOR CHILDREN, YOUNG PEOPLE AND MATERNITY SERVICES

A National Service Framework for children, young people and maternity services and child health was published in September 2004. Part 111 sets out Standard 11 for maternity services. It states:

Women have easy access to supportive, high quality maternity services, designed around their individual needs and those of their babies.

This is amplified as follows:

– Women-centred care services meet the needs of each mother and her baby, and ensure that parents are involved in the planning and evaluation of services. Women make informed choices and plan their care in partnership with profession-als. They have easy access to information and support throughout their pregnancy and post-birth, including support for women suffering from domestic violence and the opportunity to disclose it.

- Care pathways and managed care networks link maternity and neonatal services with a range of services and professionals to ensure all women and their babies have equal access to high quality care

- Improved pre-conception care includes local health promotion highlighting the importance of the health of women and their partners before conception. In pre-birth care, women are able to access a midwife as their first point of contact and all women are supported by a known midwife throughout their pregnancy. High quality ante-natal and newborn screening is offered to all women.

- Healthcare professionals are competent in identifying and addressing mental health problems for women during or after pregnancy and local perinatal psychiatric services are available for women who need them.

- Women are able to choose the most appropriate place to give birth from a range of local options including home birth and delivery in midwife-led units, with the facility for women delivering in the community to be transferred to hospital rapidly if complications arise. A consultant obstetrician is involved in any decision to offer a caesarean section, which will also depend on there being evidence of clinical benefit to either mother or baby.

- A professional skilled in neonatal resuscitation is present at every delivery, and newborn infants receive a physical examination soon after birth. Mothers receive post-birth care based on a structured assessment provided by a multidisciplinary team.

- Up-to-date information on breastfeeding and breastfeeding support for mothers is provided in line with the government's commitment to improving the health of the population.

Resources and increase in midwifery numbers will be essential to ensure the implementation of this.

Mandy Renton (2004) considers the problems of implementing the NSF in the light of the experience of Cumberlege,[54] and Heather Mellow (2005) discusses the holistic approach of the NSF in comparison with Cumberlege,[55] while Richens and Thomas (2004) see the NSF as bringing in a culture change.[56]

THE PATIENT'S CHARTER AND MATERNITY SERVICES

As part of the Patient's Charter initiative, the government's Citizen's Charter Unit published a leaflet explaining the special standards for maternity services. This set out the following rights:

- To be told the name of the midwife who will be responsible for the care

- To have the opportunity to see a Consultant obstetrician at least once during the pregnancy

- To have the opportunity to see a Consultant paediatrician if the obstetrician anticipates problems with the baby

- To have a right to see the maternity records and have the confidentiality respected

- To be given information on local maternity services

- To have an appointment system for antenatal clinics and to be seen within 30 min of the time fixed

- To have the choice of whether a partner or other friend or relative should be present during the confinement

- To have the baby identified for security reasons

- To have information on feeding the baby

- To have respect for privacy, dignity, religious and cultural beliefs

- To be able to have visitors at all reasonable times

- To have access to hospital and community services according to any special needs.

These rights are not legally enforceable by the individual client, unless there are separate rights recognised by statute or by the common law. Thus, as will be seen in Chapter 10, the mother has a statutory right of access to her health records unless certain exemption conditions exist. Similarly, if the baby requires specialist input from a paediatrician and the GP, midwife or obstetrician fails to refer the baby to a paediatrician and the baby suffers harm as a result, then there would be a breach of the duty recognised by the common law to take care of the client.

Where, however, such legal rights do not already exist to support those standards identified in the Charter, the only remedy for the client is to use the complaints system (see Ch. 11) and bring to the attention of the trust or Health Authority failures in the standards prescribed by the Charter. For example, the Charter Standard for waiting in an antenatal clinic is a maximum of 30 min after the appointment time. If a woman waits 2 hours for her examination, she has the right to complain, but it is unlikely that she can enforce this standard personally through action in the courts. The NHS Plan envisages that a new Citizen's Charter is to be published.

DEVELOPMENT OF MATERNITY SERVICES

In May 2001[57] the Government announced that £100 million was being made available to transform maternity services: an extra 2000 midwives would be appointed by 2005 (former midwives would be offered £1500 to help them through a retraining period and also help with childcare worth up to £150/week); there would be a wholesale refurbishment of maternity wards so that they became a home away from home, rather than a clinical environment and there would be greater freedom for women to choose a home birth. A further allocation of £100 million was made in October 2001[58] (see Ch. 21). It was anticipated that the National Service Framework (NSF) being prepared for child and maternity services (see above) will set out how the target of ensuring that every woman will have access to a dedicated midwife when in established labour 100% of the time can be achieved. This target was described as the 'gold standard'. In June 2001[59] the Department of Health gave further details of these plans, including improving facilities for fathers and for bereaved parents in maternity units. It is intended that women who lose their babies are not placed in postnatal wards with new mothers.

THE RIGHT TO A HOME BIRTH

As an example of the weakness of rights which are not legally enforceable in the area of midwifery and child care, we will take the example of a woman who wishes to have a home birth. It is clear that government policy as set out in the Cumberlege Report and in the NHS Plan favours the right of patient decision making and maximum involvement of the patient in the care they obtain. If, however, a woman was to request that she had a home birth, it appears that there are considerable pressures against her. The report of the National Birthday Trust confidential enquiry in 1994 showed that there was considerable anecdotal evidence that GPs refused to allow women to book for home birth. Other evidence showed that some women have been struck off the GP practice for insisting on home birth.[60] Obstacles are placed in the way of a home birth. It takes a very assertive and strong woman to overcome these obstacles and insist upon a home confinement. The National Birthday Trust Report[61] quoted earlier showed that 'women booking home births were of a higher social class, had continued in education for longer and were more likely to breastfeed'. The vast majority of women would probably be defeated by the first refusal and accept hospital confinement even if the stay is only a few hours.

There is evidence that the average uncomplicated vaginal birth costs 68% less in a home than in a hospital.[62] There is also some evidence that, following careful selection for home birth, the risks are lower.[63] However, there is evidence that bullying to deter women from seeking home births exists[64] (see the case of Paul Beland below). It will be noted from the discussion above that the courts in the past have been reluctant to become involved in decisions against the Secretary of State where resource issues arise. If a woman were to bring a court action against the trust to compel provision for a home birth, the court may be reluctant to issue an order for specific performance requiring arrangements to be made for her home confinement, since there is a general reluctance for the court to order persons to carry out particular activities when the court cannot itself supervise them. However, payment of compensation may be seen as an alternative for not having a home birth. In theory, there may well be a legal right for the woman to insist upon a home confinement, if she can show that it is in her best interests and that the resource implications benefit the NHS, but in practice it may be very difficult for her to secure this. (In Ireland an attempt by four home birth mothers to force the state to recognise the right to home births failed.)[65,66]

Many organisations have worked strenuously to support the woman's right to have a home birth, if clinical conditions permit. The National Childbirth Trust, the Association for the Improvement in Maternity Services, the Association of Radical Midwives, Royal College of Midwives, the Association of Community Based Maternity Care and the International Home Birth Movement have all promoted the provision of information to women so that they have clear choices over the place of birth. Over 12 years have passed since the publication of Changing Childbirth and there is little evidence that the situation for women has significantly altered. Sheila Kitzinger (2005) has argued strongly that it is a woman's right to have a home birth.[67] The legal and ethical issues are explored by Jones (2003).[68] Liz Stephens (2005) discusses some of the hurdles to providing a woman with a real choice of a home birth and how these could be overcome.[64]

The UKCC published a position statement on supporting women who wish to have a home birth[69] and updated this on 31 August 2001.[70] This clarified the situation where an employer says that it is unable to provide a planned home birth service, because there are insufficient midwives available to support both the hospital and the home birth services. The UKCC stated its position as follows:

It is the Council's expectation that a practising midwife will be competent to provide midwifery care in any setting and that women who wish to have their baby at home can be supported to achieve this by a midwife who is able to practise within the home environment. The Council supports women having choice in the method and place of birth . . . While the employed midwife has a contractual duty to her employer, she also has a professional duty to provide midwifery care for women and would not wish to leave a woman in labour at home unattended, thus placing her at risk at a time when competent midwifery care is essential.

The UKCC noted that across the four countries of the UK there is no statutory duty to provide any specific aspect of the maternity services. It also recognised that an employed midwife has a primary contractual duty to carry out the wishes of her employer, although the employer would not expect an employee to do anything illegal, including anything which contravenes the Midwives Rules. It stated:

A midwife would not be in breach of her professional duty if unable to attend a woman requesting a home birth by reason of her employer's decision not to provide such a service. In an emergency situation, the midwife has a professional responsibility to provide midwifery care to the best of her ability.

The UKCC emphasised that a midwife should not refuse to continue to provide care for a woman on the basis of where the woman intends the birth to take place.

The midwife must ensure that her supervisor is brought in if there are such difficulties.

The Supervisor of Midwives must be mindful of the woman's right to choose and so has a key role to play in providing professional support for the midwife.

An example of the problems which can arise when an employer instructs its midwives that there are not the resources to employ midwives to attend home births, can be seen from the following news report.[71]

Paul Beland, a community midwife has been sacked for attending a home birth when instructed not to do so. Peterborough and Stamford Hospitals NHS Foundation Trust suspended its home birth service in June 2004 because of staff shortages, but Paul subsequently attended a home birth. He was initially suspended but was dismissed following a hearing. He stated that the ban breached the NMC's rules, stating that if a woman insists on giving birth at home a midwife must not withdraw care. The Trust stated that it had suspended its service because of reduced staffing levels due to maternity and sick leave. "It is our view that providing this (i.e. home birth) service may compromise the care offered to other women in the maternity unit." (Helen Clark MP took the case up in the House of Commons.)

He lost his internal appeal against his dismissal and decided not to pursue the case in an employment tribunal. His case has received considerable comment.[72,73] In October 2004 the Trust announced that it was planning to resume a home birth service by 31 October 2004 since more midwives had been recruited.[74]

In the future, the National Institute for Health and Clinical Excellence may publish recommendations on research-based practice and the clinical effectiveness of home confinements. The establishment of primary healthcare trusts may assist women in having a real choice and may encourage home confinements. However, to secure these changes general practitioners will have to become convinced that home births are, where clinically possible, the preferred option, and midwives will have to have the confidence that they will not be penalised as a result of supporting the woman's choice. A news item in the RCM Journal suggested that the increasing number of women being encouraged to request home births is affecting hospital-based midwives and resources.[75]

INEQUALITY IN MATERNITY SERVICES

In 2003, the House of Commons looked at two aspects of maternity care: its 8th report[76] looked at inequalities in maternity services and its 9th report[77] considered choice in maternity services. Both reports make fundamental and significant recommendations for the future provision of services. The 8th report recommended that the Government investigate the RCM's concerns about the recruitment of midwives from minority ethnic communities and its final recommendation was:

We recognise the potential of midwives and of maternity services to play an expanded role in promoting public health. However, maternity care staff must have access to appropriate levels of training and support if they are to be effective in this role. We recommend that the Department should facilitate the implementation of the proposals in Making a Difference by making a detailed assessment of the training and support needs of staff who provide maternity care.

The ninth report on choice in maternity care considered that the current delivery of maternity services . . .

over-medicalises birth. Barriers to home births were wholly unacceptable. Women should know that they have a right to have a home birth without seeking "the GP's permission".

Its final recommendation was that the Government should consider allocating some one-off resources to maternity units to make changes to their practice so that they could carry out the work recommended in the Report, the money going to staff rather than buildings (in contrast to the 2001 allocation).

The Royal College of Midwives has reaffirmed its support for home births[78] and the Welsh Assembly Minister for Health and Social Services declared at the RCM conference in 2004 her aim of securing 10% home births.[79]

THE RIGHT TO A CAESAREAN

Of considerable controversy has been whether a woman has a right to insist on having a caesarean even when there are no clinical grounds to support such a decision. Almost 1 in 4 births are now by caesarean section and this increase has been due partly to the result of increasingly defensive practice by obstetricians but also because of pressure from women. The author has argued that there is no legal right for a patient to demand care when there is no clinical justification.[80] However, a midwife may come across a situation where a Consultant, although he or she does not personally see a clinical need for a caesarean section to take place, is prepared to support the woman's request. In such circumstances, the midwife has no alternative other than to provide the woman with all the appropriate care which she would have if the caesarean was clinically indicated.

A warning about the dangers of believing too easily that the figures showing an increase in the rate of caesarean sections result from pressure of patients' choice is given by Tricia Anderson (2001).[81] Anderson comments on an article[82] which suggested that maternal choice accounts for 49% of the decision-making process when deciding whether to opt for an elective caesarean section. She warns of the danger of obstetricians creating a view that caesarean section is best and urges the importance of women being given full information about the risks inherent in a caesarean section. She sees the increase in the rate of caesarean section as the result of 30 years of hospitalised, medicalised birth, as recommended in the Peel Report of 1970.[83]

A National Sentinel Caesarean Section Audit was carried out by the RCOG, the RCM, the Royal College of Anaesthetists and the National Childbirth Trust funded by the Department of Health through NICE.[84] The results were presented at a launch meeting in October 2001[85] and showed that the caesarean section rate overall in England was 21%, and 24% in Wales and Northern Ireland. (This compares with the 10–15% range recommended by the World Health Organization in its consensus statement in 1985.)[86] The Sentinel Report was discussed by the All-Party Parliamentary Group on Maternity on 6 November, 2001 and a conference was held in January 2002. NICE guidelines on caesarean section were published in 2004[87] and included key priorities for implementing them, covering: woman-centred care; planned CS; factors affecting the likelihood of CS; procedural aspects; care of the new born and mother; recovery and vaginal birth after caesarean section. NICE has also issued guidance especially for pregnant women, their partners and the public.[88] NICE recommends that health professionals should counsel women about the relative merits and demerits of cae-sarean section, rather than allow automatic compliance with caesareans on request and that maternal request alone is not an indication for caesarean section.[89,90] The guidelines were not received with unanimous approval.[91] The Chief Executive of NICE highlighted some of the challenges in the implementation of NICE guidelines generally and how he hopes the work of NICE will overcome them.[92] The RCM has provided an information paper on caesarean sections without health indications.[93] This explores the reasons why women are opting for non-medically indicated cae-sarean sections and the relative risks of CS compared with vaginal delivery. In March 2005, the Royal College of Midwives[94] stated that it was disappointed with the cae-sarean section figures published on 31 March 2005, which showed that 22.7% of deliveries in England in 2003–2004 were by caesarean section, a slight increase on the previous year. Its general secretary stated that 'we believe that caesarean delivery is appropriate and beneficial in only 10–15% of all births as specified by the World Health Organization'. The RCM[95] launched a campaign for normal birth in 2005, seeking a decline in unnecessary intervention rates. The Court of Appeal decision in the Burke case (which is discussed in Ch. 9), where it held that a patient does not have the right to insist upon specific treatment which the health professional does not consider is in his or her best interests, has significant implications for those women who wish to have a caesarean section, when there are no clinical grounds for such an operation.

In Chapter 13, the legal significance of NICE guidelines in the law of negligence is considered.

BREASTFEEDING

The Scottish Parliament has passed the Breastfeeding etc. (Scotland) Act 2005 which makes it a criminal offence to deliberately prevent or stop a woman breastfeeding.[96] It is an offence to deliberately prevent or stop a person in charge of a child from feeding milk to that child in a public place or on licensed premises. An exception to this offence is if the child, at the material time, is not lawfully permitted to be in the public place or on the licensed premises otherwise than for the purpose of being fed milk. The Act also places a duty on the Scottish Ministers to make arrangements to such extent as they consider necessary to meet all reasonable requirements, for the purpose of supporting and encouraging the breastfeeding of children by their mothers. The Scottish Ministers are given the power to disseminate, by what ever means, information promoting and encouraging breastfeeding. It is hoped that the implementation of the Act will be monitored to determine whether similar provisions should be made across the rest of the UK.

RCM MANIFESTO

A manifesto published by the RCM in March 2005[97] sets out six key priorities for maternity services:

1. Choice in maternity services

2. A well-staffed service

3. A fair deal for midwives

4. Supporting teenage mothers

5. Support for breastfeeding mothers

6. Providing a smoke-free environment.

CONCLUSIONS

This chapter has looked at the rights set out in the European Convention on Human Rights, the statutory duty to provide maternity services, the Cumberlege Report and changes in the establishing of standards within the NHS, including clinical governance, CHAI, NICE and the National Service Frameworks and the RCM Manifesto. The Cumberlege Report concluded that the mother should have a major role in the determination of the care she receives. The House of Commons (Winterton) Report (Para. 52) stated:

We conclude that there is a widespread demand among women for greater choice in the type of maternity care they receive; and that the present structure of the maternity services frustrates, rather than facilitates, those who wish to exercise this choice.

As we noted, however, the legal entitlement of the woman to receive services and to be involved in the choices relating to her care depends upon the existing laws relating to the provision of statutory services, trespass to the person, consent to treatment, the duty in negligence to provide information and the Articles of the European Convention on Human Rights as set out in the Human Rights Act 1998.

As we shall see in subsequent chapters, there are many deficiencies and weaknesses in the law in relation to the pregnant woman, and cases show that there is no clear legal basis at present to the concept of woman-centred care. Nor would there appear to have been comprehensive implementation of the 'know your midwife concept'.[98] The proposals in the NHS Plan to strengthen patient representation and advocacy are considered in Chapter 11. The Report of the Bristol Inquiry[99] into children's heart surgery recommended that the patient should be at the centre of healthcare and that there should be an equal partnership between patient and healthcare professional. The implementation of its recommendations could have significant consequences for woman-centred care. The Report is considered in Chapter 21. In September 2001, the Department of Health published plans to give patients suffering from chronic conditions more control over managing their own illness.[100] There is no reason why the philosophy and principles behind this initiative should not become incorporated into midwifery practice, since that was at the heart of the Changing Childbirth proposals.

However, it is evident, especially from the failure to secure a right for all suitable mothers to be offered a home birth, that there is still more rhetoric than action in securing the implementation of the principles set out in Changing Childbirth.

QUESTIONS AND EXERCISES

1. Consider the targets set out in Box 6.2 in the light of your own practice and determine what steps would be needed to implement them.

2. Do you consider that a woman should have a legally enforceable right to receive the kind of care which she wants?

3. What effect does a National Service Framework for maternity care have on your practice and the rights of your clients?

References

1 A National Health Service Trust v. D. Times Law Report, 19 July 2000; [2000] Lloyd's Rep Med 411.

2 NHS Trust A v. Mrs M and NHS Trust B v. Mrs H. Family Division, 25 October 2000; [2001] 1 All ER 801.

3 Re A (Minors) (Conjoined Twins: Separation) [2000] Lloyd's Rep Med 425.

4 NHS Trust A v. M; NHS Trust B v. H [2001] Fam 348; A National Health Service Trust v. D. Times Law Report, 19 July 2000; [2000] Lloyd's Rep Med 411.

5 R (Pretty) v. Director of Public Prosecutions and another, Medical Ethics Alliance and others, interveners. Times Law Report, 23 October 2001.

6 R (on the application of Pretty) v. DPP [2001] UKHL 61; [2001] 3 WLR 1598.

7 Pretty v. UK ECHR Current Law 380, June 2002; 2346/02 [2002] 2 F.L.R. 45.

8 Osman v. United Kingdom 2000 29 EHRR 245.

9 A v. The United Kingdom (100/1997/884/1096) judgement on 23 September, 1998.

10 Z. v. UK 1999 28 EHRR CD 65.

11 News item. The Times, 28 April 1994.

12 News item. RCM response to prison service apology. Midwives Chronicle 1994; 107:219.

13 News item. Handcuffing pregnant prisoners. Bull Med Ethics 1994; 98:9.

14 Walker A. The shame I felt in chains. The Guardian, 11 January 1996.

15 Home Office. News item. Health Service J 1996; 106:6.

16 Travis A. Manacles policy loosened. End to chains for pregnant prisoners. The Guardian, 16 January 1996.

17 Beech BAL. Shackled prisoner wins compensation. AIMS J 1998; 10:13.

18 McGlinchey and others v. United Kingdom, Lloyd's Rep Med [2003] 264.

19 Cading-Paull C. Mothers in prison. Mod Midwife 1994; 4:26.

20 Price S, Ridge H. Pregnant and in prison. MIDIRS Midwifery Digest 2001; 11:325–328.

21 News item. Pregnant woman shackled to radiator for five hours. RCM Midwives J 1998; March:2.

22 Kitzinger S. Pregnant prisoners. NHS Magazine 2004; November:10–11.

23 Price S. Women in prison. MIDIRS Midwifery Digest 2004; 14:295–298 and Maternity services for women in prison: a descriptive study. Br J Midwifery 2005; 13:362–368.

24 Farrant F. An age of innocence? MIDIRS Midwifery Digest 2004; 14:298–299.

25 R v. Bournewood Community and Mental Health NHS Trust ex parte L [1998] 3 All ER 289.

26 L. v United Kingdom (Application No 45508/99) Times Law Report, 19 October 2004.

27 Department of Health Bournewood Consultation: The approach to be taken in response to the judgement of the European Court of Human Rights in the "Bournewood" case. DoH; March 2005.

28 Re F (Adult: Court's Jurisdiction) [2000] 2 FLR 512 Court of Appeal; [2000] Lloyd's Rep Med 381.

29 Tehrani v. UKCC [2001] IRLR 208.

30 Nurses, Midwives and Health Visitors (Professional Conduct) (Amendment) Rules 2001 Approval Order 2001. SI 2001 No 536.

31 R v. Secretary of State for the Home Department ex parte Mellor. Times Law Report, 31 July 2000.

32 R v. Secretary of State for Health ex parte Lally. Times Law Report, 11 October 2000.

33 Kitzinger S. Birth in prison: the rights of the baby. Practising Midwife 1999; 2:16–18.

34 R (P) v. Secretary of State for the Home Department; R (Q) v. the same. Times Law Report, 1 June 2001; [2001] 2 FLR 1122.

35 R (on the application of N) v. Ashworth Special Hospital Authority [2001] EWHC Admin 339; The Times, 26 June 2001.

36 Halford v. UK 1997 24 EHRR 523.

37 Gunn-Russo v. Nugent Care Society and the Secretary of State for Health [2002] 1 FLR 1.

38 Bale J. Beckham family affairs are fair game for public. The Times, 25 April 2005:11.

39 Audit Commission Human Rights: Improving Public Service Delivery, September 2003.

40 R v. Secretary of State for Social Services ex parte Hincks and others. 29 June 1979 [1979] 123 Solicitors Journal 1979:436.

41 R v. Central Birmingham Health Authority ex parte Walker [1987] 3 BMLR 32; The Times 26 November, 1987.

42 R v. Cambridge HA ex parte B [1995] 2 All ER 129.

43 R v. North West Lancashire HS ex parte A, D, and G [1999] Lloyd's Law Reports Medical 399; [1999] 53 BMLR 148 CA.

44 NHS Executive Letter: EL (95)97.

45 House of Commons. Second report of Health Committee Session 1992/92 on maternity services: Winterton Report.

46 Changing Childbirth: Report of the Expert Maternity Group, Department of Health. London: HMSO; 1993.

47 King's Fund Centre for Health Services Development. Consensus statement on maternity care: choice, continuity and change. London: King's Fund Centre.

48 Department of Health. Changing childbirth. London: HMSO; 1993.

49 Department of Health. The NHS Plan: a plan for investment, a plan for reform Cm 4818-1 July 2000. London: HMSO; 2000.

50 Department of Health. Delivering the Best. London: HMSO; 2003.

51 Department of Health. The New NHS: Modern, dependable. London: HMSO; 1997.

52 Catherine Eden at the National Childbirth Trust: 020 8992 2616. Online. Available: c_eden@national-childbirth-trust.co.uk

53 Department of Health report to the DH Children's Taskforce from the Maternity and Neonatal Workforce Group, 2003.

54 Renton M. The NSF – use it or lose it. The Practising Midwife 2004; 7:4–5.

55 Mellows H. A framework for change. The Practising Midwife 2005; 8:4–5.

56 Richens Y, Thomas M. Service framework calls for cultural shift. Br J Midwifery 2004; 12:668–670.

57 Department of Health. Milburn announces £100 million boost for maternity units and 2000 extra midwives by 2005. Press release 2001/0212; 2 May 2001.

58 Department of Health. Maternity units receive £100 million to modernise and improve facilities. Press release 2001/0470; 10 October 2001.

59 Department of Health. Health Minister sets out plans to modernise maternity services. Press Release 2001/026214; June 2001.

60 Carlisle D. Laboured relations. Nursing Times 1995; 91:16.

61 National Childbirth Trust. GPs block home births. Health Visitor 1995; 68:87.

62 Anderson RE, Anderson DA. The cost effectiveness of home birth. J Nurse-Midwifery 1999; 44:30–35.

63 Chamberlain G, Wraight A, Crowley P, eds. Home Births: the report of the 1994 confidential enquiry by the National Birthday Trust Fund. Carnforth: Pantheon Publishing Group; MIDIRS abstract in MIDIRS Midwifery Digest 1997; March:109.

64 Stephens L. Worrying truth behind home birth figures. Br J Midwifery 2005; 13:4–5.

65 O'Connor M. Medical monopoly – a short lived triumph? Midwifery Matters 2004; 100:38–39

66 O'Brien B. Homebirth. Home Birth Association of Ireland Newsletter 2003; 21:7–9.

67 Kitzinger S. Home birth: a social process, not a medical crisis. Practising Midwife 2005; 8:26–29.

68 Jones S. Ethico-legal issues in home birth. RCM Midwives J 2003; 6:126–128.

69 UKCC. Position Statement: Registrar's Letter 20/2000.

70 UKCC. Position Statement: Registrar's Letter 21/2001.

71 News Item. Midwife sacked for attending homebirth. Practising Midwife 2004; 7:8.

72 Flint C. Maternity hospitals and suspensions. Br J Midwifery 2004; 12:558.

73 Walsh D. Home birth, staffing and acute service. Br J Midwifery 2004; 12:616.

74 News item. Midwife appeals against sacking. The Practising Midwife 2004 7:11.

75 News item. R Coll Midwives J 2004; 7:54.

76 United Kingdom Parliament. Online. Available: www.publications.parliament.uk/pa/cm200203/cmselect/cmhealth/696/69602.htm

77 United Kingdom Parliament. Online. Available: www.publications.parliament.uk/pa/cm200203/cmselect/cmhealth/796/79602.htm

78 News item. R Coll Midwives J 2004; 7:235.

79 News item. Practising Midwife 2004; 7:20–24.

80 Dimond B. Is there a legal right to choose a caesarean? Br J Midwifery 1999; 7:515–518.

81 Anderson T. Commentary. MIDIRS Midwifery Digest 2001; 11:368–370.

82 Marx H, Wiener J, Davies N. A survey of the influence of patients' choice on the increase in the caesarean section rate. J Obstet Gynaecol 2001; 21:124–127.

83 Central Health Services Council. Standing Maternity and Midwifery Advisory Committee. Domiciliary midwifery and maternity bed needs. (Chairman Sir John Peel.) London: HMSO; 1970.

84 Thomas J, Paranjothy S. Royal College of Obstetricians and Gynaecologists Clinical Effectiveness Support Unit. The National Sentinel Caesarean Section Audit Report. London: RCOG Press; 2001. Online. Available: www.rcog.org.uk

85 Royal College of Midwives and National Childbirth Trust. The rising caesarean rate: causes and effects for public health. Conference Report November 2000; London: RCM and NCT; 2001.

86 World Health Organisation. Appropriate technology for birth. Lancet 1985; 2:436–437.

87 National Institute for Clinical Excellence. Clinical Guidelines on Caesarean Section. NICE; 28 April, 2004.

88 National Institute for Clinical Excellence. Caesarean section – understanding NICE guidance: information for pregnant women, their partners and the public. NICE; 28 April 2004.

89 Kmietowicz Z. NICE advises against caesarean section on demand. BMJ 2004; 328:1031.

90 Page L. Caesarean sections: NICE guidelines. Br J Midwifery 2004; 12:76.

91 Nock S. What the papers said. AIMS J 2004; 16:9–10.

92 Dillon A. NICE clinical guidance: supporting implementation. Focus 2004; July:10–11.

93 Royal College of Midwives. Information paper: caesarean sections without health indications. RCM; December 2004.

94 Royal College of Midwives. RCM disappointed with caesarean section figures. News item, 31 March 2005.

95 Royal College of Midwives. Campaign for normal birth. RCM 2005.

96 The Scottish Parliament. Online. Available: www.scottish.parliament.uk

97 Royal College of Midwives. RCM Manifesto sets out priorities for maternity services on new website. March 2005.

98 Flint C, Poulengeris P. The Know Your Midwifery Report 1987. Obtainable from 49 Peckarmans Wood, Sydenham Hill, London SE26 6RZ.

99 Bristol Royal Infirmary. Learning from Bristol: the report of the public inquiry into children's heart surgery at the Bristol Royal Infirmary 1984–1995. Command Paper CM 5207; 2001. Online. Available: www.bristol-inquiry.org.uk

100 Department of Health. Patients to become the key decision-makers in their own care. Press release 2001/0421, 14 September 2001.

Chapter 7
CONSENT

In the main, two legal actions can arise in relation to consent. The first is an action for trespass to the person, where there is no consent to the touching of another person or other legal justification, or there has been fraud or duress. In this action, harm need not be proved: merely the touching or apprehension of touching. The other action is one for negligence where the person has not been informed of significant information. In this action, the claimant would have to prove that harm has been suffered which would not have been suffered if the information had been given. This chapter considers the action for trespass to the person and the defences including the defence of consent.

The next chapter (Ch. 8) looks at the information which must be given and the duty of care which includes the duty to inform.

Guidance has been provided by the Department of Health on consent, which can be accessed via the Internet and is intended to be updated on a regular basis.[1] There are separate guidelines for use by adults, children and young persons, those with learning disabilities, parents and relatives and carers. The Department of Health identifies 12 key points on consent which are expanded upon in the Reference guide. These cover the following areas:

– When is consent needed?

– Can children consent for themselves?

– Who is the right person to seek consent?

– What information should be provided?

– Is the patient's consent voluntary?

– Does it matter how the patient gives consent?

– Refusals of treatment

– Adults who are not competent to give consent.

MIDWIFERY INTERVENTIONS

First, what are the various kinds of treatment and diagnostic procedures over which the woman might wish to exercise choice?

Box 7.1 sets out a few of the decisions which may be made during the course of a pregnancy.

Box 7.1 Decisions during pregnancy

*Caesarean section	Vitamin K injections
*Episiotomies	Syntometrine
*Epidurals	*Anaesthetic
*Admission to obstetric unit	Tubal ligation
Home confinement	Seeing the doctor
*Fetal monitoring	*Blood transfusion
Induction	Screening for syphilis and HIV
*Artificial rupture of membranes	Anti-D injections
Water birth	Examination by students
Catheterisation	Fetal blood sampling
*Blood tests	Suppositories
*Forceps	Enemas
*Intravenous infusion/treatment	*Intrauterine monitoring
*Suturing	*Fetal scalp electrodes
Vaginal examinations	Rectal examinations
Removal of jewellery	Ultrasound scanning

The list shown in Box 7.1 is not exhaustive but it shows the many decisions which may have to be made during the pregnancy. Those procedures marked with an asterisk (*) are ones which could lead to serious harm to the mother or baby, if the mother refused to give consent for them. Those without an asterisk are not of a life-saving necessity, either for the mother or baby, and the mother could refuse most of these procedures without any major disadvantages healthwise. However, to carry out any of these tasks or procedures without consent would, in the absence of lawful justification, be regarded as a trespass to the person.

TRESPASS TO THE PERSON

The definition of trespass to the person is shown in Box 7.2.

Box 7.2 Trespass to the person

An act of the defendant which directly and intentionally causes either some physical contact with the person of the claimant without the claimant's consent (this is known as a battery) or causes the claimant immediately to apprehend a contact with his person (this is known as an assault).

The claimant is the person suing for compensation in the civil courts, formerly known as the plaintiff. Like its fellow causes of action, trespass to goods and trespass to land, no harm has to be proved. The action is known as 'actionable per se', i.e. actionable in its own right, and is unlike an action for negligence where harm must be established. The mere fact that there is a touching of a person's body without authorisation is sufficient to constitute a trespass. Social touching would not normally however constitute a trespass in the absence of unusual factors.

This means that, even where the midwife has acted out of good will and in the best interests of the mother, if she has failed to obtain consent and in the absence of any of the other defences mentioned below, she could be liable to an action for trespass to the person. (In practice, the claimant would sue the midwife's employer who is vicariously liable for the actions of an employee who is acting in the course of employment (see Ch. 13), unless of course the midwife was self-employed.) The following case illustrates the principle that if a person is mentally competent, then providing treatment contrary to her wishes is a trespass to her person.

CASE OF RE B[2]

Miss B suffered a ruptured blood vessel in her neck which damaged her spinal cord. As a consequence, she was paralysed from the neck down and was on a ventilator. She was of sound mind and knew that there was no cure for her condition. She asked for the ventilator to be switched off. Her doctors wished her to try out some special rehabilitation to improve the standard of her care and felt that an intensive care ward was not a suitable location for such a decision to be made. They were reluctant to perform such an action as switching off the ventilator without the court's approval. Miss B applied to court for a declaration to be made that the ventilator could be switched off.

The main issue in the case was the mental competence of Miss B. If she were held to be mentally competent, then she could refuse to have life saving treatment for a good reason, a bad reason or no reason at all. She was interviewed by two psychiatrists who gave evidence to the court that she was mentally competent. The judge therefore held that she was entitled to refuse to be ventilated. The judge, Dame Elizabeth Butler-Sloss, President of the Family Division, held that Miss B possessed the requisite mental capacity to make decisions regarding her treatment and thus the administration of artificial respiration by the trust against her wishes amounted to an unlawful trespass. Dame Elizabeth further found that there had been a trespass to her person and awarded Miss B a nominal amount as compensation. The judge restated the principles which had been laid down by the Court of Appeal in the case of St George's Healthcare Trust[3] (see facts of this case below).

– There was a presumption that a patient had the mental capacity to make decisions whether to consent to or refuse medical or surgical treatment offered.

– If mental capacity was not an issue and the patient, having been given the relevant information and offered the available option, chose to refuse that treatment, that decision had to be respected by the doctors; considerations of what the best interests of the patient would involve were irrelevant.

– Concern or doubts about the patient's mental capacity should be resolved as soon as possible by the doctors within the hospital or other normal medical procedures.

– Meanwhile the patient must be cared for in accordance with the judgement of the doctors as to the patient's best interests.

– It was most important that those considering the issue should not confuse the question of mental capacity with the nature of the decision made by the patient, however grave the consequences. Since the view of the patient might reflect a difference in values rather than an absence of competence the assessment of capacity should be approached with that in mind and doctors should not allow an emotional reaction to, or strong disagreement with, the patient's decision to cloud their judgement in answering the primary question of capacity.

– Where disagreement still existed about competence, it was of the utmost importance that the patient be fully informed, involved and engaged in the process, which could involve obtaining independent outside help, of resolving the disagreement since the patient's involvement could be crucial to a good outcome.

– If the hospital was faced with a dilemma which doctors did not know how to resolve that must be recognised and further steps taken as a matter of priority. Those in charge must not allow a situation of deadlock or drift to occur.

- If there was no disagreement about competence, but the doctors were for any reason unable to carry out the patient's wishes, it was their duty to find other doctors who would do so.

- If all appropriate steps to seek independent assistance from medical experts outside the hospital had failed, the hospital should not hesitate to make an application to the High Court or seek the advice of the Official Solicitor.

- The treating clinicians and the hospital should always have in mind that a seriously physically disabled patient who was mentally competent had the same right to personal autonomy and to make decisions as any other person with mental capacity.

It was reported on 29 April 2002 that Miss B had died peacefully in her sleep after the ventilator had been switched off.

DEFENCES TO AN ACTION FOR TRESPASS TO THE PERSON

These are set out in Box 7.3.

Box 7.3 Defences to an action for trespass to the person

- Consent to treatment by patient (and/or in the case of a person under 18 by the parent or guardian)

- Necessity

- Statutory authorization, e.g. Mental Health Act 1983

- Declaration of the court

CONSENT

This is the main defence to an action for trespass to the person, i.e. that the individual who was touched, or feared a touching, gave consent to that action.

What, however, is meant by consent? Are there any factors which could invalidate an apparently valid consent? What capacity is required of the person in order to give a valid consent? Does the law require it to be given in any specific form?

REQUIREMENTS OF A VALID CONSENT

ABSENCE OF DURESS OR FRAUD

To be valid as a defence to an action of trespass to the person, the consent which the defendant is relying upon must be given freely and without duress and without fraud, by a mentally competent person. Evidence of compulsion or fraud would invalidate the consent. However, where prisoners claimed that the very nature of their confinement in a prison institution made consent invalid, they failed in their action for trespass to the person.[4] The Court of Appeal stated that they were not incapable in law of giving a valid consent by reason of the fact they were in prison, and that refusal might adversely affect prison privileges or even parole.

RELEVANT TO THE DEFENDANT'S ACTION

Clearly, the consent must be relevant to the act of the defendant. Consent to a caesarean would not be a defence to carrying out a hysterectomy, though other defences (e.g. necessity) might be relevant. This is an important area for the midwife since it must be clear whether or not the mother has given consent to an intimate examination and the midwife must protect the mother against any unauthorised intimate examinations.[5] When consent is given, the person should have a general idea as to the purpose of the contact proposed. However, absence of sufficiently detailed information is more likely to be grounds for an action for negligence, for failure on the defendant's part to fulfil the duty of care in informing the patient, and would not invalidate the consent for the purpose of defending an action of trespass. This was explained clearly by the High Court in the case of Chatterton v. Gerson.[6]

The claimant ran kennels with her twin sister. When her sister became a nurse, she worked as a universal aunt. In 1973, she went into hospital for treatment of varicose veins and she was advised at that time that a hernia repair operation should be carried out. Unfortunately, afterwards she suffered intractable and chronic pain as the result of the ileo-linguinal nerve being trapped. After various unsuccessful treatments, she was referred to Dr Gerson, a pain specialist, and was given treatment, which unfortunately resulted in her right leg becoming completely numb, considerably impairing her mobility. She claimed damages against the defendant, alleging that he had not given her an explanation of the operations and their implications so that she could make an informed decision about whether to risk them, and that:

(a) he had committed a trespass to the person since her consent to the operation was vitiated by the lack of prior explanation, and

(b) he had been negligent in not giving an explanation as he was required to do as part of his duty to treat a patient with the degree of professional skill and care expected of a reasonably skilled medical practitioner.

She failed on both counts: point (a) is considered here; point (b) is discussed in the next chapter.

In deciding that her action for trespass to the person failed, Judge Bristow said:

In my judgement once the patient is informed in broad terms of the nature of the procedure which is intended, and gives her consent, that consent is real, and the course of action on which to base a claim for failure to go into risks and implications is negligence, not trespass . . . In this case Miss Chatterton was under no illusion as to the general nature of what an intrathecal injection of phenol solution nerve block would be, and in the case of each injection her consent was not unreal.

METHODS OF EVIDENCING CONSENT

The agreement of the person that the touching may take place can occur in various ways, as shown in Box 7.4.

Box 7.4 Methods of giving evidence of consent

- In writing (this may or may not be on a specially designed consent form)

- By word of mouth

- By implication.

WRITTEN CONSENT

Forms have been issued by the Department of Health[7] as part of its Good Practice in Consent implementation guide, replacing those issued by the NHS Management Executive in 1990 and updated in 1992.

Box 7.5 shows more details about the new forms.

Box 7.5 Consent forms issued in the Department of Health's Good Practice in Consent implementation guide

Consent Form 1: Patient agreement to investigation or treatment

- Name of treatment and brief explanation

- Health professional's statement

▶

▶

- Intended benefits

- Serious/frequently occurring risks

- Any extra procedures which may become necessary during the procedure

- Leaflets/tapes provided

- Anaesthesia/sedation required

- Health professional's name, signature and contact details

– Statement of interpreter (where appropriate)

– Statement of patient

  - I agree to the procedure.

  - I understand that you cannot give me a guarantee that a particular person will perform the procedure. The person will, however, have appropriate experience.

  - I understand that I will have the opportunity to discuss the details of anaesthesia with an anaesthetist before the procedure, unless the urgency of my situation prevents this. (Only applies to patients having general or regional anaesthesia.)

  - I understand that any procedure in addition to those described on this form will only be carried out if it is necessary to save my life or prevent serious harm to my health.

  - I have been told about additional procedures which may become necessary during my treatment. I have listed below any procedures which I do not wish to be carried out without further discussion.

There are also provisions made for a witness to sign where an adult is unable to do so but has indicated his consent, and for a person with parental responsibility to sign. Consent Form 4 is for adults who are unable to consent to investigation or treatment, and includes:

– Details of the procedure or course of treatment proposed

– Assessment of the patient's capacity

▶

- Assessment of the patient's best interests

- Details of the involvement of the patient's family and significant others.

Consent Form 2 is for treatment on children and provides for parents, and (where appropriate) for the child him or herself, to give consent in writing).

Consent Form 3 can be used for treatments where there is no loss of consciousness.

Only on rare occasions is there a statutory requirement for consent to be given in writing or for consent to be evidenced in writing. Box 7.6 lists such circumstances.

Box 7.6 Statutory requirements relating to the giving of consent

- The Abortion Act 1967 requires forms to be completed by the doctors who confirm that the statutory requirements are met (except in an emergency).

- The Mental Health Act 1983 Part IV covers the giving of treatment for mental disorder. The responsible medical officer has to confirm, in specified circumstances, that the patient is capable of understanding the nature, purpose and likely effects of the treatment and has given consent.

- The Human Fertilisation and Embryology Act 1990 sets out specific requirements on consent, preceded by counselling in relation to the use of gametes and embryos (see Ch. 27).

The Department of Health has suggested that consent should be evidenced in writing:

- For any significant procedure such as a surgical operation or when the patient participates in a research project or a video recording (even if only minor procedures are involved).[1]

Where special forms are not required, written consent which is not on one of the recommended forms will not be invalid, provided that it clearly indicates the object of the consent and gives the signature of the person consenting. It must be remembered that the form is not the actual consent, but evidence that consent was given.

The forms may incorporate a phrase such as 'I also give consent to any other procedure deemed necessary'. This would be interpreted in the light of the treatment or procedure for which consent has been given. It would not cover a procedure unrelated to the treatment. For example, if a mother has signed such a statement in relation to a caesarean, it would not necessarily cover a sterilisation. If such a procedure were considered to be life-saving, it would be better for the professionals to rely on the defence of acting in the best interests of a mentally incapacitated patient (see below) than assume that actual consent has been obtained for this.[8] Diana Brahams, a medical lawyer, stated that in her view when the consent form included permission for such surgery as the surgeon thinks necessary, there should have been a discussion with the patient over those further options that might arise during the agreed procedure.

'Otherwise a catch-all form may not constitute consent, and a dissatisfied patient may seek remedy via the police or by civil proceedings against the surgeon for compensation.'

In certain circumstances, failure by the surgeon to obtain consent to a procedure could be treated as a criminal offence of battery and assault.

CONSENT BY WORD OF MOUTH

This consent may be just as valid as consent in writing, but in the event of dispute, it is very much more difficult for the fact that consent was given to be proved. Unless witnesses were present, it may be a case of the mother's word against that of the midwife. It is therefore recommended that for cases where the procedure is risky or hazardous, and where there could be a controversy as to whether consent was ever given, the midwife should attempt to obtain consent in writing.

IMPLIED CONSENT

The view has been taken that simply coming into hospital or seeing a midwife automatically implies that the woman agrees to all the treatments and procedures which they recommend. In the light of the variety of treatments and procedures now available and the emphasis upon the involvement of the mother in decision making, it would be better to confine the term 'implied consent' to those circumstances where the mother indicates by her non-verbal behaviour that she agrees that certain treatment can be given. For example, she raises her sleeve for blood pressure readings to be taken or for an injection to be given, she lies on the couch for a physical examination; such actions denote an agreement for the midwife or other professional to proceed.

Care however must be taken that the action carried out is that to which the implied consent refers. This shows the weakness of relying upon the implied consent of the mother, and the problems of misinterpretation. Where any risky procedure is contemplated, written consent (preferably) or consent by word of mouth should be obtained.

WHO CAN GIVE CONSENT?

MENTALLY COMPETENT PERSONS OVER 18 YEARS

Each mentally competent adult has the right to give or withhold consent. The courts respect the autonomy of the individual. This was clearly stated by the Court of Appeal in the case of Re T[9] (see below). Competence would be defined in relation to the procedure/treatment which is proposed. Thus, in relation to a woman with learning disabilities, she might have the competence to give consent to having stitches for a wound, but not to give consent for an abortion or caesarean section. The determination of capacity is considered below.

THE 16- AND 17-YEAR-OLD

These young persons have a statutory right to give consent under the Family Law Reform Act 1969 s.8. Consent can be given for surgical, medical and dental treatment and the definition of treatment covers any procedure undertaken for the purposes of diagnosis and any ancillary procedures such as administration of anaesthetic.

The parents also have the right to give consent on behalf of the 16- and 17-year-old. This is preserved by s.8(3) of the Family Law Reform Act 1969. Where there is a clash between the parent and the minor, the professional would normally follow the wishes of the minor. However, much depends upon the circumstances. In the case of Re W 1992,[10] a 16-year-old who suffered from anorexia refused to go to a specialist unit for treatment and the courts decided that she could be compelled to go against her wishes since it was in her best interests to receive treatment. The case is important to the midwife who is caring for pregnant minors of 16 and 17, since although they have a statutory right to give consent to treatment (including ancillary and diagnostic procedures), their refusal can in certain circumstances be overruled. The case would usually be referred to the court.

The following is a decision by the House of Lords over the sterilisation of a 17-year-old girl.

Re B (1987)[11]

A 17-year-old girl, who had a mental age of 5–6 years, was in the care of the local authority. It was established that she would have no understanding of sexual intercourse, pregnancy and birth. The local authority applied for her to be made a ward of court and for leave to be given for the operation of sterilisation to be carried out.

The House of Lords held that the paramount consideration for the exercise of its wardship jurisdiction was the welfare and best interests of the child. The Court held that it was in the best interests of the minor for the sterilisation to proceed and permission was given to the operation.

LEGAL ASPECTS OF MIDWIFERY | CHAPTER 7

THE CHILD UNDER 16 YEARS

While children under 16 years of age do not have a statutory right to consent to treatment, the right to give consent at common law (i.e. judge-made law) was recognised by the House of Lords in the Gillick case.[12]

If a child has the maturity to understand the nature, purpose and likely effects of any proposed treatment, then she could give a valid consent without the involvement of the parents. This has given rise to the expression 'Gillick competent', which is also known as the test of competence according to Lord Fraser's guidelines (Lord Fraser was one of the judges in the House of Lords which decided the Gillick case). Lord Fraser stated that:

Provided the patient, whether a boy or a girl, is capable of understanding what is proposed, and of expressing his or her own wishes, I see no good reason for holding that he or she lacks the capacity to express them validly and effectively and to authorise the medical man to make the examination or give the treatment which he advises.

While the Gillick case itself was concerned with family planning and treatment, the principle applies to other forms of treatment, including abortion, and can apply to boys as well as girls. The principle that the ascertainable wishes and feelings of the child concerned (considered in the light of his age and understanding) should also be taken into account is also stated in the Children Act 1989 s.1(3a) as one of the factors to which the court shall have regard in determining what if any orders should be made or varied. Again, this right of the child is paralleled by a right and even duty of the parent to give consent. In addition, s.3(5) of the Children Act 1989 enables a person who:

(a) does not have parental responsibility for a particular child; but

(b) has care of the child

to do what is reasonable in all the circumstances of the case for the purposes of safeguarding or promoting the child's welfare.

Thus, if the midwife were caring for a pregnant minor, and if the patient did not have the competence to give consent herself, a person caring for her could do so.

If the parent or guardian of a minor under the age of 16 refused to give consent to treatment which was necessary in the best interests of the minor, the doctor could act out of necessity in the best interests of the minor according to the principle set out in Re F (see below). Alternatively, the authority of the court could be sought for treatment to proceed against the parents' wishes. Should the parents fail to give consent to essential treatment or arrange for the treatment to take place, they can face prosecution in the event of harm befalling the child. For example, a Rastafarian couple who had refused on religious grounds to allow their diabetic daughter who was 9 years old to be given insulin were convicted of manslaughter on 28 October 1993, in Nottingham. The father was given a sentence of imprisonment and the mother a suspended sentence.[13]

An example of a clash between parents and under-age daughter is seen in the following case which related to abortion.

Re P (1982)[14]

A girl of 15 who had already given birth to a boy, and was in the care of the local authority, became pregnant again. Her parents wished to prevent her having an abortion and refused to give consent. The girl herself wished to have an abortion and the requirements of the Abortion Act 1967 were satisfied. The judge, Mrs Justice Butler-Sloss, using the test that the welfare of the girl was of paramount importance, decided that the termination should proceed.

THE MENTALLY INCOMPETENT ADULT

Until the Mental Capacity Act 2005 (see below) is brought into force (expected to be April 2007), the present law applies. Where an adult is mentally incompetent no person is authorised in law to give consent on her behalf. Her parents cannot give consent once the minor has attained the age of majority (i.e. 18 years). An example of the problem of consent to abortion and sterilisation arose in the following case of T v. T.

T v. T (1988)[15]

T was 19 years old and pregnant. She was doubly incontinent, had a mental age of two-and-a-half years and could barely communicate. Her mother and doctors applied for a declaration that it would be lawful to abort the baby and then sterilise her. The judge granted the declaration stating that the doctor was justified in taking such steps as good medical practice demands and that in her case, her mental abnormality was such that she would never be able to give a valid consent. It should be noted that the court did not itself give permission for the operation to proceed.

Until the Mental Capacity Act 2005 is brought into force, the common law (i.e. judge made law/case law) covers decision making on behalf of mentally incapacitated adults. Health professionals and others have the power to act in the best interests of the mentally incapacitated adult out of necessity.

COMMON LAW POWERS

Until the Mental Capacity Act 2005 is brought into force, decisions on the care and treatment of the mentally incapacitated adult must be on the basis of the decision in Re F,[16] with reference to the court where necessary.

In Re F the House of Lords held that if a patient is incapable of giving a valid consent, the professional must act in the patient's best interests and follow the approved accepted practice of the reasonable professional, i.e. the Bolam Test[17] (see Ch. 13 for discussion of this Test). Acting in the best interests of a mentally incapacitated adult is known as the 'defence of necessity' (see below). In a more recent case, also known as Re F, the Court of Appeal held that the Court had the inherent power to make day-to-day decisions on behalf of the mentally incapacitated adult.[18]

THE MIDWIFE AND THE MENTALLY INCAPACITATED MOTHER

The midwife may become involved in such judicial hearings to make decisions where she is caring for a mentally impaired adult or a person who becomes unconscious. For example, it is likely that one of the special category procedures for which the judicial forum would have to make a decision would be whether a mentally impaired woman should be sterilised following a pregnancy. If a pregnant woman becomes unconscious following a road accident, decisions on whether the mother should be kept alive on a ventilation machine during the pregnancy might also be considered by the judicial forum. Other decisions which may be left to the professional might be the decision to induce a mentally incompetent person and the management of her confinement.

VALIDITY OF A REFUSAL

Where the patient refuses life-saving treatment, the Court of Appeal has emphasised that the professional has a duty to ensure that the refusal is valid.

Re T (1992)[9]

The patient was a 20-year-old pregnant woman who had been brought up by her mother who was a Jehovah's Witness. She was injured in a road accident and when admitted to hospital told the nurse that she would not wish to have a blood transfusion. At that stage, it seemed highly improbable that one would be required. However, her condition deteriorated and she went into labour. She was transferred to the maternity unit and told the midwife that she was a Jehovah's Witness and would not accept a blood transfusion. The midwife got her to put her name on a form which she had not read and of which she probably did not understand the significance. Her condition worsened until it was realised that a blood transfusion was essential. At this stage, the father and the co-habitee referred the case to court.

The judge hearing all the facts decided that her refusal was not valid and the transfusion should proceed. His decision was upheld shortly afterwards by the Court of Appeal which, while it stated that the adult mentally competent person has a right to refuse treatment, emphasised that professionals must ensure that a refusal of life-saving treatment is given by a person who is mentally competent and who is not overborne by the views of another or under the influence of drink or drugs.

WITHDRAWAL OF CONSENT

It is a necessary corollary that where treatment is being given on the basis of consent, then that consent can be withdrawn at any time. This could of course pose problems. For example, a woman who may initially have given agreement to an epidural, might change her mind as it is being done and it may not be possible to stop the procedure part-way through. Where however it is possible to stop the procedure without causing harm to the woman, then this should happen if consent is withdrawn. If it is not possible, presumably the professional must continue to give the treatment and rely upon one of the other defences to an action for trespass to the person, such as necessity.

NECESSITY

It has long been recognised at common law (i.e. judge-made law) that there may be circumstances where urgent action needs to be taken in the interest of a person, where his/her consent is lacking. It may be for example in a situation where the person is unconscious. It may be because the person lacks the mental capacity to give consent. In such circumstances the House of Lords has laid down the following principle:

A doctor may lawfully operate on or give treatment to a person who lacks capacity to give consent provided that it is in the best interests of the patient, being necessary to save life, or to prevent a deterioration, or ensure an improvement, in his physical or mental health.

Re F (1989)[16]

A severely mentally impaired woman had formed an attachment with a fellow patient in a hospital for the mentally handicapped. It was clear that she did not have the capacity to understand or cope with a pregnancy and it was considered that it would be advisable if she were sterilised. However, since she was over 17, no one had in law the right to give consent on her behalf. A declaration was therefore sought from the courts that she could be sterilised. In giving the required declaration, the court recommended that while most day-to-day activities by professionals on behalf of mentally incapacitated adults could take place under the doctrine of necessity, it wished applications in relation to sterilisations to come before the courts and a Practice Direction covering this has subsequently been published.

Two points should be emphasised about the decision in Re F (1989). One is that the court stated that in acting in the best interests of the patient, the professional should follow the Bolam Test (see Ch. 13). The other is that the decision refers to the patient who lacks capacity or for some reason is unable to give consent. Where the patient has the capacity to give consent but refuses, Re F does not justify compulsory treatment.

THE DETERMINATION OF MENTAL CAPACITY

In order to give a valid consent, a person must have the requisite mental capacity. How is the capacity of the patient determined? This was the issue before the court in a case involving a Broadmoor patient who obtained a court injunction prohibiting doctors from amputating his leg.

Re C (1994)[19]

C, a 68-year-old patient suffering from paranoid schizophrenia, developed gangrene in a foot during his confinement in a secure hospital while serving a 7-year term of imprisonment. He was removed to a general hospital where the Consultant surgeon diagnosed that he was likely to die imminently if the leg was not amputated below the knee. The prognosis was that he had a 15% chance of surviving without amputation. He refused to consent. The hospital authorities considered whether the operation could be performed without C's consent and made arrangements for a solicitor to see him concerning his competence to give a reasoned decision. Treatment with antibiotics and conservative surgery averted the immediate threat of imminent death but the hospital refused to give an undertaking to the solicitor that in recognition of his repeated refusals it would not amputate in any future circumstances. An application was made to the High Court for an injunction restraining the hospital from carrying out an amputation without his express written consent. The hospital contended that C's capacity to give a definitive decision had been impaired by his mental illness and that he had failed to appreciate the risk of death if the operation was not performed.

The High Court, exercising its inherent jurisdiction, granted the declaration sought by C. It held that although C's general capacity to make a decision had been impaired by schizophrenia, the evidence failed to establish that he lacked sufficient understanding of the nature, purpose and effects of the proposed treatment, but instead showed that he had understood and retained the relevant information, believed it and had arrived at a clear choice. It followed that the presumption in favour of his right to self-determination had not been displaced.

There were three tests of capacity laid down by the court:

1. Could the patient comprehend and retain the necessary information?

2. Was he able to believe it?

3. Was he able to weigh the information, balancing risks and needs, so as to arrive at a choice?

Applying these tests to the patient, the court decided that he did have the necessary capacity to refuse the amputation and issued the injunction to stop any doctor operating without his consent.

REFUSAL OF TREATMENT IN A CAESAREAN CASE

In a much disputed case, Re S,[20] a woman who refused to give consent to a caesarean on religious grounds was compelled by the Family Division court to have one (see below). This decision is difficult to reconcile with the case of the Broadmoor patient and is now discredited.

Re S (1992)

The Health Authority applied for a declaration to authorise the surgeons and staff of a hospital to carry out an emergency caesarean operation upon a patient, referred to as Mrs S. She was 30 years old and was in labour with her third pregnancy. She was admitted to hospital on 10 October 1992, with ruptured membranes and in spontaneous labour, and continued in labour. She was 6 days overdue beyond the expected date of birth and she refused, on religious grounds, to submit herself to a caesarean section operation. She was supported in this by her husband and they were described as 'born-again Christians' and were considered quite sincere in their beliefs.

The obstetrician in charge of the patient gave evidence of the condition of the patient, which was described by the President of the Family Division as follows:

Her situation is desperately serious, as is also the situation of the as yet unborn child. The child is in what is described as a position of "transverse lie", with the elbow projecting through the cervix and the head being on the right side. There is the gravest risk of a rupture of the uterus if the section is not carried out and the natural labour process is permitted to continue. The evidence of the obstetrician is that we are concerned with "minutes rather than hours" and it is a "life and death" situation.

The obstetrician and other staff had done their best to persuade the mother that the only means of saving her life, and also the life of her unborn child, was to carry out a caesarean section operation. The obstetrician stated that it was absolutely the case that the baby could not be born alive if a caesarean operation was not carried out.

The President of the Family Division made the declaration in the knowledge that there was no English legal authority directly in point. The timing shows the speed of the decision. The application came to the notice of court officials at 1.30 p.m. It came on for hearing just before 2.00 p.m. and at 2.18 p.m., the declaration was made. No appeal was brought against the decision and it is understood that the mother accepted the ruling and the caesarean section was performed. The baby died but the mother survived.

Had the reasoning for this decision been supported in subsequent cases, there would have been major implications in terms of the rights of the mother, and the possibility that a slippery slope would commence, where interventions could be made against the will of a competent mother, in the interests of the baby, thus treating the pregnant woman as lacking the ability to make decisions.

One of the implications of the decision in Re S was that the mother could be forced to recognise the potential harm and action could be taken against her. Drugs, smoking, alcohol, eating unwisely, dangerous sporting and leisure activities have all been shown to have the potential to cause underweight or premature babies. On the basis of Re S, action could have been taken to restrict a mother's activities in the interests of the unborn child.

Cases after Re S

There was considerable outcry as a result of the Re S decision. The Ethics Committee of the Royal College of Obstetricians and Gynaecologists published guidelines which commented adversely on the decision and made the conclusions set out in Box 7.7.

Box 7.7 Conclusions of the RCOG Ethics Committee on Re S

1. The aim of those who care for pregnant women is to foster the greatest benefit to both mother and fetus with the least risk.

2. Occasionally problems arise when a pregnant woman and her doctor fundamentally disagree over action believed to be in the best interest of mother and fetus or when advice is in conflict with her religious scruples.

3. Although obligations to the fetus *in utero* increase as it develops, UK law does not grant it personal legal status. This comes from the moment of birth.

4. The law provides no restriction on a woman's freedom on account of her pregnancy. Any medical action requires her informed consent.

5. A pregnant woman has a natural duty and moral obligation to the welfare of her fetus as a future person and member of society.

6. Society should provide all the necessary services and incentives to help the pregnant woman to fulfil her obligation.

7. It is rare for a doctor to be faced with a conflict where judicial intervention on behalf of the fetus might be considered.

8. Such circumstances are usually unexpected and the requirement of haste leaves little time for the case to be properly prepared and decided.

9. Doctors must recognise that medical advice is based on evidence that is seldom infallible. It is the doctor's duty to provide appropriate information so that the pregnant woman can make an informed and thoughtful decision.

10. Where conflict arises, the doctor should seek help and advice from other professional colleagues and, with the patient's agreement, it may be appropriate to involve other members or friends of her family.

11. A doctor must respect the competent pregnant woman's right to choose or refuse any particular recommended course of action while optimising care for both mother and fetus to the best of his or her ability. A doctor would not then be culpable if these endeavours were unsuccessful.

12. We conclude that it is inappropriate, and unlikely to be helpful or necessary, to invoke judicial intervention to overrule an informed and competent woman's refusal of a proposed medical treatment, even though her refusal might place her life and that of her fetus at risk.

SUBSEQUENT DECISIONS SINCE Re S

Re S was followed by several other cases where compulsory caesarean operations were carried out, without the consent of the woman. In one case[21] the patient suffered from paranoid schizophrenia, was detained in a psychiatric hospital under Section 3 and was refusing to have a caesarean operation. The consultant psychiatrist gave evidence that if there were a stillbirth, that would lead to a profound deterioration of the patient's mental health and once the pregnancy was over, the woman could have the anti-psychotic medication which had been discontinued during the pregnancy because of dangers to the fetus. The judge declared that the operation could proceed under s.63 of the Mental Health Act 1983 as being treatment for mental disorder (s.63 enables treatment (not coming under 57 brain surgery for mental disorder or 58 medication after 3 months or electro convulsive therapy) to be given without the consent of the patient as being treatment for mental disorder, if the treatment is given by or under the direction of the responsible medical officer: see Ch. 33). This decision could be criticised on the grounds that treatment for mental disorder was given too wide a definition: if a caesarean section is considered to be treatment for mental disorder, it would be difficult to find any treatment which by reason of some benefits to the mental state, would not come within the definition of treatment for mental disorder.

In a second case,[22] a pregnant woman had a history of psychiatric treatment and had had three previous children who were delivered by caesarean section. A Consultant psychiatrist examined her and declared that she was not suffering from mental disorder at the time, but she was unable to balance the information given to her. The application was made to the court for a forceps delivery to take place, and if necessary a caesarean section. The judge decided that in the light of the evidence, she lacked the mental competence to make a decision about treatment. A declaration was made on the lines sought.

After these decisions, which received much adverse publicity in the press, there was a need for clarification by the Court of Appeal and this came in the case of Re MB.

Re MB (1997)[23]

Miss MB required a caesarean section in order to save her fetus. However, while she gave consent to the operation, she suffered from a needle phobia which caused her to panic and refuse the preliminary anaesthetic. The trust applied for a declaration that the caesarean could take place on the grounds that the needle phobia rendered her mentally incapacitated and therefore the operation should proceed in her best interests.

The judge held that the woman was mentally incapacitated as a result of the phobia and the operation could therefore proceed in her best interests.

The same day the Court of Appeal upheld that decision. In a reserved judgement, it set out how capacity was to be determined (see Box 7.8) and the general principles which apply to the refusal of treatment (see Box 7.9).[24]

Box 7.8 Determining capacity: Re MB

A person lacks capacity if some impairment or disturbance of mental functioning renders him unable to make a decision on whether to consent to or to refuse treatment. That inability to make a decision will occur when:

(a) The patient is unable to comprehend and retain the information which is material to the decision, especially as to the likely consequences of having or not having the treatment in question

(b) The patient is unable to use the information and weigh it in the balance as part of the process of arriving at the decision.

Box 7.9 Principles laid down in Re MB and incorporated in guidance issued by the Department of Health[24]

1. The court is unlikely to entertain an application for a declaration unless the capacity of the patient to consent to or refuse the medical treatment is in issue.

2. For the time being, at least, the doctors ought to seek a ruling from the High Court on the issue of competence.

▶

3. Those in charge should identify a potential problem as early as possible so that both the hospital and the patient can obtain legal advice.

4. It is highly desirable that, in any case where it is not an emergency, steps are taken to bring it before the court, before it becomes an emergency, to remove the extra pressure from the parties and the court and to enable proper instructions to be taken, particularly from the patient, and where possible give the opportunity for the court to hear oral evidence, if appropriate.

5. The hearing should be inter parties.

6. The mother should be represented in all cases, unless, exceptionally, she does not wish to be. If she is unconscious she should have a guardian *ad litem*.

7. The Official Solicitor should be notified of all applications to the High Court . . .

8. There should in general be some evidence, preferably but not necessarily from a psychiatrist, as to the competence of the patient, if competence is in issue.

9. Where time permits, the person identified to give the evidence as to capacity to consent to or refuse treatment should be made aware of the observations made by the Court of Appeal in this judgement.

10. In order to be in a position to assess a patient's best interests the judge should be provided, where possible and if time allows, with information about the circumstances of and relevant background material about the patient.

The Court of Appeal emphasised that every person is presumed to have the capacity to consent to or to refuse medical treatment unless and until that presumption is rebutted. A competent woman who has the capacity to decide may, for religious reasons, other reasons, for rational or irrational reasons or for no reason at all, choose not to have medical intervention, even though the consequence may be the death or serious handicap of the child she bears, or her own death. In that event, the courts do not have the jurisdiction to declare medical intervention lawful and the question of her own best interests, objectively considered, does not arise.

St George's Healthcare NHS Trust v. S[25]
This case reaffirmed the principles set out by the Court of Appeal in the case of Re MB. A woman who was about 36 weeks pregnant was diagnosed as suffering from severe pre-eclampsia, severe oedema and proteinuria. She was advised to have early induction of labour as a life-saving necessity. She refused, on the grounds that she would prefer to let nature take its course. She was then examined by an approved

social worker and two doctors and was detained in hospital under Section 2 of the Mental Health Act 1983. From there she was transferred to St George's Hospital for obstetric treatment. She was advised by a solicitor that she had the right to refuse treatment. The hospital applied in an *ex parte* application to the High Court judge stating that it was a life and death situation and the patient had gone into labour. This latter information was incorrect, and the judge was not informed that the patient had instructed solicitors. The judge made the declaration that S's consent could be dispensed with. S was then given a caesarean section. She was transferred back to the psychiatric hospital where a doctor decided that she was not suffering from mental disorder and ended the detention under Section 2, following which she took her own discharge.

The case eventually came before the Court of Appeal which emphasised the pregnant woman's right of self-determination, that the Mental Health Act should not have been used when a person was refusing treatment for hypertension, and that an unborn child is not a separate person from its mother.

Lord Justice Judge held that:

(A pregnant woman) is entitled not to be forced to submit to an invasion of her body against her will, whether her own life or that of her unborn child depends on it. Her right is not reduced or diminished merely because her decision to exercise it may appear morally repugnant. The declaration in this case involved the removal of the baby from within the body of her mother under physical compulsion. Unless lawfully justified, this constituted an infringement of the mother's autonomy. Of themselves, the perceived needs of the fetus did not provide the necessary justification.

STATUTORY AUTHORISATION

Certain Acts of Parliament justify actions which would otherwise be regarded as a trespass to the person. Thus, the Mental Health Act 1983 has provisions which enable treatment for mental disorder to be given to a detained patient under specific conditions without the person's consent. The care of those with a mental disorder is considered in Chapter 33.

The Police and Criminal Evidence Act 1984 enables a citizen to carry out a lawful arrest in certain circumstances, and if the specified circumstances exist, an action for trespass to the person would not succeed.

DECLARATION OF THE COURT

If there is doubt over the capacity of the woman to give consent, and life-saving action is required, a declaration can be sought from the court. The issue before the court will be whether or not the person has the mental capacity to make their own decisions. If the person is deemed to lack the appropriate mental capacity (and evidence would have to be given of the incapacity) then a declaration could be issued, where appropriate, that treatment could proceed in the person's best interests. In the case of Re C (the Broadmoor patient, see above) the patient succeeded in obtaining an injunction preventing the doctors from operating upon him.

BIRTH PLANS

It would be wrong to see birth plans as written consent to treatment. Rather they result from discussions between midwife and mother over the options available and reflect the mother's wishes at a given moment in time. Where the philosophy behind Changing Childbirth is implemented, then there is likely to be far greater usage of birth plans as the outcome of the discussions. Where, however, consent is required to specific procedures, it is preferable to obtain this consent in writing, and the usual consent form should then be completed.

WHAT IS THE LEGAL SIGNIFICANCE OF BIRTH PLANS?

If the above view of the birth plan is taken, then it is seen not as a legal document binding upon the midwife but rather as the expression of the mother's wishes if all goes according to plan. If the mother and midwife agree at the beginning of the pregnancy on the preferred choices for the mother, but in the event it is not clinically possible for these preferences to be followed without harm to mother or child, what is the midwife's position? Could she still carry out those procedures to which the mother has not consented? Ideally, of course, in obtaining the mother's involvement in the treatment and confinement agreement it should be made clear that the plan is subject to the clinical situation. In some situations, the clinical needs of the mother may conflict with her original wishes and the preferences she expressed. For example, the mother might have expressed a wish to have a natural birth but after protracted labour and fetal distress, it might be essential for her own life and that of the child for her to have a caesarean. Should problems arise then it is highly recommended that the midwife should have the freedom to act in the mother's best interests at the time. It is preferable that a restraint is not placed upon the professional judgement of the midwife and obstetrician. If the mother accepts this, then there is every justification for the midwife in departing from the birth plan, should this be clinically necessary. If the mother refuses to accept the possibility of variations from the birth plan, and she is mentally competent, she has the right to refuse any recommended procedure. However, the mother should be given the opportunity to change her mind at a later stage. Care should be taken to ensure that the mother is fully informed about all the risks which could occur if the proposed treatment does not go ahead. Where there is reason to believe the woman lacks the necessary mental competence to make a valid refusal, then the fact of that incompetence and the issue of what is in the mother's best interests would be referred to court.

The Maternity Alliance has published a booklet, 'Your Baby, Your Choice', as a guide to planning labour. It makes it clear that 'the birth plan is best used in an antenatal class, as a trigger for discussion'. It thus gives information on various procedures before confinement, positions for labour and delivery, checking the baby's heartbeat, pain relief, induction and acceleration, cuts and tears after the birth, caesarean sections, special care and breastfeeding. The birth plan form it provides enables the mother to consider which options she would prefer. However, there is no legal status to the document and it recognises that what the mother wants is not always possible.

Many of us will plan one kind of birth and end up with another, either because the labour proved more difficult than we had hoped or possibly because some forms of pain relief are not available locally.

When the Mental Capacity Act 2005 (see below) is brought into force, the woman would have power to create a lasting power of attorney whereby a donee is given power to make specific decisions at a time when the woman lacks the necessary mental capacity. Greater use of advance directions may also be made (see Ch. 9).

IMPLICATIONS OF THE EUROPEAN CONVENTION ON HUMAN RIGHTS

The articles of the Convention are discussed in Chapter 6 and can be found in Appendix 1. While there is no explicit right to give consent recognised in the Convention, failure to obtain consent would be a breach of Article 3, 'Not to be subjected to inhuman or degrading treatment'. There may also be a breach of Article 5 and the 'right to liberty and security of person if a woman is held against her will without lawful authority'. The House of Lords held that a person with learning disabilities could be held in a psychiatric hospital without his consent and without being placed under the Mental Health Act 1983.[26] This decision was however overruled by the European Court of Human Rights which held that such detention was contrary to Article 5(1) of the Convention.[27] At the time of writing, the Department of Health is consulting on options to fill the gap created by the Bournewood case.[28] Article 8 is also relevant to maternity care, since it recognises the individual's right to private and family life, home and correspondence.

MENTAL CAPACITY ACT 2005: BACKGROUND

The problems created by the statutory vacuum on decision making on behalf of adults who lack mental capacity have been considered by the Law Commission in a series of consultation papers on decision making and the mentally incapacitated adult.[29] The Law Commission issued its final report on Mental Incapacity in 1995.[30]

It included draft legislation for a Mental Incapacity Bill, which envisaged that there should be new courts which would have the jurisdiction for decision-making on behalf of mentally incapacitated adults. In 1997, the Lord Chancellor issued a consultation[31] which led to the publication of a white paper.[32] A draft Mental Incapacity Bill was introduced which was subjected to pre-parliamentary scrutiny by a Joint Committee of Parliament.[33] The Bill was redrafted in the light of the recommendations of the Joint Committee, including the title which was changed to Mental Capacity Bill and the Bill received the Royal Assent on 7 April 2005. It is due to be brought into force in April 2007.

MENTAL CAPACITY ACT 2005: CONTENTS

There are two basic concepts which underpin the new statutory provisions. The one is the concept of mental capacity; the other of acting in the best interests. Both concepts receive statutory definition.

MENTAL CAPACITY

An adult person is presumed to have the necessary mental capacity to make their own decisions. However, this presumption can be rebutted. A person lacks capacity for the purposes of the statute in relation to a matter:

– If at the material time he is unable to make a decision for himself in relation to the matter because of an impairment of, or a disturbance in the functioning of, the mind or brain.

– The impairment or disturbance can be permanent or temporary. A lack of capacity cannot be established merely by reference to: a person's age or appearance or a condition of his, or an aspect of his behaviour, which might lead others to make unjustified assumptions about his capacity.

This is known as a functional definition: capacity is determined in the light of the particular decision to be made. It follows that a person may have the mental capacity to make certain decisions, but not others. The decision as to whether the necessary capacity exists must be decided on the balance of probabilities.

A person is unable to make a decision for himself if he is unable:

a. to understand the information relevant to the decision

b. to retain that information

c. to use or weigh that information as part of the process of making the decision, or

d. to communicate his decision (whether by talking, using sign language or any other means).

A person is not to be regarded as unable to understand the information relevant to a decision if he is able to understand an explanation of it given to him in a way that is appropriate to his circumstances (using simple language, visual aids or any other means).

The fact that a person is able to retain the information relevant to a decision for a short period only does not prevent him from being regarded as able to make the decision.

BEST INTERESTS

Anyone who makes decisions on behalf of a person who lacks mental capacity must make those decisions in the best interests of that person. The person making the determination must consider all the relevant circumstances. The decision must not be made merely on the basis of: a person's age or appearance or a condition of his, or an aspect of his behaviour, which might lead others to make unjustified assumptions about what might be in his best interests.

The considerations of the decision maker are then identified as including in particular: whether the incapacity is temporary or permanent; how the person can be encouraged to participate in decision making; (in the case of life-sustaining treatment) assuming that it will be in the person's best interest for his life to continue; taking into account the person's present and past wishes and feelings, including the beliefs and values that would have been likely to influence his decisions had he the necessary capacity, and other factors the person would have considered. The views of others must be taken into account, if it is practicable and appropriate to consult them.

PRINCIPLES OF THE ACT

The Joint Committee recommended that the Bill should contain basic principles which should apply to decision making on behalf of the adult who lacks mental capacity, comparable with those set out in the Adults with Incapacity (Scotland) Act 2000. The Act contains the following principles:

– Every adult must be assumed to have capacity unless it is established that he lacks capacity.

– A person is not to be treated as unable to make a decision unless all practicable steps to help him have been taken without success.

– A person is not to be treated as unable to make a decision merely because he makes an unwise decision.

- An action done, or decision made, under this Act for or on behalf of a person who lacks capacity must be done, or made, in his best interests.

- Before the act is done, or the decision is made, regard must be had to whether the purpose for which it is needed can be effectively achieved in a way that is less restrictive of the person's rights and freedom of action.

COURT OF PROTECTION

A revamped Court of Protection with new powers to cover welfare and treatment decisions (in the past it has been confined to property and affairs) will be able to appoint *deputies* who will have the responsibility of making decisions on behalf of a mentally incapacitated adult. The deputies can be given specific powers in relation to where the person is to live; what contact, if any, he or she is to have with any specified person; powers in relation to decisions on healthcare and treatment.

The Court of Protection will be supported by a new Officer known as the *Public Guardian*, whose functions include establishing and maintaining registers of lasting powers of attorney and of orders appointing deputies; supervising deputies appointed by the court and directing a *Court of Protection Visitor* to visit.

LASTING POWER OF ATTORNEY

Provision is made for a person (the *donor*), who has the requisite mental capacity, to draw up a *lasting power of attorney* to a *donee*, who can act on behalf of that person, should they lose their capacity.

ADVANCE DIRECTIONS

Living wills are also given statutory recognition and enable a person when mentally capacitated to refuse treatments in the future if they then lack capacity.

CODES OF PRACTICE

The whole Act is underpinned by the duty of the Secretary of State to prepare Codes of Practice covering most of the statutory provisions. These will give detailed guidance for those responsible for acting on behalf of mentally incapacitated persons.

OVERVIEW

The Mental Capacity Act 2005 puts into statutory form many of the principles which are already recognised by the common law. When it is brought into force, it is likely that there will be a growing number of cases which give further interpretation to the principles and provisions relating to the care of those adults who lack mental capacity.

CONCLUSIONS

In the months before the Mental Capacity Act 2005 is brought into force, the decisions of the Court of Appeal in the case of Re MB and St George's are to be welcomed, since they have clarified the legal situation where a pregnant woman is refusing life-saving treatment. They have emphasised that a mentally competent pregnant woman, like any other mentally competent adult, can validly refuse life-saving treatment. If the refusal of a mentally competent adult were overruled, this would constitute a trespass to the person, as well as possibly a criminal act.

QUESTIONS AND EXERCISES

1. The mental capacity of a woman to refuse life-saving treatment is central to the question of whether action can be taken in the best interests of the woman and the baby. What arrangements do you have for determining the mental capacity of a mother?

2. Do you consider there are any dangers or advantages in making birth plans legally enforceable?

3. Analyse your practice and during a week of work consider the different ways in which you obtain the consent of the mother to treatments proceeding. What proportion of the total number are obtained in writing?

References

1 Department of Health. Reference Guide to Consent for Examination or Treatment. London: HMSO; 2001. Online. Available: www. doh.gov.uk/consent

2 In Re B (Consent to treatment: Capacity) The Times Law Report, 26 March 2002; [2002] 2 All ER 449.

3 St George's Healthcare NHS Trust v. S [1998] 3 All ER 673.

4 Freeman v. Home Office [1984] 1 All ER 1036.

5 Caswell A. Medical rape. Med J Austr 1993; 157:561–562.

6 Chatterton v. Gerson [1981] 1 All ER 257.

7 Department of Health. Good practice in consent implementation guide. London: DH; November 2001.

8 Brahams D. Medico-legal J 1993; 62:225–226.

9 Re T. [1992] 4 All ER 649; [1992] 3 WLR 782.

10 Re W (a minor) (medical treatment) [1992] 4 All ER 627.

11 Re B (a minor) (wardship: sterilisation) [1987] 2 All ER 206.

12 Gillick v. W. Norfolk and Wisbech Area Health Authority [1986] 1 AC 112.

13 News item. The Times, 29 October 1993.

14 Re P (a minor) [1982] 80 Local Government Reports 301.

15 T v. T [1988] 1 All ER 613.

16 Re F v. West Berkshire HA [1989] 2 All ER 545.

17 Bolam v. Friern HMC QBD [1957] 2 All ER 118.

18 Re F (adult: court's jurisdiction) [2000] 2 FLR 512 Court of Appeal.

19 Re C (adult: refusal of medical treatment) Family Division [1994] 1 All ER 819.

20 Re S (adult: refusal of medical treatment) [1992] 9 BMLR 69; [1993] FAM 123.

21 Tameside and Glossop Acute Services Trust v. CH [1996] 31 BMLR 93.

22 Norfolk and Norwich Healthcare (NHS) Trust v. W [1996] 2 FLR 613.

23 Re MB (an adult: medical treatment) [1997] 2 FLR 426.

24 Department of Health Circular EL (97)32 1997.

25 St George's Healthcare NHS Trust v. S; R v. Collins *ex parte* S [1998] 44 BMLR 160 CA.

26 R v. Bournewood Community and Mental Health NHS Trust *ex parte* L [1998] 1 All ER 634 HL.

27 L. v. United Kingdom (Application No 45508/99). Times Law Report, 19 October 2004.

28 Department of Health. Bournewood Consultation: The approach to be taken in response to the judgement of the European Court of Human Rights in the "Bournewood" case. London: DH; March 2005.

29 Law Commission. Paper 119 (1991) and papers 128, 129 and 130 (1993). London: HMSO.

30 Law Commission. Report No 231 (1995). Mental incapacity. London: HMSO.

31 Lord Chancellor. Who decides? Making decisions on behalf of mentally incapacitated adults. London: Lord Chancellor's Office; 1997.

32 Lord Chancellor. Making decisions. London: Lord Chancellor's Office; 1999.

33 House of Lords and House of Commons Joint Committee on the Draft Mental Incapacity Bill Session 2002–3 HL paper 189-1; HC 1083-1.

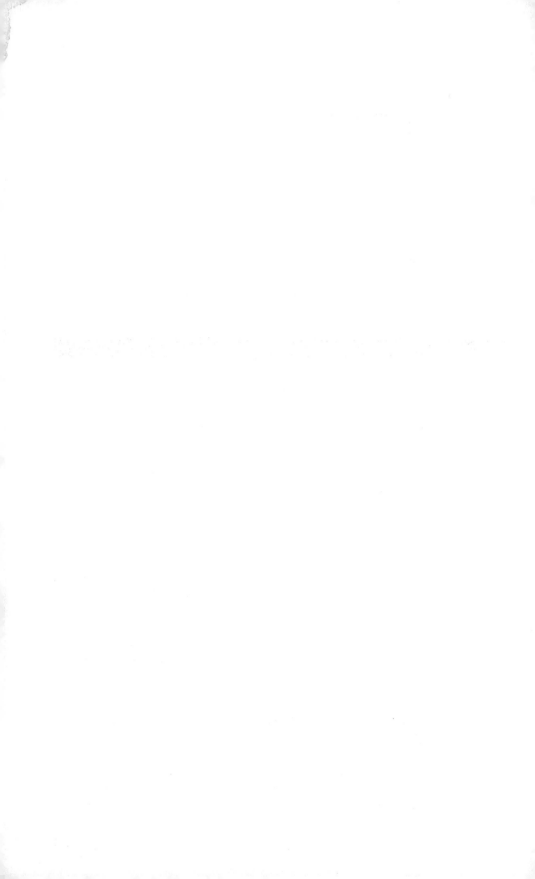

Chapter 8
THE DUTY TO INFORM

In Chapter 7, we considered an action of trespass and the defences available if an apparent trespass has been committed. Of increasing importance in the field of consent is, however, the extent and nature of the information which should be given to the mother before she decides to go ahead with certain procedures. It will be recalled that in the case of Chatterton v. Gerson the distinction was made between the action for trespass, which will not succeed if a valid consent has been given, and an action in negligence on the basis that insufficient information has been given. See the statement of the judge in Box 8.1.

Box 8.1 Chatterton v. Gerson: Judge's statement

The court has to ask, was there real consent? I think justice requires that in order to vitiate the reality of consent there must be a greater failure of communication between doctor and patient than that involved in a breach of duty if the claim is based on negligence. When the claim is based on negligence the plaintiff must prove not only the breach of duty to inform but that had the duty not been broken she would not have chosen to have the operation. Where the claim is based on trespass to the person, once it is shown that the consent is unreal, then what the plaintiff would have decided if she had been given the information which would have prevented vitiation of the reality of her consent is irrelevant.

What standard is applied to the giving of information to the patient? Is there a difference where the patient asks questions compared to situations where the patient does not ask for further information? Is it ever lawful to withhold information from the patient?

These questions will be considered in the light of the cases of Sidaway v. Bethlem Royal Hospital Governors and others, and Blythe v. Bloomsbury Health Authority.

SIDAWAY v. BETHLEM ROYAL HOSPITAL GOVERNORS AND OTHERS[1]

In this case, the plaintiff suffered chronic and intractable pain following an operation for a hernia repair. She was eventually referred to a specialist in pain relief who warned her of the possibility of disturbing a nerve root and the possible consequences of so doing, but did not mention the possibility of damage to the spinal cord. The risk of spinal cord damage was less than 1%.

She consented to the operation, which was carried out by the surgeon with due care and skill. However, in the course of the operation she suffered injury to her spinal cord which resulted in her being severely disabled. She sued the surgeon for breach of his duty of care to warn her of all possible risks inherent in the operation.

The different judges in the House of Lords all had different bases for their views, but they agreed that in general, she had failed in her action. Lord Diplock applied the Bolam principle to the duty of care to inform. Lord Bridge distinguished between two extremes: warning the patient of all possible risks and, once the treatment has been decided upon in the patient's best interests, not warning the patient of any risks, in order not to alarm the patient. Between these two extremes, Lord Bridge suggested that the Bolam Test should be applied, but this did not mean handing over to the medical profession the entire question of the scope of the duty of disclosure. There will be circumstances where the judge could come to the conclusion that disclosure of a particular risk was so obviously necessary to an informed choice on the part of the patient that no reasonably prudent medical man would fail to make it. Lord Templeman stated:

In my opinion, if a patient knows that a major operation may entail serious consequences, the patient cannot complain of lack of information unless the patient asks in vain for more information or unless there is some danger which by its nature or magnitude or for some other reason required to be separately taken into account by the patient in order to reach a balanced judgement in deciding whether or not to submit to the operation.

Lord Scarman supported a 'prudent patient test', a concept derived from an American case, Canterbury v. Spence.[2] In this case, it was recognised that there were four principles:

1. Every human being of adult years and of sound mind has a right to determine what shall be done with his own body.

2. The consent is the informed exercise of a choice and that entails an opportunity to evaluate knowledgeably the options available and the risks attendant on each.

3. The doctor must therefore disclose all 'material risks'; what risks are 'material' is determined by the 'prudent patient' test, which is as follows: A risk is . . . material when a reasonable person, in what the physician knows or should know to be the patient's position, would be likely to attach significance to the risk or cluster of risks in deciding whether or not to forgo the proposed therapy.

4. The doctor has, however, a therapeutic privilege. This exception is that a reasonable medical assessment of the patient would have indicated to the doctor that

disclosure would have posed a serious threat of psychological detriment to the patient.

The House of Lords accepted that English law did not recognise the doctrine of informed consent. Risks should be disclosed to enable the patient to make a rational choice whether to undergo the particular treatment recommended by a doctor. This duty was subject to the doctor's overriding duty to have regard to the best interests of the patient. Accordingly, it was for the doctor to decide what information should be given to the patient and the terms in which that information should be couched.

The claimant therefore lost her appeal.

HOW MUCH INFORMATION SHOULD BE GIVEN?

The ruling in the Sidaway case was followed in a subsequent case by the Court of Appeal, where the issue arose as to how much information should be given to a patient.

BLYTHE V. BLOOMSBURY HEALTH AUTHORITY AND ANOTHER[3]

Mrs Blythe, a nurse, became pregnant in May 1978 and was referred to University College Hospital for antenatal care. She saw a Consultant who diagnosed that she had no or insufficient immunity to rubella. She could not be vaccinated against rubella because she was at a late stage of her pregnancy and the vaccine, if given, could have had an adverse effect on a fetus if she became pregnant again within 3 months. However, it was necessary that steps be taken to provide her with contraceptive protection. The general practice at the hospital was to use Depo-Provera (a progesterone-only contraceptive), unless countervailing factors existed or the patient did not want it.

In December 1978 she was admitted to the hospital for the birth of her baby where she received

a. a rubella vaccination, and

b. an injection of Depo-Provera.

She did not object to the prescription or the administration of Depo-Provera.

On 18 December, she was admitted to the labour ward where she subsequently gave birth to a healthy son.

On 19 December, the rubella vaccine was prescribed by a senior house officer (the vaccination being administered on 23 December by a nursing sister).

On 23 December she was seen by a senior house officer who discussed the Depo-Provera drug with the plaintiff (a dose was subsequently administered by injection on the following morning 24 December). On her discharge from hospital she was given a leaflet detailing the drug's effects on the human body, how long the injection lasted, and advised that she should consult her GP.

On 31 January 1979, she saw two doctors at the hospital's baby clinic.

On 27 March 1979, she saw her GP who prescribed 'Micronor'.

In June 1979, a further dose of Depo-Provera was prescribed.

In April 1980, she had a miscarriage.

In July 1980, she sought the advice of a professor of medicine, who was strongly opposed to the use of Depo-Provera; shortly afterwards she had a miscarriage.

In April 1981, she gave birth to a second child.

She initiated an action for negligence on 16 December 1981 on the grounds shown in Box 8.2.

Box 8.2 Grounds for Mrs Blythe bringing an action

1. The assurances that she had received from the senior house officer concerning Depo-Provera were wrong and inaccurate.

2. She would not have agreed to the injection if she had been told of all the drug's side-effects.

3. She had suffered damages as a consequence.

Subsequent amendments were added:

4. The Health Authority was negligent in failing to adopt a system or practice which enabled patients to receive skilled counselling, warning, or advice regarding the drug's side-effects.

5. Alternatively, if there was a system, that such a system or practice was not adhered to in the plaintiff's case.

The High Court dismissed Mrs Blythe's allegations against the senior house officer, but ruled that there was a case against the Health Authority on the grounds that although it had a system or practice whereby patients who received the Depo-Provera drug could receive skilled counselling, warning and/or advice in relation to the drug's side-effects, the Health Authority had failed to put its system into operation in relation to the plaintiff. She was awarded £3600.

The Health Authority appealed to the Court of Appeal against the findings of negligence.

The Court of Appeal allowed the appeal because:

1. There was no obligation to pass on to the plaintiff all the information available to the hospital, i.e. all the information contained in the senior house officer's files.

2. What a claimant should be told in answer to a general enquiry could not be divorced from the Bolam Test any more than when no such enquiry was made.

3. Answers given must depend upon the circumstances, the nature of the enquiry, the nature of the information which was available, its reliability, relevance, and the condition of the patient.

4. The extent of the duty to give information was to be judged in the light of the state of medical knowledge in December 1978.

5. There was no rule of law that, where questions were asked or doubts expressed by a patient, a doctor was under an obligation to put the patient in possession of all the information on the subject which may be available in the files of a Consultant, who may have made a special study of the subject.

6. The amount of information to be given must depend on the circumstances; it must be governed by the Bolam Test.

INFORMATION TO THE PATIENT

From the House of Lords decision in the Sidaway case, although the different appeal judges had different bases for their reasoning, the basic ruling was that the amount of information which should be given to the patient would be judged according to reasonable professional practice, i.e. the Bolam Test (see Ch. 13). In the Sidaway case, the House of Lords also recognised that there could be exceptional circumstances, where a doctor could exercise a right of therapeutic privilege and withhold information from the patient because it would have an undue influence upon the decision making of the patient. The Blythe decision shows that there is no legal expectation that a person can receive all the information which a hospital or doctor has about a particular treatment. However, the fact that the mother cannot necessarily enforce through a court of law the right to receive all relevant information should not be seen as relieving the midwife of the duty to give as full information as possible to the mother.

PEARCE v. UNITED BRISTOL HEALTHCARE NHS TRUST[4]

Mrs Pearce was expecting her sixth child. The expected date of delivery was 13 November 1991. On 27 November, the baby had still not arrived, when she saw the Consultant. She begged the doctor to induce her or carry out a caesarean. He preferred to let nature take its course, and explained to her the risks from induction and a caesarean section. The baby died *in utero* sometime between 2 and 3 December. The delivery of a stillborn baby was induced on 4 December. Mrs Pearce brought an action alleging that the Consultant should have advised her of the increased risk of stillbirth as a result of the delay in delivery between 13 November and 27 November.

The trial judge dismissed her claim, holding that there had been no negligence on the part of the Consultant in not advising Mrs Pearce of the small risk attached to waiting for natural labour to begin. The Court of Appeal held that the experts had agreed that the risk of the child being stillborn was not a significant risk; possibly 0.1–0.2%. The Court of Appeal stated that it would not interfere with the clinical opinion of the expert medical man responsible for treating Mrs Pearce. It accepted that there would be occasions in which the courts could decide that the expert opinion is not acceptable to the court.

In the recognition of this exception, the Court of Appeal was following the ruling in the Bolitho case,[5] where the House of Lords held that there would be occasions where the courts could find that the expert opinion presented to it was not acceptable. The House of Lords in the Bolitho case held that:

The use of the adjectives "responsible, reasonable and respectable" (in the Bolam case) all showed that the court had to be satisfied that the exponents of the body of opinion relied upon could demonstrate that such opinion had a logical basis.

Overruling experts was seen, however, as an extreme situation.

It would seldom be right for a judge to reach the conclusion that views held by a competent medical expert were unreasonable.

INFORMATION ABOUT SPECIFIC RISKS

Where certain procedures are being contemplated, such as ultrasound, other screening procedures and other high technology investigations and treatment, the midwife needs to be aware of current knowledge relating to any significant risks from such procedures. Her duty is to give to the woman the information which any reasonable midwife following approved accepted practice would give, or to refer her to a person who did have the necessary information. Giving information in relation to Vitamin K is discussed in Ch. 14.

WITHHOLDING INFORMATION

The House of Lords in the Sidaway case recognised the right, in exceptional circumstances, to withhold information from a patient. These exceptional circumstances would include when the information would constitute a serious threat of psychological detriment to the patient. There is therefore no recognition at common law (i.e. judge-made law) that a patient has an absolute right to obtain all information from health professionals. This is comparable with the situation under the Data Protection Act 1998 and the statutory instruments under that Act, which permits access to health records to be refused if there is a reasonable fear that serious harm would be caused to the physical or mental health or condition of the applicant or of another patient (this is considered in Ch. 10). Clearly any midwife who, in exceptional circumstances, deliberately withheld information from a patient, should have very clear justification for this decision and should ensure that there is full documentation of her actions and their justification.

CAUSATION AND CHESTER CASE

Where the claimant is alleging that he or she was not given all the necessary information, then the claimant must prove that had the appropriate information been given, including information about the risks of harm, then failure to provide that information caused the claimant to suffer from that harm. What however if there is no evidence that the claimant would have refused that particular treatment had he or she known of the problems? This is the issue which has recently been considered by the Court of Appeal which held that there was negligence by the doctor even if the claimant had not shown that she would have followed the advice anyway (Chester v. Ashfar [2002]).[6] The case was then heard in the House of Lords. The facts of the case are shown in Box 8.3.

Box 8.3 Facts of Chester v. Ashfar [2002] CA [2004] HL

The defendant, a neurosurgeon, advised the claimant to undergo lumbar surgery. She consented and following the operation suffered partial paralysis. The judge found that although the defendant had not performed the operation negligently, he had failed to warn the claimant of the small risk of partial paralysis inherent in the operation. The judge also found that, had she been warned, the claimant would not have consented to the operation taking place then but would have sought further advice before deciding what to do.

The House of Lords,[7] in a majority ruling, dismissed the appeal against the Court of Appeal decision. The House of Lords held that the defendant owed a duty to the claimant to inform her of the risks inherent in the proposed surgery, including that of paralysis, so that she could make her own decision. Lord Hope stated:

This duty to inform gave the claimant a right to be informed before she consented to it (the operation). It was unaffected in its scope by the response she would have given had she been told of those risks. The problem of causation arose in the present case, since how could causation be established when the patient could not have refused absolutely ever to undergo the operation if told of the risks but would have postponed her decision until later. The matter raised an issue of legal policy in which a judge had to decide whether justice required the normal approach to causation to be modified.

The law which imposed the doctor's duty to warn had at its heart the patient's right to make an informed choice as to whether and if so when and by whom to be operated on. Patients may have and were entitled to have different views about those matters. All sorts of factors might be at work: the patient's hopes and fears and personal circumstances, the nature of the condition to be treated and, above all, the patient's own views whether the risk was worth running for the benefits which might come if the operation was carried out. For some the choice might be easy: simply to agree or to decline the operation. But for many it would be difficult, requiring time to think, to take advice and to weigh up the alternatives.

The duty was owed as much to the patient who, if warned, would find the decision difficult as to the patient who would find it simple and could give a clear answer to the doctor one way or the other immediately. To leave the patient who would find the decision difficult without a remedy, as the normal approach to causation would indicate, would render the duty useless in the cases where it might be needed most.

That would discriminate against those who could not honestly say that they would have declined the operation once and for all if they had been warned.

The result would be unacceptable. The function of the law was to enable rights to be vindicated and to provide remedies when duties had been breached. Unless that was done, the duty was a hollow one, stripped of all practical force and devoid of all content.

On policy grounds therefore, the test of causation was satisfied and justice required that the claimant be afforded the remedy she sought, as the injury she suffered at the defendant's hands was within the scope of the very risk which he should have warned her about when obtaining her consent to the operation which resulted in that injury.

The effect of the House of Lords ruling is that in future it should be easier for a claimant to establish that compensation should be payable following failure to inform him/her of the risks of a particular procedure, if those risks actually occur and the patient is harmed. Only in clear cut cases where the patient makes it clear that they agree to an operation proceeding whatever the untold risks may be, would the patient fail. The implications for the midwife are that it must be clear what information should be given to the woman prior to any risky treatment being offered and a record should be kept of what has been said and what has been given in writing.

Information about services available

One of the key themes in Changing Childbirth (see Ch. 6) is the importance of ensuring that the mother has full information about the range of local services and her options in relation to antenatal care, delivery and postnatal care. The specific midwife allocated to the mother (the named midwife) should ensure that she herself is conversant with the local facilities and services and gives this information to the mother. The midwife might also be involved in talking to local groups such as the National Childbirth Trust and others about the choices available, and obtaining their feedback on the services provided.

The right of the woman to access information about public services is strengthened by the Freedom of Information Act 2000 which was brought into force between 2000 and 2006. Under s.1 of this Act, there is a general right of access to information held by public authorities. There are many exceptions to this right, including access to personal information which comes under the Data Protection Act 1998. Section 40 of the Freedom of Information Act 2000 exempts access to personal information from the Act, and the provisions of the Data Protection Act would then apply (see Ch. 10).

Written information and leaflets

There are considerable benefits in putting in writing information which is given to the mother. This has several advantages:

– It can be useful evidence that the information was given.

– It supports information given by word of mouth and enables the woman to read through more complex information at her leisure.

– It enables the woman to follow up the information with questions on points about which she is unsure.

The midwife should have an input into the information which is provided to the mother at different stages of pregnancy. A study carried out by Brighton Health Authority into the written material provided for patients[8] showed that many of the leaflets and general information were considered unacceptable (of 356 in-house publications produced by the Department concerned, 246 items were unacceptable). They cited as a particularly poor example a leaflet for women going home after a hysterectomy, which featured on the front cover an inappropriate tasteless cartoon of a chicken wearing an apron and a chef's hat stirring a pot with the title, 'Your recipe for home'. Vital information was missing and there were many misprints. As a result of the research, a code of good practice was prepared and advice from a public relations officer made available. The Code recommended the guidelines shown in Box 8.4.

Box 8.4 Brighton Health Authority

Information for patients should:

1. have the department heading, the date and the Health Authority logo

2. have an introduction and a list of contents with page numbers if appropriate

3. have all text in sentences, without abbreviations, jargon, or complicated medical terms

4. be professionally printed or at least produced on a word processor

5. have short paragraphs with double spacing between them. Numbering of paragraphs may be helpful

6. be photocopied from the original material

7. be assessed by as many medical and non-medical people as possible before reproduction.

Rather than produce variable quality in-house leaflets, it is possible to take advantage of leaflets produced nationally. For example, MIDIRS the Midwifery research and information service has produced informed choice leaflets covering many different aspects of care, including mode of delivery, postnatal depression, anti-D-Rhesus, vitamin K, haemoglobinopathies and caesarean section. They are available online.[9]

THE MOTHER IN CUSTODY

Some pregnant women receive custodial sentences and therefore may give birth while still in custody. The midwife may find that her professional practice is circumscribed by the conditions of the custodial arrangements. However, she should ensure through discussions with her supervisor during the antenatal period that the welfare of the mother and baby is not prejudiced by the security concerns. (The handcuffing of women prisoners during childbirth is discussed in Ch. 6 in relation to Article 3 of the European Convention on Human Rights.) The High Court has held that a woman in prison is entitled to the same standard of care in relation to her pregnancy as a woman at liberty.[10]

CONCLUSION

The midwife has a responsibility as part of her duty of care to the mother to ensure that she provides to her the information which any reasonable midwife following the approved standard of care would give. She must answer the woman's questions honestly and as fully as possible and ensure that she keeps up to date with the information which is available. She must also be aware of her ignorance and ensure that where she does not have sufficient information to answer a woman's questions, she can refer the woman to someone who does.

QUESTIONS AND EXERCISES

1. Look at three procedures or treatments which may have to be carried out during pregnancy and confinement in the light of any possible side-effects, and look carefully at the information which is given to the mother before consent is obtained.

2. Consider the information which your unit provides for the mother when pregnancy is first diagnosed. Do you consider that it is clear and sufficiently informative? Is there any additional information which you consider should be given?

3. It was held in the Sidaway case that there may be exceptional circumstances where there exists a therapeutic privilege to withhold information from a patient before consent is obtained. What circumstances do you consider relevant in the case where a caesarean operation is being discussed?

References

1 Sidaway v. Bethlem Royal Hospital Governors and others [1985] 1 All ER 643.

2 Canterbury v. Spence 464 F 2d 772 (DC, 1972).

3 Blythe v. Bloomsbury Health Authority and another Court of Appeal [1993] 4 Medical Law Report 151.

4 Pearce v. United Bristol Healthcare NHS Trust (1998) n48 BMLR 118 CA.

5 Bolitho v. City and Hackney HA [1997] 4 All ER 771.

6 Chester v Afshar. Times Law Report, 13 June 2002; [2002] 3 ALL ER 552 CA.

7 Chester v Afshar. The Times Law Report, 19 October, 2004 HL; [2004] UKHL 41; [2004] 3 WLR 927.

8 Bennett J, Bridger P. BMJ 1992; 305:1294, and reported in MIDIRS Midwifery Digest March 1993; 3(1).

9 MIDIRS the Midwifery research and information service. Online. Available: www.infochoice.org

10 Brooks v. Home Office. Times Law Report, 17 February 1999.

Chapter 9
LETTING DIE AND EUTHANASIA

In Chapters 7 and 8, we looked at different aspects of consent. In this chapter, we look at the law relating to the letting die of another individual, in relation to both the mother and the baby.

The care of neonates can give rise to legal issues or sometimes present midwives with the problem of whether there is a duty in law to carry out every possible procedure known to science in order to save the life of the baby, or whether the law allows a person to be allowed to die. In addition, the midwife needs to know what if any rights the parents have in such circumstances: if they wish the baby to be allowed to die, would the professionals be acting illegally to go against their wishes? This chapter also looks at the law relating to euthanasia and the duty of care in keeping a patient alive.

VOLUNTARY EUTHANASIA

Voluntary euthanasia means the killing of a person with that person's consent. This is unlawful. It could amount to murder which is punishable on conviction by life imprisonment. Alternatively, if the act amounts to assistance in a suicide bid, then it is illegal under s.2(1) of the Suicide Act 1961, which is shown in Box 9.1.

Box 9.1 Assisting a person to commit suicide

A person who aids, abets, counsels or procures the suicide of another or an attempt by another to commit suicide, shall be liable on conviction on indictment to imprisonment (up to 14 years).

The High Court has stated in the Diane Pretty case that the Director of Public Prosecutions has no power to pardon in advance a person who wished to aid and abet the suicide of another.

Mrs Pretty was suffering from motor neurone disease and had very little movement left. She wanted her husband to be given permission to assist her in ending her life,[1] so that she would be spared the suffering and indignity that she would otherwise have to endure. She was unable to take her own life without assistance. The High Court held that Articles 2 and 3 of the European Convention on Human Rights did not give a right to procure one's own death or confer a right to die. In addition, Articles 8 and 9 were not absolute rights and did not give her a right to die. There was no incompatibility between the provisions of the Suicide Act 1961 and the articles of the European Convention on Human Rights in these circumstances. On 1 November 2001 she was given leave to appeal to the House of Lords. She lost her appeal. The House of Lords held that the refusal to grant immunity was not an infringement of Articles 2, 3, 8, 9 or 14 of the European Convention on Human Rights. Any change in the law relating to aiding and abetting a suicide must be enacted through Parliament.[2] She also lost her application to the European Court of Human Rights in Strasbourg.[3]

Even where the parents wish a grossly handicapped baby to die, any professional who intentionally speeded up the process of death could be guilty of causing the death of the child. In the case of R v. Arthur[4] a paediatrician was prosecuted for attempting to cause the death of a grossly handicapped baby who was suffering from Down's Syndrome and who had other disabilities when he prescribed dihydrocodeine and nursing care only. The judge stated that:

There is no special law in this country that places doctors in a separate category and gives them extra protection over the rest of us . . . Neither in law is there any special power, facility or license to kill children who are handicapped or seriously disadvantaged in an irreversible way.

Dr Arthur was acquitted.

THE CASE OF DR NIGEL COX[5]

Dr Nigel Cox, a rheumatologist in Winchester, was convicted of causing the death of a patient to whom he had administered potassium chloride. He was given a suspended prison sentence. The patient was in crippling pain, and terminally ill, and her relatives were concerned at her condition. Dr Cox was also brought before his employers, the Wessex Regional Health Authority, to face disciplinary proceedings, but retained his post. He was also brought before professional conduct proceedings of the General Medical Council, but stayed on the Register.

PAIN RELIEF AND CAUSING DEATH

THE CASE OF DR BODKIN ADAMS

In contrast to the case of Dr Cox, Dr Bodkin Adams was acquitted following a trial where it was alleged that he had caused the death of Mrs Morell, a resident in a nursing home in Eastbourne, by giving her excessive morphine.

The trial judge, Mr Justice Patrick Devlin, directed the jury that:

There has been a good deal of discussion about the circumstances in which a doctor might be justified in giving drugs which would shorten life in cases of severe pain. It is my duty to tell you that the law knows of no special defence of this character. But that does not mean that a doctor aiding the sick or dying has to calculate in minutes or hours, or perhaps in days or weeks, the effect on a patient's life of the medicines which he administers. If the first purpose of medicine – the restoration of health – can no longer be achieved, there is still much for the doctor to do, and he is entitled to do all that is proper and necessary to relieve pain and suffering, even if the measures he takes may incidentally shorten life . . . It remains a law, that no doctor has the right to cut off life deliberately . . . What counsel for the defence was saying, was that the treatment that was given by the doctor was designed to promote comfort, and if it was the right and proper treatment of the case, the fact that incidentally it shortened life does not give any grounds for convicting him of murder.[6]

This ruling still applies today. However, note would be taken of what is 'right and proper treatment'. It could be that a very high dose of morphine was justified for a patient who needed that level to achieve pain relief, whereas that dose for a person who had not become resistant to morphine would be lethal and grossly reckless, and justify a criminal conviction. 'Right and proper treatment' must also take into account current research on effective pain management.

Annie Lindsell, a sufferer from motor neurone disease, brought a court action for a declaration that her GP could administer palliative drugs which could have the effect of shortening her life. She was told that a responsible body of medical opinion supported her doctor's treatment plan and she then withdrew her application for the court's intervention.[7] She died a few months later.

DISTINCTION BETWEEN KILLING AND LETTING DIE

Do these cases mean that it is never lawful to permit a patient to die, whatever the circumstances of his/her condition? The answer is that the law does not expect constant medical intervention whatever the prognosis, and that in certain circumstances it is legally permissible to let die. A distinction is however drawn between letting die and killing. Examples from decided cases will illustrate the difference.

RE B (1981)[8]

A child was born suffering from Down's syndrome and an intestinal blockage. She required an operation to relieve the obstruction if she was to live more than a few days. If the operation were performed, the child might die within a few months, but it was probable that her life expectancy would be 20 to 30 years. Her parents, having decided that it would be kinder to allow her to die rather than live as a physically and mentally handicapped person, refused to consent to the operation. The local authority made the child a ward of court and, when a surgeon decided that the wishes of the parents should be respected, they sought an order authorising the operation to be performed by other named surgeons. The judge decided that the parents' wishes should be respected and refused to make the order. The local authority appealed to the Court of Appeal which allowed the appeal. It stated that:

1. The question for the court was whether it was in the best interests of the child that she should have the operation and not whether the parents' wishes should be respected.

2. since the effect of the operation might be that the child would have the normal span of life of a mongol, and

3. since it had not been demonstrated that the life of a mongol was of such a nature that the child should be condemned to die,

4. the court would make an order that the operation be performed.

Crucial to the decision in this case was the prognosis of the child.

RE C (1989)[9]

In a contrasting case, a baby was born suffering from congenital hydrocephalus and had been made a ward of court for reasons unconnected with her medical condition. The local authority sought the court's determination as to the appropriate manner in which she should be treated, should she contract a serious infection, or her existing feeding regimes become unviable. A specialist paediatrician assessed C's condition as severely and irreversibly brain-damaged, the prognosis of which was hopeless. He recommended that the objective of any treatment should therefore be to ease suffering rather than prolong life. While not specifying the adoption or discontinuance of any particular procedures, he further advised consultation with C's carers as to the appropriate method of achieving that objective. The judge accepted this report and approved the recommendations as being in her best interests. Paragraph 3 of his order is shown in Box 9.2, but subsequently on reflection the judge amended it to that shown in Box 9.3.

Box 9.2 Judge's initial order in Re C

The hospital authority shall be at liberty to treat the minor to die and . . . shall administer such treatment to the minor as might relieve her from pain, suffering and distress inter alia by sedation . . . but it shall not be necessary either

(a) to prescribe and administer antibiotics to treat any serious infection which the minor might contract or

(b) to set up intravenous or nasal feeding regimes for the minor.

Box 9.3 Amendment to judge's order in Re C

For the words 'to die'

(To treat the minor) 'to allow her life to come to an end peacefully and with dignity'.

The official solicitor who had been appointed guardian *ad litem* of the child appealed to the Court of Appeal on the grounds that the judge had no jurisdiction and was plainly wrong in the exercise of his discretion to make an order that the hospital be at liberty to treat the minor to die. He also appealed on the grounds that by Para. 3 of his order the judge had seemed to provide that in no circumstances should certain treatments be undertaken, such direction being inconsistent with Para. 4.

The Court of Appeal changed the wording of the order by the deletion of Para. 3 but otherwise upheld the judge's decision (Box 9.4).

Box 9.4 Court of Appeal's decision in Re C

1. Whole of Para. 3 to be deleted because it was inconsistent with Para. 4

4. Para. 4 to stand

> *The hospital to continue to treat the minor within the parameters of the opinion expressed by [the specialist paediatrician] in his report of 13.4.1989 which report is not to be disclosed to any person other than the health authority.*

This case raised many issues:

1. What is meant by the best interests of the child?

2. What is the role of the doctor?

3. What is the role of the registered midwife/nurse?

4. What rights do the parents have?

5. What is the role of the courts?

1. The best interests of the child are determined by what the professionals, following the Bolam Test, would consider appropriate in the light of the specific circumstances of that individual child. It is clear that heroic surgery and medical intervention will not necessarily always be in the best interests of the child, and the court is unwilling to direct specialists over what should be done, preferring to leave the actual decisions to the clinical judgement (see below, the case of Re J 1992).

2. The doctor has a duty to make a clinical assessment, following the reasonable standard of care.

3. The role of the midwife/neonatal nurse is to ensure that she provides all the relevant information to the doctor and takes a full part in the multi-disciplinary discussions relating to the future of the baby. She is likely to have greater contact with the parents and should ensure that they have support and if necessary counselling to cope with the decisions which are made.

4. The parents do not have the right to insist that treatment ends for the child, or even that treatment is commenced. Their participation in the clinical decisions which are made is, however, essential and the midwife/neonatal nurse will have an important role to play in this.

5. There has recently been a spate of referrals of decisions relating to neonates to the court.

RE J (1990)[10]

The baby was a ward of court. In contrast with the case of Re C, the baby was not at the point of death. However, the prognosis was not good and although he was expected to survive a few years he was likely to be blind, deaf, unable to speak and have serious spastic quadriplegia. The judge made an order that he should be treated with antibiotics if he developed a chest infection, but if he were to stop breathing he should not receive artificial ventilation. The official solicitor on behalf of the child appealed against the order on the grounds that unless the situation was one of terminal illness, or it was certain that the child's life would be intolerable, the court was not justified in approving the withholding of life-saving treatment. The court held that the court can never sanction positive steps to terminate the life of a person. However, the court could direct that treatment, without which death would ensue, need not be given to prolong life, even though he was neither on the point of death nor dying. The Court had to undertake a balancing exercise in assessing the course to be adopted in the best interests of the child, looked at from his point of view and giving the fullest possible weight to his desire, if he were in a position to make a sound judgement, to survive, and taking into account the pain and suffering and quality of life which he would experience if life was prolonged, and the pain and suffering involved in the proposed treatment.

CAN THE COURT ORDER DOCTORS TO TREAT?

RE J (1992)[11]

J was born in January 1991 and suffered an accidental fall when he was 1 month old, with the result that he was profoundly handicapped both mentally and physically. He was severely microcephalic, his brain not having grown sufficiently following the injury. He also had severe cerebral palsy, cortical blindness and severe epilepsy. He was in general fed by a nasal gastric tube. Medical opinion was unanimous that J was unlikely to develop much beyond his present functioning, that that level might deteriorate and that his expectation of life, although uncertain, would be short. The paediatrician's report stated that given J's condition it would not be medically appropriate to intervene with intensive procedures such as artificial ventilation if he were to suffer a life-threatening event. The baby was in the care of foster parents with whom the local authority shared responsibility. The local authority applied to the court under s.100 of the Children Act 1989 to determine whether ventilation should be given to the child. The judge had regarded J's best interests as well as the interests of justice in preserving his life as both pointing in favour of the grant of an interim injunction requiring such treatment to take place. The mother supported the requirement that the hospital and doctors should be forced to put the baby on a life support machine.

Lord Donaldson, Master of the Rolls, stated that he could not at present conceive of any circumstances in which to require a medical practitioner, or Health Authority acting by a medical practitioner, to adopt a course of treatment which in the bona fide clinical judgement of the practitioner was contraindicated as not being in the patient's best interests, that would be other than abuse of power as directly or indirectly requiring the practitioner to act contrary to the fundamental duty he owed to his patient.

Lord Donaldson said that the order of the judge, ordering specific treatment to take place, was wholly inconsistent with the law as stated in Re J and in Re R and could not be justified on the basis of any known authority. It was also erroneous on two other substantial grounds:

a. its lack of certainty as to what was required of the Health Authority, and

b. its failure adequately to take account of the sad fact of life that Health Authorities might on occasion find that they had too few resources, either human or material or both, to treat all the patients whom they would like to treat in the way they would like to treat them. It was their duty to make choices. The court would have no knowledge of competing claims to a Health Authority's resources and was in no position to express any view on their deployment.

The Court of Appeal thus held that where a paediatrician caring for a severely handicapped baby considered that mechanical ventilation procedures would not be appropriate, the court would not grant an injunction requiring such treatment to take place.

The effect of the Court's decision to set aside the judge's ruling was to leave the Health Authority and its medical staff free, subject to consent not being withdrawn, to treat J in accordance with their best clinical judgement. That did not mean that in no circumstances should J be subjected to mechanical ventilation.

– The Court of Appeal affirmed the freedom of doctors to decide for themselves what is the best treatment.

– The Court showed its reluctance to interfere in medical practice.

RECENT CASES

The Portsmouth NHS Trust sought permission to decline to give invasive medical treatment to prolong the life of a profoundly disabled baby. Charlotte had been born at 26 weeks' gestation, weighing about 1 pound. She had chronic respiratory and kidney problems and brain damage that had left her blind, deaf and incapable of voluntary movement or response. She was capable of experiencing pain. The dispute was over what should be done should she deteriorate and required artificial ventilation. The unanimous medical advice was that to give such treatment would not be in her best interests. However, her parents' view was that such treatment should at least be instituted and that the treatment could best be prepared for by the carrying out of an elective tracheotomy. They believed that it was their duty to maintain life as they did not believe that C was yet ready to die. The court granted the application, that any further aggressive treatment, even if necessary to prolong life, was not in C's best interests. The doctors still had a duty of care to C. The order only authorised the doctors not to send C for artificial ventilation or similar aggressive treatment. The court asked the doctors to give further consideration to an elective tracheotomy on the basis of its possible contribution to her palliative care.

Subsequently, when she appeared to be making good progress, the parents asked the court to review its decision. The judge decided on 21 April 2005 that the decision should stand but it was subject to review.[12]

LETTING DIE AND HUMAN RIGHTS

In a recent case it was argued that letting a baby die was contrary to Article 3 of the European Convention on Human Rights (see Ch. 6 and Appendix 1). The court, however, held that it was not contrary to the human rights of a severely handicapped baby to allow him to die.[13] Where parents disagree with the medical decision that it is in the interests of a grossly handicapped child to let him die, the case should be referred to the court.

DISPUTE OVER TREATMENT[14]

David Glass, a boy of 13, was severely disabled with only a limited life span. The mother wished him to receive whatever medical treatment was necessary to prolong his life. Following an incident in which the hospital gave the child diamorphine against the mother's wishes, family members resuscitated the child and prevented him from dying. The relatives fought with staff over the treatment proposed, believing that the doctors had decided that the child should be allowed to die. There was a complete breakdown of trust between the family and the hospital. His mother, Ms Glass sought a declaration as to the course doctors in the hospital should take if the boy were admitted for emergency treatment and disagreements arose as to the treatment to be given to or withheld from the child. The judge refused the mother's application for judicial review and she appealed to the Court of Appeal.[15] The Court of Appeal refused to give an advance order over what should be decided at a future time, but stated that in the event of a dispute between parents and doctors there should be an application to court to determine what was in the best interests of the child. Subsequently, the relatives were convicted of assault.

Decision of the European Court of Human Rights in the Glass case[16]
However, Ms Glass won her appeal to the European Court of Human Rights. The Court held unanimously that the right to respect of private life, as guaranteed by Article 8 of the European Convention on Human Rights (ECHR), was breached where hospital authorities decided to override an applicant's objection to the treatment proposed for her severely disabled son in the absence of authorisation by a court. Ms Glass argued that both the decision to administer diamorphine to the boy against his mother's wishes and to place a DNR notice in his notes without her knowledge interfered with both their rights under Article 8. She also alleged that leaving the decision to involve the courts to the discretion of doctors was a wholly inadequate basis on which to ensure effective respect for the rights of vulnerable patients. The ECHR looked at the justifications for an interference with Article 8 rights under para. 8.2 and held that the interference was in accordance with the law and that there was a regulatory framework in the UK which was firmly based on the duty to preserve the life of a patient, save in exceptional circumstances. The same framework prioritised the requirement of parental consent and, save in emergency situation, required doctors to seek the intervention of the courts in the event of parental objection. The ECHR considered that the action taken by the hospital staff pursued a legitimate aim and was intended as a matter of clinical judgement to serve David's interests. It rejected any suggestion that it was the doctor's intention unilaterally to hasten David's death whether by administering diamorphine to him or placing a DNR notice in his case notes. The ECHR held that it had not been explained to its satisfaction why the NHS trust did not, at the time of the dispute over the diamorphine, seek the intervention of the court and held that the onus was on the trust to take the

initiative and to defuse the situation in anticipation of a further emergency. The ECHR noted that the trust was able to secure the presence of a police officer to oversee the negotiations with Ms Glass but, surprisingly, did not consider making a High Court application even though it would have been possible at short notice.

It therefore came to the unanimous conclusion that the decision of the authorities to override Ms Glass's objection to the proposed treatment in the absence of authorisation by a court resulted in a breach of Article 8. The ECHR awarded Ms Glass 10 000 Euros for non-pecuniary damage and 15 000 for costs and expenses.

The implications of the Glass case is that in the exceptional cases where there are disputes between parents and clinicians over the proposed treatment which cannot be resolved, it is essential that there should be an application to the court, thereby protecting the rights of the child, the parents and the practitioners.

GUIDANCE ON LETTING DIE

The Royal College of Paediatrics and Child Health has published guidelines on when it is appropriate to withhold or withdraw medical treatment.[17] The guidelines distinguish between the following clinical situations:

- The brain dead child

- The permanent vegetative state

- The 'no chance' situation

- The 'no purpose' situation

- The 'unbearable' situation.

In all these situations, the possibility of withholding or withdrawal of curative medical treatment might be considered. The guidance emphasises the importance of the fundamental principles of the duty of care and partnership of care and the respect for the rights of the child as set out in the United Nations Convention on the Rights of the Child.[18] The guidelines of the Royal College of Paediatrics and Child Health represent its interpretation of the law, but are not the law itself. Further advice has been published by the British Medical Association.[19] Reference could also be made to Chapter 6 in the BMA's book on consent and the rights of children and young people.[20]

AIREDALE NHS TRUST V. BLAND (1993)[21]

The House of Lords had to decide if it was lawful to permit artificial feeding to be discontinued in the case of a patient in a persistent vegetative state. The patient was a victim of the football stadium crush at Hillsborough and it was established that although he could breathe and digest food independently, he could not see, hear, taste, smell or communicate in any way and it appeared that there was no hope of recovery or improvement. The House of Lords decided that it would be in the best interests of the patient to discontinue the nasal gastric feed and he was later reported as having died. The House of Lords recommended that if any similar decisions were required to be made in the future, there should be application before the courts.

In two cases it was argued on behalf of women in a persistent vegetative state that it was contrary to their right to life under Article 2 of the European Convention on Human Rights for artificial feeding to be discontinued. The President of the Family Division, Dame Elizabeth Butler-Sloss, held that the withdrawal of life-sustaining medical treatment was not contrary to Article 2 of the Human Rights Convention and the right to life, where the patient was in a persistent vegetative state. The ruling was made on 25 October 2000 in cases involving Mrs M, aged 49 years, who suffered brain damage during an operation abroad in 1997 and was diagnosed as being in a persistent vegetative state (PVS) in October 1998 and Mrs H, 36, who fell ill in America as a result of pancreatitis at Christmas 1999.[22]

In 1994 the Select Committee of the House of Lords reported[23] that there should be no change in the law to permit euthanasia. The report's recommendations are shown in Box 9.5.

Box 9.5 Recommendations of Select Committee of House of Lords on Medical Ethics

1. No change in law to permit euthanasia.

2. Right of competent patient to refuse consent to any medical treatment is strongly endorsed.

3. Full reasons must be given if an individual refusal of treatment by a competent person is overruled by the courts.

4. Development and growth of palliative care services in hospitals and in the community strongly commended.

5. Withholding of treatment which would give relief is not justified, as long as the doctor acts in accordance with responsible medical practice with the objective of relieving pain or distress, and without the intention to kill.

6. Treatment-limiting decisions should be made jointly by all involved in the care of a patient.

7. Definition of PVS and the development of a code of practice relating to its management.

▶

8. Development and acceptance of the idea that, in certain circumstances, some treatments may be inappropriate may make it unnecessary to consider the withdrawal of hydration and nutrition.

9. Treatment-limiting decisions should not be determined by considerations of resource availability.

10. Rejection of euthanasia as an option for the individual entails a compelling social responsibility to care adequately for those who are elderly, dying or disabled.

11. Palliative care should be made more widely available.

12. Research into pain relief and symptom control should be adequately supported.

13. Training for healthcare professionals should prepare them for ethical responsibilities.

14. Long-term care of dependent people should have special regard to maintenance of individual dignity.

15. Proposal for the creation of a new judicial forum with power to make decisions about medical treatment for incompetent patients.

16. The creation of a new offence of mercy killing is not recommended.

17. Mandatory life sentence for murder should be abolished.

18. No change in the law on assisted suicide is recommended.

19. Commends the development of advance directives, but concludes that legislation for advance directives generally is unnecessary.

20. Code of practice on advance directives should be developed.

21. Do not favour the more widespread development of a system of proxy decision making.

An Assisted Dying Bill which would have legalised euthanasia in the UK failed to complete all stages before the 2005 dissolution of Parliament. A House of Lords report on the Assisted Dying Bill was published in 2005.[24] It is available on the internet.[25]

LIVING WILLS/ADVANCE REFUSAL OR DIRECTIVE

A mentally competent person can decide in advance that at a subsequent time he or she would not wish to have treatment. At present we do not have any statutory provision (i.e. Act of Parliament) recognising living wills, however when the Mental Capacity Act 2005 comes into force in April 2007 there will be statutory provision for living wills or advance directions. Before that time Living Wills are recognised at common law (i.e. judge-made law, or case law). This was stated by the House of Lords in the Tony Bland case.[21] Living wills, also known as advance refusals, or advance directions, are designed to convey the wishes of an adult, when mentally competent, to cover a future occasion when mental competence is lacking. The British Medical Association has published a Code of Practice for its members on advance statements about medical treatment.[20] It gives guidance on the law in relation to consent to medical treatment and advance statements, and advice on the drafting and contents of an advance statement. It emphasises that there must be no pressure on patients. It also gives guidance about determining the patient's capacity to make decisions. The responsibility for storing an advance directive is upon the individual but it is suggested that a copy should be given to the general practitioner. Finally, a checklist is provided for making an advance directive and this is shown in Box 9.6.

Box 9.6 BMA checklist for writing advance directive

An advance statement:

In drawing up an advance statement you must ensure, as a minimum, that the following information is included:

– Full name

– Address

– Name and address of general practitioner

– Whether advice was sought from health professionals

– Signature

– Date drafted and reviewed

▶
- Witness signature

- A clear statement of your wishes, either general or specific

- The name, address and telephone number of your nominated person, if you have one.

AN ADVANCE DIRECTIVE OVERRULED

In the case of The NHS Trust v. T[26] the High Court held that an interim declaration authorising the Trust to treat the patient by way of a blood transfusion in order to save or preserve her life or to avoid imminent risk of serious injury to her health was valid. The patient was self-harming and had signed an advance directive refusing blood transfusion. She did not want to continue to live and believed that her blood was evil and a transfusion of blood would result in contamination by her evil blood. An emergency situation had arisen because she had lost so much blood. The psychiatrist held that she was mentally disordered and did not have the capacity to refuse blood transfusions. At an earlier court hearing, an order was granted permitting blood to be given to her in an emergency. The NHS Trust subsequently sought a declaration over future treatment to be given to her including further blood transfusions.

In another case,[27] a father applied to court for a blood transfusion to be given to his daughter; the daughter had been a Muslim until the parents separated, at which point she became a Jehovah's Witness. The daughter signed an advance medical directive refusing a blood transfusion and stating that the directive could only be revoked in writing. The daughter suffered from a congenital heart condition, fell seriously ill, was hospitalised and needed a blood transfusion. The mother stated that the treatment should not proceed because the advance directive was in force. The father said that his daughter would, if not unconscious, have revoked the directive since she was now engaged to a Muslim man. The court held that the proposed treatment could be provided. It was not necessary for the advance direction to be in writing and it could therefore be revoked by word of mouth. The burden of proof was on the mother to show that the directive was still in force and any doubt had to be resolved in favour of the preservation of life. The daughter's change of faith had been a deliberate, implemented decision that was sufficient to effectively revoke and invalidate the directive.

MENTAL CAPACITY ACT AND ADVANCE DECISIONS

Sections 24, 25 and 26 of the Mental Capacity Act 2005 make provision for advance decisions. Section 24 defines and recognises the validity of an advance decision, which may be valid even though expressed in layman's terms. A withdrawal or subsequent alteration to an advance decision need not be in writing.

Under s.25, an advance decision does not affect the liability which a person may incur for carrying out or continuing a treatment in relation to the patient, unless it is valid and applicable to the treatment. An advance decision is not valid:

– if the patient has withdrawn it, when he had the capacity to do so

– has under a lasting power of attorney, created after the advance decision was made, conferred authority to give or refuse consent to the treatment covered by the advance decision or

– done anything else inconsistent with the advance decision.

An advance decision is not applicable to the treatment in question if the treatment is not specified in the advance decision or if any circumstances specified in the advance decision are absent or if there are reasonable grounds for believing that circumstances exist which the patient did not anticipate at the time the advance decision was created and which would have affected his decision. An advance decision is not applicable to life-sustaining treatment unless the patient has stated that it is to apply to that treatment even if his life is at risk. Such a statement must be in writing, signed by the patient or by a person on behalf of him, the signature is made or acknowledged by the patient in the presence of a witness, and the witness signs it or acknowledges his signature in the patient's presence.

The legal effect of a valid, relevant advance decision is that the decision has effect as if it had been made when the question of whether the treatment should be or not be given arises. A person does not incur liability for carrying out or continuing treatment unless at the time, he is satisfied that a valid, applicable advance decision exists. A person is not liable for withholding or withdrawing treatment, if he reasonably believes that a valid, applicable advance decision exists. The court can make a declaration on the validity and applicability of an advance decision and action can be taken to provide life-sustaining treatment or doing any act he reasonably believes to be necessary to prevent a serious deterioration in the patient's condition, while seeking a declaration from the court. This last point would cause considerable problems if there was uncertainty as to the validity or applicability of an advance decision drawn up by a Jehovah's Witness refusing blood, since while waiting for the court declaration on its validity or applicability, the only way of preventing a serious deterioration in the patient may be to give blood. If the court were then to declare the advance decision to be valid, the patient would already have been given the very treatment he or she was refusing.

'NOT FOR RESUSCITATION' INSTRUCTIONS

It follows from what has been said that a competent adult patient can request that there should be no resuscitation. This can be made either by means of an advance refusal or by refusing resuscitation when admitted for that particular course of treatment. For example, a man of 19 years[28] who was suffering from motor neurone disease sought a declaration from the court that it would be lawful to comply with his request to discontinue, 2 weeks from the date that he lost the ability to communicate, the artificial ventilation and the artificial nutrition and hydration which was being provided to him. He was able to communicate solely by the movement of one eyelid but this movement would shortly cease. The judge granted the declaration, holding that a patient's refusal to consent to medical treatment had to be observed where that patient was an adult of full capacity. In this case, the man was of full capacity and had clearly communicated his wishes. Such a decision was not contrary to the Human Rights Act 1998.

However, where the patient is mentally incompetent and has made no advance refusal, then the professional has a duty to take all reasonable care of the patient, and in certain cases this may involve providing resuscitation. If the prognosis is good, and there is no valid refusal of treatment by the patient, failure to resuscitate could in certain circumstances be a criminal act. Where, however, the clinician is of the view that the prognosis is extremely poor, a Not For Resuscitation (NFR) or Do Not (Attempt) Resuscitate(ion) (DN(A)R) instruction is valid.

Difficulties can arise, where such instructions are not given in writing by doctors to nursing staff or where nurses have not had an input into the decision making and are not aware of, or disagree with, the basis of the NFR/DN(A)R instruction. The views of relatives may be relevant to the decision and certainly any evidence they can give of the patient's wishes will be important, but the relatives do not have the right in law to give or withhold consent to resuscitation.

Burke case[29]

A patient suffering from cerebellar ataxia, a progressive degenerative condition, and who was of full capacity, challenged the General Medical Council guidelines on 'Withholding and Withdrawing Life-prolonging Treatments: Good Practice in Decision-making'. He argued that their guidelines were contrary to the Articles of the European Convention on Human Rights. He applied for judicial review and sought clarification as to the circumstances in which artificial nutrition and hydration (ANH) would be withdrawn. He did not want ANH to be withdrawn until he died of natural causes.

The judge granted a judicial review holding that once a patient had been admitted to an NHS hospital there was a duty of care to provide and go on providing treatment, whether the patient was competent or incompetent, or unconscious. This duty of care, which could not be transferred to anyone else, was to provide that treatment which was in the best interests of the patient. It was for the patient if competent to determine what was in his best interests. If the patient was incompetent and had left no binding and effective advance directive, then it was for the court to decide what was in his best interests. To withdraw ANH at any stage before the claimant finally lapsed into a coma would involve clear breaches of both Articles 8 and 3 because he would thereby be exposed to acute mental and physical suffering. The

GMC guidelines were therefore in error in emphasising the right of the claimant to refuse treatment, but not his right to require treatment.

The GMC appealed against this ruling and the Court of Appeal's reserved judgement was given on 29 July 2005.[30] The Court of Appeal held that doctors are not obliged to provide patients with treatment that they consider to be futile or harmful, even if the patient demands it. Autonomy and the right of self-determination do not entitle the patient to insist on receiving a particular medical treatment regardless of the nature of the treatment. However, where a competent patient says that he or she wants to be kept alive by the provision of food and water, doctors must agree to that. Not to do so would result in the doctor not merely being in breach of duty but guilty of murder. Mr Burke is considering an appeal to the House of Lords.

The implications of the Court of Appeal decision in the Burke case are significant for midwives, since the decision confirms the view that midwives cannot be compelled to provide care and treatment for a woman or child, which they consider is not in their best interests. For example if there are no clinical reasons for a caesarean section to be carried out, the woman could not, on the basis of the Burke decision, insist that one was provided.

PROFESSIONAL ADVICE AND GUIDANCE ON NFR

Prior to the implementation of the Human Rights Act 1998 the Department of Health drew attention to guidance which had been drawn up by the Resuscitation Council, the Royal College of Nursing and the British Medical Association.[31] This guidance was commended to NHS Trusts in September 2000 by the NHS Executive[32] in an NHS circular. By this circular, Chief Executives of NHS Trusts are required to ensure that appropriate resuscitation policies which respect patients' rights are in place, understood by all relevant staff, and accessible to those who need them and that such policies are subject to appropriate audit and monitoring arrangements. The action required to be taken by NHS trusts is shown in Box 9.7. The Commission for Health Improvement (CHI) (predecessor of CHAI) was asked by the Secretary of State to pay particular attention to resuscitation decision-making processes as part of its rolling programme of reviews of clinical governance arrangements put in place by NHS organisations. Guidance emphasises that there must be no blanket policies, each

---

Box 9.7 Resuscitation policies: Action to be taken by NHS trusts

- Patients' rights are central to decision making on resuscitation

- The trust has an agreed resuscitation policy in place which respects patients' rights

▶

▶

- The policy is published and readily available to those who may wish to consult it, including patients, families and carers

- Appropriate arrangements are in place for ensuring that all staff who may be involved in resuscitation decisions understand and implement the policy

- Appropriate supervision arrangements are in place to review the resuscitation decisions

- Induction and staff development programmes cover the resuscitation policy

- Clinical practice in this area is regularly audited

- Clinical audit outcomes are reported in the trust's annual clinical governance report

- A non-executive Director of the trust is given designated responsibility on behalf of the Trust Board to ensure that a resuscitation policy is agreed, implemented, and regularly reviewed within the clinical governance framework.

According to the guidelines, cardiopulmonary resuscitation (CPR) should only be withheld in the following four situations:

1. The mentally competent patient has refused treatment.

2. A valid living will covering such circumstances has been made by the patient.

3. Effective cardiopulmonary resuscitation (CPR) is unlikely to be successful.

4. Successful CPR is likely to be followed by a length and quality of life which would not be in the best interests of the patient to sustain.

individual patient must be assessed personally and policy cannot depend solely on the age of the patient.

The court considered the validity of a DNR instruction in the case of a seriously disabled boy with malformation of the brain and cerebral palsy who had developed severe epilepsy, was blind, incontinent, and had other major disabilities, who at the time of the hearing was 23 years old.[33] The court held that in the light of the medical evidence the overriding principle was that the boy's life was so afflicted as to be intolerable and that it was not in the best interests of the boy to be subjected to cardiopulmonary resuscitation in the event of his suffering a cardiac arrest. This view was supported by the boy's parents. The court held that the DNR instruction was justifiable since CPR was unlikely to be successful.

In 2001, the BMA, the Resuscitation Council (UK) and the RCN issued a joint statement.[34] It emphasised the importance of each health organisation having a resuscitation policy according to the principles set out in the guidance.

The laws relating to the removal, retention and storage of body parts and tissue are considered in Chapter 25.

CONCLUSIONS

The difference between giving a patient potassium chloride, as Dr Cox did, which is declared unlawful, and doctors being permitted lawfully to disconnect the feeding tube of a patient such as Tony Bland, is not always easy to understand. In fact, to some philosophers there is no moral difference.

However, the House of Lords in enabling the tube-feeding to be discontinued allowed the natural situation of the patient to take over. In contrast, in the Cox case, the administration of the drug was an unlawful act.

Failure to act, or an omission, could be evidence of negligence or a crime when there is a recognised legal duty to act. In the Bland case, the House of Lords considered that, given the best interests of the patient, the duty to continue active treatment had ended. Any such decisions should be brought before the court to ensure that the best interests of the patient are identified and that the patient is represented. The Burke case has established that health professionals cannot be compelled to act contrary to what they think is in the best interests of the patient. Nor however could they deny a competent patient artificial nutrition and hydration, if that is the wish of the patient.

QUESTIONS AND EXERCISES

1. In which circumstances do you consider that it should be lawful to let a baby die?

2. Do you consider that a lack of resources could be a justifiable reason for letting a baby die?

3. An abortion of a fetus suffering from congenital disabilities results in a live birth. Do you consider that there should be a duty to keep that baby alive? What is the law? (Refer also to Ch. 26.)

4. A woman wishes to draw up an advanced refusal of clinical interventions during her pregnancy and labour. What should such a statement contain to be lawfully valid?

5. Women who have been injured while pregnant have been kept on life support systems in order that the baby can survive. Do you consider that this practice raises any legal issues?

References

1 R (Pretty) v. Director of Public Prosecutions and another, Medical Ethics Alliance and others, interveners. Times Law Report, 23 October 2001.

2 2. R (on the application of Pretty) v. DPP, Secretary of State for the Home Department intervening. Times Law Report, 5 December 2001 [2001] UKHL 61; [2001] 3 WLR 1598.

3 Pretty v UK ECHR Current Law 2002; 380 June 2346/02 [2002] 2 FLR 45.

4 R v. Arthur. The Times, 6 November 1981.

5 R v. Cox. The Times, 22 September 1992; [1992] 12 BMLR 38.

6 R. v. Adams (Bodkin) Crim Law Rev 1957:365; Bedford S. The best we can do. Harmondsworth: Penguin; 1961.

7 Wilkins E. Dying woman granted wish for dignified death. The Times, 29 October 1997.

8 Re B (a minor) (wardship; medical treatment) [1981] 1 WLR 1421.

9 Re C (a minor) (wardship; medical treatment) [1989] 2 All ER 782.

10 Re J (a minor) (wardship; medical treatment) [1990] 3 All ER 930.

11 Re J. Times Law Report, 12 June 1992.

12 News item. Parents lose in sick baby case. The Times, 22 April 2005.

13 A National Health Service Trust v. D. Times Law Report, 19 July 2000; [2000] Lloyd's Rep Med 411.

14 R. v. Portsmouth Hospitals NHS Trust *ex parte* Glass [1999] 2 FLR 905; [1999] Lloyd's Rep Med 367.

15 R v. Portsmouth Hospitals NHS Trust *ex parte* Glass [1999] 50 BMLR 269.

16 Glass v. United Kingdom. The Times Law Report, 11 March 2004. ECHR; Lloyd's Rep Med [2004] 76.

17 Royal College of Paediatrics and Child Health. Withholding or withdrawing life saving treatment in children, 2nd edn. London: RCPCH; 2004.

18 United Nations. Convention on the Rights of the Child. UN; 1989.

19 British Medical Association. Withholding and withdrawing life-prolonging medical treatment, 2nd edn. London: BMJ Books; 2000.

20 British Medical Association. Advance Statements about medical treatment: Code of Practice. BMA; 1995.

21 Airedale NHS Trust v. Bland House of Lords [1993] 1 All ER 821.

22 Gibb F. Rights Act does not bar mercy killing. The Times, 26 October 2000; NHS Trust A v. Mrs M and NHS Trust B v. Mrs H Family Division [2001] Lloyd's Rep Med 27.

23 Report of the Select Committee on Medical Ethics: House of Lords Session 1993–4. London: HMSO.

24 Assisted Dying for the Terminally Ill Bill (HL) Report, Select Committee Session 2004–5 HL Paper 86-1.

25 The United Kingdom Parliament. Online. Available: www.parliament.uk

26 The NHS Trust v. Ms T. Lloyd's Rep Med [2004] 433.

27 HE v. A Hospital NHS Trust [2003] EWHC 1017, [2003] 2 FLR 408.

28 Re AK (adult patient) (medical treatment: consent) [2001] 1 FLR 129.

29 R. (on the application of Burke) v. General Medical Council and Disability Rights Commission and the Official Solicitor to the Supreme Court [2004] EWHC 1879; [2004] Lloyd's Rep Med 451.

30 R. (on the application for Burke) v. General Medical Council [2005] EWCA Civ 1003 CA, 28 July 2005.

31 British Medical Association, Resuscitation Council (UK) and the Royal College of Nursing, 1999. Decisions relating to cardiopulmonary resuscitation. London: BMA; updated 2001.

32 NHS Executive. Resuscitation Policy. HSC 2000/028.

33 Re R (adult: medical treatment) [1996] 31 BMLR 127.

34 British Medical Association, Resuscitation Council (UK) and the Royal College of Nursing. Decisions relating to cardiopulmonary resuscitation: A joint statement from the BMA, Resuscitation Council (UK) and the RCN. London: BMA; 2001.

Chapter 10
CONFIDENTIALITY AND ACCESS TO RECORDS

This chapter deals with two aspects of record keeping: the duty to maintain the confidentiality of information obtained by and about the client; and the right of the client to access information held about her. They are both regulated by the Data Protection Act 1998 and statutory instruments made under that Act. Guidance is provided by the NMC for its registered practitioners.[1]

DATA PROTECTION LEGISLATION

The European Directive on Data Protection[2] was implemented in this country by the Data Protection Act 1998. Member states were required to comply with its provisions by 24 October 1998, although the UK did not meet this target. Under the legislation, members had to establish a set of principles with which users of personal information must comply. The legislation also gives individuals the right to gain access to information held about them and provides for a supervisory authority to oversee and enforce the law. NHS guidance on the Act was provided by a circular in March 2000[3] and the NHS Information Authority action plan for the NHS is available on its website to ensure the processing of personal data within the organisation is in compliance with the Act.[4]

The Data Protection Act 1998 made significant changes to the 1984 Act. The most important change is that the 1998 Act applies to certain manual records (if they form part of a relevant filing system) as well as to computerised records. This was defined in the case of Durant v. Financial Services Authority[5] as a system in which files are structured in such a way as to clearly indicate whether specific information capable of amounting to personal data is included therein and individual files can be readily accessed. Most health records would therefore come under Data Protection legislation provisions. A possible exception to manual records not coming under Data Protection provisions are the supervision records kept by the supervisor of records in which specific patients are named. These would not come under the provisions of the Data Protection Act according to that definition of a relevant filing system. The Information Commissioner has published a statement and commentary on the case.[6] In 2001, an Information Commissioner was appointed to fulfil duties under both the Freedom of Information Act 2000 (see below) and the Data Protection Act 1998.

HUMAN RIGHTS

The Data Protection Act 1998 must, after 2 October 2000, be read in conjunction with the Human Rights Act 1998 (see Ch. 6 and Appendix 1), since Article 8 of the European Convention on Human Rights, which is set out in Schedule 1 of the Act, recognises an individual's right to private and family life, subject to specific qualifications. The right to respect for private life is to be balanced against Article 10 and the right to freedom of expression (see Ch. 6).

DATA PROTECTION ACT 1998

The main provisions of the Act are shown in Box 10.1.

Box 10.1 Data Protection Act 1998

- Part 1 Preliminary: basic interpretative provisions; sensitive personal data; the special purposes; data protection principles; application of Act; Commissioner and Tribunal

- Part 2 Rights of data subjects and others:

  - Rights of access

  - Rights to prevent processing likely to cause damage or distress

  - Rights to prevent processing for direct marketing

  - Rights in relation to automated decision-taking

  - Compensation for failure to comply with certain requirements

  - Rectification, blocking, erasure and destruction

- Part 3 Notification to the Data Controller: duty to notify; register of notifications; offences; preliminary assessment by Commissioner; power to make provision for appointment of data protection supervisors; duty of certain data controllers to make certain information available; functions of Commissioner in relation to making of notification regulations; fees regulations.

- Part 4 Exemptions:

  - National security

  - Crime and taxation

- Health, education and social work

- Regulatory activity

- Journalism, literature and art

- Research, history and statistics

- Information available to the public by or under enactment

- Disclosure required by law or made in connection with legal proceedings

- Domestic purposes

- Powers to make further exemptions by order

– Part 5 Enforcement

– Part 6 Miscellaneous and general: Functions of the Commissioner

– Schedule 1 Data protection principles

– Schedule 2 Conditions for processing any personal data

– Schedule 3 Conditions for processing sensitive personal data

– Schedule 4 Cases where the 8th principle does not apply

– Schedule 5 Data Protection Commissioner and Data Protection Tribunal

– Schedule 6 Appeal proceedings

– Schedule 7 Miscellaneous exemptions

– Schedule 8 Transitional relief

– Schedule 9 Powers of entry and inspection

– Schedule 10 Assistance under s.53

– Schedule 11 Educational records

– Schedule 12 Accessible public records

– Schedule 13 Modifications of Act having effect pre 24 October 2007.

TERMINOLOGY

The following are definitions of terms used in the Data Protection Act 1998.

– The 'data subject' is 'the individual who is the subject of personal data'. Under the 1998 provisions, the law applies only to living people and if the information is anonymous, then the person will not be considered to be identifiable, unless it is possible to link together separate items of information in order to identify an individual. If that is possible, the Act would then apply.

– 'Processing' under the 1998 Act includes any operation involving personal data including the holding of the information.

– The term 'data user' (from the 1984 Act) is replaced by the term 'controller' and is the person who determines the purposes for which and the manner in which any personal data are to be processed.

– 'Computer bureaux' is replaced by 'processor'.

– The 'Data Protection Registrar', who is the national officer responsible for the oversight of the implementation of the law, is now to be known as the Commissioner.

DATA PROTECTION PRINCIPLES

The 1998 Act slightly amends the Data Protection Principles and the new wording is shown in Box 10.2.

Box 10.2 Data Protection Principles 1998 Schedule 1 Part 1

1. Personal data shall be processed fairly and lawfully and, in particular, shall not be processed unless:

   (a) at least one of the conditions in Schedule 2 is met; and

   (b) in the case of sensitive personal data, at least one of the conditions in Schedule 3 is also met.

2. Personal data shall be obtained only for one or more specified and lawful purposes, and shall not be further processed in any manner incompatible with that purpose or those purposes.

3. Personal data shall be adequate, relevant and not excessive in relation to the purpose or purposes for which they are processed.

▶

---

4. Personal data shall be accurate and, where necessary, kept up-to-date.

5. Personal data processed for any purpose or purposes shall not be kept for longer that is necessary for that purpose(s).

6. Personal data shall be processed in accordance with the rights of data subjects under this Act.

7. Appropriate technical and organisational measures shall be taken against unauthorised or unlawful processing of personal data and against accidental loss or destruction of, or damage to, personal data.

8. Personal data shall not be transferred to a country or territory outside the European Economic Area unless that country or territory ensures an adequate level of protection for the rights and freedoms of data subjects in relation to the processing of personal data.

Interpretation of these principles is provided in Part 2 of Schedule 1 of the 1998 Act.

Principle 1 refers to Schedule 2 conditions and these include:

– The consent of the data subject

– The processing is necessary:

  - for the performance of a contract to which the data subject is a party

  - for taking steps, at the request of the data subject, to enter a contract

– The processing is necessary for compliance with a legal obligation of the data subject

– The processing is necessary to protect the vital interests of the data subject

– The processing is necessary:

  - for the administration of justice

  - for the exercise of functions conferred by any enactment

  - for the exercise of a function of the Crown, Minister or government department, or

  - for the exercise of other functions of a public nature

– The processing is necessary to meet the legitimate interests of the data controller or a third party.

Clearly patient records are covered by several of these conditions, only one of which is needed to legitimise the processing.

SENSITIVE PERSONAL DATA

Sensitive personal data are defined in s.2 (see Box 10.3).

Box 10.3 Section 2 Data Protection Act 1998

Sensitive personal data means personal data consisting of information as to:

– The racial or ethnic origin of the data subject

– His political opinions

– His religious beliefs or other beliefs of a similar nature

– Whether he is a member of a Trade Union

– His physical or mental health or condition

– His sexual life

– The (alleged) commission of any offence by him, or

– Any proceedings for any (alleged) offence, disposal of such or sentence.

Records relating to physical or mental health come within the definition of sensitive personal data and Schedule 3, conditions for disclosure of such information, is shown in Box 10.4.

Box 10.4 Schedule 3 Conditions for disclosure of sensitive personal data

1. The data subject has given his explicit consent to the processing of personal data.

2. (1) The processing is necessary for the purposes of exercising or performing any right or obligation which is conferred or imposed on the data controller in connection with employment.

▶

(2) The Secretary of State may exclude the application of sub-para. 1 in such cases as may be specified, or specify further conditions for satisfaction.

3. The processing is necessary:

   (a) to protect the vital interests of the data subject or another person, in a case where:

      i. consent cannot be given by or on behalf of the data subject, or

      ii. the data controller cannot reasonably be expected to obtain the consent of the data subject, or

   (b) in order to protect the vital interests of another person, in a case where consent by or on behalf of the data subject has been unreasonably withheld.

4. The processing:

   (a) is carried out in the course of its legitimate activities by any body or association which:

      i. is not established or conducted for profit, and

      ii. exists for political, philosophical, religious or trade union purposes

   (b) is carried out with appropriate safeguards for the rights and freedoms of the data subject

   (c) relates only to individuals who either are members of the body or association or have regular contact with it in connection with its purposes, and

   (d) does not involve disclosure of the personal data to a third party without the consent of the data subject.

5. The information contained in the personal data has been made public as a result of steps deliberately taken by the data subject.

6. The processing:

   (a) is necessary for the purpose of, or in connection with, any legal proceedings (including prospective legal proceedings)

   (b) is necessary for the purpose of obtaining legal advice, or

(c) is otherwise necessary for the purposes of establishing, exercising or defending legal rights.

7. (1) The processing is necessary:

    (a) for the administration of justice

    (b) for the exercise of any functions conferred on any person by or under an enactment, or

    (c) for the exercise of any functions of the Crown, Minister of the Crown or a government department

    (2) The Secretary of State may by order:

    (a) exclude the application of sub-para. 1 in such cases as may be specified, or

    (b) provide that, in such cases as may be specified, the condition in sub-para. 1 is not to be regarded as satisfied unless such further conditions as may be specified in the order are also satisfied.

8. (1) The processing is for medical purposes and is undertaken by:

    (a) a health professional, or

    (b) a person who in the circumstances owes a duty of confidentiality which is equivalent to that which would arise if that person were a health professional.

    (2) In this paragraph, 'medical purposes' includes the purposes of preventative medicine, medical diagnosis, medical research, the provision of care and treatment and the management of healthcare services.

9. (1) The processing:

    (a) is of sensitive personal data consisting of information as to racial or ethnic origin.

    (b) is necessary for the purpose of identifying or keeping under review the existence or absence of equality of opportunity or treatment between persons of different racial or ethnic origins, with a view to enabling such equality to be promoted or maintained, and

(c) is c arried out with appropriate safeguards for the rights and freedoms of data subjects.

(2) The Secretary of State may by order specify circumstances in which processing falling within sub-paras 1(a) and 1(b) is, or is not, to be taken for the purposes of sub-para. 1(c) to be carried out with appropriate safeguards for the rights and freedoms of data subjects.

10. The personal data are processed in circumstances specified in an order made by the Secretary of State for the purposes of this paragraph.

CONSENT

Schedule 2 requires the consent of the data subject or one of the other conditions to be satisfied for processing to be carried on.

Schedule 3 requires the explicit consent of the data subject and the fact that processing is necessary to protect the data subject's vital interests, where consent cannot be given by or on behalf of the data subject or the data controller cannot be reasonably expected to obtain the consent of the data subject. This latter situation would obviously cover records relating to the mentally incapacitated adult and children. Another condition of Schedule 3 is that the processing is necessary for medical purposes (defined as including the purposes of preventative medicine, medical diagnosis, medical research, the provision of care and treatment and the management of healthcare services) and is undertaken by a health professional or a person who owes a duty of confidentiality which is equivalent to that which would arise if that person were a health professional. Satisfaction of this condition would obviate the need to obtain the explicit consent of every patient, in order for their health records to be processed.

RIGHTS OF THE DATA SUBJECT

The rights of the individual under the Data Protection Act 1998 are shown in Box 10.5.

Box 10.5 Rights of the data subject under the 1998 Act

1. Right of subject access (ss.7 to 9)

2. Right to prevent processing likely to cause damage or distress (s.10)

▶

3. Right to prevent processing for the purposes of direct marketing (s.11)

4. Right in relation to automated decision-taking (s.12)

5. Right to take action for compensation if the individual suffers damage by any contravention of the Act by the data controller (s.13)

6. Right to take action to rectify, block, erase or destroy inaccurate data (s.14)

7. Right to make a request to the Commissioner for an assessment to be made as to whether any provision of the Act has been contravened (s.42).

INFORMATION COMMISSIONER

The Information Commissioner has the responsibility for promoting good practice and observance of the laws, providing an information service and encouraging the development of Codes of Practice. He has considerable powers of enforcement under Parts 3 and 5 of the Act. These include the power to serve enforcement notices and powers of entry and inspection. Information is available from the Commissioner's office free of charge.[7] An explanatory guide to the new legislation was issued in 1998 and has been updated to provide legal guidance[8] on the Act.

Offences under the Act are shown in Box 10.6.

Box 10.6 Offences under the Data Protection Act 1998

1. Offences relating to failure to notify the Commissioner or comply with his requests

2. Unlawfully obtaining personal data

3. Unlawful selling of personal data

4. Forcing a person to compel access

5. Unlawful disclosure of information by the commissioner/staff or agent.

GUIDANCE FROM THE NHS EXECUTIVE

The NHS Executive has published guidelines on the protection and use of patient information to support the implementation of the Data Protection Act.[9] It states that a Working Group at the Department of Health is developing national guidance to assist NHS bodies and local authorities on the principles and practical issues involved in sharing client/patient records for service delivery and of using such aggregated data for planning, commissioning, managing and monitoring. The Department of Health Code of Practice on Confidentiality was published in October 2003 (see below) and is available from the Department of Health's confidentiality website.[10]

CALDICOTT GUARDIANS

The Government appointed a Committee chaired by Dame Fiona Caldicott to make recommendations on how to improve the way in which the NHS managed patient confidentiality. It reported in December 1997 and included in its recommendations the need to raise awareness of confidentiality requirements, and specifically recommended the establishment of a network of Caldicott Guardians of patient information throughout the NHS. Subsequently a Steering Group was set up to oversee the implementation of the Report's recommendations. Following a consultation period the NHS Executive issued a circular on the establishment of Caldicott Guardians,[11] giving advice on the appointment of the Guardians, the programme of work for the first year for improving the way each organisation handles confidential patient information, and identifying the resources, training and other support for the Guardians.

THE GUARDIAN

Each Health Authority, Special Health Authority, NHS trust and primary care group was required to appoint a Caldicott Guardian by 31 March 1999. Ideally, the Guardian should be at Board level, be a senior health professional and have responsibility for promoting clinical governance within the organisation. The name and address of the Guardian is to be notified to the NHS Executive.[12] The Guardian is expected to liaise closely with others involved in patient information such as IM&T security officers and Data Protection Officers. In making the appointment and defining the role of the Guardian, the duties which are not to be delegated should be clarified. Guardians are responsible for agreeing and reviewing internal protocols governing the protection and use of patient-identifiable information by the staff of their organisation and must be satisfied that these proposals address the requirements for national guidance/policy and law. The operation of these policies must also be monitored. Policies for inter-agency disclosure of patient information must also be agreed and reviewed, to facilitate cross-boundary working.

In 2000, the Department of Health issued guidance to Caldicott Guardians on the method by which information flows should be reviewed in NHS organisations.[13] It provided a manual which covers the mapping of information flows, the prioritising of mapped flows for review purposes and a rolling programme of review. The specific areas which are considered include commissioning flows, clinical audit and coding, medical records and patient care services.

If issues on confidentiality arise, a healthcare practitioner can raise these with the Caldicott Guardian, who in turn can access the legal advisers to the trust.

The Department of Health is currently working on policies for Caldicott Guardians in local authorities.[14]

INFORMATION GOVERNANCE

The Caldicott principles are part of a wider strategy for information governance. This includes:

– the Data Protection Act 1998

– the Freedom of Information Act 2000

– The Confidentiality Code of Practice

– Information Security Management BS7799

– Records Management (see Ch. 15).

The Information Governance has four fundamental aims:

1. To support the provision of high quality care by promoting effective and appropriate use of information.

2. To encourage responsible staff to work closely together, preventing duplication of effort and enabling more efficient use of resources.

3. To develop support arrangements and provide staff with appropriate tools and support to enable them to discharge their responsibilities to consistently high standards.

4. To enable organisations to understand their own performance and manage improvement in a systematic and effective way.

An NHS Information Quality Assurance Consultation began in March 2004 to develop a national strategy for improving the quality of information in the NHS (see Ch. 15).

The NHS National Programme for Information Technology (NPfIT) aims to connect over 30 000 GPs in England to almost 300 hospitals and give patients access to their personal health and care information. An information governance toolkit is available from the NPfIT (see Ch. 15 on Electronic health records).

A social care information governance project (SCIG) has also been set up by the Department of Health in conjunction with the Association of Directors of Social Services.[15]

THE HEALTH AND SOCIAL CARE ACT 2001

Sections 60 and 61 of the Health and Social Care Act 2001 enable the Secretary of State to draw up regulations for the control of patient information in the interests of improving patient care or in the public interest, and to establish a Patient Information Advisory Group. Powers exercised under this Section must be compatible with the Articles of the European Convention on Human Rights. Regulations for the establishment of the Patient Information Advisory Group were published in August 2001.[16] The Advisory Group is to have between 12 and 20 members, with one of them chosen by the Secretary of State as Chairman. The Group is to meet at least four times a year.

SOURCES OF THE DUTY OF CONFIDENTIALITY

The duty to respect confidentiality arises from a variety of sources which are set out in Box 10.7.[17] Should the health professional be in breach of the duty of confidentiality, then the patient could bring an action in the civil courts and have the usual remedies for breach of trust.

Box 10.7 Sources of the obligation to respect the confidentiality of patient information

(a) Duty set out in clause 5 of the NMC Code of Professional Conduct: standards for conduct, performance and ethics[17]

(b) Duty in the contract of employment

(c) Duty as part of the duty of care owed to the patient in the law of negligence

(d) Duty set out in specific statutes, especially the Data Protection Act 1998 and Human Rights Act 1998

(e) Duty as part of the trust obligation between health professional and patient.

Duty set out in clause 5 of the NMC Code of Professional Conduct: standards for conduct, performance and ethics.

As a registered nurse or midwife, you must protect confidential information:

You must treat information about patients and clients as confidential and use it only for the purposes for which it was given. As it is impractical to obtain consent every time you need to share information with others, you should ensure that patients and clients understand that some information may be made available to other members of the team involved in the delivery of care. You must guard against breaches of confidentiality by protecting information from improper disclosure at all times.

DUTY IN THE CONTRACT OF EMPLOYMENT

Employed midwives also have a duty implied in the contract of employment that they will respect the confidentiality of information which they hear of in the course of their employment. This duty would be implied by the courts and failure to respect this duty could lead to disciplinary action being taken by the employer, with the ultimate sanction being dismissal.

DUTY AS PART OF THE DUTY OF CARE OWED TO THE PATIENT IN THE LAW OF NEGLIGENCE

There is some evidence to suggest that the duty of care owed to the patient may include a duty to respect the confidentiality of information which is learnt about the patient.[18]

DUTY SET OUT IN SPECIFIC STATUTES, ESPECIALLY THE DATA PROTECTION ACT 1998 AND HUMAN RIGHTS ACT 1998

It is clear from the principles of the Data Protection Act 1998 set out above that strict rules apply to the security of information from which a person can be identified. Other legislation also created a statutory obligation to respect confidentiality. One of the strictest rules on disclosure was the Human Fertilisation and Embryology Act 1990, which proved to be so exacting that it was necessary to pass an amending Act in 1992 (see Ch. 27).

DUTY AS PART OF THE TRUST OBLIGATION BETWEEN HEALTH PROFESSIONAL AND PATIENT

The law would recognise that a relationship of trust is created between patient and health professional, which would give the right of action to the patient if there is evidence that the health professional intends to breach confidentiality without consent or other lawful justification. Those who have given information in the expectation that its confidentiality will be respected can enforce this obligation.[19]

EXCEPTIONS TO THE DUTY OF CONFIDENTIALITY

The main exceptions to the duty of confidentiality are shown in Box 10.8.

Box 10.8 Exceptions to the duty of confidentiality

(a) Consent of the client

(b) Information to the Supervisor

(c) Information given to other professionals in the interests of the client

(d) Order from the Court before or during legal proceedings

(e) Statutory justification, e.g.

  – Notification of registration of births and stillbirths

  – Infectious Disease Regulations

  – Police and Criminal Evidence Act

(f) Public interest.

CONSENT OF THE CLIENT

The duty of confidentiality exists to protect the client and the client can therefore agree to any disclosure. Such an agreement would be a defence against any action for breach.

Clause 5.2 of the NMC Code of Professional Conduct: standards for conduct, performance and ethics[17] recognises this defence:

You should seek patients' and clients' wishes regarding the sharing of information with their family and others. When a patient or client is considered incapable of giving permission, you should consult relevant colleagues.

Care must however be taken to ensure that the client is fully aware of the implications of the consent and has the mental competence to give a valid consent.

This might be of importance if it were planned to video a delivery. If this is not at the client's instigation, e.g. where a television company wishes to televise or a recording is suggested as a training document, written consent should be obtained from the client and her capacity to consent should be certified by an appropriate professional not involved in the filming. In addition, there should be a clear understanding as to what rights of distribution there are over any material obtained and the right, if any, of the client to withhold permission at a later stage.

The consent of the client is also important where the press are anxious to obtain details of the childbirth of a client who is a well-known person, or a multiple pregnancy which would attract media interest. The client is entitled to anonymity if she so wishes and only with her consent should any information be given to the press. Agreement on this could be obtained before the admission, but the client would of course be entitled to withdraw that consent at any time.

DISCLOSURE TO THE SUPERVISOR

Midwives are the only professionals who are required by statute to have a Supervisor. As can be seen from Chapter 3, the relationship between Supervisor and midwife should be a close one with the midwife informing the Supervisor immediately she is concerned about the care of the mother. If the mother gives confidential information to the midwife, it should be made clear to the mother that the midwife must inform her Supervisor of any relevant information likely to affect her practice and the safety of the mother, and advise the mother that this disclosure would be made. The midwife is obliged under Rule 10[20] to give her Supervisor, the Local Supervising Authority and the Council every reasonable facility to monitor her standards and methods of practice and to inspect her records, her equipment and any premises. She could not refuse this inspection of records on grounds of a breach of confidentiality. The NMC in its guidance on rule 12 of the Midwives Rules advises that the midwife should have 24-hour access to a Supervisor of Midwives for advice and support.

The NMC advice clearly envisages the discussion of individual cases between midwife and Supervisor, and would be a defence against any allegation of breach of client confidentiality. The Supervisor of Midwives would clearly be bound to respect the duty of confidentiality in respect of information which she learnt from the midwife, unless one of the recognised lawful exceptions discussed here existed. The NMC guidance on Rule 12[20] notes that while the record of the annual statutory supervision meeting between midwife and Supervisor is confidential, it may be required to be disclosed as part of an LSA or NMC investigation or by order of the court.

INFORMATION TO OTHER PROFESSIONALS IN THE INTERESTS OF THE CLIENT

Clearly the midwife works as part of a multi-disciplinary team and therefore she must ensure that relevant information is given to those who are also caring for the mother and baby. This is recognised by the NMC in Para. 5.1 of the Code of Professional Conduct cited above. Sharing with the multi-disciplinary team would in particular include the General Practitioner if s/he is involved in the care of the mother, and also the obstetric team. The definition of 'relevant' might cause some difficulties. The midwife should be able justify any disclosure she makes in the interests of the mother and baby. Her records should reflect the basis of her decision where this is likely to be challenged.

In one case, the Court of Appeal accepted that a County Council could disclose confidential information about an adult medical patient to his mother, as it was necessary for her to be involved in his care.[21]

Confidential information used for research purposes is considered in Chapter 31. Midwives should ensure that the interests of the client are protected in any use of patient records, whether the stated purpose is for audit or research or for the clinical care of the individual client.

COURT ORDER BEFORE OR DURING LEGAL PROCEEDINGS

If litigation is contemplated, the court has the right to make an order requiring disclosure of information relevant to an issue arising in a case.

Before litigation

Under s.33 of the Supreme Court Act 1981, disclosure can be ordered against a person likely to be a party in a personal injury case before the writ is issued. Disclosure can be ordered to the applicant's legal advisers and any medical or other professional advisers of the applicants, or, if the applicant has no legal advisers, to any medical or other professional adviser of the applicant.

Thus if a client is suing in relation to an incident during the confinement, the records of the midwife could be ordered to be disclosed to the legal advisers or professional advisers of the client. Since the reforms of civil procedure as a result of the Woolf recommendations (see Ch. 14), a pre-action protocol exists which parties in civil litigation must follow and this enables early disclosure of information to be required.

After litigation has commenced

Under s.34 of the Supreme Court Act 1981 disclosure can be ordered against a person who is not likely to be a party to a case, after the writ has been issued, if that person has information likely to be relevant.

This could cover a situation where the client who was pregnant and involved in a road traffic accident was suing the driver of the vehicle which caused the accident and he wished to have access to information about the client held by the midwife relating to the pregnancy. If, for example, there was a fear that the baby was harmed as a result of the road accident this could affect both liability and quantum (see Congenital Disabilities (Civil Liability) Act 1976, in Ch. 17).

Disclosure can also be ordered during any court proceedings where powers of subpoena exist to compel witnesses to attend court and bring relevant documents with them. The midwife has no defence of privileged information on the grounds that it was given to her in confidence if she is ordered by the judge to disclose the information. A refusal could be punished by imprisonment for contempt of court.

The reforms in civil court procedures have led to the adoption of a pre-action protocol which requires the parties to disclose information which is relevant to the dispute at an early stage and sanctions can be imposed for failure to conform to the protocol (see Ch. 14).

The only limitations on the powers of the court to order disclosure of information are:

– where national security is at stake and a Minister of the Crown has signed a certificate to that effect (the Scott enquiry recommended that this should not be done in criminal proceedings) and

– where the communication is one between lawyer and client for the purposes of litigation and is protected by the principle of legal professional privilege. (This privilege is destroyed if there is any fraud.)[22]

OTHER INVESTIGATIONS

In a case in 2001[23] a GP relied upon Article 8 of the European Convention on Human Rights in refusing to permit a health authority to access child protection records which the HA wished to see in connection with disciplinary investigations of the GP. The court permitted disclosure on the express condition that the confidentiality of the documents was preserved and that there would be effective and adequate safeguards of the patient's confidentiality and anonymity. The Court of Appeal dismissed the appeal (see p. 194 below).

In the case of Junia Woolgar,[24] the Court of Appeal held that a registered nurse and matron could not prevent the police disclosing to the UKCC details of their investigations into her activities as matron of a nursing home. Following their investigations, the police did not charge her.

The Department of Health clarified the situation on the disclosure of patient identifiable information to Members of Parliament to assist MP investigations. A statement was given during a House of Commons adjournment debate on 27 April 2004 on NHS Trusts and the Data Protection Act 1998.

STATUTORY JUSTIFICATION

Certain Acts of Parliament require the midwife to pass on specified information and therefore would be a defence against an action for breach of confidentiality. In some situations, the midwife would face legal proceedings herself if she failed to make the appropriate notifications.

The duty in relation to the notification of births and stillbirths is discussed in Chapter 25 and the duty in relation to the notification of infectious diseases can be found in Chapter 29.

PUBLIC INTEREST

This is the most difficult area and the advice provided in the NMC Code of Professional Conduct is of assistance.

If you are required to disclose information outside the team that will have personal consequences for patients and clients, you must obtain their consent. If the patient or client withholds consent, or if consent cannot be obtained for whatever reason, disclosures may be made only where:

– *They can be justified in the public interest (usually where disclosure is essential to protect the patient or client or someone else from the risk of significant harm)*

– *They are required by law or by order of a court*

Where there is an issue of child protection, you must act at all times in accordance with national and local policies.

There have been several court cases which, though not involving midwives, are relevant to the issue of public interest.

In W. v. Egdell,[25] a detained psychiatric patient requested an independent report from a psychiatrist on his condition for the purposes of his application for discharge from the Section. The report was not favourable to him, and the doctor, against the wishes of the patient, sent a copy of the report to the Medical Director of the hospital and the Home Office. The patient lost his action against the doctor for breach of the duty of confidentiality since the doctor had a public duty to disclose this information.

In this case, the patient had been convicted of killing five people 10 years before and the possible dangers to the public from a premature release from detention were therefore clear. The case does not assist other than in providing a general statement as to when the public interest in the disclosure of information overrides the public interest in respecting the duty of confidentiality to an individual patient.

In X v. Y[26] the courts granted an injunction against a newspaper, preventing it publishing the names of two doctors working in the NHS who were suffering from AIDS. The court held that the information obtained from hospital records should be kept confidential and the public interest did not require the publication of the names (see also Ch. 29). The court did not order the disclosure by the press of their informant as the circumstances did not constitute one of the exceptional grounds on which the disclosure could be ordered against the press.

In C. v. Dr AJ Cairns[27] the claimant, born in 1963, was the victim of sexual abuse by her stepfather in 1968/69. Her mother informed the GP in 1975 that the daughter had been abused on a single occasion, but asked that he keep this information confidential and said that she would monitor the situation. The GP took no action and the abuse escalated. The claimant suffered from severe mental disorders including eating disorders, adolescent enuresis, alcohol abuse and deliberate self harm. In 1995, she received counselling by a rape and sexual abuse centre, linked her mental problems with the abuse and in 1996 reported her stepfather to the police. He was subsequently convicted and imprisoned. She sued the GP alleging breach of the duty of care, which had caused her harm. She failed in her claim, the judge holding that in 1975 the duty of confidentiality was greater than at the present time and in 1975 the understanding of child sexual abuse was such that nearly all GPs would not then have reported the situation to other agencies. She was out of time in bringing her action since all the necessary information was available to her in 1985 and it would be inequitable to use discretion under s.33 of the Limitation Act 1980 (see Ch. 13) to waive the time limit, since 25 years had expired and the delay meant that it would be impossible to reconstruct the consultation in order to analyse the GP's actions.

In the case of A health authority v. X and others[28] the Court of Appeal dismissed an appeal by a health authority against restrictions (such as that the HA could not, without the consent of the court, disclose the papers to any person other than a specified disciplinary body) which the High Court judge had placed on the disclosure of records which were to be disclosed to it by the local authority following proceedings under the Children Act 1989. The Court of Appeal held that the real issue in the case was whether the conflict in the private/public interest in the confidentiality of medical records and some other public interest should be decided by a health authority or by a judge. Since the judge in the High Court had not heard the original childcare case, he was entitled to attach conditions to the disclosure.

MIDWIVES AND DISCLOSURE IN THE PUBLIC INTEREST

Midwives should ensure that they only disclose confidential information on the justification of the public interest if they can explain and record why the public interest arises. They should be able to respond to any challenge on the disclosure.

Some possible circumstances would include:

– A concern that a client was harming her existing child(ren).

– A concern that a client may harm her baby when born.

– A concern that the client may harm herself.

What, however, if the information which the midwife wishes to be made known relates not to the individual circumstances of the client but to fears concerning the environment of care and the possibility of dangers to the client. The Code of Professional Conduct clauses 8.1, 8.2, 8.3 and 8.4 requires the practitioner to make known her fears in relation to any possible danger to the patient/client. (This duty to 'whistle blow' is discussed further in Chs 5 and 22.) Midwives should make sure that they obtain copies of the circular and follow the procedure laid down by their employer.

CONFIDENTIALITY AND THE PRESS

In a case brought by Ashworth Hospital against Mirror Group Newspapers, the judge made an order requiring the newspaper group to disclose to the hospital the identity of the source of their information about a convicted murderer who was a patient at Ashworth. The Court of Appeal upheld this judgement, holding that the protection of patient information was of vital concern to the NHS.[29] Mirror Group Newspapers disclosed that the clinical notes had been received from a freelance investigative journalist, Mr Ackroyd. He then refused to identify his sources within the hospital. The Hospital then sought an order requiring him to disclose the source of the notes. Mr Ackroyd stated that although he had been paid £1250 from the Mirror, his sources at the hospital had not received any payment and were not motivated by financial gain, but to reveal publicly the way in which Ian Brady had been treated. The Court of Appeal held that the protection of journalistic sources was one of the basic conditions of press freedom and the hospital had to establish an overriding public interest amounting to a pressing social need to which the need to keep press sources confidential should give way. The current case was different from the original MGN case, since as a journalist he was entitled to present different evidential material from a different perspective. The passage of time since the original case meant that there was no cloud of suspicion which was still blighting activity at the hospital and there had been no breach of confidentiality. The journalist succeeded in his appeal against the order to disclose his source.[30]

DEPARTMENT OF HEALTH CODE OF PRACTICE ON CONFIDENTIALITY

The Department of Health prepared a Code of Practice on Confidentiality[31] in 2003. It covers the following areas:

- Confidentiality: definition, disclosing and using confidential patient information; patient consent to disclosing, obligations on individuals working in the NHS

- Providing a confidential service

- Using and disclosing confidential patient information

- Annex A: Detailed requirements in providing a confidential service

- Annex B: Confidentiality decisions

- Annex C: Index of confidential decisions in practice: health purposes, medical purposes other than healthcare, non-medical purposes.

CLIENT ACCESS TO RECORDS

HUMAN RIGHTS ARTICLES

Article 8 of the European Convention gives a right to respect for private life and this has been held to include access to personal records. Thus in the case of Gaskin v. UK[32] the applicant sought documents from his local authority relating to the period of time when he was in care. The court recognised the need to balance the applicant's interest in obtaining information about his childhood against the importance of confidentiality of public records and held that an independent authority should have decided whether access should be granted.

The provisions for access to records are now covered by the Data Protection Act 1998, except for access to the records of those who have died, where the Access to Health Records Act 1990 still applies.

PATIENT-HELD RECORDS

Many midwifery units are now permitting mothers to hold their own records. Certainly during the antenatal stage, excellent results have been obtained by entrusting the records to the care of the patient. It has been found that patients are less likely to lose the records than a medical records department. Changing Childbirth sets as one of the targets that all clients should hold their records (see Ch. 6). One of the indicators of success identified in Changing Childbirth[33] was that within 5 years, all women should be able to carry their own notes. Antenatal records were often the earliest to be disclosed to or even kept by patients and in general midwives are able to have a more open policy of disclosure to mothers and do not require formal applications to be made under the Data Protection Act 1998 before access will be permitted.

Statutory entitlement by the patient to access health records is given by the statutory instrument enacted under Data Protection legislation. Access is also permitted to

Medical Reports obtained for employment or insurance purposes under the Access to Medical Reports Act 1988.

RIGHT OF ACCESS TO PERSONAL DATA

Section 7 of the Data Protection Act 1998 enables an individual to be informed of data held about him and to access that data. Special provisions exist in relation to health, education and social work.

Health, education and social work

Section 30 of the Data Protection Act enables the Secretary of State to draw up specific provisions setting exemptions from the statutory rights of access in relation to health, education and social work records. Statutory Instruments (SIs) have been enacted setting out details of the restrictions on access to these records.[34–36]

RIGHT TO WITHHOLD ACCESS

Access can be withheld under the Data Protection Act 1998 in the following circumstances:

– where in the opinion of the holder of the record, serious harm would be caused to the mental or physical health or condition of the applicant or of any other individual

– where the identity of a third person would be made known and this person has not consented to access. (This does not apply where the other person is the health professional caring for the patient.)

– where the reports are confidential under a statutory provision such as information supplied in a report or other evidence given to the court by a local authority, Health or Social Services Board, Health and Social Services Trust or probation officer.

The Department of Health established a Health Records and Data Protection Review Group in May 2002 to advise the Government on helping people to gain access to their health records. The minutes of its meetings are available online via the Department of Health website, which also provides the answers to frequently asked questions about accessing health records.[37]

IMPLICATIONS FOR MIDWIVES

Voluntary system

Before any statutory provisions for access were in place, many midwives and obstetric units permitted wide access to records, with many mothers being responsible for the antenatal records. The legislation does not replace this system, and open access can be permitted on a much wider basis than is required statutorily.

Standard of record keeping

Since the midwife knows that the mother has a statutory right of access, there is even more reason to ensure a high standard of record keeping. The fact that the mother can ask for corrections if she considers that the records are incomplete, misleading or inaccurate should encourage the midwife to maintain high standards to prevent possible criticisms (see Ch. 15).

PROBLEMS OF OPEN ACCESS

UNWANTED DISCLOSURE

One problem which openness can bring is shown in Box 10.9.

> **Box 10.9 Situation: unwanted information**
>
> Frances Davies had not told her husband that she had had a child when she was 15 years old, which was adopted, or that she had had a subsequent miscarriage. She was asked for details of the earlier gestation history when she booked into the antenatal clinic for her present pregnancy. In this clinic, a system was operated whereby mothers took their antenatal records home, and Frances was concerned about her husband reading the previous obstetric history. She asked if these details could be omitted from her records.

The danger of agreeing with Frances's request and editing medical history is that at a subsequent time those events may become significant, and to rely upon the patient being conscious or on there being a midwife present who remembered the missing details is clearly unsatisfactory. One possibility in such a case is to arrange for these records to be kept at the hospital and not to be taken home. Alternatively, it may be possible to devise a formula for detailing this information which would not be understood by the spouse. This cannot be done where the patient is requesting statutory right of access under the legislation since the holder of the records would have a duty to translate any jargon and decipher any illegible parts or find any missing parts so that the records are comprehensible to the applicant. Another possibility is to mark on the form that other information is held at the hospital. It would then be important for any midwife to ensure that she had both sets of records. There are obvious inherent dangers in a two-set record system. Another possibility is for the woman to be told to exercise her right of keeping the record confidential to herself and therefore secret from her husband. However, in the circumstances, this may not be a realistic possibility. Nor may the possibility of the woman making a full disclosure to the husband be realistic.

It is recognised by some midwives that some clients book late for the initial booking at antenatal clinic because their partner does not know of a previous pregnancy and they are afraid that it will become general knowledge. The midwife should reassure the client that this will be kept strictly confidential. Some midwives take the view that in order to preserve this confidentiality, there is no reason to record the fact of the previous history in the records, especially where the first birth or miscarriage was normal. There are, however, dangers in this approach, especially if the client is rhesus negative or if subsequent events make the earlier history significant.

FEAR OF LOST RECORDS

Another concern is the possibility that the records could be lost while being cared for by the mother and in the event of later litigation the midwife could suffer considerable disadvantages.

The loss of records may well be less when the mother has responsibility than when they are cared for by a medical records department. The absence of records would probably work more against the mother in litigation than in her favour, since the burden is on the claimant to show on a balance of probabilities that there has been negligence.

COMPUTERISED RECORDS

In March 2001, the government announced its intention to introduce, by March 2005, a system whereby every patient would have an electronic health record. The electronic health record is defined by the Department of Health as a record holding summarised key data about patients, such as name, address, NHS number, registered GP and contact details, previous treatments, ongoing conditions, current medication, allergies and the date of any next appointments. The stated intention is that it will be securely protected, created with patient consent, with individual changes made only by authorised staff. Pilot schemes are in operation at the time of writing but the original timetable has been revised. Clearly, any system will have to comply with data protection legislation requirements over security and control over patient access. The scheme will also have implications for record keeping, which are discussed in Chapter 15.

FREEDOM OF INFORMATION ACT 2000

The Freedom of Information Act 2000 was brought into force over a period of 5 years. It gives a right to people to obtain information from public authorities. An Information Commissioner (combining both Data Protection and Freedom of Information statutory duties) has been appointed and an Information Tribunal adjudicates on grievances under the Act. Part 2 of the Act lists many areas of information which are exempt from the access provisions. Under s.40, access to personal information will come under the Data Protection Act 1998. The Act gives a general right of access to information held by public authorities, but this right is subject to significant exceptions. The main exemptions from the duty are set out in Part 2 of the Act.

Some of the exemptions are subject to *a public interest test* and these include: Information intended for future publication; National security; Defence; International relations; Relations within the UK; The economy; Investigations and proceedings conducted by public authorities; Law enforcement; Audit functions; Formulation of government policy; Prejudice to effective conduct of public affairs; Communication with Her Majesty, etc. and Honours; Health and safety; Environmental information; Personal information; Legal professional privilege and commercial interests. The public interest test means that a public authority must consider whether the public interest in withholding the exempt information outweighs the public interest in releasing it.

Other exemptions are absolute. These include: Information accessible to the applicant by other means; Information supplied by or relating to bodies dealing with security matters; Court records; Parliamentary privilege; Prejudice to effective conduct of public affairs; Personal information where the applicant is the subject of the information. This means that for information coming under this category a public interest does not apply and the information does not have to be disclosed.

Another exception to disclosure is contained in s.14 where a request which is vexatious, or where the public authority has already complied with the request, does not have to be complied with.

CONCLUSIONS

The impact of the Articles of the European Convention on Human Rights in this area cannot at this stage be easily evaluated, but it is clear from the many cases being brought that the courts are having to determine the balance between Article 8 and the right to private and family life and Article 10 and the right of free expression. In addition the Freedom of Information Act and the qualified right to access information held by public bodies is slowly having an influence. Midwives need to ensure that they have training in electronic record keeping and are familiar with the

Department of Health's Code of Practice on confidentiality. It is hoped that the implementation of a strategy on the use of confidential information will assist in securing the rights of patients in this complex field. Further reference may be made to the author's work.[38]

QUESTIONS AND EXERCISES

1. What measures do you think could be taken to ensure higher standards of confidentiality in midwifery units?

2. Disclosure in the public interest causes considerable difficulty. In the light of the NMC guidance on confidentiality (as contained in the Guidelines for Professional Practice), draw up a protocol to be followed if disclosure in the public interest appeared to be justified.

3. There is no absolute right of access by the patient to her records. In what circumstances, if any, do you consider that the right of the client to access should be withheld?

4. Consider the provisions of the Freedom of Information Act and decide how it could work for the benefit of pregnant women.

References

1 Nursing and Midwifery Council. Code of Professional Conduct: standards for conduct, performance and ethics 2004.

2 European Directive on Data Protection, adopted by the Council of the European Union in October 1995.

3 NHS Executive. Data Protection Act 1998. HSC 2000/009.

4 NHS. Online. Available: www.standards.nhsia.nhs.uk/sdp

5 Durant v. Financial Services Authority [2003] EWCA Civ 1746.

6 Information Commissioner. Case summary, October 2004.

7 Information Commissioner. Information: Address: Wycliffe House, Water Lane, Wilmslow, Cheshire SK9 5AF. Information line: 01625 545745; Tel: 01625 545700; Fax: 01625 524510.

8 Information Commissioner. Legal Guidance on Data Protection Act 1998. Online. Available: www.dataprotection.gov.uk.

9 NHS Executive. 2000. Data Protection Act: Protection and Use of Patient Information. HSC 2000/009.

10 Department of Health. Online. Available: www.doh.gov.uk/ipu/confiden/protect

11 NHS Executive. Caldicott Guardians. HSC 1999/012.

12 Raj Kaur, NHS Executive Information: Contact: 3E58 Quarry House, Leeds LS2 7UE; Fax: 0113 254 6114.

13 Department of Health. Protection and using patient information: A Manual for Caldicott Guardians. London: HMSO; 2000.

14 Department of Health. Information contact: Carole Bell: Tel: 0207 972 4978.

15 Department of Health. Social Care Information Governance, May 2004 DoH.

16 Patient Information Advisory Group (Establishment) Regulations 2001 No 2836.

17 Nursing and Midwifery Council. NMC Code of Professional Conduct: standards for conduct, performance and ethics 2002, updated 2004.

18 Furniss v. Fitchett [1958] NZLR 396.

19 Stephens v. Avery and others [1988] 2 All ER 477.

20 Nursing and Midwifery Council. Midwives Rules and Standards. NMC; August 2004.

21 R (Stevens) v. Plymouth City Council and C [2002] 1 FLR 1177.

22 Kuwait Airways Corporation v. Iraqi Airways Co. (No 6) The Times Law Report, 25 April 2005 CA.

23 A Health Authority and another v. X and others. Lloyd's Rep Med [2001] 349.

24 Woolgar v. Chief Constable of Sussex Police and another [1999] 3 All ER 604 CA.

25 W. v. Egdell [1990] 1 All ER 835.

26 X. v. Y [1988] 2 All ER 648.

27 C. v. Dr AJ Cairns. Lloyd's Rep Med [2003] 90.

28 A Health Authority v. X and others [2001] EWCA 2014; Lloyd's Rep Med [2002] 139.

29 Ashworth Hospital Authority v. MGN Ltd [2001] 1 All ER 991.

30 Ackroyd v. Mersey Care NHS Trust [2003] EWCA Civ 663; Lloyd's Rep. Med [2003] 379.

31 Department of Health. The NHS Confidentiality Code of Practice. DoH; 2003; Online. Available: www.doh.gov.uk/ipu/confiden/protect/ (superseding HSG(96) 18 LASSL(96)).

32 Gaskin v. UK [1990] 12 EHRR 36.

33 Department of Health. (Cumberlege Report) Changing Childbirth. London: HMSO; 1993.

34 Data Protection (Subject Access Modification) (Health) Order 2000 SI 2000 No 413

35 Data Protection (Subject Access Modification) (Education) Order 2000 SI 2000 No 414

36 Data Protection (Subject Access Modification) (Social Work) Order 2000 SI 2000 No 415.

37 Department of Health. Online. Available: www.dh.gov.uk

38 Dimond B. The legal aspects of confidentiality. Wiltshire: Quay Books/Mark Allen; 2002.

Chapter 11
COMPLAINTS

There was a statutory duty for all hospitals to have a complaints procedure (Hospital Complaints Procedure Act 1985) and the Secretary of State has requested that this duty should be recognised also by NHS community health organisations. The duty was reinforced by the Patient's Charter, which expected all patients to have the opportunity to make known any concerns to the management. The NHS Plan published in 2000 also introduced new forms for participation and representation. New Complaints Regulations came into force on 30 July 2004.[1]

WAYS OF MAKING A COMPLAINT

At present there are many ways in which complaints can be made, as shown in Box 11.1.

Box 11.1 Methods of making complaints

1. Health Authority or Primary Care Trust in respect of the services of General Practitioners, dentists, pharmacists and other primary care services

2. NHS trust in relation to hospital and community services

3. Special Health Authorities as the commissioners of healthcare services from trusts and from nursing homes

4. Local Authorities as the commissioners for community social services and residential accommodation or Care Trusts where these have been established

5. Professional registration bodies in respect of the conduct of individual practitioners

6. The Healthcare Commission (i.e. The Commission for Health Audit and Inspection, CHAI) as the independent review stage of the complaints procedure or The Health Service Commissioner as the final stage in the NHS complaints procedure

---

▶

7. The Commission for Social Care Inspection for complaints relating to care homes and the Local Authority Ombudsman where the complaints relate to local authority services

8. Litigation via solicitors

9. Complaints via the Patient Representation Organisations (see below) or Community Health Councils (in Wales)

10. Police

11. Members of Parliament, the media etc.

Midwives are increasingly likely to be involved in the hearing of a complaint, either in relation to their own practice or in being asked to give evidence about the practice of colleagues. Complaints may also be made about administrative procedures, property and other topics not directly the concern of the midwife. The midwife should, difficult though it may be, welcome complaints and regard them as an opportunity to monitor and improve the service to mothers. One of the advantages of the named midwife scheme is that some of the concerns and worries of mothers can be made known to the midwife and therefore addressed at an early stage informally, so that they do not eventually become the subject of a formal complaint. However, for this to be so, the midwife must respond positively to the mother, making it easy for her to express her concerns and be vigilant in following up the anxieties.

INFORMAL COMPLAINTS

It is recommended that where concerns are expressed to the midwife, she should keep a brief note of the details shown in Box 11.2.

Box 11.2 Recording informal complaints/concerns

– Date and time

– Mother/client

– Brief description of concern

– Action taken by midwife

A note should also be made in the mother's records

Where the midwife has had to refer the issue to a senior manager or other professional, she should follow it up to ensure that action is taken where necessary. Her regular contact with the mother should also ensure that she discovers if the concerns are now allayed.

FORMAL COMPLAINTS

The midwife should always make it clear to the client that it is always open to the client to make a formal complaint. She must ensure that she knows the procedure and who is the designated Complaints Officer for the unit/hospital. Where necessary, she should offer assistance to the complainant, particularly if the complainant has difficulty in expressing herself in writing. It should be made clear however that there is no requirement for the complaint to be put in writing by the complainant personally, and that someone else could do that on her behalf.

BACKGROUND TO DEVELOPMENT OF COMPLAINTS PROCEDURES: THE WILSON REVIEW

Because there were so many procedures and ways in which complaints could be made, and the systems which then existed were confusing and slow and could be bureaucratic, an expert committee was set up under the Chairmanship of Professor Alan Wilson to review NHS complaints procedures.[2] The report reviewed the current situation and set objectives for any effective complaints system. The principles it saw for any effective complaints system are set out in Box 11.3.

Box 11.3 Principles of an effective complaints system set by the Wilson Report

- Responsiveness

- Quality enhancement

- Cost effectiveness

- Accessibility

- Impartiality

- Simplicity

▶

▶

- Speed

- Confidentiality

- Accountability

The report recommended that these principles should be incorporated into an NHS complaints system and it made extensive recommendations.

The recommendations of the Wilson Committee were implemented in the NHS Complaints procedure. There were three stages: local resolution; second stage, i.e. independent review panel, and health service commissioner (Ombudsman).

REVIEW OF COMPLAINTS PROCEDURE

Research was commissioned by the Department of Health on the effectiveness of the complaints system set up under the Wilson recommendations. In the light of the results of that research, the Department of Health published a document suggesting a number of ways to improve the current procedure.[3] It also issued a consultation document[4] on which feedback was invited. Subsequently, Regulations on Complaints introduced a statutory complaints procedure which came into force in England on 30 July 2004.

NEW COMPLAINTS REGULATIONS[1]

These cover the topics shown in Box 11.4.

Box 11.4 Contents of the Complaints Regulations 2004

Part I Introduction

1. Citation, commencement and application

2. Interpretation

Part II Handling and consideration of complaints by NHS bodies

3. Arrangements for the handling and consideration of complaints

4. Responsibility for complaints arrangements

▶

SUMMARY OF THE PROCEDURES

Each NHS body has a statutory duty to make arrangements in accordance with the Regulations for the handling and consideration of complaints. These arrangements must be accessible and such as to ensure that complaints are dealt with speedily and efficiently and that complainants are treated courteously and sympathetically and as far as possible involved in decisions about how their complaints are handled and considered. The arrangements must be in writing and a copy must be given free of charge to any person who makes a request for one. Where the NHS Trust or primary care trust makes arrangements for the provision of services with an independent provider, then it has a duty to ensure that that organisation has in place arrangements for the handling and consideration of complaints and any matter connected with its provision of services as if the Regulations applied to it.

The NHS organisation has a duty to designate one of its members (in the case of an NHS Trust, a member of its board of directors), who has two statutory responsibilities:

1. to take responsibility for ensuring compliance with the Regulations and

2. to ensure that action is taken in the light of the outcome of any investigation.

COMPLAINTS MANAGER

This is a person designated by the NHS organisation to manage the procedures for handling and considering complaints and in particular:

1. to perform the functions of the complaints manager as set out in the Regulations and

2. to perform such other functions in relation to complaints as the NHS organisation may require.

The complaints manager can delegate the functions to any person authorised by the NHS organisation to act on his behalf.

SUBJECT OF COMPLAINTS

Under the statutory procedures, a complaint to an NHS body can be about any matter reasonably connected with the exercise of its functions in providing services or commissioning healthcare or other services, either under an NHS contract or provision by an independent provider or NHS foundation trust.

Excluded from the consideration of complaints under these statutory arrangements are the following:

1. A complaint made by an NHS body which relates to the exercise of its functions by another NHS body.

2. A complaint made by a primary care provider which relates either to the exercise of its functions by an NHS body or to the contract or arrangements under which it provides primary care services.

3. A complaint by an employee of an NHS body about any matter relating to his contract of employment.

4. A complaint made by an independent provider or an NHS foundation trust about any matter relating to arrangements made by an NHS body with that independent provider or NHS foundation trust.

5. A complaint which relates to the provision of primary medical services under the transitional arrangements between PCT and strategic health authority.

6. A complaint being investigated by the Health Service Commissioner.

7. A complaint arising out of an NHS body's alleged failure to comply with a data subject request under the Data Protection Act 1998 or a request for information under the Freedom of Information Act 2000.

8. A complaint about which the complainant has stated in writing that he intends to take legal proceedings.

9. A complaint about which an NHS body is taking or is proposing to take disciplinary proceedings in relation to the substance of the complaint against a person who is the subject of the complaint.

COMMENT ON THESE EXCLUSIONS

In the past, there has been a discretion about investigating complaints where there is a declared intention of the complainant to take legal action. However, in the consultation document 'Making Amends'[5] on a new clinical negligence compensation scheme it was suggested that the rule that an investigation of a complaint should be halted if the complainant commenced a claim should be removed, since the investigation should automatically take place as part of the initial local response to a complaint and even if the patient subsequently decided to pursue litigation, the complaints process should continue to provide the explanations required by patients and families. This seems to a more positive attitude, since many complaints which could lead to litigation may be prevented if early investigation or mediation could resolve the issues.

WHO CAN MAKE A COMPLAINT

The complainant must be either the patient or any person who is affected by or likely to be affected by the action, omission or decision of the NHS body which is the subject of the complaint. A complaint can also be made by the personal representative acting on behalf of a person:

– who has died,

– is a child or

– is unable by reason of physical or mental incapacity to make the complaint himself or

– the patient has requested the representative to act on his behalf.

Where the patient is a child or unable to act by reason of physical or mental incapacity, the representative must be a relative or a person who in the opinion of the complaints manager has or had a sufficient interest in his welfare and is a suitable person to act as representative. Where the complaints manager concludes that the person is unsuitable to act as a representative, he must notify that person in writing stating his reasons. Where the complaint is on behalf of a child, the representative must be a parent, guardian or other adult who has care of the child or a person authorised by a local authority or a voluntary organisation where the child is in the care of the LA or the voluntary organisation.

METHOD OF MAKING THE COMPLAINT

The complaint can be made to the complaints manager or any other staff member of the NHS body and can be made orally or in writing (including electronically). The complaints manager must make a written record of a complaint made orally, and include the name of the complainant and the date on which it was made. Where it is made in writing, the complaints manager must make a written record of the date on which it was received.

ACTION ON RECEIPT OF COMPLAINT

The complaints manager must send to the complainant a written acknowledgement of the complaint within two working days of the date on which the complaint was made, which includes information of the right to assistance from the independent advocacy services provided.

Where the complaint was made orally, the acknowledgement must be accompanied by the written record drawn up by the complaints manager, with an invitation to the complainant to sign and return it. A copy of the complaint must be sent to any person identified in the complaint as the subject of the complaint.

INVESTIGATION

The complaints manager must investigate the complaint to the extent necessary and in the manner which appears to be most appropriate to resolve it speedily and efficiently. Where the complaints manager thinks it appropriate to do so, and where the complainant agrees, he may make arrangements for conciliation, mediation or other assistance for the purposes of resolving the complaint, and in such a case the NHS body must ensure that appropriate conciliation or mediation services are available. The complaints manager must take such steps as are reasonably practicable to keep the complainant informed about the progress of the investigation.

RESPONSE

A written response must be prepared by the complaints manager which summarises the nature and substance of the complaint, describes the investigation and summarises its conclusions. This response must be signed by the chief executive of the NHS body, except in cases where for good reasons the chief executive is not himself able to sign it, in which case it is signed by a person acting on his behalf. The response must be sent within 20 working days, beginning on the date on which the complaint was made, or where that is not possible, as soon as reasonably practicable. The response must notify the complainant of his right to refer the complaint to the Healthcare Commission and a copy of the response must be sent to any person who received a copy of the complaint.

TIME LIMITS

A complaint must be made within 6 months of the date on which the matter which is the subject of the complaint occurred or 6 months of the date on which the matter which is the subject of the complaint came to the notice of the complainant. Complaints outside these time limits can be investigated if the complaints manager is of the opinion that having regard to all the circumstances, the complainant had good reasons for not making the complaint in time and notwithstanding the time that has elapsed it is still possible to investigate the complaint effectively and efficiently.

ROLE OF THE HEALTHCARE COMMISSION IN HANDLING COMPLAINTS

Where a complainant is not satisfied with the result of an investigation by an NHS trust, primary care trust or independent provider or for any reason an investigation has not been completed within six months of the date on which the complaint was made, or the complaints manager has decided not to investigate the complaint because it was outside the time limits, then the complainant may request the Healthcare Commission to consider the complaint. This right also applies to a person who has complained about a primary care provider and is not satisfied with the outcome of the investigation. The application to the Healthcare Commission can be made either orally or in writing (including electronically) and must be made within 2 months of, or where that is not possible, as soon as reasonably practicable after, the date on which the response was sent to the complainant.

Where a person has made a complaint to an NHS foundation trust, and is not satisfied with the outcome of the investigation or the NHS foundation trust has no complaints procedures, then he can apply to the Healthcare Commission for his complaint to be considered. In the case of foundation trusts, the Healthcare Commission's role is limited to the consideration of a complaint which is made by a patient and is reasonably connected with the provision of healthcare or other services to patients by or for the NHS foundation trust; Para. 15(2).

EXCLUDED FROM THE JURISDICTION OF THE HEALTHCARE COMMISSION IN RELATION TO FOUNDATION TRUSTS

The following complaints cannot be considered by the Healthcare Commission:

Where the complaint:

– is one about which the complainant has stated in writing that he intends to take legal proceedings

– is one about which the NHS foundation trust has stated in writing that it is taking or proposing to take disciplinary proceedings in relation to the substance of the complaint against a person who is the subject of the complaint

– arises out of the foundation trust's alleged failure to comply with a data subject request under the Data Protection Act 1998 or a request for information under the Freedom of Information Act 2000

– is being or has been investigated by the Health Service Commissioner.

The Healthcare Commission must refer the complaint to the Independent Regulator (i.e. for NHS foundation trusts; see Ch. 21) where he decides that it does not come within the provisions of Para. 15(2). The same time limits for applying to the Healthcare Commission about complaints from NHS trusts and primary care trusts apply to complaints about NHS foundation trusts. The Healthcare Commission must send a copy of a complaint about an NHS foundation trust to the Independent Regulator within two working days of its receipt and with the consent, express or implied, of the complainant, and invite his views.

PROCEDURE FOR HEALTHCARE COMMISSION

The Healthcare Commission must assess the nature and substance of the complaint and decide how it should be handled, having regard to:

– the views of the complainant

– the views of the body complained about

– the views of the Independent Regulator (where appropriate)

– any investigation of the complaint and action taken as a result

– any other relevant circumstances.

DECISIONS OF THE HEALTHCARE COMMISSION

As soon as is reasonably practicable, the Healthcare Commission must notify the complainant as to whether it has decided:

– to take no further action

– to make recommendations to the body which is the subject of the complaint as to what action might be taken to resolve it

– to investigate the complaint further

– to consider the subject matter of the complaint as part of or in conjunction with any other investigation or review which it is conducting or proposes to conduct in the exercise of its functions (see Ch. 21)

– to refer the complaint to a regulatory body

– to refer the complaint to the Independent Regulator or

– to refer the complaint to the Health Service Commissioner.

Different parts of a complaint can be dealt with in different ways.

THE INVESTIGATION BY THE HEALTHCARE COMMISSION

Under Regulation 17 there are rules relating to how the Healthcare Commission should investigate, including time limits for giving notice of its intention. It can request, in writing, information and documents from any person or body it considers necessary to enable a complaint to be considered properly. It cannot request information which is confidential and relates to a living individual unless that person gives consent to the disclosure and use for the purpose of the investigation.

The Healthcare Commission must prepare and keep up to date a list of people who, in its opinion, are suitable to be members of an independent lay panel to hear and consider complaints. Excluded from the list are members or employees of an NHS body and any person who is or has been a healthcare professional or employee of a healthcare professional. Procedures for the panel are set out in Regulation 18.

REPORT OF INVESTIGATION BY THE HEALTHCARE COMMISSION

As soon as reasonably practicable after an investigation, the Healthcare Commission must prepare a written report of its investigation which:

- summarises the nature and substance of the complaint

- describes the investigation and summarises its conclusions including any findings of fact, the Healthcare Commission's opinion of those findings and its reasons for its opinion

- recommends what action should be taken and by whom to resolve the complaint

- identifies what other action, if any, should be taken and by whom.

The report may include suggestions which it considers would improve the services of an NHS body, an NHS foundation trust or a primary care provider, or which would otherwise be effective for the purposes of resolving the complaint.

The report is sent to the complainant with a letter explaining his right to take his complaint to the Health Service Commissioner, to the NHS body complained about, the commissioner of services from an independent provider, the primary care trust (in the case of complaint about a primary care provider), any relevant strategic health authority and the Independent Regulator (where appropriate).

The report must be adapted to prevent any breach of confidentiality of a living person without his or her consent.

GENERAL PROVISIONS

There are requirements relating to the publicity of the complaints procedures, and in ensuring that specified persons such as patients and carers, visitors, staff, independent providers are informed of the complaints procedures, the name of the complaints manager and the address at which he can be contacted.

Under the monitoring arrangements, each NHS body must prepare a report for each quarter of the year for consideration by its Board. The reports must:

- specify the numbers of complaints received

- identify the subject matter of those complaints

- summarise how they were handled including the outcome of the investigations and

- identify any complaints where the recommendations of the Healthcare Commission were not acted upon, giving the reasons why not.

In addition, each NHS body must prepare an annual report on its handling and consideration of complaints and send a copy to specified organisations.

HEALTH SERVICE COMMISSIONER

Legislation which came into force on 1 April 1996 widened its jurisdiction to include the investigation of matters concerned with the exercise of clinical judgement and the investigations of complaints about family practitioner services. The HSC has a duty to prepare a report which is submitted to Parliament, under s.14(4) of the Health Service Commissioners Act 1993. The Select Committee of the House of Commons has the power to investigate further any complaint reported by the HSC, if necessary summoning witnesses to London for questioning. The HSC is completely independent of the NHS and the Government and has the jurisdiction to investigate complaints against any part of the NHS about:

– a failure in service, or

– a failure to purchase or provide a service one is entitled to receive, or

– maladministration (administrative affairs).

The Health Service Commissioner has retained the role of the ultimate forum of appeal in relation to complaints within the NHS. However, since the Healthcare Commission has now undertaken the role of independent review and has powers of investigation, it may mean that far fewer complaints result in an investigation by the Health Service Commissioner.

NHS PLAN[6]

Chapter 10 of the NHS Plan envisaged giving patients more say in their own treatment and more influence over the way the NHS works. To achieve this, the following initiatives were planned:

– Greater information to empower patients

– Greater patient choice

– Patient advocates and advisers in every hospital

– Redress over cancelled operations

– Patients' forums and citizens' panels in every area

– New national panel to advise on major reorganisations of hospitals

– Stronger regulation of professional standards.

These are considered briefly below.

GREATER INFORMATION TO EMPOWER PATIENTS

This is provided through the publication of patient-friendly versions of NICE guidelines, the establishment of NHS Direct online, Digital TV and NHS Direct Information points in key public places. Better communication between clinicians and doctors is secured by letters between clinicians about an individual patient being copied to the patients as of right; by smart cards for patients allowing easier access to health records (see Ch. 15 on Electronic patient records).

GREATER PATIENT CHOICE

Patients have a choice of GP and this will be supported by more information being given to patients about the GP practices in their area. By 2005, the Department of Health anticipated that patients would be able to book hospital appointments and choose to be admitted at times which are convenient to them. This has been implemented in some areas, but it is by no means universal.

PATIENT ADVOCACY AND LIAISON SERVICES (PALS)

An NHS-wide Patient Advocacy and Liaison Service (PALS) has been set up in every trust. Patient advocates act as independent facilitators to handle patient and family concerns. A patient advocacy team, usually situated in the main reception areas of hospitals, acts as a welcoming point for patients and carers and a clearly identifiable information point. Patient advocates act as an independent facilitator to handle patient and family concerns, with direct access to the chief executive and the power to negotiate immediate solutions. They work with other organisations such as the Citizens Advice Bureau. Special provision is made in respect of patient and advocacy services for the purposes of the Mental Health Act 1983 s.134, which concerns the withholding of correspondence. Under Regulations of 2003, correspondence with a patient advocacy and liaison service is exempt from the provisions of s.134.[7]

REDRESS OVER CANCELLED OPERATIONS

If a hospital operation is cancelled on the day of surgery by the hospital for non-clinical reasons, the hospital must offer the patient an appointment within a maximum of 28 days or fund the patient's treatment at the time and hospital of the patient's choice.

PATIENTS' AND PUBLIC INVOLVEMENT FORUMS AND CITIZENS' PANELS IN EVERY AREA

Under s.15 of the NHS Reform and Health Care Professions Act 2002, the Secretary of State has a duty to set up in every trust and primary care trust a body to be known as a Patients' and Public Involvement Forum. The members of each Patients' Forum are appointed by the Commission for Patient and Public Involvement in Health (see below). The statutory functions[8] laid down for them are to:

1. monitor and review the range and operation of services provided by, or under arrangements made by, the trust for which it is established

2. obtain the views of patients and their carers about those matters and report on those views to the trust

3. provide advice, and make reports and recommendations, about matters relating to the range and operation of those services to the trust

4. make available to patients and their carers advice and information about those services

5. in prescribed circumstances, perform any prescribed function of the trust with respect to the provision of a service affording assistance to patients and their families and carers

6. carry out such other functions as may be prescribed.

The Forums are required to cooperate together when appropriate. They also have the responsibility for providing independent advocacy services to persons in the trust's area or who have been provided with services by the trust; for giving advice to patients and carers about the making of complaints and representing the views of members of the public about matters affecting their health (s.16 NHS Reform and Health Care Professions Act 2002).

They are also expected to promote the involvement of members of the public in the area of the trust in consultations about decisions and the formulation of policies which would affect the health of those members of the public.

Regulations give rights to patients' forums to inspect any premises where NHS patients go to receive healthcare. Each patient forum must prepare an annual report and this must include details of the arrangements maintained by the forum in that year for obtaining the views of patients (s.18 of 2002 Act). Regulations have been enacted on the functions, membership and procedures for patient forums.[9,10]

In November 2004, it was announced[11] that every NHS trust and PCT area had a forum and over 5000 volunteers had been recruited to the Patient and Public Involvement Forums by the Commission for Patient and Public Involvement in Health (CPPH).[12]

Financial rewards to trusts will be linked to the results of the annual National Patients' Survey. A new NHS Charter will replace the current Patients' Charter. A National Charter on long-term care was published in 1999[13] and local charters have been commissioned by the Department of Health covering long-term care.[14]

Independent local advisory forums chosen from residents of the area to provide a sounding board have been appointed. Local government will be given the power to scrutinise NHS plans locally.

The Community Health Councils were abolished in England. (The Welsh Assembly decided in favour of the retention of CHCs.) Under the NHS plan, patients will be represented at all levels within the NHS.

INDEPENDENT COMPLAINTS AND ADVICE SERVICES (ICAS)

Under s.12 of the Health and Social Care Act 2001, the Secretary of State has a responsibility to provide independent advocacy services to assist patients in making complaints against the NHS. The Independent Complaints Advisory Services[15] were available nationally from September 2003. A consultation paper 'Involving patients and the public in healthcare'[16] was issued by the Department of Health in September 2001 for consultation on proposals for greater public representation to replace the CHCs.

ICAS focus on helping individuals to pursue complaints about NHS services. They aim to ensure complainants have access to the support they need to articulate their concerns and navigate the complaints system – maximising the chances of their complaint being resolved more quickly and effectively. ICAS work alongside the trust-based Patients Forums and Patient Advocacy and Liaison Services (see above). The Commission for Patient and Public Involvement in Health (CPPH) (see below) identifies and disseminates quality standards on ICAS, sets criteria for its provision and provides a national assessment. Information about ICAS and the current range of pilot services is available on the Department of Health website.[17] A report of the first year of ICAS activity was published in January 2005.[18]

These organisations replace CHCs, which as noted above were abolished in England in September 2003.

PATIENT REPRESENTATION

'Involving Patients and the Public in Healthcare'[19] was issued by the Department of Health in September 2001 for consultation on proposals for greater public representation to replace the CHCs. In a press release on 3 September 2001[20] the Department of Health announced that a new independent body was to be established. There were to be two levels: at national level, a new national body – the Commission for Patient and Public Involvement in Health – and at local level bodies called Voice which would report patients' concerns from PALS and Forums to the new Strategic Health Authorities. Voice would set national standards and monitor local services, helping to ensure communities had an effective say in their local NHS. Voice would work alongside the trust-based Patients' Forums and Patient Advocacy and Liaison Services.

Subsequently, the concept of 'Voice' appears to have been dropped but the CPPH and the local Patients' Forums were established.

COMMISSION FOR PATIENT AND PUBLIC INVOLVEMENT IN HEALTH (CPPH)

This Commission was established under s.20 of the NHS Reform and Health Care Professions Act 2002 as a corporate body with the following statutory functions:

– The appointment of members of Patients' Forums (see above)

– Advising the Secretary of State and other prescribed bodies about arrangements for public involvement in and consultation on matters relating to the health service

– Advising the Secretary of State about arrangements for the provision of independent advocacy services

– Representing to the Secretary of State and advising him on the views of and arrangements for Patients' Forums

– Providing staff to Patients' Forums established for primary care trusts and advice and assistance to Patients' Forums and facilitating the coordination of their activities

– Advising and assisting providers of independent advocacy services

– Setting quality standards relating to any aspect of the way Patients' Forums exercise their functions and the services provided by independent advocacy services; monitoring how successfully they meet those standards and making recommendations to them about how to improve their performance against those standards.

– Any other functions which may be prescribed.

In addition, the CPPH was required to promote the involvement of members of the public in consultations or processes leading to decisions or the formulation of policies which might affect the health of those members of the public. The CPPH was also expected to review the annual reports of the Patients' Forums and as a consequence make reports and recommendations to the Secretary of State on matters arising. If the Commission became aware of any matter connected with the health service which in its opinion gave rise to concerns about the safety or welfare of patients and was not satisfied that the matter was being dealt with, then the Commission must report this to the appropriate body.

Subsequently, in July 2004 the Secretary of State for Health announced that he was intending to abolish the CPPH in order to reduce bureaucracy in the NHS and a consultation exercise was initiated to consider the arrangements which would replace it.[21] The consultation exercise ended on 30 January 2005. Supporting the patient and public involvement in health, the Department of Health set up a research programme, 'Health in Partnership', involving 12 separate research projects. A report of the findings is available from the Department of Health.[22] A separate piece of research has been carried out by Christine Hogg, an independent consultant, focussing on the views of representatives of organisations involved in patient and public involvement.[23]

In May 2005 the Secretary of State called for NHS leaders to listen to patients to help improve family health services.[24] She wanted the National Leadership Network for Health and Social Care (which replaced the NHS Modernisation Board) to play a central role in ensuring public engagement in the process of redesigning family health services. A White Paper on Health outside Hospitals is to be published at the end of 2005.

STRONGER REGULATION OF PROFESSIONAL STANDARDS

New quality standards have been introduced into the NHS. There is now a mandatory national scheme for adverse incident reporting known as the National Patient Safety Agency (see Ch. 19) and the Chief Medical Officer's proposals[25] for improving standards of doctors, including annual appraisal and clinical audit, have been implemented. A National Clinical Assessment Authority has also been established with the role of reviewing an individual doctor's performance if concerns have arisen. The NHS Tribunal has been abolished and new procedures introduced for the removal or suspension of doctors from practice. New regulatory machinery for registration bodies has been introduced. A Council for the Regulation of Health Care Professionals was established under the NHS Reform and Health Care Professions Act 2002, which is responsible for the oversight of the workings of the regulatory bodies such as the NMC and the GMC (see Ch. 3).

CONCLUSIONS

Major innovations have been introduced into the NHS as a consequence of the Health Act 1999, the NHS Reform and Health Care Professions Act 2002, the Health and Social Care (Community Health and Standards) Act 2003 and the NHS Plan (see Ch. 21). These changes include the new complaints system discussed above. The Bristol Royal Infirmary Inquiry[26] following the deaths of children during heart surgery recommended that patients must be given the opportunity to pass on views on the service which they have received, and emphasised there is a duty of candour, i.e. a duty to tell a patient if adverse events have occurred, which is owed by all those working in the NHS to patients. The Inquiry recommends:

Complaints should be dealt with swiftly and thoroughly, keeping the patient (and carer) informed. There should be a strong independent element, not part of the trust's man-

agement or board, in any body considering serious complaints which require formal inves-
tigation. An independent advocacy service should be established to assist patients (and
carers).

The implementation of the many recommendations contained in the Inquiry Report
should have significant implications for the standards of care of every midwifery patient, including how complaints are handled. The Government published a response to the Kennedy Report which was considered by the author.[27]

The Health Service Commissioner[28] recently published a withering attack on the
present complaints system, identifying five key weaknesses including fragmentation
of the complaints system within the NHS and between public and private healthcare
systems and inadequate investigation by incompetent staff. Similar criticisms were
also made by the Healthcare Commission in June 2005. It called upon the health
service to improve its dealings with dissatisfied patients. Its figures showed that more
than 25% of complaints are referred back by the Healthcare Commission to the NHS
organisations because the trust had not done enough to resolve the issue. Clearly
significant reforms must take place if the complaints system is to be brought up to
standard.

QUESTIONS AND EXERCISES

1. Consider the complaints relating to midwifery services over the past year and
   discuss the extent to which these could be used to improve the services
   provided.

2. Consider the complaints procedure drafted by your employer in the light of the
   new Complaints Regulations and consider how this is implemented in your
   department.

3. To what extent do you consider that complaints relating to community services
   need to be handled differently from those relating to hospital services?

4. Obtain a copy of Chapter 10 of the NHS Plan. How would you ensure that your
   clients were encouraged to be positively involved in the provision of services
   and the quality assurance mechanisms?

5. How are women involved in the provision of midwifery services in your
   organization?

6. Obtain a copy of the Inquiry into the Bristol children's heart surgery, study the
   recommendations under the heading Respect and Honesty and consider the
   extent to which your department complies with its proposals.

References

1 The National Health Service (Complaints) Regulations 2004, SI 2004 No 1768.

2 Department of Health. Being heard. The report of a review committee on NHS Complaints procedures. London: HMSO; 1994.

3 Department of Health. The NHS complaints procedure: National evaluation. London: HMSO; 2001.

4 Department of Health. Reforming the NHS complaints procedure: a listening document. London: HMSO; 2001.

5 Department of Health. Making amends. A consultation paper setting out proposals for reforming the approach to clinical negligence in the NHS. CMO June 2003.

6 Department of Health. NHS plan: A plan for investment, a plan for reform. London: HMSO; 2000.

7 Mental Health. (Correspondence of patients, patient advocacy and liaison services) Regulations 2003, SI 2003 No 2042.

8 NHS Reform and Health Care Professions Act 2002, s.15(3).

9 Patients' Forums (Functions) Regulations 2003 SI 2003 No 2124.

10 Patients' Forums (Membership and Procedure) Regulations 2003, SI 2003 No 2123.

11 Department of Health. Patient and public involvement – a brief overview. London: DoH; 4 November 2004.

12 Department of Health. Patient and public involvement forums go live. London: DoH; Press release 2003/0483 28 November 2003.

13 Department of Health. Better care, higher standards. London: DoH; 1999.

14 Department of Health. Meeting the standard? Analysis of the first round of local 'Better Care, Higher Standards' Charters.

15 Department of Health. Information on ICAS. Online. Available: www.doh.gov.uk/complaints

16 Department of Health. Involving patients and the public in healthcare. London: DoH; September 2001.

17 Department of Health. Online. Available: www.doh.gov.uk/complaints/advocacyservice.htm

18 Department of Health. Independent Complaints Advocacy Service (ICAS). The first year of ICAS, 1 September 2003–31 August 2004. London: DoH; 2005.

19 Department of Health. Involving patients and the public in healthcare. London: HMSO; 2001.

20 Department of Health. New voice for patients to shape local services. London: DoH; 2001: Press release.

21 Department of Health. Consultation on the future support arrangements for patient and public involvement in health (PPI), November 2004.

22 Department of Health. Patient and public involvement in health: the evidence for policy implementation, May 2004. Online. Available: www.dh.gov.uk/ppi

23 Department of Health. Christine Hogg Report on Patient and Public Involvement. London: DoH; 2005.

24 Department of Health. Press release 2005/0182, 19 May 2005.

25 Chief Medical Officer of the DoH. Supporting doctors, protecting patients. London: HMSO; 2000.

26 Bristol Royal Infirmary. Learning from Bristol: the report of the public inquiry into children's heart surgery at the Bristol Royal Infirmary 1984–1995 (The Kennedy Report). Command paper CM 5207; 2001. Online. Available: www.bristol-inquiry.org.uk

27 Dimond B. After Bristol: government support and rejection. Br J Midwifery 2002; 10(3):169–171.

28 Health Service Ombudsman. Making things better? A report on Reform in the NHS Complaints Procedure in England. London: The Stationery Office; 2005.

Chapter 12
TEENAGE PREGNANCIES

INTRODUCTION

A chapter devoted to this topic seemed justified because many legal concerns arise from the high level of under-age pregnancies in this country. This chapter should be read in conjunction with Chapter 32 on Child protection, Chapter 7 on Consent and Chapter 26 on Termination of pregnancy. In 2001, the Department of Health launched a campaign to bring the teenage pregnancy rate down and provide advice on sex and relationships. In November 2001, the Department of Health[1] announced the launch in 2002 of a national information campaign to promote sexual health as part of its National Strategy for sexual health and HIV. Teenage pregnancies place greater demands upon midwives, for which they require support and training.[2] Midwives should also be aware of the possibility of teenagers sharing prescription medication.[3]

This chapter considers the following topics:

- Legal position of the 16- and 17-year-old

- Legal position of the under 16-year-old

- Refusal to have treatment by a 16- or 17-year-old

- Refusal to have treatment by a child or young person under 16 years

- Human Rights

- Determining competence

- Decisions during the pregnancy and labour

- Rights of under-age parents to take decisions on behalf of their children

- Consent by an under-age girl to abortion

- Powers of parents: overruling a girl who wants to keep the child

- Confidentiality and keeping information away from the parents

- Young persons with learning disabilities

- Giving information about risks and sexual diseases

- Social services and the police, and the child under 13 years

- NSF for children, young people and maternity services

- Government and other initiatives and teenage pregnancy

LEGAL POSITION OF THE 16- AND 17-YEAR-OLD

A young person of 16 or 17 has a statutory right to give consent to treatment under s.8(1) of the Family Law Reform Act 1969. The definition of treatment under s.8(2) is comprehensive and covers medical, surgical, dental treatments and diagnostic and anaesthetic procedures. This would include termination of pregnancy. Under s.8(3), the right of a parent to give consent on behalf of a young person of 16 or 17 is preserved. However, it would be unwise to rely upon parental consent if the young person was opposed to the treatment offered. If there were a dispute between parents and a young person, it would be preferable to seek a declaration of the courts. There is a presumption in law that a young person of 16 or 17 has the capacity to give consent, but this presumption can be overruled if there is evidence to the contrary.

LEGAL POSITION OF THE UNDER 16-YEAR-OLD

A mentally competent girl, who understands the information given to her and appreciates the risks and benefits, can make treatment decisions for herself, without parental involvement. The decisions must be made in her best interests. This is the principle which was established by the House of Lords in the Gillick case,[4] from which the term 'Gillick competent child' came (an alternative term is 'competent according to Lord Fraser's guidelines', see Ch. 7). The level of capacity must relate to the nature of the decision to be made. The evidence that consent has been given could be shown by the use of Form 2 of the forms recommended by the Department of Health in its 'Good Practice in Consent Implementation Guide'.[5] The child as well as the parents could sign this form.

DETERMINING COMPETENCE

For an adult and a young person of 16 or 17, there is a presumption of capacity. This can be rebutted, if there is evidence to the contrary. The Court of Appeal in the case of Re MB[6] laid down the following test for the competence of the patient:

A person lacks the capacity (to give a valid consent) if some impairment or disturbance of mental functioning renders the person unable to make a decision whether to consent to or to refuse treatment. That inability to make a decision will occur when:

a. *The patient is unable to comprehend and retain the information which is material to the decision, especially as to the likely consequences of having or not having the treatment in question;*

b. *The patient is unable to use the information and weigh it in the balance as part of the process of arriving at the decision.*

The test in Re MB will be replaced by a statutory definition of capacity when the Mental Capacity Act 2005 is brought into force, which is expected to be April 2007 (see Ch. 7).

REFUSAL TO HAVE TREATMENT BY A YOUNG PERSON OF 16 OR 17 YEARS

The fact that the young person of 16 or 17 has a statutory right to give consent to treatment does not mean that they cannot be compelled to have treatment or that their refusal cannot be overruled. The Court of Appeal in the case of Re W[7] upheld the decision of the High Court judge to order a child of 16 years who was suffering from anorexia nervosa to undergo medical treatment against her will. Clearly over-ruling a child or young person's refusal is an extremely significant step to take and would only occur in very serious circumstances of a life-saving kind. In the case of a young person of 16 or 17, Form 1 of the forms recommended for use by the Department of Health in its publication 'Good Practice in Consent Implementation Guide'[5] could be completed.

Many factors will influence the answer to Jane's situation in Scenario 1 (Box 12.1). They include:

Box 12.1 Scenario 1: Refusal by the 16- or 17-year-old

Jane, aged 16 years, has become a member of a religious group which does not believe in surgical intervention. She is pregnant and has made it clear that she will refuse any surgical intervention said to be required. Late on in the pregnancy it is found that the fetus is in a transverse lie and only a caesarean section will save the life of the child and that of Jane. Jane is adamant that she will not agree to such a procedure.

– an assessment of her competence to refuse treatment

– her rights under the European Convention (especially Articles 3, 8, 9 and 14: see below)

– the fact that in the UK a fetus does not have a legal personality until it is born, and

– the power of the Court to make an order declaring that action can be taken to overrule the refusal of a young person, if that is in that person's best interests.

REFUSAL BY A CHILD OR YOUNG PERSON UNDER 16 YEARS

If a young person of 16 and 17 cannot in law refuse life-saving treatment if the treatment is in her best interests, it is even less likely that a child or young person under 16 years can refuse recommended treatment. In the case of Re M[8] a girl of 15 years refused to have a heart transplant which was essential for her survival. The parents sought an injunction from the court that the transplant operation could proceed, and this was granted in the best interests of the child.

HUMAN RIGHTS

Under the Human Rights Act 1998, a person is entitled to have their Rights as set out in the European Convention on Human Rights to be respected by public authorities. Article 3 is an absolute right and states that:

No one shall be subjected to torture or to inhuman or degrading treatment or punishment

It could be argued that overruling the refusal of a young person of 16 and 17, when the refusal of an adult would not be overruled, is inhuman and degrading. The point has yet to be established by the House of Lords.

Article 8 is a qualified right. It states that:

Everyone has the right to respect for private and family life, his home and his correspondence

This right is subject to the following qualifications:

There shall be no interference by a public authority with the exercise of the right except such as is in accordance with the law and is necessary in a democratic society in the interests of national security, public safety or the economic well-being of the country, for the prevention of disorder or crime, for the protection of health or morals, or for the protection of the rights and freedoms of others.

It could be argued that failure to respect the refusal or confidentiality of a young person and involving her parents is inhuman treatment and a breach of privacy. However, the age of the child would have to be taken into account and it could be argued that such rights are subject to the overriding duty to ensure that her life is protected and her parents informed of her condition.

Article 9 recognises the right to freedom of thought, conscience and religion. Jane belongs to a particular religious group and is entitled to have the practice of her beliefs protected. However, like Article 8 this is not an absolute right and is subject to several qualifications (see Appendix 1).

The extent to which a young person's refusal (on religious grounds) to have life-saving treatment is protected by the Articles of the European Convention on Human Rights has yet to be determined by the courts of this country. At present, the decision of the Court of Appeal in Re W is still valid. The BMA has published guidance on the rights of the child and young person, which considers both the legal and ethical issues[9] and the human rights dilemmas.

Even where the child and parents agree that treatment should not be given, as in the case of a Jehovah's Witness family, the court can order treatment to proceed if it is considered to be in the best interests of the child (Case of Re E).[10]

DECISIONS DURING THE PREGNANCY AND LABOUR

If a teenager requires interventions during the pregnancy, who should give consent?

If the teenager is 16 or 17 then she has a statutory right to give consent under s.8(1) of the Family Law Reform Act 1969, quoted above.

A teenager below 16 years can, if she is Gillick competent, give consent to treatment under the common law principles recognised by the House of Lords in the Gillick case. If however she is refusing necessary treatment, then her refusal can be overruled under the principle of Re W.[11] This is in contrast to the legal position where a mentally competent adult refuses treatment. The law states that an adult with the requisite mental capacity can refuse to give consent to life-saving treatment for a good reason, a bad reason or no reason at all.[12] Parents can give consent where a daughter is refusing life-saving treatment which is in her best interests. However, it is unlikely that health professionals would rely upon parental consent to overrule a refusal by a mentally competent teenager: it would be preferable to seek a declaration from the court. In the case of Glass[13] the European Court of Human Rights emphasised the importance of a court hearing in a dispute over the appropriate treatment for a child (see Ch. 9).

RIGHTS OF UNDER-AGE PARENTS TO TAKE DECISIONS ON BEHALF OF THEIR CHILDREN

If the mother in Scenario 2 (Box 12.2), even though she is under 16 years, is competent to make decisions on behalf of her child, then it is her wishes which will prevail. This is subject to her acting in the best interests of her child. Step-parents and grandparents (and others such as midwives and other health professionals or teachers) who do not have parental responsibilities but have temporary care of the child can make certain decisions in the interests of the child under s.3(5) of the Children Act 1989. This may well include giving consent to treatment in situations where those with parental responsibilities are unlikely to disagree. However, where there is clear conflict between the wishes of the mother and the grandmother, the wishes of the mother should prevail, provided that the best interests of the baby are served.

Box 12.2 Scenario 2: Who makes the decisions?

Grace is 14 years old and has a child of 6 months. She has decided that she does not want her daughter to have the triple vaccine. Grace's mother disagrees with her and wants to take her grandchild to have the vaccine. Who has the right to make the decision?

PARENTAL RESPONSIBILITIES

Where parents are married, both have decision-making powers in relation to the child and these continue unless the child dies or is adopted, even though the parents are divorced or separated. The unmarried father has no parental rights (even though he may be paying child maintenance) unless he has completed the appropriate forms. However, from December 2003, an unmarried couple have been able to register the birth together, in which case they both obtain parental rights.

GRANDPARENTS AND THEIR RIGHTS AND RESPONSIBILITIES

Where a teenager has a child and lacks the capacity to make her own decisions, her parents are asked to make decisions both on behalf of their daughter and also on behalf of their grandchild. Clearly any such decisions must be made in the best interests of both the young person and the child and if it was feared that this was not the case, then action should be taken under the Children Act 1989 to ensure that the best interests of both were being considered. The basic principle at the heart of the Children Act 1989 is that the welfare of the child is the paramount consideration. Parents have a responsibility under the Children Act 1989 to take action for the welfare of their children. They also have powers at common law and recognised by the Family Law Reform Act 1969 s.8(3) to give consent on behalf of their children until they become adults at 18 years (see above).

CONSENT BY AN UNDER-AGE GIRL TO ABORTION

It follows from Scenario 3 (Box 12.3) that a competent girl of 14 years could make a decision to have a termination of pregnancy. Clearly any counselling preceding the termination should have included information on how the termination would take place, what the procedure would be and how it would be preferable if the parents were informed. The young person's confidentiality should be respected. However, in Avril's case there are considerable dangers if she leaves hospital, unaccompanied, in the middle of the termination and her parents are ignorant of her condition. Since she is only 14, it is suggested that nursing staff would have a responsibility to ensure that steps are taken in her best interests to prevent serious harm to her, and this may mean informing the parents or ensuring that she is accompanied home. In Scenario 3, the parents are not aware of the situation of Avril, who has asked for them to be kept in ignorance. As soon as Avril refuses to accept the necessity of completing the termination under the supervision of health professionals, she puts her life at risk. Action can then be taken lawfully to save her life. In spite of Avril's fears, it is preferable for her parents to be notified: they could give consent for treatment to be continued in her best interests. If, on the other hand, Avril's parents as Roman Catholics would have wished the termination to be halted (if this is practicable), then a court hearing under the Children Act 1989 may be necessary to determine what action should be taken to protect the welfare of Avril. The court would act on the principle that 'the welfare of the child is the paramount consideration' and this may result in the court agreeing that the termination could proceed in Avril's best interests, despite the opposition of the parents, as the case below illustrates.

Box 12.3 Scenario 3: Under-age abortion

Avril, a girl of 14, had agreed to a termination of her pregnancy without the consent or knowledge of her parents. The termination was to be carried out in two stages. She took the required medication for the first stage and then was admitted to hospital for an estimated 12 hours for the termination to take place. At nine o'clock in the evening after she had been in hospital for 6 hours, she stated that she was now going home. The nurses strongly advised her to stay since she could haemorrhage, which could be life-threatening. Avril said that her mother was not aware that she was having a termination, that her parents were devout Roman Catholics and would turn her out if they knew about it, and it was essential that she returned home before they found out.

MOTHER IGNORANT OF DAUGHTER'S ABORTION

In a highly publicised case in May 2004, a mother only discovered by chance that her daughter was having an abortion.[14] The mother spoke of her horror at the situation and said, 'I feel like my right as a parent has been taken away from me. I feel like I've had my heart ripped out'.

The facts suggest that the mother only found out by chance from a passer-by in the street that the girl had had a pill to commence the termination. The mother then talked to her daughter about it and brought the unborn child's father and his mother into the discussion. The girl changed her mind about the termination and they contacted King's Mill Hospital in Sutton-in-Ashfield, which initially was reported to have told them that the pregnancy could be saved, but next day it was found that the situation was irretrievable. The mother later said that had she not found out about the situation the girl would have gone to hospital to undergo an abortion without a member of the family with her. A trustee of the charity Life is reported to have said that teachers should consult parents in confidence if they are the first to know. 'This incident has got at least three victims – the girl, her mother and the unborn baby'. (It was subsequently reported on 22 July 2005 that the girl later had a baby boy 13 months after the termination of her earlier pregnancy.)

There is no doubt that on the basis of the Gillick judgement in the House of Lords, the teachers who respected the confidence of the girl and failed to tell her parents were acting within the law, if they assessed her as Gillick competent. A test of competence would have been applied to the ability of the girl to decide upon the termination of pregnancy and also to respecting her confidentiality and not informing the parents. If this test of competence is satisfied, then it is lawful for the termination to take place if the statutory provisions are present. The mother of the girl in the reported case has said that she wishes to challenge the law. If this occurs, then the House of Lords may eventually be revisiting the grounds it considered in the Gillick case in 1985. Many however would feel that, in spite of possible criticisms, to accept that children and young persons below 16 years can make appropriate treatment decisions and have their confidentiality respected is a significant aspect of the rights of the child.

PARENTAL RIGHTS AND RESPONSIBILITIES

It could be said that there are ambiguities in our present laws: parents who fail to ensure that their under-age child attends school could be imprisoned for the truancy of their child, yet those same parents could be kept in ignorance that the child was attending an abortion clinic. Clearly any person counselling a teenager before an abortion would strongly recommend that the girl tells her parents, but if the girl is adamant that she wishes her confidentiality to be respected and she appears to have the necessary competence, it would be a breach of confidentiality to contact the parents contrary to her wishes. Only if there were serious child protection issues arising or serious harm were feared to the mental or physical health of the girl would a breach of confidentiality be justified.

PARENTS WISHING TO PREVENT TERMINATION PROCEEDING

It does not follow that, because parents can give a valid consent for treatment in the best interests of the children, they have the right to forbid a termination of pregnancy taking place. In the case of Re P,[15] a girl of 15 who had already given birth to a boy, and was in the care of the local authority, became pregnant again. Her parents wished to prevent her having an abortion and refused to give consent. The girl herself wished to have an abortion and the requirements of the Abortion Act 1967 were satisfied. The judge, Mrs Justice Butler-Sloss, using the test that the welfare of the girl was of paramount importance, decided that the termination should proceed (see Ch. 26). Roman Catholic parents do not therefore have a right to stop a termination of pregnancy going ahead: as long as the provisions of the Abortion Act 1967 are satisfied and the girl has the mental competence to give a valid consent, the termination can proceed.

TO GIVE CONSENT ON BEHALF OF THEIR CHILDREN

Parents have a responsibility under the Children Act 1989 to take action for the welfare of their children. They also have powers at common law and recognised by the Family Law Reform Act 1969 s.8(3) to give consent on behalf of their children until they become adults at 18 years.

POWERS OF PARENTS: OVERRULING A GIRL WHO WANTS TO KEEP THE CHILD

If the girl decided to keep the baby, she would of course be dependent upon parental support to keep it. If there is evidence that there is a conflict between the young girl who wishes to keep the baby and the parents who wish her to have a termination, the midwife and other health professionals should ensure that the girl's wishes are bolstered.

Where the teenager decides to continue with the pregnancy, many issues arise in relation to the rights of the parents of the teenager (and future grandparents of the baby) and the teenager, as is illustrated in Scenario 4 (Box 12.4).

Box 12.4 Scenario 4: Rights of decision making in a teenage pregnancy

Karen is 14 years old and pregnant. Her mother wishes her to live in the family home and intends to bring her grandchild up as her own child. Karen wants to make the decisions about the baby for herself. What legal principles apply?

If Karen is Gillick competent, then she can give consent both on her own account and also for the care of her child, as long as the decision is in the best interests of the child. However, Karen is only 14 years old; she is entitled to protection under the Children Act. She will clearly be the responsibility of the social services. It may be that social services will provide her with accommodation for her and her child, but if her parents are willing to look after her and her baby, there would have to be an agreement between social services, the parents and Karen as to what is in the best interests of Karen and her baby.

CONFIDENTIALITY AND KEEPING INFORMATION AWAY FROM THE PARENTS

There is no doubt that on the basis of the Gillick judgement in the House of Lords, the midwife or other health professionals who respected the confidence of the girl, and failed to tell her parents about a termination taking place, would be acting within the law. A test of competence would have been applied to the ability of the girl to decide upon the termination of pregnancy and also to respect her confidentiality by not informing the parents. If this test of competence is satisfied, then it is lawful for the termination to take place if the statutory provisions are present, without informing the parents.

Avril (in Box 12.3) has asked that her parents should not be informed of the termination. If she is Gillick competent and there is no danger to herself or other people, this confidence can be kept. However, an exception to the duty of confidentiality recognised by the Courts[16] and in the Code of Practice of the NMC is disclosure in the public interest, for example where serious harm to physical or mental health of the patient or other persons is feared. Notifying parents about Avril's situation may therefore be a justifiable exception to the duty of confidentiality. Clearly such a decision must be in the best interests of Avril.

YOUNG PERSONS WITH LEARNING DISABILITIES

When 16 years old, the young person with severe learning disabilities would not be able to benefit from the statutory right to make treatment decisions under s.8 of the Family Law Reform Act 1969 because the presumption of mental capacity would be rebutted. Decisions could still be made on the young person's behalf by the parents. These decisions must be in the best interests of the young person and an appropriate declaration could be sought from the court. Parents can give consent to treatment on behalf of their children up to 18 years.

When the young person becomes an adult at 18 years old, parents no longer have the right in law to make decisions on behalf of their child. In England, Wales and Northern Ireland, there has been a vacuum in the statute law (in Scotland, the Adults with Incapacity (Scotland) Act 2000 applies) which has been filled by a decision of the House of Lords in Re F.[17] In this case, the House of Lords said that there was power at common law (judge-made law or case law) for health professionals to act in the best interests of a mentally incapacitated adult. In the actual case, the House of Lords declared that carrying out a sterilisation operation on a woman with severe learning disabilities would be lawful if the operation was in her best interests and carried out according to the reasonable standards of professional care. Where it is recommended that treatment should be carried out in the best interests of a mentally incapacitated adult, Form 4 in the Department of Health's Good Practice in Consent implementation guide could be used as evidence of the fact that the decision was taken in the best interests of the mentally incapacitated adult, and that relatives were advised about the need for such treatment and were aware that the patient was incapable of giving consent him or herself.

The Mental Capacity Act 2005 (see Ch. 7) is due to be brought into force in April 2007. It will establish a statutory framework for the making of decisions on behalf of mentally incapacitated adults.

The Sexual Offences Act 2003 (see below and Ch. 32) creates offences under ss.30–33 designed to give protection to persons with a mental disorder which impedes choice, so even though a young person is over 13 years and does not come under those offences which rule out the consent of a child under 13 as a defence, the young person may still be a victim of a criminal offence. Sections 34, 35, 36 and 37 create offences in relation to providing inducements to persons with a mental disorder to engage in sexual activity and ss.38–43 create offences in relation to care workers and sexual activity with a person with a mental disorder.

GIVING INFORMATION ABOUT RISKS AND SEXUAL DISEASES

The duty of care includes the duty to inform the patient of all significant risks of substantial harm which could arise from any treatment which is recommended. Information giving is part of the duty of care of health professionals and therefore in order that both the child/young person or the parent can understand the implications of giving consent to treatment, they need to be told the significant risks of substantial harm which could occur and also the existence of alternative treatments or even of no treatments. The British Medical Association publication[18] which considers the rights of the child emphasises the importance of ensuring that appropriate information is given to the child or young person. Unless information is shared with a child, the child will become disempowered and their understanding of their condition will be reduced. Clearly, it is essential that this sharing of information takes place sensitively and appropriately according to the level of maturity of the child. Children with long-term chronic conditions often develop an understanding and maturity beyond their physical years, but this will only occur if information is shared with them.

The answer to Scenario 5 (Box 12.5) relating to Mavis depends upon her capacity. If she is capable of understanding the implications of the genetic disorder and make an appropriate decision, then to withhold that information from her prevents her from realising her options. Under the amended Abortion Act (see Ch. 26), a termination can be carried out without limitation of time if two registered medical practi-

Box 12.5 Scenario 5: Duty to inform

Mavis, aged 15, is pregnant and her parents agree with the midwife that she should not be informed that there is a danger that the baby could suffer from a genetic disorder for which the grandparents are carriers. After the birth of the baby, it is discovered that the baby is a sufferer, and Mavis is then furious that she was not warned, since she says that she would have preferred to have had a termination. The parents say that that is why they decided to withhold the information.

tioners are of the opinion formed in good faith that there is substantial risk that if the child were born it would suffer from such physical or mental abnormalities as to be seriously handicapped.

SOCIAL SERVICES AND THE POLICE AND THE CHILD UNDER 13 YEARS

The social services authority has statutory duties under the Children Act 1989 to act in the protection of children. If there is any concern about the welfare of a child and the need to refer a child to court, then social services must be informed. The Sexual Offences Act 2003 (see Ch. 32) makes it a criminal offence for a person to penetrate with a penis, any other body part or object the vagina, anus or mouth of a child under 13 years and the consent of the child is no defence. Other offences are created in relation to causing or inciting a child under 13 years to engage in sexual activity. Whether or not the police should be informed when it appears that an offence has been committed is often left to health professionals to determine, normally in consultation with social services. A prosecution does not always follow the reporting of the offence: it all depends upon the circumstances. However, these new offences with the express provision that the consent of a child under 13 years is no defence raises major issues of public policy for those providing contraceptives to girls below 13 years (refer also to Ch. 32 on Child Protection).

CHILDREN, YOUNG PEOPLE AND MATERNITY SERVICES NATIONAL SERVICE FRAMEWORK (NSF)

In September 2004 the NSF for Children, Young People and Maternity Services was published. Standard 4 relates to growing up into adulthood and states:

All young people have access to age-appropriate services which are responsible to their specific needs as they grow into adulthood.

This comprises the following subsections:

- Services implement policies and good practice guidelines on consent and confidentiality policies for young people.

- Health promotion for young people is targeted to meet their needs and, in particular, to reduce teenage pregnancy; smoking, substance misuse, sexually transmitted infections and suicide. Young people are actively involved in planning and implementing health promotion services and initiatives.

- Services support young people to achieve their full potential by providing targeted support through coordinated working, for example, Connexions and Youth Services. This includes addressing their social and emotional needs as well as assisting their educational and career development.

- There is improved access to services and advice for young people – in particular, addressing the needs of disabled young people, young people in special circumstances and those who live in rural areas.

- Transition to adult services for young people is planned and coordinated around the needs of each young person to maximise health outcomes, their life chance opportunities and their ability to live independently – this is particularly important for disabled young people or those with long-term or complex conditions.

- Additional support is available for looking after children leaving care and other young people in special circumstances.

COMMENT ON THE NSF

Midwives who are involved in the care of young women should find that the NSF is of assistance in attracting resources to implement the stated standards. Strategic planning of the services for teenagers should take account of the NSF and other Department of Health guidance.

GOVERNMENT AND OTHER INITIATIVES AND TEENAGE PREGNANCY

A National Strategy for Sexual Health and HIV implementation plan was published in June 2002,[19] which set out details of how the interventions proposed in the strategy would be delivered. A cross-Government unit located within the Department of Education and Skills has set up a teenage pregnancy unit with its own website.[20] The unit was set up to implement the Social Exclusion Unit's report on Teenage Pregnancy. The Teenage Pregnancy Unit website contains lists of other useful websites for teenagers and parents, providing advice on sexual health and related issues. An overview of the research to support those engaged in implementing the national teenage pregnancy strategy has been provided by the Health Development Agency.[21]

An Independent Advisory Group (IAG) on Sexual Health and HIV established in 2003 was part of the implementation Action Plan for the National Strategy for Sexual Health and HIV. In 2004, this IAG published its response to the Health Select Committee on Sexual Health.[22] It considered access to services, capacity, commissioning and prioritisation, funding prevention, education and sexual health promotion, and the patient voice. It agreed with the Select Committee's conclusions on the six key factors which were the principal causes of the current situation:

1. A failure of local NHS organisations to recognise and deal with this major public health problem

2. A lack of political pressure and leadership over many years

3. The absence of a patient voice

4. A lack of resources

5. A lack of central direction to suggest that this is a key priority

6. An absence of performance management.

It believed that sexual health and HIV must be explicitly prioritised at both a local and national level. A news item in the Royal College of Midwives Journal warns that the teenage pregnancy strategy contributes to a rise in sexually transmitted diseases.[23]

The British Medical Association published a report in December 2003 on adolescent health and highlighted weaknesses in controlling the epidemic of sexually transmitted infections.

Figures were released by the Office for National Statistics (ONS) in February 2005 which showed that teenage pregnancies had fallen to their lowest rate since 1995, with about 4% of girls aged under 18 years becoming pregnant in a year. The most common factors in teenage pregnancies were poverty, truancy and low educational achievement.[24] A government spokesman stated that the new certificate in sexual health for teachers and schemes to train midwives and health visitors in giving advice on second pregnancies were having an impact on bringing down the pregnancy rate. The ONS figures also showed that abortions were at an all-time high (see Ch. 26).

CONCLUSIONS

At the time of writing, the law is unclear on the extent to which the Articles of the European Convention on Human Rights protect the refusal of a Gillick competent child to have life-saving treatment. Presently, we need a House of Lords decision on whether a young person's right to refuse life-saving treatment can be upheld under Articles 3, 8 and 9 and when that refusal can be overruled in the best interests of the young person. Midwives are often caught up in conflicts: the rights of the teenager against the powers of her parents; her right to confidentiality against the need to act in the best interests of her safety and that of her child; the right to privacy of the teenager and the public interest in bringing to justice those who have committed criminal offences. Experienced senior staff and supervisors should be consulted over the action to be taken, and when it is necessary to seek the advice of the NHS trust lawyer and seek a declaration of the court. The fact that it is legally no longer a defence that a child under 13 gave consent to sexual activity must be taken into account in determining the action which should be taken in protecting young persons. It is essential that comprehensive records should be kept of the action taken and the justification for that action.

Legal issues relating to abortion are considered in Chapter 26 and pregnancy in Chapter 14. For some of the complex legal issues which can arise in this field see Dimond (2002).[25]

The Maternity Alliance has produced an updated version of its leaflet 'Money for teenage parents 2004, your benefits and entitlements'. This covers recent changes in benefits which affect young parents, including the education maintenance allowance.[26]

References

1 Department of Health press release 2001/0579 29 November 2001.

2 Shakespeare D. Exploring midwives' attitude to teenage pregnancy. Br J Midwifery 2004; 12(5):320–326, 329.

3 Daniel KL, Honein MA, Moore CA. Sharing prescription medication among teenage girls: potential danger to unplanned/undiagnosed pregnancies. Pediatrics 2003; 111(5):1167–1170.

4 Gillick v. West Norfolk and Wisbech Area Health Authority [1986] 1 A.C. 112.

5 Department of Health. Good practice in consent implementation guide: consent to examination or treatment. London: The Stationery Office; 2001.

6 Re MB (caesarean Section) (1997) 2 FLR 426.

7 Re W (A Minor) (Medical Treatment: Court's Jurisdiction) [1992] 4 All E.R. 627.

8 Re M (A Minor) (Medical Treatment) (1999) 2 FLR 1097.

9 British Medical Association. Consent, Rights and Choices in Health Care for Children and Young People. London: BMJ Books; 2001.

10 Re E (A Minor) (Wardship: Medical Treatment) (1993) 1 FLR 386.

11 Re W (A minor) (medical treatment) 1992 4 All ER 627.

12 Re MB (An Adult: Medical Treatment) [1997] 2 FLR 426

13 Glass v. United Kingdom. The Times Law Report, 11 March 2004 ECHR; 61827/00 [2004] Lloyd's Rep Med 76; [2004] 1 FLR 1019.

14 Willey J. School fix abortion for girl, 14. The Daily Express, 13 May 2004.

15 Re P (A Minor) (1982) 80 LGR 301.

16 W. v. Egdell 1989 1 All ER 1089.

17 Re F (Mental Patient: Sterilisation) (1990) 2 A.C. 1.

18 British Medical Association. Consent, rights and choices in health care for children and young people. London: BMA Books; 2000.

19 Department of Health. National Strategy for Sexual Health and HIV implementation action plan, June 2002.

20 Department of Health. Online. Available: www.info.doh.gov.uk/tpu/tpu.nsf/vwWebHome?OpenView

21 Health Development Agency. Teenage Pregnancy: an overview of research evidence, 2004.

22 Independent Advisory Group on Sexual Health and HIV. Response to the Health Select Committee Report on Sexual Health. DoH January 2004.

23 News item. Teenage pregnancy strategy contributes to STIs. Royal College of Midwives J 2004; 7(5):184.

24 Blair A. Teenage pregnancies lowest for decade. The Times, 25 February 2005.

25 Dimond B. Teenage pregnancy and the law. Br J Midwifery 2002; 10(2):1005–1008.

26 Maternity Alliance. Contact: Tel: 020 7490 7639, ext. 134. Online. Available: www.maternityalliance.org.uk

SECTION C

LITIGATION AND ACCOUNTABILITY

In Section C of this book, aspects of the law relating to the accountability of the midwife are considered. The midwife is accountable for her practice before the Statutory Committees of the NMC (see Ch. 4) and before her employer's disciplinary machinery if she is in breach of the terms of her contract of employment (see Ch. 22). In addition, she may face criminal proceedings if she is guilty of an offence, or civil proceedings if there is a claim brought against her or her employer in respect of her alleged negligent practice. Chapter 13 considers the general principles involved in the bringing of a civil action for compensation. Chapter 14 will consider special areas, and the final chapters in this Section of the book look at cases involving negligent sterilisation and abortion, liability in the criminal law including health and safety laws and the rights of the fetus. Finally, the law relating to the administration of medicinal products and liability in negligence will be considered.

Chapter 13
NEGLIGENCE

As patients seek compensation for alleged harm, litigation is increasing and the greatest risk area is obstetrics. In a recent report of the National Audit Office,[1] it was stated that the NHS expects to pay out £5.89 billion, at today's prices, over a number of years in respect of known or expected claims . . . An additional £3.2 billion of claims are possible but unlikely. The 2001–2 NAO report[2] noted that the number and value of claims continued to rise, and they were taking on average about 5.5 years to settle. Somewhat startlingly, it was found that nearly half of the claims settled in 1999–2000 cost more in legal and other costs than the settlement itself. For settlements of up to £50 000, the costs of reaching the settlement are greater than the damages awarded in over 65% of the cases.[3] In the light of this report, the Department of Health has proposed a new compensation scheme which is considered in Chapter 14. Some of the largest sums of money are awarded in birth damage cases, with examples of claims of £2 million now being awarded or agreed.

There are concerns that the fear of litigation has led to defensive medical practice and to a reluctance to enter high-risk spheres of practice.[4] Even if the midwife is not personally at fault, she may well be involved and have to give evidence in a case brought because of alleged negligence by an obstetrician or other colleagues. It is therefore important for a midwife to understand the law relating to negligence, and her own position should an action in respect of her negligence be brought.

Midwives who are employed will rarely be the defendants, since the person seeking compensation, the claimant (formerly known as the plaintiff), will normally bring the action against the employer on the basis of its vicarious liability for the negligent actions of its employees while acting in course of employment. Independent midwives, who have no employer, would however be sued personally (see Ch. 23). Employed midwives who act as a midwife for friends and relatives outside the course of employment could also be sued personally. This is further explained below.

NEGLIGENCE

An action for negligence is the most frequent civil action brought in order to obtain compensation. It is one of a group of civil wrongs known as 'torts'. An action would be brought in the county court where less than £50 000 was being claimed. Claims above that amount would be brought in the High Court – the Queen's Bench Division (see Ch. 1). Other torts which the midwife may come across are set out in Box 13.1.

> ## Box 13.1 Civil actions known as 'torts'
>
> – Action for negligence
>
> – Action for breach of statutory duty
>
> – Action for trespass to the person, goods or land (this is considered in Ch. 7 on Consent)
>
> – An action for nuisance
>
> – An action for defamation (which includes libel and slander).

This chapter covers the following topics:

– The elements which the claimant must establish to prove liability in negligence

– Vicarious liability of the employer compared with personal liability of the employee

– How compensation is calculated

– Defences to an action for negligence

– The NHS Litigation Authority and the Clinical Negligence Scheme for Trusts.

In Chapter 14, detailed facts from decided cases will be considered, together with some specialist areas of litigation and the procedure for litigation in the civil courts.

LIABILITY IN NEGLIGENCE

To obtain compensation in an action for negligence, the claimant must establish the elements shown in Box 13.2.

> ## Box 13.2 Elements in an action for negligence
>
> 1. The defendant owed a duty of care to the claimant.
>
> 2. The defendant was in breach of that duty of care, and
>
> 3. as a reasonably foreseeable result of that breach,
>
> 4. harm recognised by the courts as subject to compensation was caused.

The burden is on the claimant to establish on a balance of probabilities that each of the four elements shown in Box 13.2 is present.

DUTY OF CARE

Usually it is fairly clear if the law would recognise a duty of care as being owed to an individual in the context of healthcare. The midwife clearly has a duty of care towards all her clients. This may include others for whom she is not directly responsible but whom she is asked to care for. It may also, depending upon her contract of employment, require her to return from off duty in a crisis. The duty will certainly involve the need to communicate with the mother and relatives and colleagues. The duty to inform the mother about significant risks is as much a part of the duty of care as treatment and midwifery procedures. The duty to inform is considered in Chapter 8.

The definition of the duty of care was raised in a House of Lords case in 1932.[5] It was concerned with the question of whether a manufacturer owed a duty of care to the ultimate consumer, regardless of who had paid for the product.

The facts in this case were that the claimant alleged that she had drunk ginger beer which contained the decomposed remains of a snail, and held the manufacturers liable for the harm she suffered. The case went to the House of Lords over the issue of whether the manufacturers owed a duty of care to her. In a majority decision, the House of Lords decided in her favour. This may seem very remote from the duty of care owed by a midwife, but the statement of Lord Justice Atkins is very important in defining duty of care. He said:

You must take reasonable care to avoid acts or omissions which you can reasonably foresee would be likely to injure your neighbour. Who then, in law, is my neighbour? The answer seems to be persons who are so closely and directly affected by my act that I ought reasonably to have them in contemplation as being so affected when I am directing my mind to the acts or omissions which are called in question.

Usually there is no dispute that a duty of care is owed by a midwife to her clients and the babies. However, there can be situations where the existence of a legal duty of care is disputed. For example, it follows from the statement quoted above that the midwife would have a duty of care to ensure that reasonable care was taken of toddlers brought by mothers to clinics: cupboards containing dangerous substances should not be left unlocked and within their reach. However, it also follows that no person has a duty to volunteer help, if a duty of care does not already exist.

Is there a duty to volunteer?
The law does not require an individual to volunteer help unless there is a pre-existing duty. Thus, if a midwife were on holiday in Brighton, sunning herself on the beach, and she noticed that a heavily pregnant woman a few yards away had gone into

labour, the law would not require her to rush to the woman saying 'I am a midwife. Let me help.' So if in such circumstances the midwife were to refuse assistance and if the pregnant woman, realising that there was a midwife on the beach who could have assisted her and prevented harm arising, were to sue the midwife for breach of a duty to care, it is probable that such an action would fail. The existence of a duty of care owed by the holidaying midwife to the pregnant woman would not be established in law. However, the NMC has made it clear in its Code of Professional Conduct: standards for performance, conduct and ethics[6] that there is professional duty upon the registered practitioner at all times. Para. 8.5 states:

In an emergency, in or outside the work setting, you have a professional duty to provide care. The care provided would be judged against what could reasonably be expected from someone with your knowledge, skills and abilities when placed in those particular circumstances.

This means that failure to volunteer help in certain situations could be seen as evidence of lack of fitness to practise. Of course, once a practitioner volunteers to take on a duty of care, then she is required in law to follow the reasonable standard of care and could be held accountable for any failures. It is unlikely that her employer would accept vicarious liability for such Good Samaritan acts, so a midwife would require professional indemnity insurance cover (see below).

Of what does the duty consist?

The duty of care would include not only duties in relation to treatment and care, and in giving information, but also duties relating to the keeping of satisfactory records, duties in relation to management of the situation, of supervision and delegation to other staff, and all actions necessary to ensure that the mother and baby will be reasonably safe. A duty would also be held to exist in relation to colleagues, to ensure that they are reasonably safe. All those elements identified by the WHO and the EC and discussed in Chapter 2 as activities of the midwife would be considered to be part of the duty of care.

The Court of Appeal has held that an ambulance service could owe a duty of care to an individual member of the public, once an emergency phone call providing personal details of that person had been accepted by the service.[7] The London Ambulance Service was held liable when the ambulance took 38 min to arrive to assist a pregnant woman who was asthmatic. The time of arrival had been falsely recorded. As a result of the delay, the woman suffered respiratory arrest with catastrophic results, including substantial memory impairment, personality change and a miscarriage.

Would there be a duty in relation to the children of the client?

Certainly, if in preparing for the delivery, whether at home or in hospital, the midwife is aware that there are young children who should be supervised, she would probably have a responsibility to ensure that a person took over the care of the children, and to take any other action which would be reasonably required in the circumstances. The duty of the occupier to visitors is considered in Chapter 19.

In 2005, the Court of Appeal ruled that council education officers were professionals who owed a duty of care towards the child with special educational needs[8] if it was established that damage was reasonably foreseeable, the test of proximity was satisfied and the situation was one in which it was fair, just and reasonable that the law should impose a duty of care. On the facts of the case, however, the Court of Appeal held that there was no evidence of a breach of that duty of care.

DUTY TO PARENTS

The House of Lords (in a majority verdict) has held that healthcare and other childcare professionals did not owe a common law duty of care to parents against whom they had made unfounded allegations of child abuse and who, as a result, suffered psychiatric injury (see Ch. 32).[9]

The House of Lords has also held[10] that the police owed no duty of care to victims or witnesses. It confirmed an earlier decision[11] in a case brought by the mother of one of the Yorkshire Ripper's later victims, that while ethically, police should treat victims and witnesses properly and with respect, this ethical duty was not converted into a legal duty of care. The prime function of the police was the preservation of the Queen's peace.

STANDARD OF CARE

The claimant (formerly known as the plaintiff, i.e. the person suing for compensation) has to show that the defendant acted in breach of the duty of care. This is the 'fault element' which is required under the present laws to obtain compensation. In order to show that there has been a breach, it is first necessary to establish what standard should have been followed and how the defendant's actions differed, if at all, from what it was reasonable to expect.

The courts use a test known as the 'Bolam Test' to determine the standard expected from professionals. The name derives from a case heard in 1957[12] where a psychiatric patient was given electro-convulsive therapy without any relaxant drugs or restraint. He suffered several fractures and claimed compensation against Friern Hospital Management Committee. Mr Justice McNair, in deciding how to determine the standard which should have been followed, said:

When you get a situation which involved the use of some special skill or competence, then the test as to whether there has been negligence or not is . . . the standard of the ordinary skilled man exercising and professing to have that special skill. A man need not possess the highest expert skill; it is well-established that it is sufficient if he exercises the ordinary skill of an ordinary competent man exercising that particular art.

He added later:

He is not guilty of negligence if he has acted in accordance with a practice accepted as proper by a responsible body of medical men skilled in that particular art.

The Bolam Test has since been applied to a variety of professions including solicitors, architects, surveyors, etc. It relates to the standards which were reasonably expected at the time the alleged negligent act took place. It thus enables the standards applied by the courts to change, and for professionals to be judged against the standards of the time of the alleged negligent acts, not the standards which existed at the time of the court hearing which may be many years later.

In the actual case of Bolam, the patient lost his claim. However, were the same facts to occur in the twenty-first century, there would probably be an offer to settle without any attempt to defend the case, since standards are much higher now.

The Bolam Test was applied by the House of Lords in a case involving a brain-damaged baby (Whitehouse v. Jordan 1981).[13]

The facts (in brief – the full facts are discussed in Ch. 14) of this case were as follows:

Stuart Whitehouse was born in January 1970 with severe brain damage. His mother alleged that the brain damage was caused because the doctor pulled too hard and too long with forceps, as a consequence of which the baby was severely disabled. The doctor denied the allegations. The mother won the case in the High Court and £100 000 was awarded.

The doctor appealed, and this was allowed by the Court of Appeal, on the grounds that an error of judgement was not negligence. The mother then appealed to the House of Lords. Among the issues the House of Lords had to decide was the extent to which an error of judgement was or was not negligence. In applying the Bolam Test to the facts, the House of Lords made it clear that there was no absolute rule relating to errors of judgement; they may or may not constitute negligence depending on the circumstances and what would have been the standard of the ordinary skilled man exercising and professing to have that special skill.

If a surgeon failed to measure up to that, in any respect ('clinical judgement' or otherwise) he had been negligent and should be so adjudged.

Further discussion of this case can be found in Chapter 14.

What if there are different opinions over the standard which should be followed?

Mr Justice McNair in the Bolam case referred to the fact that there are sometimes differences of opinion, and quoted from an earlier case (Hunter v. Hanley 1955)[14]:

In the realm of diagnosis and treatment there is ample scope for genuine difference of opinion, and one man clearly is not negligent merely because his conclusion differs from that of other professional men, nor because he has displayed less skill or knowledge than others would have shown. The true test for establishing negligence in diagnosis or treatment on the part of a doctor is whether he has been proved to be guilty of such failure as no doctor of ordinary skill would be guilty of, if acting with ordinary care.

This principle was followed in the case of Maynard v. West Midlands Regional Health Authority (Box 13.3).[15]

Box 13.3 Maynard v. West Midlands Regional Health Authority

Mrs Maynard had been advised to have a biopsy in order to establish whether she was suffering from Hodgkin's Disease. It seemed likely that her symptoms were those of TB, but because of the possibility of the prognosis of recovery from Hodgkin's Disease being improved with earlier treatment, it was important to eliminate that possibility as soon as possible. The operation of mediastinoscopy to provide a biopsy was performed and unfortunately caused damage to her left laryngeal nerve. The biopsy was found to be negative and the patient was diagnosed as suffering from TB. She was then advised that her condition was clearly one of TB and there was no need for the biopsy to have been performed. She therefore sued the Regional Health Authority and the doctor.

Mrs Maynard lost the case, the House of Lords holding the following:

It was not sufficient to establish negligence for the plaintiff (i.e. claimant) to show that there was a body of competent professional opinion that considered the decision as wrong, if there was also a body of equally competent professional opinion that supported the decision as having been reasonable in the circumstances.

The lessons of this are clear for midwives:

– First, the midwife must ensure that she understands what are the present standards of care which would be provided by a reasonable midwife in any specific circumstances. This means that she must be aware of the protocols, guidelines and procedures which have been drawn up both nationally and locally.

- Second, she must also have an understanding as to the circumstances in which any reasonable midwife would depart from the agreed protocols because of the particular circumstances of the situation. This means that midwifery will never become simply a book of regulations which must be followed. There will always be a need for professional judgement and discretion to be exercised.

- Third, the midwife should ensure that her records show accurately the particular circumstances which provided the justification for departing from the agreed procedure. Should harm occur to the mother and/or child and the midwife be challenged on what she had done, she would require comprehensive clear records to defend her actions.

- Fourth, she must keep up-to-date and ensure that her knowledge, skill and experience is constantly updated, since the standards improve and she would be judged against those expected of her at the time, not those which applied several years before.

- Fifth, in any area of development where standards are not certain, she should obtain as much information as possible to ensure that she can care for the mother and baby safely. This is a particular issue with waterbirths, which are discussed in Chapter 6.

How do local standards relate to national standards?

The courts are concerned with applying what it is reasonable for a claimant to expect from the professionals. Expert witnesses would give evidence for both claimant and defence (there are new rules for expert evidence, see below) on what standards could have been expected. If local standards are lower than that which could be expected nationally, they would not suffice. Local standards may however be higher than national standards, where a specialist service is offered. For example, it may be that a trust advertises itself as being able to provide a specific form of childbirth not generally available, and has referrals on that basis. If in carrying out this special procedure, harm occurs as a result of negligence by a member of staff, it would not be acceptable as a defence for the trust to say that no other hospital could have performed the technique better.

How do protocols relate to the Bolam Test?

Many trusts have now devised their own protocols for midwifery practice. For example, antenatal protocols may be devised for identifying risk factors at the initial antenatal booking. If these protocols conformed to what would be the reasonable practice of a midwife following the practice accepted as proper by a responsible body of midwives, then in normal circumstances it would be expected that these protocols should be followed. However, there may well be circumstances in which the midwife would be acting reasonably in not following the protocol to the letter. Her independent professional judgement can never be replaced by reliance upon a set procedure. Compliance levels in conforming to protocols may vary for a variety of reasons.[16]

A useful consideration of the legal implications of guidelines, policies, protocols and procedures is given by Brian Hurwitz.[17] He discusses the circumstances where it is negligent not to follow guidelines and also those situations where it is negligent to follow the guidelines absolutely. Professional judgement and discretion are required and clear documentation must record the full circumstances as to why the guidelines were not entirely appropriate for the specific circumstances which existed.

Standard setting, the National Institute of Health and Clinical Excellence (NICE) and National Service Frameworks (NSF)

As the work of NICE (see Ch. 21) develops, it is likely that there will be more guidance on clinically effective practice and medication. Such guidance will probably be absorbed into the Bolam Test, so that a claimant may argue that there has been a failure to follow a reasonable standard of care as indicated in the published research findings and publications of NICE. For example, in June 2001, NICE published the Clinical Guidelines on the Induction of Labour.[18] A National Guideline on fetal heart surveillance was published by NICE in May 2000.[19] Neither met with unqualified acceptance.[20,21] While it is accepted that there may be situations where these guidelines would not be appropriate, it is likely that in the event of harm occurring, the claimant would use failure to follow the guidelines as evidence of negligence and therefore the professional would have to give evidence of the circumstances which made following the guidelines inappropriate. This is also true of the findings of such bodies as the National Evidence-based Midwifery Network. As their work develops in promulgating good practice, so their recommendations will be absorbed into what is considered to be reasonable practice, according to the Bolam Test[22,23] (see also Ch. 21). NICE recognises[24] that they are based on the best available evidence and help healthcare professionals in their work, but they do not replace their knowledge and skills.

The National Service Framework (NSF) for children and maternity care published in 2004 should lead to the establishment of minimum standards which should be made available for mothers and children. This may increase litigation if harm can be shown to result from a failure to follow such recommended standards (NSFs are discussed in Ch. 21). The Department of Health announced[25] that the NHS Clinical Governance Support Team is working in partnership with the Royal College of Obstetrics and Gynaecology, the Royal College of Midwifery and the NHS Litigation Authority to develop a targeted multi-disciplinary, task-orientated programme involving 12 maternity units. They will produce a working model for safe and high-quality care. Evidence of failure to implement such standards will inevitably be used by claimants in litigation.

Under its powers under s.46 of the Health and Social Care (Community Health and Standards) Act 2003 to prepare and publish statements of standards, 'Standards for Better Health' were published in July 2004 by the Department of Health.[26] These identify the seven domains of:

– Safety

– Clinical and cost effectiveness

- Governance

- Patient focus

- Accessible and responsive care

- Care environment and amenities

- Public health.

Outcomes are specified for each domain which identifies two types of standards: core and developmental. They will be used by the Healthcare Commission in its inspections. In addition, they are likely to be used by litigants who allege that they have suffered harm as a result of a failure to ensure that these standards were implemented.

Through the Clinical Governance initiative, case studies (performance enhancing stories, PENS) on service improvements are published by the Department of Health which could be a useful resource for midwives. For example a case study on midwifery-led care for low-risk women in labour in Dudley showed the change from treating all women as high-risk to a midwifery-led low-risk service.[27]

The Confidential Enquiry into Stillbirths and Deaths in Infancy (CESDI) was merged in 2003 with the Confidential Enquiry into Maternal Deaths (CEMD) into the Confidential Enquiry into Maternal and Child Health (CEMACH) funded by NICE.[28] This Enquiry also provides information from its analysis of the causes of death which can lead to higher standards of care. For example, in the CESDI seventh Annual Report,[29] it reviewed deaths following breech presentation and found that the single and most avoidable factor was suboptimal care given in labour rather than the conduct of the delivery itself. It made strong recommendations to trusts on the conduct of a breech presentation.

The Clinical Negligence Scheme for Trusts (CNST) has also laid down standards to be followed by those trusts who belong to the scheme, some specifically relating to midwifery and obstetrics (see below). Other sources of guidance, for example professional associations and government departments, could also recommend procedures and policies which could eventually be incorporated within a Bolam Test of the reasonable standard of care. For example, the Chief Medical Officer commissioned a review of the use of catheters for the intravenous feeding of sick newborn babies, following the death of four babies in the Greater Manchester area in 2000. The review made 14 recommendations, including the advice that the tip of the catheter should not be positioned in the heart.

Expert evidence
Unfortunately, expert evidence has not always been based on a detached, objective view of the facts, and the House of Lords ruled in the Bolitho case[30] that experts should be sure that their evidence related to the facts of the case. In this case the House of Lords stated that:

The court had to be satisfied that the exponents of the body of opinion relied on can demonstrate that such opinion has a logical basis. In particular, in cases involving, as they often do, the weighing of risks against benefits, the judge, before accepting a body of opinion as being responsible, reasonable or respectable, will need to be satisfied that, in forming their views, the experts had directed their minds to the question of comparative risks and benefits and had reached a defensible conclusion on the matter.

The use of the adjectives 'responsible, reasonable and respectable' (in the Bolam case) all showed that the court had to be satisfied that the exponents of the body of opinion relied upon could demonstrate that such opinion had a logical basis.

It would seldom be right for a judge to reach the conclusion that views held by a competent medical expert were unreasonable.

Following the Woolf Reforms (see below), parties to personal injury litigation are expected to agree upon an expert witness. The new civil procedure rules emphasise that the principal duty of the expert witness is to the court.

It follows from the Bolitho judgement that there may be exceptional cases where a judge decides that expert opinion given by a defendant is not reasonable. This occurred in the case of Marriott v. West Midlands Health Authority 1999.[31]

Standards of care in prison
In a recent decision (Box 13.4)[32] it was argued by the defence, unsuccessfully, that women in prison could not expect the same standards of maternity care as those outside.

Box 13.4 Brooks v. Home Office

A woman who was pregnant with twins was remanded in custody at Holloway prison, where the prison medical service had responsibility for her care. Her pregnancy was classified as high risk, requiring regular monitoring by ultrasound scans and clinical examination. A scan at the prison revealed that twin 1 was 20% smaller than twin 2 and had not grown sufficiently within the previous 2 weeks. Following the death of the baby and her suffering psychiatric injury, the mother sued, claiming that there had been a breach of the duty of care owed to her since the doctor in charge of her care had insufficient obstetric expertise, failed to seek immediate specialist obstetric advice and permitted a 5-day delay before she received specialist attention.

The High Court disagreed with the proposition put by the defendants that a pregnant woman in prison was not entitled to expect the same careful standard of obstetric care and observation as if she was at liberty. However, on the facts, the woman's action failed, since it was held that the baby had died before expert opinion could reasonably have been expected to have been obtained. The loss could not therefore have been caused by the breach of duty, i.e. the baby would have died anyway, even if the reasonable standard of care had been followed.

▶
> Even though the action failed, the case has established an important principle in terms of the standard of care owed by the prison service to pregnant women and mothers, and it may be that in the future a pregnant woman who suffers harm as a result of failures within the prison service may obtain compensation. It might surprise some midwives that the defendant would have put forward a contrary proposition: how could it ever be justifiable to give a pregnant woman a lower standard of maternity care just because she is imprisoned?

In March 1996 the Royal College of Midwives[33] published a paper emphasising the duty of all those providing maternity services to ensure that the dignity of every pregnant woman is preserved, regardless of her situation or the way in which care is delivered. It was concerned that maternity care which is both safe and appropriate should be available to women in prison. The role of the midwife is to attend to women during pregnancy and childbirth and it is the midwife's responsibility to ensure high standards of care throughout that time, whatever the woman's circumstances. The subject of pregnant women in prison is considered in Chapter 6.

CAUSATION

It is not enough for the claimant to show that the duty of care which was owed was broken; the claimant must also show that there was a causal link between that duty and the harm which has occurred. This is known as 'causation'. There must be factual causation as well as the link being reasonably foreseeable. Factual causation was lacking in the case shown in Box 13.4 above.

Factual causation

If the baby would have been harmed anyway, then the fact that there has been negligence by the midwife would not, in itself, be sufficient to enable the claimant to obtain compensation. For example, a mother might be able to show that a midwife failed to act appropriately when fetal distress was identified. However, if the child would have been born brain-damaged as a result of a congenital defect inherited from its parents, and the midwife's negligence has not caused any additional harm, then no compensation would be payable.

In one decided case,[34] three night watchmen drank tea which made them vomit. They went to the casualty department of the local hospital. The casualty officer, on being told of the complaints by a nurse, did not see the men, but told them to go home and call in their own doctors. Some hours later, one of them died from arsenical poisoning. The court held that:

– The casualty department officers owed a duty of care in the circumstances.

– The casualty doctor had been negligent in not seeing them, but

– even if he had, it was improbable that the only effective antidote could have been administered in time to save the deceased, and

– therefore the defendants were not liable. The patient would have died anyway.

The onus is on the claimant to establish that there is this causal link between the breach of the duty of care and the harm which occurred.

In the following case (Box 13.5),[35] the claimants failed to establish causation and the House of Lords ordered a new hearing on the issue of causation.

Box 13.5 Wilsher v. Essex Area Health Authority[35]

A premature baby was being treated with oxygen therapy. A junior doctor mistakenly inserted the catheter to monitor the oxygen intake into a vein rather than an artery. A senior registrar, when asked to check what had been done, failed to notice the error. The baby was given excess oxygen. The parents claimed compensation for the retrolental fibroplasia that the baby suffered, but failed to prove that it was the excess oxygen which had caused the harm. They therefore failed in their claim. It was agreed that there were several different factors which could have caused the child to become blind, and the negligence was only one of them. It could not been presumed that it was the defendant's negligence which had caused the harm. The House of Lords ordered the case to be reheard on the issue of causation. In the event, the parties settled.

It has also been difficult for claimants to establish causation when suing for compensation for harm which it is claimed has resulted from vaccine damage.[36] This is further discussed in Chapter 28.

In a case where a boy suffering from meningitis was given an overdose of penicillin, the parents claimed compensation for loss of hearing. The House of Lords, however, held that it had not been established that the deafness was caused by the overdose of penicillin, and the parents therefore lost their claim.[37] Factual causation between a brain-damaged baby and negligent care at birth may be difficult to establish, and of crucial importance will be the evidence of early fetal distress.

Causation was not established in a case[38] where a baby was placed in an incubator in a special care baby unit suffering from respiratory distress syndrome (RDS). It was argued on the baby's behalf that he should have been transferred to a hospital with ventilation facilities sooner than he was, before his condition became acute and that had he been, the baby would not have suffered brain damage. The judge held that the standard of care was not below the standard to be expected as reasonable in 1977 and the staff were justified in waiting before requesting the transfer. However, had they been wrong in that and there had been a breach of the duty of care, then it was not this breach which caused the brain injuries. There was no evidence that ventilation reduced the incidence of intraventricular haemorrhage (IVH). In fact the most significant cause of death in ventilated babies was IVH. Therefore transferring the baby earlier would not have prevented his IVH from occurring.

A baby who had a stroke at birth failed in her claim for compensation.[39] On her behalf it was contended that signs of fetal distress should have been noted much earlier from the CTG, that oxytocin was administered for too long and that the resultant hypoxia had led to her stroke. The defendants conceded that the caesarean should have been carried out earlier, but contended that the risk of a stroke did not come within its duty of care and that causation had not been proved. The High Court judge ruled that the management of the labour was mishandled and fell below the required standard of care; however, the claimant had not proved that it had led to her stroke. None of the medical research evidence submitted came close to showing that neonatal stroke was likely to result from hypoxia. Without establishing such a likelihood, the claimant could not prove that one or more of the events in labour which would not have occurred but for the negligence actually caused the stroke, and the necessary causal link had not been made out.

An intervening cause, which breaks the chain of causation, may also prevent causation being established and therefore cause the claimant to fail in her claim.

LOSS OF A CHANCE

The House of Lords (in a majority ruling) ruled in January 2005[40] that where a doctor negligently failed to refer for investigation a patient with possible symptoms of cancer, with the result that there was a 9-month delay in treatment for the condition, the patient (whose chances of survival during that delayed period had fallen from 42% to 25%) could not recover damages for that loss of chance. The delay had not deprived that patient of the prospect of a cure because on a balance of probability he could probably not have been cured anyway, and loss of a chance was not in itself a recoverable head of damage for clinical negligence.

HARM

To obtain compensation for negligence it must be established that harm has resulted from the negligent act. Harm includes personal injury and death, loss and damage of property. What types of harm do the courts recognise as being subject to compensation? Some of the forms of harm are shown in Box 13.6.

Post-traumatic stress syndrome

Where psychiatric harm has occurred as well as physical injury, then that is compensatible if a breach of the duty of care and causation can be established. However, where nervous shock (or post-traumatic stress syndrome as it is now known) has

Box 13.6 Harm recognised as subject to compensation in the civil courts

- Personal injury, pain and suffering

- Death

- Loss of the ability to have children

- Loss of the opportunity to have an abortion

- Having a child after being sterilised

- Post traumatic stress syndrome or nervous shock

- Loss or damage of property.

occurred on its own, compensation will only be paid if a duty of care can be established. The principles of liability for nervous shock were outlined by the House of Lords in the case of McLoughlin v. O'Brian 1982.[41] More recently, the House of Lords has set out the principles in a series of cases, some involving post-traumatic stress syndrome suffered by those who witnessed or assisted at the Hillsborough football stadium disaster. In Alcock v. Chief Constable of South Yorkshire Police[42] the House of Lords held that a person who suffers reasonably foreseeable psychiatric illness as a result of another person's death cannot recover damages unless he can satisfy three requirements:

1. that he had a close tie of love and affection with the person killed, injured or imperilled

2. that he was close to the incident in time and space, and

3. that he directly perceived the incident rather than, for example, hearing about it from a third person.

In Page v. Smith[43] the House of Lords made a distinction between primary and secondary victims: a claimant who was within the range of foreseeable injury was a primary victim, all other victims must satisfy the requirements set out above.

This was applied by the House of Lords in the case of White v. Chief Constable of South Yorkshire Police and Others[44] where it decided by a majority that police officers who had assisted in the aftermath of the Hillsborough disaster could not obtain compensation because they were not primary victims since they were not in the zone of danger, nor did they satisfy the requirements set out above of being secondary victims. In contrast, a girl who witnessed her mentally-ill brother stab their mother to death was given £500 000 compensation by the NHS trust who admitted liability for her severe mental breakdown.[45] An independent inquiry had found that he had been allowed to leave the ward, even though medical staff realised that he posed a danger to himself and others.

In one case,[46] the claimant suffered psychiatric illness after her daughter died following an operation for the removal of her wisdom teeth. Due to negligence on the part of the defendant, the daughter never regained consciousness and was pronounced dead 48 hours after the operation had taken place. The mother failed in her claim on the basis that there was no evidence showing that the events at the hospital had induced a post-traumatic stress syndrome and the overwhelming factor in her psychiatric illness was the fact of the death of her daughter, rather than the events at the hospital. The claim therefore failed on the ground of causation.

The way in which compensation for nervous shock was calculated in a case involving brain damage at birth is discussed below.

The rights of the child to bring an action are considered in Chapter 32. It should be noted here however that the law does not recognise a child's right of action for being born (e.g. where a sterilisation or abortion has failed) as opposed to a right of action for being born disabled.[47]

Harm may also include financial losses such as loss of earnings. The way in which the compensation is calculated is shown below.

Establishing the facts: 'The thing speaks for itself'
The claimant (formerly known as the plaintiff), i.e. the person bringing the action, normally has the burden of proving that there was negligence by the defendant which caused harm to her. The standard of proof in the civil courts where an action for compensation would take place is 'on a balance of probabilities'. This contrasts with the standard of proof in a criminal case, which is 'beyond reasonable doubt'.

However, where certain circumstances arise it is possible for the claimant to argue that 'the thing speaks for itself' and the defendant has the task of showing that he was not negligent. This is known as a *res ipsa loquitur* situation. The circumstances which have to be shown by the claimant are:

– the events were under the control of the defendant

– something has occurred which would not normally occur if all reasonable care were taken

– the defendant has not offered any explanation which shows he was not negligent.

A typical example of a *res ipsa loquitur* situation would be where a swab is left in a patient after surgery, or where the wrong limb is amputated. If these elements can be shown by the claimant, then he has made out a *prima facie* case that there is evidence of negligence by the defendants. The burden of proof, however, remains with the claimant to satisfy on a balance of probabilities.[48]

An example of the application of the doctrine of *res ipsa loquitur* from obstetrics is given in Box 13.7.[49]

Box 13.7 Brown v. Merton, Sutton and Wandsworth Area Health Authority (Teaching)[49]

In the course of preparation for giving birth, the claimant underwent epidural anaesthesia in a hospital. She developed severe pain when receiving the second dose of epidural and, as a result, developed quadriplegia. She brought an action against the defendants, a Hospital Authority, who admitted that they were responsible for the management of the hospital, that the claimant was, at all material times, a patient at that hospital and that the anaesthetic was administered by their servants or agents, for whose acts they were, in law, vicariously responsible. They denied that they had been negligent and specifically denied that the claimant was able to rely upon the doctrine of *res ipsa loquitur*. At a preliminary hearing, it was ordered that the number of expert medical witnesses who might be called at the trial should not be limited. On appeal by the claimant, the judge ordered that the number should be limited to five for each party. The claimant appealed to the Court of Appeal.

The Court of Appeal held that the pleadings (the documents which pass between the parties in the run-up to the hearing) showed that the defendants now admitted that the treatment was wholly under the management of the defendants and that this type of accident does not happen in the ordinary course of epidural anaesthesia when proper care is used. That is an admission of liability on the pleadings, and it is not in any way protected by the optimistic proposition that inquiries are still being made in an endeavour to find out whether the defendants can hereafter dispute liability. There was therefore no issue as to liability, only as to damages. The Court of Appeal therefore amended the order by deleting any reference to the doctors who were to give evidence on the treatment, and limited it purely to the condition and prognosis of the claimant. In total, the sum of £398 629 was awarded. (It must be remembered that this was 1982 and considerably more would be awarded today.)

VICARIOUS LIABILITY

It would be usual in the case of an employed midwife for her employer to be sued in the event of her being negligent. For obvious reasons, the employer is more likely to be able to pay the compensation due as a consequence of any harm caused by her negligence. This applies even though the employer has not been negligent in any way. In order to ensure that an innocent victim obtains compensation for injuries caused by an employee, public policy dictates that the doctrine of vicarious liability applies. Under the doctrine of vicarious liability, the employer is responsible for compensation payable for the harm.

For vicarious liability to be established, the elements shown in Box 13.8 must be established.

Box 13.8 Elements in vicarious liability

– There must be negligence, i.e. a duty of care which has been breached and, as a reasonably foreseeable consequence, has caused harm, or some other failure by the employee.

– The negligent act or omission or failure must have been by an employee.

– The negligent employee must have been acting in the course of employment.

EMPLOYEE

Normally there is no difficulty in defining who is an employee for the purposes of vicarious liability. The term may well include bank or agency midwives, but much would depend upon the contractual relationship established between them and the NHS trust or hospital. Independent midwives are not employees. They may have an honorary contract to work in hospital premises. This is unlikely to make the hospital legally liable for their actions. If the hospital were prepared to pay out compensation in respect of the negligence of an independent midwife, it would probably be subject to the right of indemnity by the trust against the midwife. The situation relating to independent midwives is considered in Chapter 23.

An employer is not liable for the actions of an independent contractor unless he has authorised them or is at fault in his choice of contractor. Thus, if decorators come on site and harm is caused by the negligence of one of their employees, the occupier of the site or the person who arranged for the decorators to be contracted will not normally be responsible for their activities (see Ch. 19). Similarly, if independent midwives have an agreement that they can come into the hospital managed by an NHS trust and deliver the mother, it is unlikely that the NHS trust will consider itself to be vicariously liable for the actions of the independent midwife, though it may be vicariously liable for its own staff, or it may be directly liable through failing to provide a safe system of work, safe premises and equipment and competent staff. Much, however, depends upon the independent midwife's contract with the NHS trust and she may agree that whilst she is working on the trust's premises, she works as an employee of the trust.

COURSE OF EMPLOYMENT

Not only must the negligent person be an employee but this person must have been acting in the course of employment. This phrase is wider than 'within the job description' or 'within the rules' or 'following procedures'. Even where the employee is deliberately disobeying the orders of the employer, that action could still be construed as being in the course of employment if it is part of the work that an employee is authorised to do. Thus, a midwife who failed to follow the procedures relating to water births in a domiciliary setting would be acting in the course of employment. In contrast, a midwife who supervised the delivery of a friend or relative who was not her client would be acting outside the course of employment. Even if the midwife were failing to obey the instructions of the employer, or working contrary to agreed protocols and procedures, the courts may still hold that the employer is vicariously liable for her actions. The House of Lords (in the case of Lister and Others v. Helsey Hall Ltd) has held that school owners, who were the employers of a warden, could be held liable for acts of sexual abuse committed by the warden of a school boarding house against pupils.[50] The reasoning was that the acts of abuse were sufficiently connected with the work that he had been employed to do that they could be regarded as having been committed within the scope of his employment, i.e. in the course of his employment.

Even where the employer is held to be vicariously liable, the midwife who is responsible for harm, such as the death of a woman or baby, could be found guilty of manslaughter for her gross negligence which led to the death; could lose her job following disciplinary action and could also be struck off the register following an NMC fitness to practise hearing. A schoolmaster was sentenced to a year's imprisonment following the death of a boy on a school trip in the Lake District. The judge held that he was unbelievably foolhardy and negligent in allowing the boy to jump into a turbulent mountain pool.[51]

EMPLOYER'S RIGHT OF INDEMNITY

While the doctrine of vicarious liability enables the victim of negligence to obtain compensation, it does not necessarily deprive the employer of his rights against the negligent employee. If an employee has been negligent then she is in breach of her contract of employment, which requires her to take all reasonable care and skill. This breach gives the employer a right to be indemnified against the negligent employee. The House of Lords confirmed this principle in the case of Lister v. Romford Ice and Cold Storage Co. Ltd.[52]

In the health service, hospital doctors and dentists, even though employees, accepted that they were personally liable for their negligent acts and were covered by membership of the medical defence unions. However, in 1990, Health Authorities agreed to pay the compensation resulting from the negligence of employed doctors and dentists.[53] It is therefore unlikely that NHS trusts would seek to enforce their right of indemnity against midwives and other professional staff.

INDEMNITY AND THE MIDWIFE

Following a consultation the NMC decided to introduce a new clause relating to indemnity into its Code of Professional Conduct: standards for conduct, performance and ethics. Clause 9 is set out in Chapter 23.

It is unfortunate that the NMC uses the phrase 'employers accept vicarious liability', since in practice whether an employer is vicariously liable or not is determined by the courts, as can be seen by the case of L. and Others v. Helsey Hall Ltd, discussed above. Certainly where the midwife works outside the course of her employment by undertaking a Good Samaritan act as required by the NMC (see discussion of Clause 8.5 of the NMC code above), the courts are unlikely to hold the employer vicariously liable and the midwife should secure her own personal indemnity cover, which is usually provided by relevant health professional associations. It should also be noted that Clause 9 makes a recommendation, rather than a requirement, and appears in 9.3 to be accepting the fact that some independent midwives may not have sufficient indemnity cover. This is discussed in Chapter 23 on the independent midwife.

CALCULATION OF COMPENSATION: QUANTUM (HOW MUCH?)

In some cases of negligence, liability might be accepted by the defendant, but there might be disagreement between the parties over the amount of compensation. In other cases, there might be agreement over the amount of compensation but liability is in dispute. In others, both liability and quantum might be in dispute.

If, as a result of negligence, the child has died, then the parents can only recover a sum for bereavement under the Fatal Accidents Act 1976. This currently stands at £10 000. (This sum is not payable if the fetus dies, since the unborn child does not have legal status; see Ch.17.)

In one case where the child died, parents were able to recover for the nervous shock which they suffered as a result of the midwife's negligence (Box 13.9).[54]

Box 13.9 Re W (1993)[54]

The first claimant gave birth to a child on 23 July 1989, who suffered from cerebral palsy. The baby died on 19 November 1989. The mother sued in her own right in respect of her claim for post-traumatic stress disorder and on behalf of the estate of her baby for general damages and the costs of care.

▶

The second claimant was the baby's father, who also claimed for post-traumatic stress disorder. The birth was managed by midwives who failed to highlight the potential problems of delivery in advance, given:

– the mother's short stature

– that the previous children were small at birth

– that in her second labour she had a precipitate delivery of a severely distressed child

– the failure to recognise and act upon signs of fetal distress

– the failure to carry out an episiotomy

– the failure to undertake a forceps delivery, and

– the failure to maintain or properly use resuscitation equipment.

Total damages came to £40 000 which was apportioned as follows:

Mother, general damages	£8500
Bereavement damages[a]	£3500
Cost of care	£10 925
Father, general damages	£7500

The balance was made up of interest.

[a]The amount now payable for bereavement has been increased to £10 000.

An example of the payments in a case of a brain-damaged baby is given below. The details of the negligence are shown in Chapter 14. In the case of Inman v. Cambridge Health Authority[55] damages were assessed as follows:

General damages	£125 000
Interest	£12 500
Past care	£58 000

Accommodation	£50 000
Other past expenses	£139 000
Future care	£600 000
Claimant's loss of earnings	£115 000
Accommodation	£40 000
Other future expenses	£225 000
Education	£50 000
Total	£1 415 000

A structured settlement was eventually agreed between the parties. The sum of £689 000 was returned to the defendants to provide £20 000 per annum to the claimant to the age of 19 years and thereafter £35 000 p.a. A contingency fund of £300 000 was set up under a trust with the parents as co-trustees. The judge approved the settlement and scheme.

DEFENCES

The main defences to an action for negligence are set out in Box 13.10.

Box 13.10 Defences

- Dispute over facts

- One of the elements of negligence is not present, e.g. no duty, no breach, no causation, no harm

- Limitation of time

- Contributory negligence

- Exclusion of liability

- Voluntary assumption of risk.

GENERAL POINTS ON DEFENCES

An action may be commenced by the claimant who might, at any stage before or during the hearing, realise that the facts of negligence and causation cannot be established, so abandon the claim. Alternatively, the defendant might find that it is difficult to dispute the claimant's claim. In such a case the defendant might either offer the claimant an *ex gratia* payment in the hope that the claim can be settled speedily, or if the case commences, the defendant might make a payment into court offering to settle the claim. If the claimant accepts the payment, the case will be ended at that point and the defendant will usually be liable to pay the claimant's costs up to that stage. If the claimant refuses the offer of the payment, the case continues with the claimant at risk, i.e. if the judge either finds against the claimant or awards a sum equal to or less than the defendant's payment into court, the claimant will have to pay the defendant's costs from the time that payment was made. This is because, had the claimant accepted what was clearly a reasonable sum, there would have been no wasted time and costs in having a court hearing. Case management has been introduced under new civil procedural rules which are considered in Chapter 14.

DISPUTE OVER THE FACTS

Often a case will be determined by proof of the facts. It is therefore important to understand how facts are established before a court. For the most part, facts are proved through witnesses of fact who give evidence and may then be cross-examined by the other side. Documentary evidence will also be used, but usually such documents, with exceptions, are not taken as proof of the truth of the facts contained in them. The writer of the document would give evidence so that the judge could decide the weight which could be given to them as evidential value.

Since most cases are determined by the facts, and may take many years to come to court, the importance of the records can be understood. This is further discussed in Chapter 15.

Expert witnesses would be called to give evidence on such issues as the standard which should have been followed, and on whether the alleged fault caused the harm, and also on the amount of compensation payable.

ELEMENTS OF AN ACTION FOR NEGLIGENCE NOT PRESENT

Even where the facts are agreed, the defendant might still be able to defeat a claim by showing that one of the essential elements in an action for negligence is not present. There may, for example, be a situation where there is no duty of care, or the claimant is unable to establish that the reasonable standard of care was not followed.

Even where a duty of care can be shown and a breach of duty is established, it might still be impossible for the claimant to show that there was causation.

DEFENCE OF LIMITATION OF TIME

One possible defence is for the defendant to show that the claimant was out of time in bringing the action.

In cases of personal injury or death, the claim form should be issued within 3 years of the negligent act taking place, or within 3 years of the claimant's date of knowledge of the injury, whichever is the later. Under s.14 of the Limitation Act 1980, 'knowledge' means that the claimant must know the following:

- that the injury was significant
- that the injury was attributable in whole or in part to the alleged wrongful act or omission
- the identity of the defendant
- the identity of any other person who caused the act or omission, if that person was not the defendant (e.g. the employee, where the employer is the defendant being sued for vicarious liability).

The fact that the claimant does not know that the act was wrong as a matter of law does not prevent knowledge, for the purposes of the limitation of time, arising. However, it is not necessary for the claimant to have actual knowledge of the facts. If it would be reasonable for the claimant to have acquired this knowledge from facts observable or ascertainable by her, or from facts ascertainable by her with help from experts which it would have been reasonable for her to have consulted, then she would be deemed to have constructive knowledge such that time will then start to run against her.

There are two main exceptions to the 3-year time limit from the date of the knowledge (actual or constructive) of the injury and wrong: those under a mental disability and children.

Those under a mental disability
Time does not run against such persons until the disability ends or the person dies. In most cases (e.g. brain damage at birth), the disability may never end until death, when the time limit starts to run.

Children
Time does not run against a child until the child becomes an adult at 18 years. This of course has profound implications in a childbirth case. Time might run against the

mother immediately (in respect of harm which she has suffered), if she has the requisite knowledge, but will not run against the child until the child becomes an adult at 18 years. Where, however, the child has suffered brain damage, there is no time limit for bringing an action until the death of that person. The implications can be seen in the case of Bull and Wakeham v. Devon Area Health Authority (Box 13.11).[56]

Box 13.11 Bull and Wakeham v. Devon Area Health Authority

In this case Stuart, one of twins, was born on 21 March 1970. The mother alleged that he was brain damaged because of failures in the care provided. The mother commenced an action on her own behalf and also, as next friend, in the name of the child, which was heard on 9 April 1987 (17 years after the birth). The writ was issued on 23 April 1979.

The mother's claim
The judge found that the mother knew all the facts relevant to her own claim as soon as they occurred on 21 March 1970, so that was the date from which the 3-year period ordained by s.11(4) of the Limitation Act 1980 ran. The judge refused to exercise his discretion to exclude the time limits under s.33 of the 1980 Act (see below). The mother's action was therefore held to be statute barred.

The child's claim
Time did not run against the child until he was an adult, i.e. 18 years. However, as a brain damaged person, time would not run against him until his disability ceased.

Stuart's claim was therefore not out of time, and could be heard, and was upheld.

From the case of Bull and Wakeham, it would be apparent to midwives that records of childbirth must be kept for at least 25 years after a birth, and even longer where the child is brain damaged or mentally disordered. The implications for record keeping are discussed in Chapter 15.

Judge's discretion
Under s.33 of the Limitation Act 1980, the judge has the right to exclude the time limit, if he considers it equitable to do so, having regard to the degree to which the ordinary limitation rules prejudice the claimant and any exercise of the power would prejudice the defendant. As has been seen in the Bull and Wakeham case, the judge refused to exercise his power to exclude the time limit in the mother's favour. He

said it would not be equitable to allow her action to proceed having regard to the prejudice to the Authority.

In a more recent case, the judge exercised his discretion under s.33 to enable a woman to pursue her claim.[57] In this case, the mother of a child, who was born in 1995 with severe brain damage and cerebral palsy and who died in 2003, brought an action against the trust for damages for pain, suffering and loss of amenity in continuing with her pregnancy and for the cost of bringing up her child. The judge held that she was out of time in bringing the action since she had knowledge of her child's condition before she made a decision on a termination of pregnancy. However, he held that it was appropriate and equitable to disapply the time limits and allow her action to proceed both in relation to the personal injury claim and in relation to the costs incurred in supporting her child (see also the case of Das v. Ganju[58] discussed in Ch. 16 and the case of C. v Dr AJ Cairns[59] considered in Ch. 10).

In contrast, the Court of Appeal overturned a decision to exercise discretion under s.33[60] where the claimant alleged that the local authority had failed in its duty to ameliorate his condition of dyslexia. The Court of Appeal held that he was aware of the injury within the time limits and although he did not have the knowledge that he might have a legal action (the case of Phelps v. Hillingdon LBC[61] not being decided till later), that was irrelevant for the purposes of s.14. He had the requisite knowledge when he reached his majority and his claim was time barred. Nor were his Article 6 rights under the European Convention on Human Rights violated.

CONTRIBUTORY NEGLIGENCE

The claimant owes a duty of care to herself. This means that if the harm which has occurred is partly her own fault as well as the fault of the defendant, then the compensation which is payable can be reduced by the extent to which the claimant was responsible for the harm. The apportionment is entirely one of fact and is required by the Law Reform (Contributory Negligence) Act 1945. Section 1(1) reads as follows:

Where any person suffers damage as the result partly of the fault of any other person or persons, a claim in respect to that damage shall not be defeated by reasons of the fault of the person suffering the damage, but the damages recoverable in respect thereof shall be reduced to such extent as the court thinks just and equitable having regard to the claimant's share in the responsibility for the damage.

In determining contributory negligence, the court would take into account the extent to which it would have been reasonable to expect the claimant to have taken care of herself. Less care would be looked for in a child than in an adult.

In the case of Beverley Pidgeon v. Doncaster Health Authority[62] the claimant had been given a cervical smear test in 1988 which was mistakenly reported as negative.

Between 1988 and 1997, she had numerous urgings from both the GP and the FHSA to have further smear tests, which she refused. In 1997, a smear was taken following withdrawal bleeding and she was found to have cervical carcinoma at Stage 2A or 2B. She underwent treatment which included a resection of her bowel. It was agreed that if the result had been noted and acted upon in 1988, the abnormal cells could have been removed by less invasive surgery. She sued for the negligence of the defendants and the court held that she was two-thirds responsible and so was therefore entitled to only one-third of the compensation payable.

In a midwifery case, contributory negligence could be seen in a client failing to comply with suggestions for medication and treatment. There may be circumstances where the contributory negligence is so extensive that minimal compensation by the defendant is payable. At the other extreme, the contributory negligence may be so minor that no reduction in compensation is justifiable.

The contributory negligence of the mother is not attributable to any claim brought in the name of the child (thereby reducing the child's claim to compensation), unless the claim is brought under the Congenital Disabilities Act. For further discussion on this, see Ch. 17.

EXCLUSION OF LIABILITY

A person may attempt to exclude his/her liability for causing loss or damage by reference to a notice or ticket, or in some other way. Is this exclusion valid? Reference must be made to the effects of the Unfair Contract Terms Act 1977.

The effect of this Act, which applies to actions for tort as well as breach of contract, is that in business situations, a person cannot by reference to a contract term or notice given to persons specifically or generally exclude his liability for death or personal injury. Business includes a profession and the activities of any government department or local or public authority.

The significance for the midwife is that if a mother wishes to have a particular form of delivery which is considered hazardous, the midwife could not say, 'Well, provided I am excluded from liability, I will deliver you in the manner you wish.' It has been suggested, for example with waterbirths, that the mother should be able to choose that form of birth, but agree that the midwife should not be liable for any harm which occurs. If the midwife is negligent, she cannot exclude her liability because of the effects of the 1977 Act. This also applies to the independent midwife.

In contrast, liability for loss or damage to property may be excluded, provided that it is reasonable to do so. The requirement of reasonableness is satisfied if it would be fair and reasonable to allow reliance upon the term, having regard to all the circumstances obtaining when the liability arose or (but for the notice) would have arisen. It is for the person claiming that the term satisfies the requirement of reasonableness to show that it does.

This may be of importance in the care of patients' property. If a notice is placed in an antenatal clinic that the NHS trust is not responsible for loss or damage to property however caused, this may be effective in relieving the NHS trust of liability, even if one of their employees is at fault. It would be for the trust to prove that it was reasonable for it to rely upon the notice excluding liability.

VOLUNTARY ASSUMPTION OF RISK

Another defence on which a defendant may sometimes rely is that even though duty, breach, causation and harm can be shown, the claimant voluntarily agreed to waive the right to bring an action for negligence. This is known as *volente non fit injuria*, i.e. 'to the willing, there is no wrong'.

It has been suggested that where a mother wants to have a waterbirth, which might be contrary to the policy of the hospital, she could, by signing a document, state that she voluntarily took on the risks involved and would not hold the midwives in any way responsible should harm occur to her or the baby. In this way, the midwife could enable the mother to have the confinement she wanted, without the risks of being sued for compensation. If the mother voluntarily assumes the risk of being injured through negligence, and the unborn child is harmed by that negligence and is subsequently born alive, if an action were to be brought in the name of the child under the Congenital Disabilities Act this could be used as a defence (see Ch. 17).

There are, however, several dangers for the midwife in relying upon this defence to cover for her failure to provide a reasonable standard of care.

- In the first place, it is only effective as a defence against the risks of which the claimant is made aware. Were other risks to occur, the mother could argue that she had not voluntarily agreed to waive a right to sue in respect of the harm caused by negligence.

- Second, if there is evidence that the mother was placed in a situation where she really had no real choice, it is unlikely that the defence would succeed.

- Third, even if the defence were effective in defeating a claim of negligence, the midwife might still be accountable to the NMC for evidence of lack of fitness to practise (see Ch. 4) and to her employer for breach of the contract of employment (see Ch. 22).

The Road Traffic Act prevents a driver requiring a passenger to travel at his own risk. Thus if a midwife offered a pregnant woman a lift on the understanding that she travelled at her own risk, this would be illegal, and would not be a valid defence for the midwife to bring were the mother to sue her.

Employers have in the past claimed that employees who worked in particularly dangerous conditions voluntarily assumed the risk of being injured. The courts are however extremely reluctant to allow such a defence to prevail against the negligence of the employer who caused harm. Thus a midwife, whose back was injured as the result of the employer's failure to take care of her health and safety and to use hoists and provide training, should not be defeated in her claim for compensation on the grounds that she knew that the practice of midwifery caused back injuries (see Ch. 19 on health and safety law).

THE CLINICAL NEGLIGENCE SCHEME FOR TRUSTS AND NHS LITIGATION AUTHORITY

The Clinical Negligence Scheme for Trusts (CNST)[63] was established by the NHS Executive in 1994, to provide a means for trusts to fund the cost of clinical negligence litigation and to encourage and support effective management of claims and risk. The scheme covers claims arising from incidents on or after 1 April 1995. The NHS Litigation Authority (NHSLA), a Special Health Authority (see below), administers the scheme. Membership is voluntary and open to all NHS trusts in England. Each trust can choose its own level of self-retention, and the scheme will contribute to the cost of claims in excess of this figure. Funding is on a 'pay as you go' non-profit basis. Actuaries appointed by the NHSLA analyse the available data and predict the total amount expected to be paid to the member trusts in respect of damages, costs and other expenses which will be incurred in the ensuing financial year. This amount is then apportioned between the member trusts. Individual trust contributions are based on a range of criteria, such as activities, budget, numbers of doctors by discipline, nurses and other professionals. These contributions can be reduced if a trust meets certain risk management criteria (the CNST Risk Management Standards). As the scheme matures, it is possible that other criteria such as claims experience will influence individual trust contributions.

STANDARDS OF CNST

The assessment is based on nine 'core' standards. In addition, there are separate standards for maternity care, mental health and ambulance services, which are applicable only to trusts which provide such services. There are three levels of criteria: level one criteria represent the basic elements of a clinical risk management framework; levels two and three are more demanding. Many are concerned with the implementation and integration into practice of policies and procedures, monitoring them and acting on the results.

Advice on the standards and general aspects of risk management is given in the 'NHSLA Review', and at workshops and seminars.

The separate clinical risk management standards which have been drawn up for maternity services[64] contain eight core standards:

1. Organisation

2. Learning from experience

3. Communication

4. Clinical care

5. Induction, training and competence

6. Health records

7. Implementation of clinical risk management

8. Staffing levels.

These standards cover all aspects of maternity services whether they are provided in an acute, primary or community care setting and include antenatal services, intrapartum services, postnatal services midwifery-led care, obstetric anaesthetics and obstetric ultrasonography. Each standard identifies the criteria required to meet this standard at the specified level and sets out the source of the criterion and guidance which is available. It stipulates the verification and identifies links with other standards and the scoring available. An example is given in Box 13.12, for level 1 criterion 3.1.1 for the standard on communication.

Box 13.12 Criterion 3.1.1

There is information available to women and their partners, which describes the alternatives, risks and benefits of their proposed treatment in pregnancy care, treatment and delivery.

Level   1

Source   NICE clinical guidelines 2001; CNST

               UK National Screening Committee 2001;

               HSC 2001/023 Good Practice in Consent. Department of Health, November 2001 (see Ch. 7)

               Toolkit for producing patient information. Department of Health 2003.

Guidance   Leaflets and other printed material should be provided to women well before proposed treatment, informing them about their condition and the proposed treatment. At higher levels of CNST assessment it is expected that the Trust will audit that provision of information is documented.

The Assessor will expect to see some of eight specified leaflets, including place of delivery (home or hospital), mode of delivery (instrumental and caesarean section).

Commercially produced material must reflect actual practice.

Verification   Information covering a minimum of five areas.

Links   Standard 7 Implementation of clinical risk management.

Scoring   10

The maternity clinical risk management standards document sets out full details of the assessments and the pre-assessment visits to maternity services, the procedure which is followed and the documentary evidence for every standard which will be required for each level of assessment. It also provides contact details of the CNST officers.

There are clear advantages for all midwives to have access to the CNST standards, whether or not the trust in which the midwife is employed is a participant of the CNST. The standards, criteria and verification data can be used to ensure that a strategy is in place to secure minimum levels of care. If there is clear inconsistency between the recommended standards and the situation within a specific department, then midwives can discuss means of improving services, supported by the provisions of the Public Interest Disclosure Act 1998, if there appears to be inaction or even indifference on management's part.

NHS LITIGATION AUTHORITY (NHSLA)

A litigation authority has been set up for the NHS.[65] The NHS Litigation Authority (NHSLA) exercises functions in connection with the establishment and the administration of the scheme for meeting liabilities of health service bodies to third parties for loss, damage or injury arising out of the exercise of their functions. Membership and claims issues of the CNST are dealt with by the NHSLA. Risk management matters are dealt with on behalf of the NHSLA, by the CNST assessment team at Willis Ltd, working closely with and overseen by the NHSLA. Further information on the activities of the NHSLA and risk management programme can be found on its website[66] and in its annual reports.

Guidance on NHS indemnity for clinical negligence claims has been issued by the NHS Executive.[67]

In the 2001 report of the National Audit Office,[2] recommendations were made that the NHS Litigation Authority and the Legal Services Commission should work together to speed up the completion of cases; the Department of Health, the Lord Chancellor's Department and the Legal Services Commission to resolve the smaller and medium-sized claims with a wider range of non-financial remedies; and for the Department of Health to give clear guidance to NHS trusts on what information should be given to patients who have suffered adverse incidents. The RCM has provided an update of its guide on litigation in midwifery.[68]

The significant changes to the process of civil litigation resulting from the Woolf Reforms are considered in Chapter 14, together with proposed changes to the system for obtaining compensation for clinical negligence claims.

CONCLUSION

This chapter has set out the basic principles of liability in civil actions for negligence and considered the context of litigation and indicated the duty placed in law upon the midwife and the legal requirement that she practises a reasonable standard of care. Chapter 14 looks at some special situations involving the midwife.

QUESTIONS AND EXERCISES

1. Take any incident at work which could have led to an action for compensation and consider the extent to which each of the required elements was established.

2. What evidence would you consider was relevant if you were the defendant in a negligence case?

3. To what extent do you consider that an employer should be able to determine the policies to be followed by professional staff?

4. Examine the publications of NICE and the CNST on maternity standards and consider the extent to which these are reflected in your own practice.

References

1 National Audit Office. NHS Summarised Accounts 2002–3 HC 505 28 April, 2004. Report of the Controller and Auditor General. House of Commons. Online. Available: www.nao.gov.uk

2 National Audit Office. Handling clinical negligence claims in England: Report of the Controller and Auditor General. House of Commons Session 2000–2001.

3 Dimond B. Litigation in the NHS: Recommendations for change. Br J Midwifery 2001; 9(7):443–446.

4 Venkatesan Ranjan, for example. MROG. Obstetrics and the fear of litigation. Professional Care of Mother and Child 1993; 3(1), who quotes research where only 146 of 1300 senior house officers in obstetrics wished to continue in that field.

5 Donoghue v. Stevenson [1932] AC 562.

6 Nursing and Midwifery Council Code of Professional Conduct: standards for performance, conduct and ethics 2004.

7 Kent v. Griffiths (No 3) [2001] QB 36.

8 Carty v. Croydon London Borough Council. The Times, 3 February 2005 CA.

9 D. v. East Berkshire Community Health NHS Trust and Another; MAK and Another v. Dewsbury Healthcare NHS Trust and Another; RK and Another v. Oldham NHS Trust and Another. The Times Law Report, 22 April 2005 HL.

10 Brooks v. Commissioner of Police of the Metropolis and Others. The Times Law Report, 26 April, 2005 HL.

11 Hill v. Chief Constable of West Yorkshire [1989] AC 53 HL.

12 Bolam v. Friern Hospital Management Committee [1957] 1 WLR 582.

13 Whitehouse v. Jordan [1981] 1 All ER 267.

14 Hunter v. Hanley [1955] SLT 213.

15 Maynard v. West Midlands Regional Health Authority [1985] 1 All ER 871.

16 Young AFE, Lim J, Hudson CN *et al*. Audit of compliance with antenatal protocols. Br Med J 1992; 305(6863):1184–1186, for example.

17 Hurwitz B. Clinical Guidelines and the Law. Abingdon: Radcliffe Medical Press; 1998.

18 NICE. Induction of labour: Inherited clinical guideline D. London: NICE; 2001. Online. Available: www.nice.org.uk

19 NICE. The use of electronic fetal monitoring: Inherited clinical guideline C. London: NICE; 2001.

20 Thornton J. Not so NICE guidelines. Br J Midwifery 2001; 9(8):470–472.

21 Spiby H. NICE guidelines on electronic fetal monitoring. Br J Midwifery 2001; 9(8):489.

22 Foundation for Nursing Studies. Contact: 32 Buckingham Palace Road, London SW1W 0RE; Tel: 0207 233 5750. Online. Available: www.fons.org

23 Hunt G, Monro J. First National Evidence-Based Midwifery Network Conference. Br J Midwifery 2001; 9(10): 676–677.

24 National Institute for Clinical Excellence. About clinical guidelines. Online. Available: www.nice.org.uk

25 Department of Health. Building a safer NHS for patients. London: HMSO; 2001, press release, 17 April 2001, 2001/0190.

26 Department of Health. Standards for better health. London: DoH; July 2004.

27 Department of Health. Clinical Governance case studies. London: DoH; 2004.

28 NICE. Online. Available: www.nice.org.uk

29 Confidential Enquiry into Stillbirths and Deaths in Infancy. 7th Annual Report. London: Maternal and Child Health Research Consortium; 2000.

30 Bolitho v. City and Hackney Health Authority [1997] 3 WLR 1151.

31 Marriott v. West Midlands Health Authority [1999] Lloyd's Rep Med 23.

32 Brooks v. Home Office. Times Law Report, 17 February 1999; [1999] 2 FLR 33.

33 Royal College of Midwives. Caring for pregnant prisoners. London: RCM; 1996.

34 Barnett v. Chelsea HMC [1968] 1 All ER 1068.

35 Wilsher v. Essex Area Health Authority HL [1988] 1 All ER 871.

36 Loveday v. Renton and another. The Times, 31 March 1988.

37 Kay v. Ayrshire and Arran Health Board [1987] 2 All ER 417.

38 Ball v. Wirral H A [2003] Lloyd's Rep Med 165.

39 Dowson v. Sunderland Hospitals NHS Trust [2004] Lloyd's Rep Med 177.

40 Gregg v. Scott. The Times Law Report, 28 January 2005 HL.

41 McLoughlin v. O'Brian [1982] 2 All ER 298.

42 Alcock v. Chief Constable of South Yorkshire Police [1992] 1 AC.

43 Page v. Smith [1996] AC 155.

44 White v. Chief Constable of South Yorkshire Police and others [1999] 1 All ER 1 HL.

45 Frean A. 2001. Sister who saw killing wins record trauma sum. The Times, 5 November 2001:5.

46 Ward v. The Leeds Teaching Hospitals NHS Trust [2004] EWHC 2106.

47 McKay v. Essex AHA [1982] 2 All ER 771.

48 Ratcliffe v. Plymouth and Torbay HA, Exeter and Devon HA [1998] Lloyd's Rep Med 162 CA.

49 Brown v. Merton, Sutton and Wandsworth Area Health Authority (Teaching) [1982] 1 All ER 650.

50 L. and Others v. Helsey Hall Ltd. Times Law Report, 10 May 2001; [2001] UKHL 22; [2001] 2 WLR 1311.

51 Jenkins R, Owen G. Jailing of teacher may spell the end for school trips. The Times, 24 September 2003.

52 Lister v. Romford Ice and Cold Storage Co Ltd. [1957] 1 All ER 125.

53 Health Service Circular (89)34.

54 Re W [1993] Association for the victims of medical accidents. Med Leg J Summer 1993.

55 Inman v. Cambridge Health Authority. In: Kemp and Kemp. Quantum of damages, Vol 2. London: Sweet and Maxwell; 1998.

56 Bull and Wakeham v. Devon Health Authority [1989] CA 2 February 1989 Transcript; [1993] 4 Med LR 117 CA.

57 Godfrey v. Gloucester Royal Infirmary NHS Trust [2003] EWHC 549; [2003] Lloyd's Rep Med 398.

58 Das v. Ganju (1998) 42 BMLR 28 QBD.

59 C. v. Dr AJ Cairns Lloyd's Rep Med [2003] 90.

60 Rowe v. Kingston upon Hull City Council [2003] EWCA Civ 1281 [2003] ELR 771 CA.

61 Phelps v. Hillingdon LBC [1997] 3 FCR 621, [1997] CLY 2142.

62 Beverley Pidgeon v. Doncaster Health Authority. Lloyd's Rep Med [2002] 130.

63 CNST. A disc setting out standards information is available from the CNST: Contact helpline: 0845 300 12230.

64 NHS Litigation Authority. Clinical negligence scheme for trusts: Maternity Clinical Risk Management Standards, April 2004. Online. Available: www.nhsla.com

65 NHS Litigation Authority (Establishment and Constitution) Order 1995, SI No 2800, as amended by SI 2005 No 1445.

66 NHS Litigation Authority. Online. Available: www.nhsla.com

67 Health Service Circular (96)48 NHS Indemnity: Arrangements for Clinical Negligence Claims in the NHS.

68 Hardman L, Bates C, eds. Litigation: a risk management guide for midwives. London: RCM; 2005.

Chapter 14
SPECIFIC SITUATIONS IN NEGLIGENCE AND CIVIL COURT PROCEDURE

In Chapter 13 we considered the outline of the law relating to liability for negligent actions, the elements which have to be shown and the defences available. In this chapter, certain specific situations will be considered which are of particular relevance to the midwife and in addition some cases relating to midwifery and obstetric practice, together with the procedure which is followed in the civil courts, will be discussed.

This chapter covers the following areas:

– Liability for failures in communication

– CTG and litigation

– Identification of the newborn and security against intruders and bogus professionals

– Protection against dangerous professional staff (Allitt situation)

– Examples of decided cases in midwifery and child care

– Conditional fee system

– Woolf Reforms of civil procedures.

LIABILITY FOR FAILURES IN COMMUNICATION

The duty of care in the law of negligence may include the duty to give information. In Chapters 7 and 8, failures in communicating to the mother important information relating to treatment and care are considered in relation to the laws relating to trespass to the person and negligence, and it is seen that even though the mother has agreed in principle to have particular treatment, she may still be able to claim compensation if she is able to show that had certain risks been explained to her, she would not have agreed to that treatment and that as a result of having that treatment, the risks have occurred and she has been harmed. In Chapter 28, the midwife's duty to give information about vaccinations is discussed.

In this chapter, we look at the wider duty possessed by the midwife in relation to the giving of information. The importance of communication cannot be over-estimated, and communication between midwife and mother is at the heart of the Cumberlege proposals and the National Service Framework (NSF) for maternity services (see Ch. 6). It is also central to the philosophy of equal partnership between patient and professional advocated in the report which followed the Inquiry into the children's heart surgery in Bristol.[1]

The Bristol Report recommends that:

> Patients should always be given the opportunity and time to ask questions about what they are told, to seek clarification and to ask for more informa-tion. It must be the responsibility of employers in the NHS to ensure that the working arrangements of healthcare professionals allow for this, not least that they have the necessary time.

It also recommends that staff should be given the training necessary to ensure good communication skills. Recommendation 59 states:

> Communication skills include the ability to engage with patients on an emotional level, to listen, to assess how much information a patient wants to know, and to convey information with clarity and sympathy.

In Recommendation 60, the report states:

> Communication skills must also include the ability to engage with and respect the views of fellow healthcare professionals.

Communication between mother and midwife is only one of the many forms of communication by the midwife. She must also communicate with professionals, with the public, with the children of clients and with her colleagues.

Liability for negligence in communicating can arise when it can be shown that there exists:

– a duty of care

– failure to follow a reasonable standard, and

– as a reasonably foreseeable result of the failure to communicate,

– harm arises.

The potential litigant must show that the midwife has failed to communicate appro-priately and also that it is as a reasonably foreseeable result of that failure that harm has occurred. The claimant will have the burden of proving all of the required elements on a balance of probability and sometimes it might be one person's word against another's.

It may be preferable in certain situations that the word of mouth should be supported by written instructions. For example, if specific instructions are given to the client during the antenatal stage, not only is it of value for the mother to receive this in written form for future reference, it will also support the midwife's case that the necessary information was given.

Communication, however, means listening as well as speaking and it is essential that the midwife listens carefully to what the mother says. For example, the mother may express fears which the midwife discounts as being insignificant, not realising that the mother's own perceptions and background affect the significance which she attaches to symptoms and problems. This perception may be very different from the midwife's. The midwife should make sure that she asks the mother carefully about any particular worries that the mother has and takes full note of them. Clearly, if the midwife gets to know the mother well, she will be aware of the mother who makes light of incidents which may in fact be of great significance.

Dr Sweeney reported[2] that one study found that a group of patients with diabetes who were taught to be more assertive in questioning their doctor about their disease were found to manage their condition better than those who were not. The doctors in the study were uncomfortable about the greater degree of control these patients exercised during consultations. Midwives must learn to encourage full involvement and discussion with the mothers of all aspects of the pregnancy and confinement if the Cumberlege and Bristol proposals are to be implemented in spirit as well as by the letter.

Failure to advise about the risk of a Down's syndrome baby led to a successful action in a case in 2003.[3] In this case expert evidence suggested that it should have been routine practice for a woman of 37 to be counselled about the possibility of Down's syndrome, and the fact of the counselling and the woman's response would have been recorded. The three witnesses for the defence, the GP, the midwife and the obstetrician, said that she had been counselled, but none of them had recorded that. The claimant said that had she been so advised, she would have had a termination.

INADEQUATE INFORMATION AVAILABLE

Often the midwife's task of giving information is impeded by an absence of clear professional opinion over what is the best practice. The history of guidance over vitamin K is a good example of confusion in the early stages over what was the best advice to give to mothers. Professor Jean Golding of the Institute of Child Health, Bristol, told a conference in 1992 that she had found a link between childhood cancers and administration of intramuscular (but not oral) vitamin K to newborn babies.[4] As a consequence, midwives did not know if they should be recommending that vitamin K should be taken orally rather than intramuscularly. There was evidence that oral administration was less effective than intramuscular administration, and oral administration had not been licensed. Were the risks of not recommending it greater than the risks involved in taking it? What was the legal position of the midwife if she continued to recommend it but the patient suffered harm as a result? Could the midwife be held personally liable for the resulting harm? Such were the uncertainties until the British Paediatric Association issued definitive guidelines in the report of an expert committee.[5] Sara Wickham shows that there are continuing concerns over Vitamin K[6] and raises the issue as to whether babies are born with less vitamin K than they need, and whether babies of women receiving medical management in hospitals should be treated in the same way as those born to women in home births. The Department of Health has issued information for parents-to-be on vitamin K.[7]

In such circumstances, the midwife can only obtain the best possible advice at the time and advise the women of the controversy. Similar problems currently arise over recommending the triple vaccine; this is discussed in Chapter 28. Clearly it is important for the midwife to document the advice which was available and which she gave, and to ensure that as new guidance is published from respected organisations, this is also passed on to the women.

CTG AND LITIGATION

In a multiple pregnancy it would be current practice (in contrast to the case of Bull v. Wakeham (discussed in Ch. 13 and the record-keeping aspects considered in Ch. 15, where CTG recordings were not made) to apply continuous electronic fetal monitoring. Where such electronic monitoring is in place, the midwife finds it useful to record upon the graph itself significant events. The advantage of this is that the graph is timed and the midwife does not need to write in the time again. In addition, some of the equipment allows the machine itself to record significant events if the appropriate buttons are pressed. The Royal College of Midwives' booklet on litigation recommends that the name of the woman, the date and the time of commencement should be recorded on the CTG trace.

> If the machine is one that automatically records the time, the clock on the machine must be checked. In addition, there should be a record on the trace or in the notes to show when the trace ends, otherwise it may be said that part has gone missing.

It would also be of value for computer-held records to be signed and dated when they are printed out. Recent cases have shown the importance attached to CTG records where these are available.

Central to many cases alleging negligence at birth is the reading or misreading of the CTG. Williams and Arulkumaran explore the medico-legal issues which have arisen from cardiotocography.[8] They show that compulsory education and training in the interpretation of CTGs and in best practice are key factors in minimising the threat of litigation. They have analysed claims for alleged negligence and have identified the following recurring factors:

- Misinterpretation of CTG tracing

- Inappropriate action or delayed response

- Technique and equipment problems

- Inappropriate use of oxytocin

- Record keeping and communication issues

- Poor supervision

- Inadequate staffing.

IDENTIFICATION OF THE NEWBORN AND SECURITY AGAINST INTRUDERS AND BOGUS PROFESSIONALS

In the early 1990s, there were several cases where there were mistakes in giving the wrong baby to the mother, and where intruders entered midwifery units and stole babies. Each maternity unit has, as part of its duty of care, to ensure the implementation of a system to prevent any mix-up of babies occurring, and to prevent the admission of intruders and bogus professionals. The system must be constantly monitored and reinforced.

The system would include:

- tagging of baby and mother

- checking to ensure that tags are put in place correctly.

If a baby were to be given to the wrong mother, could that mother be forced to hand over the baby when the mistake was realised? The answer is probably yes, but it may depend upon the age of the children when the error was discovered and the welfare of the child would be the fundamental consideration.

In 1994, Abbie Humphries, a 4-hour-old baby, was handed to a person pretending to be a nurse and claiming that she wished to take the baby for a hearing test.[9] Such an event would raise a *prima facie* case of negligence by the trust and its employees. In its defence, the trust would have to show that all reasonable care was taken to prevent such an occurrence. In determining whether there had been a breach of duty, the following facts would be considered:

- What is the risk of harm?

- How serious would the harm be if it were to occur?

- What is the cost of avoiding harm?

- What were the circumstances of the defendant's business?

Such precautions as the use of electronic tags, locks on all entrances, and identity tagging for all staff working in the unit would be seen as reasonable measures to be taken to prevent the harm arising. What was reasonable for a specific trust would depend upon the hospital layout and geography.

Precautions against bogus professionals operating in the community might include:

– identity cards

– identification of personnel for mothers to check

– code names

– check by phone calls

– better confidentiality over visit times and names and addresses of patients.

PROTECTION AGAINST DANGEROUS PROFESSIONAL STAFF: THE ALLITT CASE

Major lessons can be learned from the events at Grantham and Kesteven General Hospital between February and April 1991, which resulted in Beverly Allitt, an enrolled nurse, being convicted of the deaths of four children and causing harm to nine others. The Regional Health Authority set up its own inquiry into the situation and an independent inquiry chaired by Sir Cecil Clothier was appointed by the Secretary of State. It reported in 1994[10] and a summary of its main recommendations is shown in Box 14.1. The recommendations relate to the recruitment and selection of staff, the role of the occupational health department and the procedures to be taken when an unexpected death of a child or untoward event takes place.

Box 14.1 Main recommendations of the Clothier Inquiry

1. For all those seeking entry to the nursing profession, in addition to routine references, the most recent employer or place of study should be asked to provide at least a record of time taken off on ground of sickness.

2. In every case, coroners should send copies of post-mortem reports to any Consultant who has been involved in the patient's care prior to death, whether or not demanded under Rule 57 of the Coroner's Rules 1984.

3. The provision of paediatric pathology services should be reviewed with a view to ensuring that such services be engaged in every case in which the death of a child is unexpected or clinically unaccountable, whether the post-mortem examination is ordered by a coroner or in routine hospital practice.

►

4. No candidate for nursing in whom there is evidence of major personality disorder should be employed in the profession.

5. Nurses should undergo formal health screening when they obtain their first posts after qualifying.

6. The possibility should be reviewed of making available to occupational health departments any records of absence through sickness from any institution which an applicant for a nursing post has attended or been employed by.

7. Procedures for management referrals to occupational health should make clear the criteria which should trigger such referrals.

8. Further consideration should be given to using in practice the criteria for detecting the presence of a personality disorder and monitoring for it (i.e. the suggestion of the Chairman of the Association of NHS Occupational Physicians).

9. Consideration should be given to how GPs might, with the candidate's consent, be asked to certify that there is nothing in the medical history of a candidate for employment in the National Health Service which would make them unsuitable for their chosen occupation.

10. The Department of Health should take steps to ensure that its guide, 'Welfare of children and young people in hospital', is more closely observed

11. In the event of failure of an alarm on monitoring equipment, an untoward incident report should be completed and the equipment serviced before it is used again.

12. Reports of serious untoward incidents to District and Regional Health Authorities should be made in writing and through a single channel which is known to all involved.

APPLICATION TO MIDWIFERY

Such events might be unthinkable, but they are not unforeseeable, and even though the possibility is remote, such incidents could occur in a midwifery unit, nursery or special care baby unit. The Inquiry admitted that even if all the recommendations were to be implemented,

> no measures can afford complete protection against a determined miscreant. The main lesson from our Inquiry and our principal recommendation is that the Grantham disaster should serve to heighten awareness in all those caring

for children of the possibility of malevolent intervention as a cause of unexplained clinical events.

What is clear is the need for far greater management control over staff, their sickness records and the knowledge of their present physical and mental health. Staff, too, should be encouraged as the result of the recent legislation on whistle-blowing (see Ch. 22) to raise their concerns with management without the fear of reprisals or victimisation. High standards of care should be identified, linked with an unwillingness to accept changes in patients' condition as an inevitable consequence of being ill.

The recommendation that persons with major personality disorders should not be employed, and that GPs should be asked to certify that there is nothing in a candidate's medical history which would make them unsuitable for employment in the NHS, should be handled with care. Unfortunately, NHS trusts and others, and GPs in determining unsuitability, may in the new scenario of risk management decide that it would be safer not to employ anyone with a history of mental illness, whatever its cause, diagnosis and prognosis. This would be a retrograde step and contrary to the Disability Discrimination Act 1995 (see Ch. 22) and Articles 3 and 14 of the European Convention on Human Rights (see Ch. 6 and Appendix 1).

In addition, it would not necessarily prevent a similar situation arising, since as the Inquiry recognised, there was no evidence at the time of employment that Allitt came into the category to be excluded.

Lessons for the midwife:

- Be aware of the possibility of an Allitt situation.
- Do not be complacent if there is an unexplained deterioration of the patient.
- Ensure new staff are closely monitored.
- Ensure appropriate delegation and supervision.
- Be prepared to raise issues of concern with senior management and pursue these issues if adequate action is not taken.

The report of the Bristol Inquiry recommends that there should be openness within the NHS: that a duty of candour, i.e. a duty to tell a patient if adverse events have occurred, must be recognised as owed to patients by all those working in the NHS. When things go wrong patients are entitled to receive an acknowledgement, an explanation and an apology.[1]

SHIPMAN

An independent public inquiry was set up following the conviction of Dr Shipman, a GP who was convicted of murdering 15 patients. The Committee has published several reports.

The first report[11] considered how many patients Shipman killed, the means employed and the period over which the killings took place.

The second report examined the conduct of the police investigation into Shipman that took place in March 1998 and failed to uncover his crimes.[12]

The third report[13] considered the present system for death and cremation certification and for the investigation of deaths by coroners, together with the conduct of those who had operated those systems in the aftermath of the deaths of Shipman's victims. The report noted that the present system of death and cremation certification failed to detect that Shipman had killed any of his 215 victims (this is considered further in Ch. 18).

The fourth report[14] on the regulation of controlled drugs is discussed in Chapter 20.

The fifth report on the general monitoring and regulation of GPs is considered in Chapter 4.[15]

EXAMPLES OF DECIDED CASES IN MIDWIFERY AND CHILD CARE

Some cases brought in the civil courts for compensation for alleged negligence will now be considered in depth, to illustrate the detail into which the courts go to establish whether or not there is liability. Two cases involving shoulder dystocia are analysed by Natasha Carr.[16] In Holly Lobb v. Hartlepool and East Durham NHS Trust,[17] the claim was dismissed since it was held that the midwife had followed the Bolam Test in deciding not to perform an episiotomy and the fact that she was not aware of the suprapubic option was irrelevant since by placing the mother in the lateral position she achieved in conduct an appropriate standard of care. The use of force was a question of clinical judgement and the judge was not satisfied that the midwife exerted force at an inappropriate time. In contrast in the other case, Sutcliffe v. Countess of Chester Hospital NHS Trust,[18] the claimant succeeded in his claim for Erb's palsy. Liability of the defendant was established on grounds that the evidence of the expert witness called for the claimant (which suggested that brachial plexus injury was caused by the application of excessive traction) was preferred to that of the defendant's expert, whose report was not supported by proper empirical evidence. In the absence of independent recollection, the registrar and the midwife were dependent on their notes and there was an absence of record about shoulder dystocia and the use of a finger to assist delivery. The cases illustrate the importance of clear, comprehensive record keeping and also the fact that protocols and procedures cannot replace clinical judgement.

In the case of Lucy Reynolds v. North Tyneside Health Authority[19] the claimant was born with cerebral palsy caused by birth asphyxia due to acute umbilical cord prolapse which resulted in a severe hypoxaemic insult immediately prior to her delivery. She succeeded in her claim for negligence. The judge held that:

– There was evidence that there was a practice of not carrying out a vaginal examination in the circumstances of the claimant's case, on admission prior to giving an enema.

– The practice of not performing a vaginal examination on admission did not constitute a body of opinion and even if there had been such a body of public opinion, this was a rare case in which it was appropriate to conclude that there was no proper basis for such a body of opinion.

– The evidence of the defendant's midwifery expert was not persuasive since she was not in practice at the relevant time and because it was based on unidentified anecdotal sources.

– The failure to perform the vaginal examination was negligent.

– Had it been performed, the emergency would not have been unforeseen and planned management of the risks could have taken place.

– Had the vaginal examination taken place, the claimant would probably have been delivered without damage.

WISNIEWSKI V. CENTRAL MANCHESTER HEALTH AUTHORITY[20]

On 15 January 1988 at about 2.50 a.m. Mrs W, 31, was admitted to St Mary's Hospital for delivery of her child. The expected date of delivery was 7 January 1988. A midwife, Sister B, carried out an abdominal examination, measured the fetal heart rate (recorded as 160 and regular), recorded the fetus's position as a cephalic presentation with the head 3–4/5ths palpable and noted contractions as irregular. She carried out a vaginal examination at 3.05 a.m. and recorded that the cervix was 1–2 cm dilated, the head was about 3 cm above the ischial spines, in the pelvic rim and not completely free. The midwife considered that Mrs W was a normal patient in early labour.

Mrs W was taken to the pre-delivery room. A CTG trace for the period 3.10 to 3.40 a.m. showed a fetal heart baseline of between 170 and 175 beats per minute (bpm), rising to 180 bpm but not dropping below 160 bpm. The beat to beat variability was 5 bpm. Between 3.10 and 3.40 a.m. there were two decelerations in the fetal heart rate when the rate fell to 130 bpm (at 3.23) and 110 bpm (at 3.40), although it rapidly recovered on both occasions. Sister B did not feel that she needed a doctor but contacted Dr R, the SHO, to inform him of the tachycardia. The Corometric monitor was disconnected shortly after 3.40 a.m. and Mrs W allowed to walk about the ward. The monitor was reconnected at 4.20 a.m. There was no written record of any monitoring. The trace showed less beat to beat variability and decelerations at 4.25 to 120 bpm, at 4.28 to 120 bpm, at 4.35 to 150 bpm, at 4.40 to 150 bpm and at 4.50 to 150 bpm, with a slow recovery. At 5.00 a.m., Sister B carried out a further abdominal examination and recorded that there were two weak to moderate contractions every 10 min and the head was still 3–4/5ths palpable. She also noted tachycardia of 170 from the CTG trace. Sister B said that she did not consider that Mrs W was in established labour at 5.00 a.m.

The vaginal examination was concluded at 5.23 a.m. and revealed that the dilation of the cervix was 5 cm and that it was thin and effaced. The head of the baby was noted as being 1–2 cm above the ischial spines. Sister B explained that it was hospital policy to carry out an artificial rupture of the membrane when the mother was in established labour and that was the reason why at that point she artificially ruptured the membrane; she made a note on the admission record: 'thick meconium-stained liquor'. A fetal scalp electrode was then attached and the fetal heart rate recorded as 160 and regular.

At 5.27 a.m. the CTG trace showed the fetal heart rate failing rapidly and the admission record showed that the fetal heart rate dipped to 60 bpm and did not pick up. Sister B said that she decided to call Dr R when she observed the meconium-stained liquor and that the fetal heart rate had dropped.

Dr R attended at once and many others were then summoned to help. There had been a rapid increase in contractions after the rupture of the membrane. Labour progressed very rapidly and at 5.40 a.m. Philip was born. His head descended rapidly and the cord tightened, depriving him of a blood supply for 13 min.

At birth, his APGAR scores were nil and he showed no signs of life. Only through the highly skilled efforts of the neonatal specialists was Philip revived and the damage to him minimised beyond that which had occurred during the 13 min prior to his birth. At the time of the hearing, Philip was 10 years old and suffered from athetoid cerebral palsy.

The judge decided in favour of the claimant. The main points of his decision were that:

1. Dr R did not attend and examine Mrs W at 3.40 a.m. and therefore did not see the CTG traces as it was not removed from the monitor.

2. It was negligent of Dr R not to attend because:

   (a) There was no supervening emergency that prevented Dr R or another doctor attending.

   (b) Dr R should have attended Mrs W at 3.40 a.m., examined her and considered the CTG trace before deciding what to do; no responsible medical practitioner should have done otherwise and there was no responsible body of medical opinion that would support a decision not to attend.

   (c) The doctor was negligent to have relied upon the midwife and not attended to make his own judgement because Sister B was over-confident in her own abilities and not in any way qualified to make the clinical judgement required at 3.40 a.m., in that her lack of ability to make the proper assessment of treatment that a patient should receive was shown:

(i) by her failure to take any action at 4.50 a.m., when it was accepted by the defendants' experts that action should have been taken, and

(ii) by her failure to ask for a doctor to attend until 5.27 a.m., particularly in the light of what she had found on the vaginal examination at 5.20 a.m.

3. (a) It could be inferred from Dr R's failure to attend at the trial that he had no answer to criticisms made and that, if he had attended at 3.40 a.m. he would, after examination of Mrs W and the CTG trace, have concluded because of the tachycardia and decelerations that it was necessary to rupture the membrane, and concluded it was safe to do so, and thereafter proceeded to a caesarean section.

(b) A competent doctor would, after examination of Mrs W, have concluded that an artificial rupture of the membrane should be performed and that it was safe to do so, and proceeded to a caesarean section because the only real risk that was entailed in carrying out a rupture of the membrane at or shortly after 3.40 a.m. was the possibility of a cord prolapse; there was no risk of accelerating labour at that time.

(c) Any competent assessment of that risk would have to take into account an examination to see if the cord could be felt, the position of the head, which was not free, and the risk of the head moving.

His failure to attend was the direct cause of the baby being born with cerebral palsy as, had he attended, he would have ruptured the membrane, noted the meconium and that would have led to a decision to perform a caesarean section.

4. Sister B was negligent in not calling the doctor and in delaying the vaginal examination, and rupturing the membranes without asking the doctor to attend was seriously negligent.

The defendants appealed to the Court of Appeal, but lost the appeal on the grounds that:

1. It was impossible for the court to hold that the views sincerely held by the defendants' experts could not logically be supported at all; accordingly, the views expressed by those experts could be supported and held by responsible doctors.

2. The judge did not err in drawing an adverse inference from the failure of Dr R to appear at the trial because the principles were:

(a) In certain circumstances, a court may draw adverse inferences from absence of a witness who might be expected to have material evidence to give on an issue.

(b) If a court were willing to draw such inferences, they might strengthen evidence adduced on that issue by the other party – or weaken evidence adduced by the party who might reasonably have been expected to call the witness.

(c) There must be a case to answer on that issue.

(d) If the reason for the witness's absence satisfied the court then no such adverse inference might be drawn.

3. The plaintiff had established a *prima facie*, if weak, case that a doctor who attended the mother at 3.40 a.m. would probably have adopted the course which the plaintiff's expert witness testified was his duty. The judge was entitled to treat Dr R's absence as strengthening the case against him on that issue.

4. As to causation, the judge correctly held that since the damage that occurred was caused by hypoxia, it made no difference that the precise mechanism by which the hypoxia arose was not foreseeable.

Many points arise from this case
1. Fault must be shown

As was noted in Chapter 13, we have at present a system of fault liability, so in order to obtain compensation for negligence it must be shown that there was a breach of the duty of care. In this case, this was established and so the claimant obtained compensation. In countries where a system of no-fault liability is in place, compensation is payable if a medical accident can be shown to have occurred, whether or not there was fault by anyone. The Department of Health is considering the possibility of introducing a system of no-fault liability in clinical claims.

2. The importance of record keeping (see Ch. 15)

Since the baby was born 10 years before the court hearing, there would have been almost total reliance on what was recorded during the labour.

3. The importance of defining the scope of professional practice

Sister B was criticised for failing to obtain the doctor's attendance. She was seen as over-confident. The judge considered that, had she asked the doctor to attend when she first phoned him, then the doctor would have ruptured the membranes, seen the stained meconium and arranged for a caesarean to have taken place immediately. The case raises the issue of what the competent midwife can be expected to do without the involvement of the doctor, and when reasonable practice requires the midwife to call in the doctor.

4. The importance of ensuring that witnesses give evidence

In this case, the doctor was, at the time of the hearing, in Australia and said that there was no point in his returning because he could not provide any further evidence. The judge criticised the failure to obtain his attendance or conduct a video interview.

5. Role and importance of expert witnesses

Experts are required to give evidence to the court on the standards which they would have expected to have been followed at the time. They may also (as in this case) give evidence on causation, i.e. whether the harm which occurred could be factually attributed to the breach of duty by the defendant (see Ch. 15 on the role of experts and witnesses of fact).

HALLATT AND HALLATT V. NORTH WEST ANGLIA HEALTH AUTHORITY[21]

Mrs H, who was 29–30 weeks into her seventh pregnancy on 8 October 1990, visited her GP, who in the light of the urine test ordered a random blood sugar test which proved to be normal. On 21 November 1990, Mrs H was examined by the clinical assistant to the Consultant obstetrician at Peterborough District Hospital. He noted the urine test showed glycosuria but was reassured by a random blood sugar result of 4.6 mmol/l. Accordingly, a glucose tolerance test (GTT) was not carried out. On 26 December 1990, Mrs H gave birth to a boy weighing 12 lbs 12 oz. Vaginal delivery was stopped because of shoulder dystocia. The baby was delivered by caesarean section, but suffered brain damage caused by oxygen deprivation and damage to the left brachial plexus. Mrs H sued for negligence on her own account and that of the baby. The High Court judge dismissed her claim on the following grounds:

- On 8 October 1990, on the balance of probabilities, she was not suffering from gestational diabetes, but she was by 21 November 1990.

- A GTT carried out on or after that date would have disclosed that fact, and good obstetric practice would have led to the baby being delivered by caesarean section, probably with no significant injuries or disabilities.

- Reliance on a random blood test could not stand up to critical analysis, but its use could be justified on grounds of ease and convenience, provided its limitations were recognised. In this case, it was relied upon in ignorance of its limitations and, to that extent, the practice at Peterborough Hospital could not be approved.

- The claimants had not shown that the decision itself was wrong and that no reasonably competent doctor would have failed to carry out a GTT in the prevailing circumstances.

Mrs H appealed against this decision. The Court of Appeal held that:

- The question which the clinical assistant had to consider was whether the single random urine sample result on 8 October converted the case from one in which no GTT was required into one where it was.

– The clinical assistant was assessing the significance of a single and isolated observation of mild glycosuria at 29 or 30 weeks. By most criteria, that did not suffice to require the GTT. The clinical assistant was entitled to be reassured by the negative result of the random blood test which could only go to confirm the assessment that this single incident of glycosuria did not alter the risk assessment.

Mrs H lost her appeal.

Comment on the case

– A distinction is drawn between best practice and reasonable practice. It would have been excellent practice for a GTT to have been taken on 21 November 1990 but it would not have been reasonable in the light of the evidence which existed.

– The case also shows that hindsight should not be used against the defendant. Clearly in hindsight, had a GTT been carried out on 21 November, the birth would have followed a very different course, but in the light of the knowledge available on 21 November 1990 it was not reasonable to have required a GTT.

– The issue of causation did not arise: the judge accepted that had a GTT been undertaken the gestational diabetes would have been diagnosed. The issue was simply what the reasonable standard would have been. Clearly had a no-fault system of compensation been in existence, Mrs H would have been able to obtain compensation.

WHITEHOUSE V. JORDAN[22]

The defendant, a senior hospital registrar, took charge of the plaintiff's delivery as a baby after the mother had been in labour for a considerable time. The notes made by the Consultant professor in charge of the hospital maternity unit identified the pregnancy as likely to be difficult and noted that a 'trial of forceps' delivery would have to be tried before proceeding to delivery by caesarean section. Trial of forceps was a tentative procedure, requiring delicate handling of the baby with forceps and a continuous review of the baby's progress down the birth canal, with the obligation to stop traction if it appeared that the delivery could not proceed without risk. Having examined the mother and read the professor's notes, the defendant embarked on a trial of forceps delivery. He pulled on the baby six times with the forceps coincident with the mother's contractions, but when there was no movement on the fifth and sixth pulls he decided, some 25 min after the commencement of the trial of forceps, to abandon that procedure and to proceed to a caesarean section. He then quickly and competently delivered the plaintiff by caesarean section. The plaintiff was found soon after the delivery to have sustained severe brain damage due to asphyxia. Acting by his mother as next friend, he claimed damages for negligence against the defendant, alleging that he had pulled too long and too hard on the plaintiff's head in carrying out the trial of forceps and thereby caused the brain damage.

At the trial the mother gave evidence that she was 'lifted off' the bed by the application of the forceps and although that description of what happened was rejected by the judge as being clinically impossible, on the suggestion of an expert witness he interpreted it to mean that the forceps were applied with such force that she was pulled towards the bottom of the bed in a manner inconsistent with a properly carried out trial of forceps.

The defendant gave evidence that when there was no progress on the fifth pull of the forceps he pulled once more to see if he could ease the head past what might have been only a minimal obstruction, but as there was no further progress he decided to proceed to caesarean section and he had easily pushed the head slightly upwards to effect the caesarean section. He denied that the head was wedged or stuck prior to the caesarean section. The judge interpreted his evidence to mean that he had pulled too long and too hard, causing the head to become wedged or stuck.

There was also in evidence a report made by the Consultant professor shortly after the delivery, from clinical notes and after discussion with the defendant, the tenor of which was that the mother had received correct and skilled treatment and that no blame attached to anyone for the plaintiff's condition. However, in the report the professor referred three times to 'disimpaction' of the head prior to the caesarean section. At the trial, the professor gave evidence that he had used that term as meaning no more than that a gentle push of the head up the birth canal was needed before proceeding to the caesarean section. There was no unanimity of opinion among the other medical experts as to the meaning of the term 'impacted' or whether it meant that there had been excessive or unprofessional traction with the forceps. The evidence of the medical experts made it clear, however, that the amount of force to be properly used in a trial of forceps was a matter of clinical judgement, although there should be no attempt to pull the fetus past a bony obstruction, and if the head became so stuck as to cause asphyxia, excessive force had been used. The judge inferred from the professor's use of the term 'disimpacted' that the plaintiff's head had become so firmly wedged or stuck, that in so doing or in getting the head unwedged or unstuck he had caused the plaintiff's asphyxia, and that in so using the forceps he had fallen below the standard of skill expected from the ordinary competent specialist and had therefore been negligent. The judge accordingly awarded the plaintiff £100 000 damages.

The defendant appealed.

The Court of Appeal reversed the judge's decision, on the following grounds:

1. If the judge's finding that the defendant pulled too long and too hard with the forceps during the trial of forceps was accepted, that amounted only to an error of clinical judgement and as such was not negligence in law.

2. In any event, the court was entitled to, and would, reverse that finding because it was based on an unjustified interpretation of the evidence.

The plaintiff appealed to the House of Lords.

The House of Lords held that although the view of the trial judge (who had seen and heard the witnesses) as to the weight to be given to their evidence was always entitled to great respect, where his decision on an issue of fact was an inference drawn from the primary facts and depended on the evidentiary value he gave to the witnesses' evidence and not on their credibility and demeanour, an appellate court was just as well placed as the trial judge to determine the proper inference to be drawn and was entitled to form its own opinion thereon. Since the judge's conclusion of fact that the defendant had pulled too long and too hard with the forceps was primarily an inference from the primary facts, no issue as to credibility was involved. Accordingly, his conclusion was open to reassessment by the appellate court and it was entitled to find that the evidence did not justify the inference that the defendant negligently pulled too hard and too long with the forceps. It followed that the Court of Appeal was entitled to reject the judge's finding of negligence.

The appeal would therefore be dismissed.

In addition, three judges stated that

> To say that a surgeon had committed an error of clinical judgement is wholly ambiguous and does not indicate whether he has been negligent, for while some errors of clinical judgement may be completely consistent with the due exercise of professional skill, other acts or omissions in the course of exercising clinical judgement may be so glaringly below proper standards as to make a finding of negligence inevitable. The test whether a surgeon has been negligent is whether he has failed to measure up in any respect, clinical judgement or otherwise, to the standard of the ordinary skilled surgeon exercising and professing to have the special skill of a surgeon.

The court also emphasised that it is necessary that expert evidence presented to the court should be, and should be seen to be, the independent product of the expert, uninfluenced as to form or content by the exigencies of litigation.

Comment

This was the only one of the cases discussed above which went before the House of Lords. The principles which were established in the judgement on the definition of the standard of care, and when, if ever, an error of judgement can be regarded as negligence are binding on all courts in the country and can only be overruled by the House of Lords itself or by Act of Parliament.

The case shows the dangers of using words loosely. One of the experts referred to the head being impacted, when there was no clear evidence that this was so. When midwives are keeping records it is essential that they should not put down information unless there is clear evidence for what they write, and that terms are not used carelessly.

KNIGHT V. WEST KENT HEALTH AUTHORITY[23]

The claimant brought a claim in respect of a number of medical problems attributed to the birth including damage to the perineum, persistent rectal and abdominal pains, dyspareunia, a cervical tear and fistula, depression, irritable bowel syndrome and a laparoscopy for a vaginal prolapse. She claimed that the obstetrician was in breach of his duty of care to her by attempting a long difficult pull in a forceps delivery and failing to abandon it when it was apparent that vaginal delivery could only be effected by very strong traction. In the High Court the mother won compensation of £64 059.20, with costs. The Health Authority appealed against the decision and succeeded. The Court of Appeal upheld their appeal on the grounds that the trial judge was wrong to conclude that the doctor had been negligent. He used no more than moderate and therefore an appropriate amount of force and exercised his clinical judgement in deciding that this was appropriate. In addition, given the size of the baby (11 lb 2 oz) the mother did not suffer any more damage than she would have had if the baby was delivered naturally. The mother did however receive compensation for the additional pain and suffering that she had endured because, on the admission of the defendants, the doctor had attended 2.5 hours later than he should have done. The amount to be paid for this was to be agreed between the parties.

Comment

It is unusual for the Court of Appeal to go against the trial judge's findings of fact, but here they were clearly of the view that the judge was wrong to conclude that the defendant was negligent. The defendants had admitted some negligence because of the delay in the doctor arriving, but compensation in respect of the harm caused by that would be much less than if the original finding of negligence in the management of the birth had been upheld.

INMAN V. CAMBRIDGE HEALTH AUTHORITY[24]

(The details of the award of compensation of this case are shown in Ch. 13.)

The mother was admitted to the maternity hospital for induction of labour for postmaturity on 21 October 1988. Contractions started at 11.10 p.m. on 22 October. A CTG scan was commenced and from 1.50 a.m. showed gross dips, but medical assistance was not sought by the midwife. From 1.58 a.m., these dips were confluent and the fetal heart rate dipped to 60 bpm. Still the midwife failed to call for medical assistance. At 2.00 a.m. there was only a thin anterior lip of the cervix. At 2.10 a.m. full dilation was recorded and the midwife summoned a paediatrician, but not an obstetrician. The CTG continued to record fetal distress with a fetal heart rate of 60 bpm, which then swung wildly from 60 to 80 bpm until the child was delivered at 2.37 a.m. He was severely acidotic and had suffered acute intrapartum asphyxia as a result of cord entanglement which had led to an increase in hypoxia as the head descended. The child sustained bilateral cerebral cortical damage resulting in spastic quadriplegic cerebral palsy.

A writ was issued in July 1992 and a defence served in March 1993 admitting negligence on the part of the midwife for failing to summon an obstetrician at about 2.00 a.m. but denying causation. An order was made for a split trial, but just prior to the case being set down for hearing, the defendants admitted liability for all of the child's cerebral palsy. The child's paediatric neurologist advised that it was too early to give an opinion on prognosis and life expectancy and therefore, pending a final settlement, a series of interim payments were made to fund his therapies and equipment, and to build a specially-designed bungalow for the child, his parents and two older brothers. The assessment of damages hearing was listed for March 1998. The claimant wished to investigate a structured settlement but the NHSLA failed to approve the annuity figures. The NHSLA finally agreed a structured settlement when threatened with the possibility of the Chief Executive of the NHSLA being called to court to explain why it was attempting to charge the claimant extra for the structure.

Comment

Like the Wisniewski case (p. 284) this is another case of failure by the midwife to summon the obstetrician at the appropriate time. However, in this case, the defendants accepted that the midwife was in breach of her duty of care, but denied that this fault had caused the harm suffered by the baby. Shortly afterwards, however, the defendants accepted liability and the only outstanding issue was how much compensation should be paid (see Ch. 13). The case also illustrates the problems in setting up a structured settlement.

EVIDENCE BY MIDWIVES IN OTHER CASES

While midwives can anticipate having to give evidence in court if there is a claim brought by a mother on her own behalf or on behalf of her baby, the midwife might also have to give evidence in other proceedings involving colleagues such as doctors registered with the General Medical Council. For example, in January 2001 the General Medical Council heard a case of professional misconduct brought against an obstetrician and gynaecologist in Gateshead. Mothers alleged that he had used so much force in forceps deliveries that one baby was born with a black eye and another had his head swollen to twice the normal size. Midwives at the unit had to give evidence to the GMC, which decided that he should be struck off.[25] The Royal College of Obstetricians and Gynaecologists said that the case highlighted the need for trusts to employ doctors who are Members of the College and had proper practical and communication skills. The spokesman stated, 'Doctors must treat women with respect at all times, particularly during labour, when a woman is most in need of sympathetic care'.

WOOLF REFORMS OF CIVIL PROCEDURES

Lord Woolf was invited to examine the deficiencies and make recommendations for reform in our procedure for civil justice. In June 1995 Lord Woolf issued an interim report on access to justice.[26] This reported on recommendations to change our system of obtaining compensation for personal injuries. His specific proposals on medical negligence include:

– training of health professionals in negligence claims

– GMC and other regulatory bodies to consider the need to clarify the professional conduct responsibilities in relation to negligence actions

– improvement of record systems to trace former staff

– use of alternative dispute mechanisms

– a separate medical negligence list for the High Court and County Courts

– specially designated court centres outside London for handling medical negligence cases

– methods to reduce delays by improving arrangements for listing of cases

– investigation of improved training for judges in medical negligence

– standard tables to be used where possible to determine quantum

– practice guide on the new case management

– pilot study to consider medical negligence claims below £10 000.

The final report was published in July 1996[27] and led to the implementation of a new procedure for civil claims in April 1999.

Features of the scheme include:

– A new system of case management with the courts rather than the parties taking the main responsibility for the progress of cases.

– Defended cases are allocated for the purposes of case management by the courts to one of three tracks:

  - small claims (up to £5000). This provides a procedure for straightforward claims which do not exceed £5000, without the need for substantial pre-hearing preparation and the formalities of a traditional trial and where costs are kept low.

  - A new fast track with limited procedures and reduced costs (up to £10 000). Factors deciding whether a case is allocated to the fast track include: the limits likely to be placed on disclosure, the extent to which expert evidence may be necessary and whether the trial will last longer than a day. However, certain

exceptions to the fast track were recommended and these included medical negligence cases.

- A new multi-track (for more complex cases over £10 000).

The court allocates each case to one of these three tracks on the basis of information
provided by the claimant on the statement of case. If it does not have enough information to allocate the claim then it will make an order requiring one or more parties
to provide further information within 14 days.

Case management (see below) directions are given at the allocation stage or at the
listing stage.

MEDIATION

One of the results of the Woolf Reforms in civil justice is that the parties are encouraged to resolve the dispute before going to court using mediation or other forms of
resolution such as Alternative Dispute Resolution. Often such processes can be linked
with the complaints procedure (see Ch. 11) to avoid litigation. In mediation, an
independent mediator attempts to assist the parties to bring about an agreement to
resolve the dispute. Unlike arbitration, the parties are under no compulsion to accept
any ruling by the independent person. The Annual Report for 2000 of the NHS
Litigation Authority points out the low uptake of mediation: 'Virtually everyone
engaged in civil litigation pays lip service to the benefits of mediation, but in practice
it is proving extremely difficult to persuade the parties to put their words into
practice'.

CASE MANAGEMENT

The overriding principle enshrined in the new Civil Procedure Rules[28] (see Box 14.2)
is that all cases should be dealt with justly. The court must seek to give effect to this
overriding principle when it exercises any powers under the rules and when it inter-
prets any rule. The parties also have a duty to help the court to further this overriding
objective. The court in furthering this principle of dealing with cases justly must
actively manage the cases. Active management includes:

– encouraging the parties to cooperate with each other in the conduct of the
  proceedings

– identifying the issues at an early stage

– deciding promptly which issues need full investigation and trial and accordingly
  disposing summarily of the others

– deciding the order in which the issues are to be resolved

– encouraging the parties to use an Alternative Dispute Resolution procedure if the court considers that appropriate, and facilitating the use of such procedure

– helping the parties to settle the whole or part of the case

– fixing timetables or otherwise controlling the progress of the case

– considering whether the likely benefits of taking a particular step justify the cost of taking it

– dealing with as many aspects of the case as it can on the same occasion

– dealing with the case without the parties needing to attend court

– making use of technology, and

– giving directions to ensure that the trial of a case proceeds quickly and efficiently.

CLINICAL NEGLIGENCE PRE-ACTION PROTOCOL

As a consequence of the Woolf Reforms and the work of the Clinical Disputes Forum (a multi-disciplinary group formed in 1997 as a result of the Woolf recommendations) a clinical negligence pre-action protocol was drawn up which is now part of the Practice Directions which are part of the Civil Procedure Rules. This protocol requires parties to follow specific steps at the beginning of an action (3 months from the notification of the claim) and they are penalised if they fail. Times are set for the response to requests for records, etc. (Box 14.2).

Box 14.2 Overriding objective in civil proceedings

The rules are a new procedural code with the overriding objective of enabling the court to deal with cases justly. Dealing with a case justly includes, so far as is practicable:

1. Ensuring that the parties are on an equal footing

2. Saving expense

3. Dealing with the case in ways which are proportionate:

   (a) to the amount of money involved

   (b) to the importance of the case

▶

(c) to the complexity of the issues, and

(d) to the financial position of each party

4. Ensuring that it is dealt with expeditiously and fairly, and

5. Allotting to it an appropriate share of the court's resources, while taking into account the need to allot resources to other cases.

The Lord Chancellor's Department published its first review of the new Civil Procedure Rules in April 2001.[29] It concluded that there appeared to have been a drop in the number of claims issued, that the new pre-action protocols were working well, settlements were increasing, with alternative methods of resolving claims being used.

NEW SCHEME FOR OBTAINING COMPENSATION FOR CLINICAL NEGLIGENCE

In Chapter 13, the report of the National Audit Office[30] was considered. It was stated that the NHS must make provision for almost £4 billion for outstanding claims and estimated further liabilities for claims arising out of negligent episodes which had already occurred. There is no doubt that radical measures are necessary to halt the increase in the cost of litigation and the size of claims within the NHS, and the burden that this places upon NHS funds. On 10 July 2001 the Secretary of State[31] announced that the Chief Medical Officer was to chair a committee to look at possible changes to the present system for securing compensation within the NHS, with the intention of enabling a White Paper to be published in 2002 setting out the government's reforms for obtaining compensation within the NHS. Suggestions for change include:

– a no-fault liability system

– structured settlements so that patients receive periodic payments (these are already legally possible but the NHSLA (see Ch. 13) does not favour them)

– a scheme for fixed tariffs for specific injuries (comparable with the Criminal Injury Compensation scheme which is considered in Ch. 18) and

– greater use of mediation or other ways of resolving disputes.

In 2003 another consultation paper was published by the Department of Health.[32] 'Making Amends' provides a comprehensive account of the background to the present situation. It looks at the present system of medical negligence litigation and its costs. It analyses public attitudes and concerns and the earlier reviews of the negligence system by the Pearson Commission,[33] the Woolf Report on Access to Justice[27] and the National Audit Office Report in 2001.[34] It considers recent action taken to reform civil court procedures, claims handling by the NHS Litigation Authority and the use of alternative dispute resolution. It analyses systems of no-fault liability in New Zealand, Sweden, Finland, Denmark Norway and France and discusses no-fault liability as an option along with continued reform of the present tort process, a tariff-based national tribunal or a composite option drawing on all three. The scheme eventually recommended in 'Making Amends' is a composite package of reform drawing on the best elements of the three options.

An NHS Redress Scheme should be established to enable claimants, who had suffered harm, to obtain a rehabilitation, remedial and care package, explanation, apology and in certain cases financial compensation. The aim of the scheme would be that following an allegation that harm had been caused to a patient, a mechanism would exist to organise a response and in suitable cases consider whether payment for pain and suffering, for out of pocket expenses and for care or treatment provided outside the NHS should be made. The requirement of the scheme would be to reach a decision on the case within six months from the initial approach from the patient. Payment would be made to the claimant if:

– there were serious shortcomings in the standards of care

– the harm could have been avoided

– the adverse outcome was not the result of the natural progression of the illness.

Financial compensation would be limited to the notional cost of the episode of care, or up to £30 000. The hope is that while initially financial recompense may be offered, in time the emphasis should be on the provision of packages of care.

A pilot scheme would be introduced using the Bolam Test[35] of clinical negligence. Subsequently however the possibility of using a lower qualifying threshold of 'sub-standard care' would be considered. The possibility of extending the scheme to a higher monetary threshold and to primary care settings would be considered after evaluation of the scheme.

Care and compensation for severely neurologically impaired babies
At present, some babies are able to obtain substantial compensation if negligence can be proved, whilst other babies with similar disabilities are not able to obtain compensation. It is therefore recommended that within the NHS Redress scheme special eligibility criteria should be used:

– birth under NHS care

– severe neurological impairment (including cerebral palsy) related to or resulting from birth

– a claim made to the scheme within eight years of the birth

– the care package and compensation would be based on a severity index judged according to the ability to perform the activities of daily living

– genetic or chromosomal abnormality would be excluded.

The recipient would have a managed care package, a monthly payment for costs of care which cannot be provided through a care package, lump sum payments for home adaptations and equipment and an initial payment in compensation for pain, suffering and loss of amenity capped at £50 000. The scheme would be administered by a National Body using a panel of experts to review the severity of impairment and causation.

National body to administer the NHS Redress Scheme

A new National body would be created based on the NHS Litigation Authority with a wider remit to administer the NHS Redress Scheme.

NHS Redress Scheme to be part of the system for handling complaints

Each adverse event or complaint should have a full and objective investigation of the facts of the case leading to a written explanation. In addition under the NHS Redress Scheme, NHS trusts would be able to take early action to offer any remedial treatment or rehabilitation measures and payments. A new standard of care would be set for after-event/after-complaint management by local NHS providers. The Commission for Healthcare Audit and Inspection (Healthcare Commission) should assess compliance with this standard in its inspections. An individual at Board level should be identified to take overall responsibility for the investigation of and learning from adverse events, complaints and claims. The rule that an investigation of a complaint should be halted if the complainant commenced a claim should be removed, since the investigation should automatically take place as part of the initial local response to a complaint and even if the patient subsequently decided to pursue litigation, the complaints process should continue to provide the explanations required by patients and families. Training should be provided for NHS staff in communication in the context of complaints.

Retention of the right to pursue litigation through the courts and changes to the existing scheme for civil proceedings

The NHS Redress Scheme would exist alongside the existing processes for obtaining compensation through the civil courts. However, if claimants had accepted redress under the NHS scheme they would not be able to pursue a civil action through the civil courts. There are however attempts to make the NHS Redress Scheme more attractive than civil litigation. For example if claimants were to apply for legal aid to pursue civil action, whether or not they had already sought redress through the NHS scheme would be taken into account. Significant changes are also recommended for reforms to the current procedure for compensation for clinical negligence through the civil courts. For example mediation should be seriously considered before litigation for the majority of claims which do not fall within the proposed NHS Redress Scheme. Judges who hear clinical negligence cases should have special training.

Other recommendations are designed to reduce the costs of payments: for example the law will be changed to enable periodical payments to be made without the consent of the parties, so that this became the norm in clinical negligence cases; the costs of future care included in any award for clinical negligence made by the courts should no longer reflect the cost of private treatment. Instead the NHS defendant should undertake to fund a specified package of care or treatment to defined time-tables. In another attempt to reduce costs in litigation it is recommended that the Department for Constitutional Affairs and the Legal Services Commission should consider further ways to control the claimants' costs in clinical negligence cases, where they are publicly funded.

A duty of candour

A duty of candour should be introduced together with exemption from disciplinary action when reporting incidents with a view to improving patient safety: legislation should be introduced to create a duty on healthcare professionals and managers to inform patients where they become aware of a possible negligent action or omission. However, it is recommended that this should be linked with provision for an exemp-tion from disciplinary action by employees or professional regulatory bodies for those reporting adverse events, except where the healthcare professional has committed a criminal offence or it would not be safe for the professional to continue to treat patients. To provide further incentive to the reporting of adverse events it is recom-mended that documents and information collected for identifying adverse events should be protected from disclosure in court. It is recommended that this protection should only apply to reports of adverse events where full information on the event is also included in the medical record.

The consultation paper on the NHS Redress scheme ended on 17 October 2003 and a draft Bill was published in October 2005. The proposals for no-fault liability for brain-damaged babies are not included. It is unlikely that any significant changes would take place before April 2007. In the meantime new procedures for Complaints handling have been introduced (see Ch. 11) which would bar a person from using the complaints procedure if they intend to take civil action – a provision which appears to be totally contrary to the philosophy behind Making Amends.

CONCLUSION

There is no doubt that the continuing increase in claims for compensation and the burden of the current levels of payment are causing considerable anxiety to the very future and survival of the NHS. On the one hand, every reasonable action must be taken to raise standards of practice and learn from the incidents which have occurred (see the National Patient Safety Agency which is considered in Ch. 19), but on the other hand, there are very real concerns about the effectiveness of our current system for compensation, with a considerable proportion of the cost being paid to the legal professionals. Both these issues are on the agenda contained within the NHS Plan and in the wider public sector field.[36] In the meantime it is the duty of every midwife to ensure that her standards of care reflect the lessons learnt from cases of negligence analysed by lawyers[37] and researchers.[38]

QUESTIONS AND EXERCISES

1. Taking any of the cases described in detail in this chapter, consider:

   (a) whether the same standards would apply today

   (b) what evidence would be required to establish either a defence or the claimant's case

   (c) the practical lessons to be learnt for the future from such a case.

2. To what extent is your own field of practice safe from bogus professionals or the entry of strangers intent on harm?

3. What action would you take if you had concerns about a colleague's actions or omissions in relation to the safety of clients?

References

1 Bristol Royal Infirmary. Learning from Bristol: The report of the public inquiry into children's heart surgery at the Bristol Royal Infirmary 1984–1995. Command paper CM 5207; 2001.

2 The Times, 14 April 1994.

3 Enright v. Kwun [2003] EWHC 1000, The Times, 20 May 2003.

4 Pharmaceutical Journal, 16 May 1992, 641.

5 British Paediatric Association. Vitamin K Prophylaxis in Infancy: Report of an Expert Committee. London: British Paediatric Association; 1992.

6 Wickham S. Vitamin K: A flaw in the blueprint. Midwifery Today 2000; 56:39–41; reprinted in MIDIRS Midwifery Digest 2000; 11(3):393–396.

7 Department of Health. Vitamin K: Information for parents to be. London: HMSO; 2000. Online. Available: www.doh.gov.uk/vitk.htm

8 Williams B, Arulkumaran S. Best practice and research, Vol 18. London: Elsevier; 2004:457–466; reprinted as Cardiotocography and medico legal issues. MIDIRS Midwifery Digest 2004; 14(4):504–509.

9 News item. The Times, 2 July 1994.

10 Department of Health. The Allitt Inquiry. Chaired by Sir Cecil Clothier. London: HMSO; 1994.

11 Shipman Inquiry First Report. Death disguised, published 19 July 2002. Online. Available: www.the-shipman-inquiry.org.uk/reports.asp

12 Shipman Inquiry Second Report. The police investigation of March 1998, published 14 July 2003. Online. Available: www.the-shipman-inquiry.org.uk/reports.asp

13 Shipman Inquiry Third Report. Death and cremation certification, published 14 July 2003. Online. Available: www.the-shipman-inquiry.org.uk/reports.asp

14 Shipman Inquiry Fourth Report. The regulation of controlled drugs in the community, published 15 July 2004. Online. Available: www.the-shipman-inquiry.org.uk/reports.asp

15 Shipman Inquiry Fifth Report. Profession regulation safeguarding patients: lessons from the past – proposals for the future. Command Paper CM 6394. London: Stationery Office; 2004. Online. Available: www.the-shipman-inquiry.org.uk/reports.asp

16 Carr N. Litigation and the midwife: shoulder dystocia. The Practising Midwife 2004; 7(10):24–27.

17 Lobb (Holly) v. Hartlepool and East Durham NHS Trust [2002] Lloyd's Rep Med 442.

18 Sutcliffe v. Countess of Chester Hospital NHS Trust [2002] Lloyd's Rep Med 449.

19 Reynolds (Lucy) v. North Tyneside Health Authority [2002] Lloyd's Rep Med 459.

20 Wisniewski v. Central Manchester Health Authority CA [1998] Lloyd's Rep Med 223.

21 Hallatt and Hallatt v. North West Anglia Health Authority [1998] CA Lloyd's Rep Med 197.

22 Whitehouse v. Jordan [1981] 1 All ER 267.

23 Knight v. West Kent Health Authority [1998] Lloyd's Rep Med 18.

24 Inman v. Cambridge Health Authority. In: Kemp and Kemp. Quantum of damages, Vol 2. London: Sweet and Maxwell; 1998.

25 Chittenden M. Gynaecologist struck off over brutal births. Sunday Times, 14 January 2001.

26 Lord Woolf. Interim Report on Access to Justice Inquiry. London: Lord Chancellor's Office; 1995.

27 Lord Woolf. Final Report: Access to Justice. London: HMSO; 1996.

28 Grainger I, Fealy M. Introduction to the new civil procedure rules. London: Cavendish Publications; 1999.

29 Lord Chancellor's Office. Emerging findings: an early evaluation of the Civil Justice Reforms. London: Lord Chancellor's Office; 2001.

30 National Audit Office. Handling clinical negligence claims in England: Report of the Controller and Auditor General. House of Commons Session 2000–2001, 3 May 2001.

31 Department of Health. New Clinical Compensation Scheme for the NHS. Press release 2001/0313; 2001.

32 Department of Health. Making Amends. A consultation paper setting out proposals for reforming the approach to clinical negligence in the NHS. CMO June 2003.

33 Pearson Report. Royal Commission on Civil Liability and Compensation for Personal Injury. HMSO 1978.

34 National Audit Office Handling Clinical negligence claims in England; Report by the Comptroller and Auditor General HC 403 Session 2000–2001 3 May 2001. London: Stationery Office; 2001.

35 Bolam v. Friern Hospital Management Committee [1957] 1 WLR 582.

36 Better Regulation Task Force. Better Routes to Redress. London: BRTF; May 2004.

37 Jordan L. Reducing obstetric risk: Why do women sue? MIDIRS Midwifery Digest 2001; 11(1):117–119.

38 Symon A. Obstetric litigation from A to Z. Wiltshire: Mark Allen Publishing; 2001.

Chapter 15
RECORD KEEPING, STATEMENTS AND REPORT WRITING

This chapter considers the duty of keeping clear, comprehensive records, the making of statements, the compiling of reports and giving evidence in court.

DUTY OF CARE AND RECORD KEEPING

The keeping of clear comprehensive records is part of the duty of care owed to the client. Midwives have a specific statutory duty under the Midwives Rules[1] in relation to records. The duty is set out in Box 15.1.

Box 15.1 Records and the midwife

Rule 9

1. A practising midwife shall keep, as contemporaneously as is reasonable, continuous and detailed records of observations made, care given and medicine and any form of pain relief administered by her to a woman or baby.

2. The records referred to in Para. (1) of this rule shall be kept:

    (a) in the case of a midwife employed by an NHS Authority, in accordance with any directions given by her employer

    (b) in any other case, in a form approved by the local supervising authority covering her main area of practice.

3. A midwife must not destroy or permit the destruction of records which have been made whilst she is in attendance upon a woman or baby.

4. Immediately before ceasing to practise or if she finds it impossible or inconvenient to preserve her records safely, a midwife shall transfer them:

(a) If she is employed by an NHS Authority, to that authority

(b) If she is employed by a private sector employer, to that employer

(c) If she is not covered by para. a or b, to the local supervising authority in whose area the care took place.

5. Any transfer under para. 4 must be duly recorded by each party to the transfer

6. For the purpose of this rule:

'NHS authority' means:

(a) in relation to England and Wales, any body established under the NHS Act 1977 or the NHS and Community Care Act 1990 which employs midwives

(b) in relation to Scotland, any body constituted under the NHS (Scotland) Act 1978 which employs midwives

(c) in relation to Northern Ireland, any body established under the Health and Personal Social Services (Northern Ireland) Order 1972 which employs midwives.

'Private sector employer' means:

an organisation other that an NHS authority or a limited company or partnership in which the midwife or any member of her family has or has had a substantial interest.

As was emphasised in Chapter 4, the Rules are part of the law of the country and are therefore automatically binding upon the midwife.

The NMC has provided standards for the LSA and also guidance on Rule 9. The NMC guidance incorporated in its document on the Midwives Rules replaces the previous Midwives Code of Practice.[2] The NMC Guidance on Rule 9 emphasises that:

the midwives' records relating to the care of women and babies are an essential aspect of practice to aid communication between you, the woman and others who are providing care. They demonstrate whether you have provided an appropriate standard of care to a woman or baby.

The NMC suggest that all records relating to the care of the woman or baby must be kept for 25 years. This would include work diaries if they contain clinical information. Other documents, for example, duty rotas, are a matter for local resolution and where national guidelines are available, these should be followed.

Although the NMC suggests a 25-year retention period, as does the Department of Health in its guidance on the storage of records,[3] if there is any sign that the child is brain-damaged or suffers from a mental disability, those records should be kept until after the death of that person, since there is no time limit on bringing an action for compensation as long as the complainant who has a mental disability is alive (see Ch. 13).

LOCAL SUPERVISORY AUTHORITY STANDARDS ON RULE 9

The NMC requires LSAs to ensure the safe preservation of records transferred to it in accordance with the Midwives Rules, to:

- publish local procedures for the transfer of midwifery records from self-employed midwives

- agree local systems to ensure Supervisors of Midwives maintain records of their supervisory activity

- ensure Supervisors of Midwives records, relating to the statutory supervision of midwives, are kept for a minimum of 7 years

- arrange for supervision records relating to an investigation of a clinical incident to be kept for a minimum of 25 years

- publish local procedures for retention and transfer of records relating to statutory supervision.

Guidance on supervision records is considered in Chapter 3.

GUIDELINES FOR RECORDS AND RECORD KEEPING

The NMC has published Guidelines for Records and Record Keeping[4] which update the guidance which it revised in 2002. It emphasises the responsibilities of the practitioner in relation to record keeping. Record keeping must be seen as a fundamental part of nursing, midwifery and specialist community public health nursing practice. The NMC document states that:

Record keeping is an integral part of nursing, midwifery and specialist community public health visiting practice. It is a tool of professional practice and one which should help the care process. It is not separate from this process and it is not an optional extra to be fitted in if circumstances allow.

The NMC document sets out clearly the purpose of record keeping and its importance, and, on page 7, sets out guidance on the content and style (Box 15.2).

Box 15.2 NMC guidance on content and style in record keeping

Records should:

- be factual, consistent and accurate

- be written as soon as possible after an event has occurred, providing current information on the care and condition of the patient or client

- be written clearly and in such a manner that the text cannot be erased

- be written in such a manner that any alterations or additions are dated, timed and signed in such a way that the original entry can still be read clearly

- be accurately dated, timed and signed, with the signature printed alongside the first entry

- not include abbreviations, jargon, meaningless phrases, irrelevant speculation and offensive subjective statements

- be readable on any photocopies.

Additional guidance from the NMC suggests that the records should:

- be written, wherever possible, with the involvement of the patient or client or their carer

- be written in terms that the patient or client can understand

- be consecutive

- identify problems that have arisen and the action taken to rectify them

- provide clear evidence of the care planned, the decisions made, the care delivered and the information shared.

The guidance also includes assistance on audit, legal matters and complaints, access and ownership, information technology and computer-held records (see below).

Additional advice on record keeping is given in the RCM booklet on litigation[5] which though written in 1993 is still relevant. This points out the need to ensure that all timings should be recorded consistently, preferably from the same clock; the need to record warnings of risks given to the mother and refusal by the mother to consent to recommended treatment or procedures; a note that abnormalities on the trace have been observed; and the procedure which should be followed if an error has been made in the records.

Additional guidance on record keeping is provided by the NHS Executive.[3,6,7]

CONTEMPORANEOUS RECORDS

Records should be written up as soon as possible after the events described and in any event not more than 24 hours later. Courts require records to be contemporaneous if they are to be used in evidence. One of the greatest problems in midwifery is the fact that if a midwife is under pressure during a delivery (and in hospital she may be responsible for providing care to more than one woman at the same time) it is impossible for her to record events at the same time that the delivery takes place. She therefore relies upon being able to write up the delivery at a later stage. Sometimes midwives are known to use scraps of paper or even their arms or aprons for recording information which they later transfer into the proper record, destroying or washing out the original. This is not a recommended practice. It is preferable if the information is recorded on the document which will be retained in the woman's record. Mistakes can take place on transferring the information from one document to another. Midwives should ensure that even while working under pressure, they keep as complete a contemporaneous account of the events as possible.

ALTERATIONS TO RECORDS

If changes are necessary because inaccurate information has been entered, e.g. the wrong woman's name, then Tippex or correction fluid should not be used, but a line should be placed through the wrong entry and the correct entry made, signed and dated clearly. Midwives may be under pressure to amend their records to accord with the doctor's account of the events. They should not under any circumstances allow their records to be altered.

ABBREVIATIONS

In its advice, the NMC makes it clear that abbreviations should not be used. This is the ideal situation, but in practice the midwife makes considerable use of abbreviations and other signs to save time. It is essential that no misunderstandings should

arise over the intended meaning and there are advantages in an agreed list of abbreviations being approved by the trust, and enforced through disciplinary action if
anyone uses abbreviations or signs not on the list, or uses one on the list for a different meaning.[8]

STORAGE AND DESTRUCTION OF RECORDS

Advice is given in the NMC Midwives Rules and Standards[2] about keeping the records
for at least 25 years in the case of children. In addition, records relating to brain-
damaged babies should be kept until 3 years after his/her death. The Department of
Health has given advice relating to a variety of patient and office records.[3] There will
be local policies on destruction of records which will relate to storage or microfilm
facilities, but there should be senior midwifery involvement in policies relating to
the destruction of midwifery records.

OWNERSHIP OF RECORDS

NHS records are owned by the Secretary of State, but the actual management and
responsibility for them are delegated to the individual Health Authorities and trusts.
The records are not owned by those who complete them. General Practitioners are
required under their terms of service to complete the records and return them to the
NHS Primary Care Trust (in Wales, Local Health Boards) when a patient dies or leaves
that practice. In contrast, the records of the independent midwife are owned by her,
but under the Rules, on ceasing practice, she is obliged to keep them in a safe place
or transfer them to the LSA.

LITIGATION

While the first objective of record keeping is the protection of the mother, inevitably
in the event of a complaint or claim, the records become central to the evidence
available. The fact that awards of compensation in birth injuries are amongst the
highest, and that there is a greater likelihood of litigation in obstetrics and midwifery
than other specialties, may put the records kept by midwives under greater scrutiny
by the courts than those kept by any other professional group. In the event of a
complaint or litigation, the records of other groups could also be used to complement
the midwife's documentation. For example, in an emergency, if an ambulance has
been sent for, the ambulance service will have full details of the time the call was
made; they may also have tapes of any conversations; they may check drugs with
the midwife and this would also be recorded. The midwife should not, however, rely
on these records for completing her own notes of the case. This would be regarded
as second-hand evidence. The ambulance records should be independent from those
of the midwife.

USE OF RECORDS IN LITIGATION

In any legal conflict, one of the biggest areas for dispute is over the facts of what occurred. While records are not in themselves proof of the truth of what occurred (records can be changed, or written incorrectly), they are used in conjunction with the evidence of the writer of the records so that the court can determine the weight which can be attached to them. The more distant in the past the events, the more dependent the witnesses will be on the documentation which was kept at the time. This is so whether the court proceedings are related to a claim for compensation being heard in the civil courts, a prosecution in the criminal courts and inquest before the coroner, fitness to practise proceedings or disciplinary proceedings brought by the employer against the employee.

ANALYSIS OF COMMENTS ON RECORD KEEPING: IN THE CASE OF BULL AND WAKEHAM

One of the ways of examining the value and significance of the principles set out by the NMC is to examine court cases where the records have come under scrutiny and ascertain the lessons which can be learnt.

An example is the case of Bull and Wakeham[9] which was heard 17 years after the birth of twins. The facts of the case were as follows.

The mother, who already had one child, went into labour at 33 weeks' gestation on 21 March 1970. On admission at 4.30 p.m. to the maternity unit in the first stage room, two fetal hearts were detected for the first time. (This was the first time it was realised that this was a twin pregnancy.) One fetus was recorded as vertex in brim and the other as a breech presentation. At 7.27 p.m. the first twin, a boy, called Darryl, was spontaneously delivered. A blood loss was recorded as occurring at 7.55 p.m. Mrs Bull was given a general anaesthetic at 8.25 p.m. and the second twin, Stuart, was delivered by breech extraction at 8.35 p.m. Stuart was subsequently found to have been born with severe brain damage.

The mother claimed compensation for the harm caused to the baby and the child sued in his own right through his mother as 'next friend' (this is a legal term, which applies to the person who brings an action on behalf of a person who is not competent in his/her own right). The case was heard in the High Court in April 1987 and the health authority was found to be liable. The latter appealed to the Court of Appeal and the hearing took place in February 1989.

The dispute centred on several issues:

1. Did an unidentified person pull the cord and damage the placenta after Darryl was born, thereby causing oxygen deprivation to Stuart?

2. At what point did blood loss per vagina occur, and did this cause harm to the baby?

3. Was there an unreasonable delay in the delivery of the second baby, which was *prima facie* evidence of negligence?

4. Was there a failure to provide either the immediate presence or the immediate availability of someone with skill, experience and authority sufficient to bring about the delivery of the second twin?

Two important points followed from the fact that the case was heard so long after the birth:

- it was impossible to trace a student midwife who had been present at the time and who could have explained some of the records which it was presumed that she had made

- the records were of great significance in evidence. Witnesses would have little personal recall of the events.

The record keeping was criticised by the judge.

The records showed the following entry:

- 7.26 p.m. cervix fully dilated.

- 7.27 p.m. spontaneous delivery living premature male class A. (This was the actual wording in the records.)

It was stated in evidence at the hearing by both husband and wife that no midwife was present at the moment of Darryl's birth. They also stated that shortly after his birth, a nurse entered the first stage room and pulled the umbilical cord, which was uncut and still attached to the baby. These assertions were denied by that nurse, Sister Jones, who stated that she arrived just in time to deliver the baby, that she did not pull the cord and that she would not have allowed anyone else to do so. (There was no record as to whether Syntometrine was given and there is no discussion of this in the court hearings.)

Since it was impossible to trace the student midwife who was present in the maternity ward at the time and made the records, she could not be called to give evidence.

The High Court judge concluded that:

- No midwife or doctor was present at the moment when Darryl was born, though Sister Jones was there immediately afterwards.

- Sister Jones clamped and cut the cord.

- Someone, not Sister Jones, but probably the student midwife, pulled the cord shortly after the birth in an attempt to remove the afterbirth because she had not read the notes, did not realise that this was a double birth and did it before anyone in charge could stop her.

- Damage was thereby caused to the placenta.

- The person who pulled the cord was negligent.

- Since the twins were uniovular and shared the same placenta, the pulling of the cord endangered the supply of oxygen to the second baby.

- The second baby was born at 8.35 p.m. and the judge accepted the medical evidence which suggested that this delay in the birth of the second twin was unacceptably long.

Further errors were noted: entries in the hospital notes at 7.55 p.m. and 8.00 p.m. record the hearing of the fetal heart, but did not state whether it was regular or irregular.

There was no record of a fetal heart beat being listened to between 8.00 and 8.25 p.m., but at 8.25 p.m. it was noted that the fetal heart was irregular. This was the first record of any irregularity in the heart beat.

The Court of Appeal stated that they considered that the judge had put undue weight upon the absence of any statement about the regularity or otherwise of the fetal heart beat at 7.55 p.m. and 8.00 p.m. There was also confusion over the time the mother suffered a blood loss. Sister Jones had recorded 7.55 p.m. as the time of the brisk loss of blood per vaginam. The judge concluded from hearing the mother's evidence and from the notes made by the student midwife that this loss took place at 7.45 p.m.

However, the Court of Appeal saw no reason to doubt the record made by Sister Jones in the Kardex that the loss occurred at 7.55 p.m. The Kardex had been written up by Sister Jones 2.5 hours after the delivery. One of the Court of Appeal judges (Lord Mustill) held there was no reason for the Kardex to have been falsified and it seemed a more reliable guide to the meaning of the records than a reconstruction of 17 years after the event by reference to the position on the page of entries made by a person whose identity was not even known. The judges concluded that the loss must have occurred between 7.45 p.m. and 7.55 p.m.

The result of the Court of Appeal hearing was that the decision of the trial judge was upheld, though not all his findings were accepted. Of importance in deciding that there was liability by the hospital was the delay in delivering the second child, particularly after the blood loss and the apparent lack of emergency staffing cover to provide immediate assistance. Clearly in this case, the UKCC (now the NMC) guidelines were not followed: there was no index for tracing potential witnesses, and the records were ambiguous and not always meaningful.

In the Bull and Wakeham case, it was accepted that records made 2.5 hours after the birth were contemporaneous with the birth. However, if Sister Jones had made a note on a piece of paper at the time that blood loss occurred, it would have been preferable if that piece of paper had been attached to the Kardex or delivery record.

CARDIOTOCOGRAPH READINGS

Cardiotocograph readings were not taken in the Bull and Wakeham case, but now intrapartum fetal wellbeing can be assessed by electronic means or by intermittent auscultation with a Pinard's stethoscope. (CTG readings are considered in Ch. 14.)

The recommendation of the NMC, that initials should either not be used or that there should be a local index record of signatures kept, is important. One of the most difficult tasks in midwifery litigation, as seen from Bull and Wakeham, is to identify the staff who were involved in the alleged negligent incident and to track down their current whereabouts.

Another issue in midwifery is the possibility of discrepancy between the records of the midwife and those of the obstetricians. This may sometimes reveal a conflict of evidence. For example, the midwife might have called a doctor to see the mother. Subsequently, the doctor might deny that any such request has been made. In order to prevent such a dispute, the midwife might ask the doctor to sign in the record or on the CTG the fact that he has seen the mother. The midwife should not regard such a signature as relieving her of all responsibility if harm occurs. She is still accountable for her professional duty of care to the mother and child.

LEGAL STATUS OF RECORDS

The question is often asked as to when a record becomes a legal document. The answer is simple: whenever it is relevant in a court of law and is required in evidence. In this sense, there is no limit to the nature of records which could be ordered to be produced in court. Even scraps of paper which a midwife might use to remind herself of significant events in the delivery could be ordered to be produced in court, if they are still available. X-rays, pathological test results, CTG graphs, fetal monitoring traces could all be produced in court.

However, as can be seen from the case of Bull and Wakeham, records are not evidence of the truth of what is written upon them. Normally the writer of contemporaneous records would be called to give evidence of the circumstances which led to the record being made, and could be cross-examined upon them so that the court could determine the weight which should be attached to their credibility.

In midwifery cases, as the case of Bull and Wakeham shows, it may be many years before a court action is commenced. A child can bring a court action at any time before the end of 3 years of attaining his majority (i.e. 18 years + 3 years).

AUDIT

Regular audit of record keeping standards is required to ensure that there is compliance with the Midwives Rules standards and guidance. In addition, under Rule 10, the practising midwife is required to give her Supervisor of Midwives, the Local Supervising Authority and the NMC every reasonable facility to inspect her records as well as her equipment and such part of her residence as may be used for professional purposes. In addition, her standards and methods of practice can be monitored. Regular review and advice by the Supervisor of Midwives of record keeping standards could ensure that a high standard of record keeping is established and maintained. In addition, midwives might be able to establish small internal groups of colleagues who can at regular intervals examine a set of records and monitor their standard, identifying any improvements which should be made. External auditors of record keeping standards may also be brought into the organisation to assist in establishing and maintaining standards. The King's Fund in London provides such a service. In addition, the Clinical Negligence Scheme for Trusts monitors record keeping standards for its members (see below). The NMC in its guidance on records and record keeping[10] states (p. 8) that:

Audit is one component of the risk management process, the aim of which is the promotion of quality. If improvements are identified and made in the processes and outcomes of health care, risks to the patient or client are minimised and costs to the employer are reduced.

The NMC recommends that audit tools should be devised at local level to monitor the standard of the records produced and to form a basis both to discussion and measurement. It also states that whatever audit tool or system is used

it should primarily be directed towards serving the interests of your patients and clients, rather than organisational convenience.

It suggests that practitioners may wish to consider including a system of peer review in the process and reminds practitioners that the duty of confidentiality of patient and client information applies to audit just as to the record keeping process itself.

The Audit Commission, in its report on hospital records,[11] considered that patients were being put at risk because their medical records are not kept carefully and are sometimes lost. Failure to find records led to consultations being cancelled and to operations being postponed. It recommended that hospitals set up one main records library with good security.

CLINICAL NEGLIGENCE SCHEME FOR TRUSTS (CNST)

The CNST requires those trusts which belong to the scheme to maintain specified standards in relation to a range of topics (see Ch. 13), including record keeping. The CNST has identified hospital records as one of its core standards. Criteria for this standard which was published in April 2004 are shown below:

Standard 4: Health Records   Level

A comprehensive system for the completion, use, storage and retrieval of health records is in place. Record keeping standards are monitored through the clinical audit process.

4.1.1	There is a unified health record which all specialties use.	1
4.1.2	Records are bound and stored so that loss of documents and traces are minimised for in-patients and out-patients.	1
4.1.3	The health record contains clear instructions regarding filing documents.	1
4.1.4	Operation notes and other key procedures are readily identifiable.	1
4.1.5	Machine-produced recordings are securely stored using a method that will minimise deterioration.	1
4.1.6	The storage arrangements allow retrieval on a 24/7 hours/day arrangement.	1
4.1.7	There is clear evidence of clinical audit of record keeping standards for all professional groups, in at least 25% of specialties, including any high risk specialties, within the 12 months prior to the assessment.	1
4.1.8	There is a mechanism for retaining certain records which must not be destroyed.	1
4.2.1	A&E records are contained within the main record for patients who are subsequently admitted.	2
4.2.2	There is a system for ensuring that the GP is sent a copy A&E record.	2
4.2.3	Nursing, medical and other records (e.g. Physiotherapy notes, Obstetric notes) are filed together or referenced when the patient is discharged.	2
4.2.4	There is a system for measuring efficiency in the recovery for records for in-patients and out-patients.	2
4.2.5	The health record contains a designated place for the recording of hyper-sensitivity reactions, and other information relevant to all healthcare professionals.	2
4.2.6	There is clear evidence of clinical audit of record keeping standards for all professional groups in 50% of the specialties, within the 12 months prior to the assessment.	2

4.3.1   An author of an entry in a health record is clearly and easily   3
identifiable.

4.3.2   There is clear evidence of clinical audit of record keeping standards   3
for all professional groups in all of the specialties, within the 12
months prior to the assessment.

These standards can be used as the basis for a regular internal audit of documentation, even by those units which are not members of the CNST pool, to ensure that
a reasonable standard is being maintained. Each standard is accompanied by its
reference source and additional guidance.

Reference should also be made to standard 6 of the CNST Maternity Clinical Risk
Management standards which cover health records within maternity departments.
These standards were updated in April 2004 and expand on the guidance in relation
to CTG and other machine-based recordings.

PERSONAL CHECKLIST

Individual midwives might find the checklist prepared by Dot Walters for her midwifery students at the East Glamorgan District General Hospital of value. It is set out
in Box 15.3.

Box 15.3 A checklist for record keeping in midwifery

Use this practice checklist as a way of highlighting those record keeping activities
which may need critical evaluation.

It is assumed that you will have read all the relevant UKCC documents and
'Litigation, a risk management exercise guide' (RCM 1993).

This checklist is prepared only as an outline to the principles of record keeping for
midwives.

1. Do any actions or common practices prevent me from making contemporaneous records, e.g. case notes not easily accessible?

2. Do I ever make rough notes for later transcription into the client's records e.g.
   scraps of paper, on my hand or plastic apron?

3. Are clients' records always kept with the client, especially in a high-care or
   emergency situation, e.g. when a client is receiving emergency treatment
   from medical staff, do they take away the notes for completion?

▶

---

4. If giving advice by telephone, as the advisor, do I make a record of the time, date and reason for any advice given? Do I check the outcome of the case and record this too?

5. Do I regularly evaluate my personal standard of record keeping and seek peer review?

6. Have I added my signature to the local index record of signatures? Did I update the index when I changed my surname?

7. When acting as a preceptor to students, do I always check and review their standard of record keeping?

8. Do I ever use abbreviations in the description of events, actions and clinical diagnoses?

9. Do I take up opportunities (or create opportunities) for regular re-education related to record keeping in midwifery practice?

10. Have I made any necessary changes to my practice?

ELECTRONIC HEALTH RECORDS

The Secretary of State for Health, Frank Dobson, announced on 24 September 1998 that there would be £1 billion investment to put all medical files on computer.[12] The initiative will take place over 7 years enabling records to be available for access on a 24-hour basis across the country and also permitting patients access in their own home. The initiative will link into an NHS website and there will be an expansion of NHS Direct, offering the public a 24-hour telephone advice service on non-urgent health matters. £40 million is to be spent connecting GPs to the NHS Net.

On 4 February 2001, the Department of Health issued a press release which stated that by March 2005, every person in the country will have their own electronic patient record (EHR).[13] The electronic health record is defined by the Department of Health as holding summarised key data about patients, such as name, address, NHS number, registered GP and contact details, previous treatments, ongoing conditions, current medication, allergies and the date of any next appointments. It is intended that it will be securely protected, created with patient consent, with individual changes made only by authorised staff. The timetable for the electronic health record envisaged that 5 million people would have their own lifelong EHR by 2003, rising to around 25 million by 2004 and then everyone by March 2005. This target has not been reached and there is still considerable training required. In addition, as the scheme for the electronic linking of GP surgeries with hospitals has shown, many of the existing computer systems are incompatible and many GPs are concerned about the security of the systems and patient confidentiality. The National Audit Office reported in January 2005 that more than one-third of GPs will not be linked up to the system to enable patients to choose and book hospital appointments electronically from GP surgeries by December 2005, despite the Government promises.[14] Regulations to permit electronic transmission of prescriptions was passed in 2001.[15]

A consultation on national specification for an integrated care records service was initiated in February 2004 in order to identify the requirements of such a system and the national standards and specification to be used.[16] In March 2004 a consultation on a national strategy for NHS information Quality Assurance was launched with the aim of improving the quality of information in the NHS (see Ch. 10 and the Information Governance Strategy).

In May 2005, the Department of Health issued new rules relating to patients' elec-tronic records.[17] The Health Minister, Lord Warner, published the Care Record Guarantee setting out the rules governing information held in the NHS Care Records Service. Twelve commitments were made to patients about their records, including a pledge that access to records by NHS staff will be strictly limited to those having a need to know. In due course, patients will be able to block off parts of their record to stop it being shared with anyone in the NHS, except in an emergency.

While the computer records will avoid problems of illegibility, considerable care will still have to be taken. In August 1998, it was reported[18] that a student suffering from meningitis may have died as a result of her name being wrongly spelt on a computer. The omission of the letter 'P' in her surname, Simpkin, meant that her records could not be accessed, and an inquiry found that she might have lived if vital results of blood tests, entered into the computerised records under the wrong name, had been seen by staff.

WOMAN-HELD RECORDS

In midwifery care, it is increasingly the practice that women retain their own records during their antenatal care, bringing them to the clinics for their appointments. While this practice is in general very successful, there are certain concerns: what if the mother destroys the records and then sues the trust for compensation? Can the midwife leave out information, e.g. previous pregnancy or abortion, if the woman so wishes? What if the records are lost? (See also Ch. 10.) Ann Holmes and colleagues reviewed a pilot project for client-held records in a Glasgow Maternity Hospital and concluded that the new system was valued by women and appeared to have improved communication between women and staff.[19]

Destruction of records by mother

In a claim for compensation, the burden is on the claimant to show on a balance of probabilities that the defendant or its employees failed to follow a reasonable standard of care, which caused harm to the claimant. The fact that the claimant has lost the records which were in her custody would therefore work against her case.

Omission of information from the records

It would be contrary to professional practice for a midwife to omit essential information from a woman's obstetric history. Leaving out details of an earlier pregnancy could influence clinical decisions about the care of a mother. For example, if it were thought that the mother was a primigravida, dealing with her Rhesus negative state would be different than if it were known that this was a second or later pregnancy. (In July 1998, a GP who allowed a patient to destroy part of her records was found guilty of serious professional misconduct by the GMC.[20] He had allowed the patient, who was involved in an acrimonious property dispute with her children, to remove a letter in which she was described as 'bad tempered' and another document referring to her drinking.) Where a woman wishes to have information deleted, or not kept on her record, because of fears that her partner/family may discover information of which they were ignorant, then she should be offered the opportunity to have her records kept in the hospital. Alternatively, there should be a note on her records that information kept at the hospital should be consulted before any decisions are taken. (This topic is further considered in Ch. 10.)

STATEMENT MAKING

Witnesses can refer to any contemporaneous records and contemporaneous statements in giving evidence and therefore, since it takes many years for some court hearings to take place, it is vital that comprehensive, clear records have been kept and statements made. Before preparing a statement, a health professional should have advice from a senior colleague and if possible a lawyer. The elements shown in Box 15.4 should be contained in a statement.

Box 15.4 Elements to include in a statement

- Date and time of the incident

- Full name of statement maker, position, grade and location

- Full names of any persons involved, e.g. patient, visitor, other staff

- Date and time the statement was made

▶

▶

– A full and detailed description of the events which occurred

– Signature

– Any supporting statement or document attached.

The statement writer should ensure that the statement is:

– accurate

– factual

– concise

– relevant

– clear

– legible (it will usually be typed), and

– signed.

The statement maker should read it through, checking its overall impact and whether all the relevant facts are included. A copy should be kept. Advice should be sought on its clarity and comprehensiveness, and it should not be signed unless the maker is completely satisfied that it records an accurate, clear account of what took place.

REPORT WRITING

Midwives may be required to prepare reports on a variety of topics, as managers, supervisors or individual midwives. In addition, senior midwives may be invited to provide reports as an expert witness.

Expert witnesses will normally be asked to prepare a report by a solicitor representing one of the parties to the case. This report is vital since, if it is unfavourable to the party seeking it, the outcome may be that the case is settled or even withdrawn.

Box 15.5 illustrates some of the principles to be followed in report writing.

For most purposes the style likely to be of greatest use is one of simplicity, with short sentences, clear paragraphing and sub-paragraphing, and avoidance of jargon and meaningless clichés. The report should begin with a statement as to its purpose, the person(s) to whom it is addressed, and the name and status of the writer. If it is

Box 15.5 Principles to be followed in report writing

- Identify the purpose of the report, likely readership and the kind of language which can be used, and therefore the appropriate style to be used.

- Identify the main areas to be included.

- Decide the order to be followed: sometimes chronological order is appropriate, at other times subject order may be preferable.

- Sign and date it, but only after reading it through and being 100% satisfied with it.

- Identify the different kinds of information used in the report and state the source of the material, e.g. hearsay evidence, factual evidence observed or heard by the author of the report, evidence of opinion of another person, statements by others, similar fact evidence.

- Avoid the mistakes shown in Box 15.6.

Box 15.6 Common mistakes in report writing

- Lack of clarity

- Failure to follow a logical order

- Inconsistency

- Ambiguities

- Lack of signature and/or date

- Lack of dates within the report

- Wrong names included

- Confusing account

- Mix of evidence and sources

- Inaccuracies

– Opinion without facts

– Failure to cite facts to support statements

– Too complex a style for reader

– Use of inappropriate jargon

– Use of misleading abbreviations

– Failure to give conclusions

– Failure to base conclusions on the evidence

– Failure to ask someone else to read.

confidential, this should be highlighted at the beginning. Other documents which are relevant should be carefully referenced.

GIVING EVIDENCE IN COURT

As a witness of fact, the midwife may be required to give direct evidence over a matter with which she has been involved. If she is asked to give evidence, an employed midwife would be assisted by senior midwifery management and the solicitors to the trust. In giving evidence, she should ensure that she keeps to the facts and does not offer an opinion. She may need guidance and training in how to respond to cross-examination. It is vital that she does not give facts which are outside her knowledge.

The following are key points for witness of fact.

Preparation
– Ensure that the records are available, identify significant entries with post-it notes, but do not mark or staple or pin anything to the records. Read them through so that you are familiar with them.

– Try to obtain assistance from a lawyer or senior manager in preparation for the court hearing, so that you are prepared for giving evidence in chief and answering questions under cross-examination.

– Try to visit the court in advance to familiarise yourself with its location, car parking, toilets, catering facilities, etc.

At the court before the hearing

– Be prepared for a long wait, and take work to do or something to occupy yourself.

– Dress appropriately and comfortably, but not too casually.

– Try to relax.

Giving evidence

– Keep calm.

– Give answers clearly and without exaggeration.

– Tell the truth.

– Do not feel that you are there to represent only one side; you must answer the questions honestly, even though it might put the side cross-examining you in a good light.

– Take time over your answers, and do not make up replies if you are unable to answer the question raised.

– Do not answer back or allow yourself to be flustered during the cross-examination.

– If you do not understand any legal jargon which is used, ask for an explanation.

– Keep to the facts and do not express an opinion.

– Ask for time to refer to the records if this is necessary.

EXPERT WITNESS

An expert witness is invited to give evidence of opinion on any issue which is subject to dispute. This could include the standards of care which would have been expected according to the Bolam Test (see Ch. 13), or the opinion may relate to what caused the harm suffered by the mother or baby. Expert opinion may also be brought in if there is a dispute over the assessment of compensation. An article by Georgina Lessing-Turner[21] discussed the training available for a midwife who wishes to become an expert witness.

Where an expert has prepared a report for a solicitor in anticipation or in the course of litigation, that report and any correspondence connected with it are protected by legal professional privilege (see Ch. 10) and it cannot be ordered to be disclosed in court or the expert compelled to appear by the other side. However, once the report is disclosed to the court, it loses its professional privilege (which continues to attach to any correspondence between the parties which has not been disclosed). As a result of the changes in civil procedure following the Woolf Reforms (see Ch. 14) where an expert's report is used in evidence, all amendments and changes to that report must also be disclosed. The expert has a duty to the court. The court has held[22] that the expert witness had a responsibility to approach the task of giving evidence seriously and an expert should not be surprised if the court expressed strong disapproval if that was not done. In another case the Court of Appeal upheld the principle that the expert's duty was to the court rather than to the party who had instructed him.[23] The new Civil Procedure (CP) Rules set out explicitly the duty of the expert to the court. Rule 35.3 states:

1. *It is the duty of an expert to help the court on the matters within his expertise*

2. *This duty overrides any obligation to the person from whom he has received instructions or by whom he is paid.*

Under the Rules, the Court has the power to restrict expert evidence (35.4) and there is a general requirement for expert evidence to be given in a written report (35.5). The Woolf Reforms recommended that experts should be agreed between the parties prior to any hearing, in order that the time and costs of the case could be reduced. Under Rule 35.7 the court has the power to direct that evidence is to be given by a single joint expert. This is not always possible in some of the large compensation claims in obstetrics and midwifery, when several different witnesses may be called as experts in different areas of practice.

In the case of Wardlaw v. Dr Farrar[24] the Court of Appeal considered an application from the claimant that fresh evidence should be admitted by way of some additional pages from a standard medical textbook, part of which only had been before the County Court judge. The Court of Appeal dismissed the appeal, holding that such evidence could have been adduced before trial and the standard directions on the exchange of medical expert literature should have been made. It was not prepared to interfere with the decision of the trial judge who was clearly impressed by the expert evidence given on behalf of the defendant. In contrast, the Court of Appeal[25] allowed an appeal by a claimant who had requested permission to use two obstetric experts to support a claim that an obstetric registrar had been negligent in the management of her birth. The Court of Appeal held that some exceptional circumstances justified more experts: here the defence would be calling three consultants in obstetrics to respond to the claimant's single expert and under the CP Rules it was important to ensure that the parties were on an equal footing.

CONCLUSIONS

There is perhaps insufficient sharing between colleagues of the lessons learned from litigation, even when the defendant professionals and Health Authorities/NHS trusts win the case. Regular training in record keeping is essential for all professionals, particularly in midwifery where the peaks and troughs of activity are not predictable and when, in the pressure of the delivery, record keeping may be given a low priority. In addition, midwives should have training and assistance in making statements, writing reports and in giving evidence in court. The Department of Health has signalled its intention of reviewing 'For the Record' – the guidance published in 1999 – with the aim of issuing revised guidance by June 2005.

QUESTIONS AND EXERCISES

1. Discuss a strategy for keeping records while under pressure of work. Your strategy could include the use of agreed abbreviations, pre-printed forms and other devices which would be safe to adopt in speeding up record keeping.

2. With a colleague, look critically at the records kept over a 2-week period. In what ways could the standard be improved?

3. Imagine that, in 15 years' time, you are being cross-examined on the care which you have provided in a particular case. Consider to what extent the records would be satisfactory as evidence in such circumstances.

4. Prepare a checklist for a report to be used in a child abuse case conference.

5. You have been asked to appear in court next week. Identify your worst fears about this request and devise ways of overcoming them.

References

1 The Nursing and Midwifery Council (Midwives) Rules of Council 2004, SI 2004/1764.

2 Nursing and Midwifery Council. Midwives Rules and Standards, August 2004.

3 NHS Executive. For the record. Health Service Circular 1999/053, DoH; 1999.

4 Nursing and Midwifery Council Guidelines for records and record keeping August 2004, replacing the revised document of 2002, which was an update of UKCC Guidelines for records and record keeping 1998.

5 Mason D, Edwards P. Litigation: a risk management guide for midwives. London: Royal College of Midwives in conjunction with Capsticks solicitors; 1993.

6 NHS Training Directorate. Keeping the record straight. London: DoH; 1992.

7 NHS Training Directorate. Just for the Record: A guide to record keeping for healthcare professionals. London: DoH; 1994.

8 Dimond B. Abbreviations, record keeping and the midwife. Practising Midwife 1998; 1(9):10–11.

9 Bull and Wakeham v. Devon Health Authority. Court of Appeal, 2 February 1989 transcript of hearing; Bull v. Devon AHA [1993] 4 Med LR 117 CA.

10 Nursing and Midwifery Council Guidelines for records and record keeping, August 2004.

11 Audit Commission. Setting the records straight: a study of hospital medical records London: HMSO; 1995.

12 Henderson M. £1bn scheme will put all medical files on computer. The Times, 25 September 1998.

13 Department of Health. Patients to gain access to new at-a-glance Electronic Health Records. Press release, 4 February 2001.

14 Charter D. The doctor won't see you now. The Times, 19 January 2005.

15 The Prescription Only Medicines (Human Use) (Electronic Communications) Order 2001 SI 2001 No 2889.

16 Department of Health. National specification for integrated care records service, 10 February 2004.

17 Department of Health. Press release 2005/0185 23 May 2005.

18 Johnstone H. Spelling mistake may have cost student her life. The Times, 28 August 1998.

19 Holmes A, Cheyne H, Ginley M, Mathers A. Trialling and implementing a client-held record system. Br J Midwifery 2005; 13(2):112–117.

20 Forster P. GP allowed patient to tamper with records. The Times, 7 July 1998.

21 Lessing-Turner G. Midwives as expert witnesses. The Practising Midwife 2000; 3(9):29.

22 Autospin (Oil Seals) Ltd v. Beehive Spinning (A firm). Times Law Report, 9 August 1995.

23 Stevens v. Gullis. The Times, 6 October 1999.

24 Peter Wardlaw v. Dr Stephen Farrar. Lloyd's Rep Med [2004] 98.

25 ES (by her mother and litigation friend DS) v. Chesterfield and North Derbyshire Royal NHS Trust [2003] EWCA Civ 1284; Lloyd's Rep Med [2004] 90.

Chapter 16
FAMILY PLANNING AND STERILISATION

The midwife is often the health professional who will be consulted by mothers about family planning after the birth of the baby. The duty of care includes the duty of giving advice and information, and therefore the midwife should ensure that she takes care in giving advice and information and follows the reasonable standards of practice (i.e. the Bolam Test, see Ch. 13), since she could be held liable (or her employer vicariously liable) should harm result from the mother's reliance upon her negligent advice. This chapter looks at some of the issues which have arisen in the context of family planning and sterilisations. Reference should also be made to Chapter 7, relating to consent by a minor and the Gillick case, and Chapter 12 on teenage pregnancies. Further reference should be made to Chapter 26, on termination of pregnancy and the extent to which the post-coital pill could be regarded as an abortion, and the fact that it is doubtful if giving advice on abortions is covered by the conscientious objection clause; students should also see Chapter 20, on medication and contraindications.

FAMILY PLANNING

The midwife should ensure that she is familiar with local provision and facilities for family planning, and give information to the mothers when asked. The midwife herself may be involved in family planning clinics. Each Strategic Health Authority has a duty to provide information about the family planning services in its area. An independent Advisory Group on Teenage Pregnancy has been appointed by the government to guide and monitor the government's strategy for teenage pregnancy. This is considered in Chapter 12.

NEGLIGENCE AND CONTRACEPTIVES

In a case reported in the Medical Protection Society Report for 1984, a General Practitioner in South Africa prescribed Trisequens, a combination drug which was intended by the makers for use in post-menopausal hormone replacement therapy. He had intended to prescribe Logynon. The patient, who had made it clear to the doctor that she did not want to become pregnant since she was the bread winner while her husband was still a student, became pregnant before the General Practitioner realised his mistake. A settlement was offered to the patient without admission of liability. The advice given to members was that they should familiarise themselves with any pharmacologically-active substance which they prescribe.

While the midwife is unlikely herself to be prescribing contraceptives, she may be asked by patients to comment on medicines which have been prescribed by a doctor. Should this occur, and the midwife has concerns over the appropriateness of the medication, she should take this up personally with the doctor rather than commence a dialogue via the patient. If her concerns are justified, the doctor might then arrange for the treatment to be changed. Different principles would of course apply were the midwife to be responsible for administering the medication (see Ch. 20).

DIAGNOSIS OF PREGNANCY BEFORE TREATMENT

Where treatment on the reproductive organs is to be undertaken on a woman, it is essential to ensure that she is given a pregnancy test first. In a case in the MPS report for 1984, a 25-year-old woman with a history of infrequent periods was referred to a Consultant. A cervical erosion was noted and the patient listed for D&C and cautery. The registrar noted 'Please do pregnancy test prior to op'. The D&C was carried out and, 3 weeks later, the patient aborted spontaneously a 16-week fetus. A settlement was negotiated on the basis that the doctors knew, or should have known, before carrying out the D&C that the patient was pregnant.

NEGLIGENT CAUSING OF INFERTILITY

In the case of Briody,[1] a woman was given a sub-total hysterectomy at the age of 18, which led to her being deprived of any prospect of conceiving and bearing a child naturally. The hospital was held liable, but the judge had rejected a claim for the costs of an own-egg surrogacy to be carried out in California and had also rejected an alternative surrogacy proposal using donor eggs. B sought to overthrow this decision with fresh evidence that her own eggs had been successfully fertilised with her partner's sperm and that she now had the opportunity of a surrogate birth in England. The Court of Appeal dismissed her appeal, on the grounds that the chances of a successful pregnancy using the embryos created from her eggs and her partner's sperm were extremely slight. While everybody had the right under the Human Rights Act 1998 Schedule 1 Article 8 to have the chance to have a child by natural means, no one had the right to be supplied with a child.

STERILISATION

Compensation may be claimed following an operation for sterilisation in the following situations:

- Negligent advice leading to a sterilisation being performed

- A sterilisation being carried out negligently and leading to a baby being born

- A sterilisation being carried out without negligence but no warning having been given about the possibility of its being not 100% effective

- A sterilisation having been carried out with a warning.

While the midwife would not herself be responsible for carrying out the surgery for sterilisation, she may be involved in the information which is given to the patient prior to the operation.

NEGLIGENT ADVICE

On 31 October 1987, Mrs Roberta Biles won almost £55 000 from North East Thames and Barking, Havering and Brentwood Health Authorities for a sterilisation operation which should not have been carried out. The facts were that when she was 19, she was advised by a doctor that having a baby could kill her and she was therefore sterilised. She had undergone ten operations and four times had had test-tube baby treatment without success. Seven years later when she went for a routine check-up, she discovered that the sterilisation had been unnecessary. The defendants admitted liability but contested the amount of damages. Damages were awarded for probable permanent infertility, for the physical pain and suffering of various operations and painful examinations which she had undergone, and for the scarring as a result of the sterilisation. She was also awarded damages for impairment of sexual function due to the physical and emotional pain and the regime of trying for a test-tube baby.[2]

INADEQUATE PRE-OPERATION COUNSELLING

In the case of Wells v. Surrey Area Health Authority,[3] a Roman Catholic woman was sterilised in the course of a caesarean. She was given the form to sign just before she went into the operation, and was awarded £3000 compensation on the grounds that she had been inadequately counselled about the implications of the operation.

Clearly the midwife has an important role to play, where sterilisation is being contemplated during the caesarean operation, to ensure that the woman has been given all the relevant information. See also a case where the woman of 37 was not advised about the risk of Down's syndrome and the need for screening, discussed in Chapter 14.[4]

Absence of consent

Before proceeding with an operation for sterilisation, the consent of the patient must be obtained (the consent of minors and the mentally disordered is considered below).

In the case of Devi v. West Midlands Regional Health Authority 1980[5] the patient underwent a gynaecological operation with consent. She was a Roman Catholic and objected to sterilisation operations. During the operation, the surgeons discovered that she would be in danger if she were to become pregnant and therefore decided to perform a sterilisation operation. She sued for trespass to the person. Since the doctor had made no attempt to revive her and obtain her consent to the procedure, she succeeded in her claim.

NEGLIGENT STERILISATION

If it can be established that the surgeon failed to follow the accepted approved standard of care of a reasonable professional in undertaking a sterilisation operation, and that as a reasonably foreseeable consequence of that failure, harm was caused, then compensation would be payable. Damages can be awarded where the sterilisation is carried out negligently whether or not the woman goes on to have the baby. In the case of Chaunt v. Hertfordshire Health Authority 1982,[6] the claimant terminated the pregnancy which followed a negligent sterilisation but was entitled to compensation for the additional pain and suffering occasioned by the termination. There is, however, no requirement that the woman is expected to have a termination following a negligent sterilisation.

A patient was told in 1979 that the sterilisation which was carried out in 1973, when she was 19 years old, was unnecessary. She underwent many treatments to reverse the situation and suffered stress and loss of libido and was awarded £52 269 damages.[7] (See p. 329.)

Damages for an unwanted baby?
One view has been taken that while compensation would be payable for the additional pain and suffering in undergoing another pregnancy and labour, damages were not payable for the costs of bringing up a normal healthy child, since that would be contrary to public policy. This was the view taken by Judge Jupp in the case of Udale v. Bloomsbury 1983.[8] A different view was taken by Judge Peter Pain in the case of Thake v. Maurice (see below).

In the case of Emeh v. Kensington and Chelsea and Westminster Health Authority 1985,[9] following a negligently performed sterilisation, the woman refused to have an abortion and the question arose as to whether she was therefore entitled to have compensation for the costs of bringing up the unplanned child. The Court of Appeal held that she was.

The facts of Emeh were as follows:

In May 1976, the plaintiff, who had three normal children, underwent a sterilisation operation at the defendant's hospital. In January 1977 she discovered that she was about 20 weeks pregnant and she refused to have an abortion. She subsequently gave birth to a child with congenital abnormalities who required constant medical and parental supervision. She claimed for the pregnancy and the birth, and for the upkeep of the child. The trial judge held that the operation had been performed negligently and that therefore she was entitled to the damages accrued before she discovered that she was pregnant, but that she was not, by reason of her failure to have an abortion, entitled to the damages accruing thereafter, apart from the cost of undergoing a second sterilisation operation. She appealed to the Court of Appeal. This held that:

– Since the avoidance of the further pregnancy and the birth was the object of the sterilisation operation it was unreasonable, after the period of pregnancy which had elapsed, to expect the plaintiff to undergo an abortion and, therefore, the plaintiff's failure to do so was not so unreasonable as to eclipse the defendant's wrongdoing;

– it was not contrary to public policy to recover damages for the birth of the child, and therefore

– the plaintiff was entitled to recover damages for her financial loss caused by the negligent performance of the sterilisation operation.

As a result of the decision in the Emeh case, it was possible for the parents to claim the cost of educating the child privately if that was their standard of living, as well as the costs of caring for the child and the loss of future and past earnings. This ruling was followed in the case of Allen v. Bloomsbury Health Authority.[10] However, this has now changed, as a result of the House of Lords decision in McFarlane v. Tayside Health Board (Box 16.1).[11]

Box 16.1 McFarlane v. Tayside Health Board

Damages for healthy unplanned child
Mr McFarlane had a vasectomy and after 6 months was told that he was sterile and could dispense with contraceptive precautions. Subsequently Mrs M gave birth to a healthy daughter and they sued for compensation including the costs of rearing the child and for the pain and suffering caused to Mrs M in carrying and giving birth to the child. The House of Lords held that the costs of rearing a healthy child were not recoverable, but that Mrs M could recover damages for her prenatal pain and suffering and consequential financial loss.

Unplanned child who has disabilities

The ruling in the McFarlane case was not applied when the unplanned child was disabled (see however, the decision of the House of Lords in Rees v. Darlington Memorial Hospital, discussed below). In the case of Nunnerley and another v. Warrington Health Authority and another[12] (held before the decision of the McFarlane case was known), the mother was given negligent advice which led to the unwanted birth of a child who was born disabled. The High Court judge held that the claimant's claim for damages should not be limited to the costs of the care which they themselves had a legal duty to provide, but damages were payable for the cost of care beyond 18 years. The judge held that the normal principle of compensation should apply, i.e. the claimants were entitled to be put in the position that they would have been in, but for the wrong done to them.

In the case of Kerry v. Bro Taf Health Authority,[13] the claimant underwent a negligently performed sterilisation operation for which the defendants admitted liability. She gave birth to a baby with cerebral palsy, which was not the result of the defendant's negligence. At a trial of the preliminary issue, the defendant argued that the damages should be limited to the reasonable expenses which would have been within the claimant's financial means. The High Court dismissed the defendant's application.

In another case[14] the claimant was a mental patient sectioned under s.3 of the Mental Health Act 1983 and claimed that the NHS trust was negligent in failing to take reasonable care of her and as a consequence she became pregnant. The child was being brought up by the grandmother. The High Court heard a preliminary issue as to whether the costs of the grandmother in providing for the child's upbringing, maintenance and education could be claimed. The High Court turned down the application, holding that the mother was not providing the services and the grandmother was akin to a foster parent. The mother could not claim for the costs of her mother in bringing up the child.

Failure to carry out a pregnancy test pre sterilisation
In the case of Groom v. Selby,[15] the claimant underwent a sterilisation operation on 5 October 1994. No pregnancy test was carried out before the operation and in fact she had conceived on about 29 September 1994. She saw her GP on 21 November, complaining of abdominal pain and a green discharge, but she was not examined for a pregnancy, nor was she given a pregnancy test. A second GP diagnosed the pregnancy when she was 15 weeks pregnant. The claimant said that, had the pregnancy been diagnosed at an earlier stage, she would have had a termination but did not feel that she could undergo this at 15 weeks. The baby was born healthy but subsequently developed salmonella meningitis complicated by bilateral frontal brain abscesses and convulsions and episodes of septicaemia. The mother claimed against the first GP because of negligence in failing to diagnose the pregnancy or to recommend a pregnancy test.

The High Court judge held that the birth of a baby who subsequently suffered from disabilities was a reasonably foreseeable consequence of the defendant's actions and while the mother could not have successfully claimed for the costs of caring for a healthy baby, she could recover for the additional costs involved in caring for a disabled child, but not for the past and future cost of her basic maintenance. The defendant appealed to the Court of Appeal, which held that an award of compensation limited to the costs of disability would be fair, just and reasonable.[16]

The House of Lords' decision in the McFarlane case was applied by the Court of Appeal in the case of Parkinson v. St James and Seacroft University Hospital NHS Trust.[17] In this case, a woman who underwent a laparoscopic sterilisation procedure subsequently became pregnant and had a disabled baby. It was held that she was able to recover for the damages for the costs of providing for his special needs and the care relating to his disability, but that she could not recover for the basic costs of his maintenance. The Court of Appeal has recently held[18] that a disabled mother was entitled to recover damages uniquely referable to her disability when a negligently performed sterilisation led to her giving birth to a healthy child. In this case, the mother was severely visually handicapped.

The House of Lords[19] allowed the appeal and stated that the mother's compensation would be fixed at £15 000. It supported the principles established in the McFarlane case which precluded an award of damages for the additional costs of bringing up a healthy child by a disabled mother. However, it was just that there should be recognition of the parent's loss of the opportunity to life as wished for and planned. Therefore, there would be a conventional award of damages to mark the injury and loss in the sum of £15 000.

In contrast, a claimant was unable to obtain compensation for giving up her job to have an unplanned baby. In this case,[20] the claimant attended the surgery for a course of contraception by way of injection. The nurse failed to carry out a pregnancy test. It was accepted that this was negligent and that had the claimant been aware that she was pregnant, she would have had a termination. The claimant gave birth to a healthy daughter. She gave up employment to look after the child and sought to recover damages in respect of the loss of earnings consequent upon her decision to stay at home to look after the child. She failed in her action and her appeal to the Court of Appeal failed. The court applied the ruling in the McFarlane case and held that the claim for economic loss of future earnings was too remote.

Negligence in ultrasonography
A hospital was found liable when fetal abnormalities were not correctly identified during ultrasonography. The facts of the case (P v. Leeds Teaching Hospital NHS Trust 2004)[21] were as follows:

The claimant when pregnant underwent a routine anomaly ultrasound scan at her local hospital. The scan was difficult and the ultrasonographer suspected a fetal abnormality, an omphalocele, and was unable to visualise the bladder and kidneys. A decision was made to refer the claimant to a feto-maternal medicine unit. The specialist unit failed to exercise reasonable care and skill in identifying abnormalities. The claimant was not therefore advised of the potential for a physically and psychologically harrowing life for the child, and the availability of a termination. She gave birth to a son with cloacal exstrophy, a complex congenital condition, which involved extrusion of the bladder and bowel through the abdominal wall, and deformity of the genitalia. She received compensation.

This case can be contrasted with another (B. v. South Tyneside Healthcare NHS Trust)[22] where the claimant, who had given birth to a baby with serious disabilities including partial sacral agenesis, failed to establish that the ultrasonographer had been negligent. It was recognised by the court that ultrasonography was an imperfect science involving a large amount of personal judgement and the mother was not able to claim compensation.

Wrongful life: action by baby

It has been decided that the baby has no right of action to sue for the fact that had an operation to perform the sterilisation been properly performed, it would not have been born. In the following case (Box 16.2)[23] the mother was wrongly informed that the baby was not disabled and therefore she did not have an abortion.

Box 16.2 McKay v. Essex Area Health Authority[23]

Mrs McKay was pregnant and suspected that she had contracted German measles in the early weeks of her pregnancy. Blood tests were arranged to see if she had been infected. Unfortunately, she was wrongly informed that she had not been infected. She did not therefore have an abortion. When the baby was born, it was found to be disabled as a result of the effect of German measles. The Court of Appeal held that the child's claim for wrongful life (i.e. if there had been no negligence the child would have been aborted) could not be sustained. Although the child was born before the Congenital Disabilities Act 1976 was passed (see Ch. 17), the Court held that the Act would not change the situation. The child did not have an entitlement against those who failed to give the correct information which would have led to a termination of the pregnancy. The child only has a right when he/she has been disabled as the result of negligence. The decision did not affect the right of the mother to claim for the reasonably foreseeable results of the negligence, and her claim therefore proceeded.

The McKay case was considered in a case in 1998,[24] where the judge exercised his discretion under s.33 of the Limitation Act 1980 to enable her to bring an action out of time, because she had been not been advised to take action to determine whether her child was at risk of rubella and when the child was born with congenital rubella syndrome, she was negligently told that the child could bring its own action, she was not advised of her right to sue for negligent advice.

Negligent termination of pregnancy

In the case of Scuriaga v. Powell[25] doctors were negligent in terminating the pregnancy of the plaintiff. When it was discovered that the plaintiff was still pregnant with one out of two fetuses, it was too late to carry out an abortion. The mother obtained compensation for pain, suffering and loss of future and past earnings.

NO WARNING ABOUT THE STERILISATION NOT BEING 100% EFFECTIVE

Even where the sterilisation operation has been carried out with all reasonable care and skill, compensation may still be payable if the patient had not been warned that the operation might not be 100% effective. However, the burden is on the claimant to prove that there has been a breach of the duty of care to provide the appropriate information.

In the case of Thake v. Maurice 1984,[26] no warnings were given that an operation for a vasectomy might not be 100% successful. The claimant therefore sued for breach of contract. The facts were as follows:

Mr Thake, a railway guard, and his wife and four children lived in a three-bedroomed council house. When a fifth child was expected, Mr Thake discussed with a surgeon the possibility of undergoing a vasectomy. Because of the long NHS waiting list, it was agreed that the operation would be performed privately at a cost of £20. It was made clear to Mr Thake that he would become permanently sterile. Both husband and wife signed forms consenting to the operation and declaring that they had been told of its purpose and effects. Tests on Mr Thake subsequently showed him to be sterile. However, 2 years after the operation Mrs Thake became pregnant again, but did not realise her condition until it was too late to have an abortion. The couple claimed compensation. There was no suggestion that the operation had been per-formed negligently, but suitable warnings had not been given. The judge found in favour of Mr Thake, holding that on the facts the contract was not merely a contract to perform a vasectomy but was a contract to make Mr Thake irreversibly sterile and the defendants had failed to give an appropriate warning of the possibility of failure.

The defendants appealed to the Court of Appeal,[27] which by a majority verdict decided that a reasonable person would have left the consulting room believing that Mr Thake would be sterilised by the operation, but not that he had been given a guarantee that he would be absolutely sterile. Mr Thake lost his case.

Box 16.3 Gold v. Haringey Health Authority[28]

Mrs Gold decided when pregnant with her third child that she would not have any more children, and a Consultant obstetrician discussed with her the possibility of her being sterilised. He did not discuss the possibility of her husband undergo-ing a vasectomy, which had a slightly lower failure rate, nor did he discuss the risk of the operation failing. After the birth of the third child, she was sterilised. However, it was not a success and she later gave birth to a fourth child. Her claim against the Health Authority for negligence on the grounds that (a) she had not been warned of the risk of failure of the operation and (b) there had been negligent misrepresentation in giving her an assurance that the operation was irreversible, succeeded initially and she was awarded £19 000 in compensation by the trial ▶

▶

judge. However, the defendants' appeal was upheld. The Court of Appeal held that the standard of care to be followed by the doctor in giving warnings was the standard of the reasonable professional, and applied the Bolam Test. In 1979, there was a substantial body of doctors who would have given her the same advice and not warned her of the risk of failure. Nor could the statement that the operation was irreversible be regarded as a representation that the operation was bound to achieve its objectives.

A claim also failed in the case of Eyre v. Measday[29] where the plaintiff and her husband decided that they did not wish to have any more children and in consulting a gynaecologist privately, were told that the operation was intended to be irreversible. They were not advised of the very small chance of failure. The plaintiff failed in her claim for compensation following the birth of a child, the Court of Appeal deciding that it was not a contract to render her absolutely sterile but rather a contract to perform a particular operation.

Conclusions on warnings
Nowadays it would be recommended practice for the doctor discussing an operation for sterilisation to warn of the risk of failure, and to give no warranties about irreversible sterility. Consent forms for such purpose were introduced by the NHS management executive[30] but specific forms for such treatments have not been drafted under the current guidance.[31]

Do both partners have to give consent?
It will have been noticed that in the Thake v. Maurice case, both husband and wife signed the form. This is not a legal requirement: there is no necessity for one partner to give consent to a sterilisation operation proceeding on the other. Clearly counselling of both together would be good practice, but an operation should not be refused on the grounds that the partner not undergoing the procedure is refusing to give consent to the other having the operation. If there is effective counselling, then the professional should not be involved in any matrimonial proceedings between the couple.

The child or young person and sterilisation
Where it is planned to carry out a sterilisation on a child or young person, care should be taken to ensure that a valid consent is given. While the parents could give consent on the minor's behalf, the minor should have independent representation to ensure that the operation is in her/his best interests. In the case Re B (1987)[32] the House of Lords agreed that a girl of 17 years could have a sterilisation with the consent of the parents (see Ch. 7 for further discussion of this case).

The mentally incapacitated adult and sterilisation
In the case Re F (1989)[33] the House of Lords held that where the adult lacked the mental competence to make their own decisions, then the carers could act out of

necessity in the best interests of the patient and follow the reasonable standard of care (i.e. the Bolam Test). However, where a therapeutic sterilisation was being contemplated then a declaration should be sought from the court. The Mental Capacity Act 2005 will when implemented provide a statutory framework for making such decisions on behalf of mentally incapacitated adults (see Chs 7 and 33).

Sterilisation as a last resort

In the case of S (1998),[34] her mental and emotional state meant that she was unable to look after herself and she was vulnerable to sexual exploitation. Her mother applied for a declaration that it would be lawful to sterilise her. The application was refused on the grounds that the risk of pregnancy was not an identifiable risk but rather a speculative risk. Risk had to be assessed on the basis of circumstances that existed or could be reasonably foreseen to exist. The President of the Family Division (Sir Stephen Brown) held that the risk of pregnancy was not so great so as to require sterilisation, with the consequent imposition of necessary invasive procedures which carried the risk of fatality.

Lesser measures than sterilisation may be in the best interests of the patient. In the case Re S (2000),[35] the judge had to decide whether it was in the best interests of S to be fitted with an intrauterine device called Mirena, which would significantly reduce her heavy periods and which was supported by the Official Solicitor, or to have a hysterectomy, which the mother wished her to have. The judge decided that the subtotal hysterectomy was in the best interests of S, because the intrauterine device would require a series of general anaesthetics every 5 to 7 years, and her mother might not be available to provide S with support in later years. However, this decision was overruled by the Court of Appeal.[36] The Court of Appeal held that the judge had failed to give proper weight to the unanimous medical evidence which supported the less invasive Mirena coil treatment and declared that this was in the patient's best interests.

In contrast to the decisions on sterilisation of a woman with learning disabilities in Re S, the Court of Appeal decided that it was not in the best interests of a man who had Down's syndrome to be sterilised.[37] The best interests of the patient encompassed medical, emotional and all other welfare issues. The best interests of the man were not the equivalent of the best interests of a woman because of the obvious biological differences.

CONCLUSIONS

Most of the legal uncertainties in this area which existed over the last 10 years, such as liability if warnings were not given or were inadequate, the amount of compensation for birth of an unplanned but healthy child, and sterilisation of children and those with learning disabilities have now been resolved. The midwife may well continue to be involved in discussions with clients over resource issues and the availability of family planning, fertilisation services (see Ch. 27) and facilities for termination of pregnancy (see Ch. 26).

QUESTIONS AND EXERCISES

1. Review your procedures for advising and giving information to clients who have expressed a wish to be sterilised.

2. A client expecting her fourth child has been informed that she will probably have to have a caesarean operation. On hearing this, she decided that she would wish to be sterilised at the same time. Her husband has however made it clear that he would not agree to her being sterilised. What is the legal position?

3. To what extent do you consider that the midwife's role should include advice on family planning? What is the position if the midwife is opposed on religious grounds to family planning?

4. You are aware that a mother with a daughter of 14 years of age who suffers from severe learning disabilities wants her daughter to be sterilised. What is the legal position?

References

1 Briody v. St Helens and Knowsley AHA (Claim for damages and costs) sub nom Briody v. St Helens and Knowsley AHA [2001] EWCA Civ 1010 [2001] 2 FCR 481 CA.
2 Biles v. Barking Health Authority 30 October 1987 QBD Current Law 1988 1103.
3 Wells v. Surrey Area Health Authority. The Times Law Report, 29 July 1978.
4 Enright v. Kwun [2003] EWHC 1000, The Times, 20 May 2003.
5 Devi v. West Midlands RHA [1980] 80 Current Law 687.
6 Chaunt v. Hertfordshire Health Authority [1982] 132 NLJ 1054.
7 Biles v. Barking Health Authority [1988] C.L.Y. 1103.
8 Udale v. Bloomsbury [1983] 2 All ER 522.
9 Emeh v. Kensington and Chelsea and Westminster Health Authority [1985] 2 WLR 233.
10 Allen v. Bloomsbury HA [1993] 1 All ER 651.
11 McFarlane v. Tayside Health Board [1999] 4 All ER 961 HL.
12 Nunnerley and another v. Warrington Health Authority and another [2000] Lloyds' Rep Med 170; Times Law Report, 26 November 1999.
13 Kerry v. Bro Taf Health Authority. Lloyd's Rep Med [2002] 182.
14 AD v. East Kent Community NHS Trust. Lloyd's Rep Med [2002] 424.
15 Groom v. Selby [2001] Lloyd's Rep Med 39.
16 Groom v. Selby [2002] Lloyd's Rep Med 1.
17 Parkinson v. St James and Seacroft University Hospital NHS Trust [2001] Lloyd's Rep Med 309.
18 Rees v. Darlington Memorial Hospital NHS Trust. Times Law Report, 20 February 2002 [2002] 2 All ER 177 CA.

19 Rees v. Darlington Memorial Hospital NHS Trust. Lloyd's Rep Med [2004] 1 HL.

20 Greenfield v. Flather and others [2001] Lloyd's Rep Med 143.

21 P v. Leeds Teaching Hospital NHS Trust [2004] EWHC 1392; Lloyd's Rep Med [2004] 537.

22 B v. South Tyneside Health Care NHS Trust [2004] 1169; Lloyd's Rep Med [2004] 505.

23 McKay v. Essex AHA [1982] 2 All ER 771.

24 Das v. Ganju (1998) 42 BMLR 28 QBD.

25 Scuriaga v. Powell [1979] 123 Sol J 406.

26 Thake v. Maurice [1984] 2 All ER 513.

27 Thake v. Maurice [1986] 1 All ER 497 CA.

28 Gold v. Haringey Health Authority [1987] All ER 888.

29 Eyre v. Measday [1986] 1 All ER 488.

30 Department of Health. A Guide to Consent for Examination and Treatment (HSC (90/22) as amended by HSC (92)32; 1990.

31 Department of Health. Reference guide to consent for examination or treatment. Good practice in consent: implementation guide. London: HMSO; 2001. Online. Available: www.doh.gov.uk/consent

32 Re B [1987] (a minor) (wardship: sterilisation) 2 All ER 206.

33 Re F v. West Berkshire HA [1989] 2 All ER 545.

34 Re S (medical treatment: adult sterilisation) [1998] 1 FLR 944.

35 Re S (sterilisation: patient's best interests) [2000] 1 FLR 465.

36 Re S (sterilisation: patient's best interests) [2000] 2 FLR 389 CA.

37 Re A (male sterilisation) [2000] 1 FLR 549.

Chapter 17

THE STATUS AND RIGHTS OF THE UNBORN

The law protects the unborn child by making it a criminal offence to harm it (subject to exceptions under the Abortion Act 1967 as amended – see Ch. 26), but has been reluctant to recognise the unborn child as having the rights of a person, i.e. having a legal personality.

CRIMINAL LAW

The unborn child is specifically protected in the criminal law by the Infant Life Preservation Act 1929. This statute makes it a criminal offence for any person who, with intent to destroy the life of a child capable of being born alive, by any wilful act causes a child to die before it has an existence independent of its mother. There is a defence if the act which caused the death of the child was done in good faith for the purposes only of preserving the life of the mother. There is also a defence if the unborn child died during a lawful abortion (see Ch. 26).

Under s.58 of the Offences Against The Person Act 1861, it is illegal for a woman being with child unlawfully to administer to herself any poison or use any instrument unlawfully with intent to procure a miscarriage; it is also unlawful for any other person to attempt to cause a miscarriage by similar means, whether or not the woman is actually pregnant. 'Unlawfully' excludes an abortion legally carried out under the Abortion Act 1967 (see Ch. 26).

Section 59 of the Offences Against The Person Act 1861 makes it illegal for anyone to supply a poison or any instrument knowing that it is to be used unlawfully to procure the miscarriage of any woman, whether or not she is with child.

Section 60 of the 1861 Act makes it an offence to conceal the birth of a child.

These Sections are further discussed in Chapter 26, on abortion.

LEGAL STATUS OF THE FETUS

The fetus is not regarded as having an independent legal personality. As a result of this principle, actions cannot be brought in its name before its birth. Only after it is born can legal action be brought in its behalf.

HUMAN RIGHTS ACT 1998

Article 2 of the European Convention states that

Everyone's right to life shall be protected by law. No one shall be deprived of his life intentionally, save in the execution of a sentence of a court following his conviction of a crime for which this penalty is provided by law.

(The Human Rights Act 1998 (Amendment) Order 2004[1] makes amendments to the Act following the ratification by the UK of the 13th Protocol to the European Convention on Human Rights on 10 October 2003, which abolishes the death penalty in all circumstances.)

The right to life does not however apply to the unborn child, so it could not be argued successfully that termination of a pregnancy is a breach of Article 2. In contrast, in the Republic of Ireland, the Bill of Rights of the Irish Constitution recognises the right to life of the unborn child.

CRIMINAL OFFENCE IN CAUSING THE DEATH OF A FETUS

In the Scottish case of Hamilton v. Fife Health Board (1992)[2] Lord Prosser held that where a child died in consequence of injuries sustained when he was a fetus as a result of the fault of another person, he was not 'a person dying in consequence of personal injuries sustained by him' because at the time when the injuries were sustained he was not a person. This was a decision in interpreting the provisions of the Damages (Scotland) Act 1976. In a case reported in 1992[3] a woman who allegedly kicked her neighbour, who was 36 weeks pregnant, in the stomach, killing her unborn baby, was cleared of manslaughter. In the trial of Claudette Morgan, the judge told the jury that it could not convict the accused if the child was born dead. For a charge of murder or manslaughter to succeed, the baby would have to be born alive and then die of injuries sustained in the womb (Box 17.1).[4,5]

Box 17.1 Death of baby because of pre-birth injuries[5]

In a case in 1994, a violent assault with a knife was carried out on a pregnant woman. She gave birth to a premature child who did not survive. The Court of Appeal held that an intention to cause serious injury to the mother could be transferred to the child once born so that the assailant could be guilty of murder. The House of Lords however rejected the concept of 'transferred malice' and held that the accused could not be found guilty of murder of the child once born. At the time of the attack, the fetus did not have a legal personality.

▶

Lord Mustill stated:

It is sufficient to say that it is established beyond doubt for the criminal law, as for the civil law (Burton v. Islington Health Authority, De Martell v. Merton and Sutton Health Authority) [see Box 17.3 below] that the child en ventre sa mere (in his or her mother's stomach) does not have a distinct human personality, whose extinguishment gives rise to any penalties or liabilities at common law.

It is not possible to make an unborn child a ward of court (see Box 17.4 below).

THE MOTHER AND CRIMINAL OFFENCES AGAINST THE CHILD

If the mother smokes or eats or otherwise acts in such a way during the pregnancy that she harms the fetus, is she guilty of a criminal offence?

The answer is probably no, unless her actions can be brought within the Offences against the Person Act 1861 or the Infant Life Preservation Act 1929. It would probably be difficult for the prosecution to establish the requisite *mens rea* or mental element which these charges require for a prosecution to succeed.

CIVIL LAW

CONGENITAL DISABILITIES (CIVIL LIABILITY) ACT 1976

This Act, which is shown in Appendix 2, gives a right of action to the baby who is born disabled as a result of an occurrence before its birth, which affected either parent in having a healthy baby or affected the mother or the child during the pregnancy.

The main features of the Act are shown in Box 17.2.

Box 17.2 Main features of the Congenital Disabilities Act

An action is given to the child:

- if it is born alive

- for harm caused by negligent actions to the father or mother,

---

▶ – which resulted in the child being born disabled.

– The mother is only liable if she was negligent while driving a car.

Liability to the child can be excluded to the same extent and subject to the same restrictions as liability in the parent's own case.

If the disability arises from an event pre-conception, then the defendant is not liable if both parents knew of the risk of the child being born disabled. However, if the father is the defendant, this does not apply if he knew of the risk but the mother did not.

The defendant is not liable if when responsible in a professional capacity for treating or advising the parent, he took reasonable care having regard to the then received professional opinion applicable to the particular case; but this does not mean that he is answerable only because he departed from received opinion.

The mother is not liable to the child, unless she was driving a motor vehicle and was in breach of her duty of care to the unborn child and as a consequence the child is born disabled.

LIABILITY OF THE MOTHER TO THE CHILD

The mother of the child is only liable under the Act if when driving a motor vehicle and knowing (or she ought reasonably to know) herself to be pregnant she is negligent and in consequence of this negligence the child is born with disabilities. The child could then sue in respect of those disabilities. In practice, of course, the child would be suing the insurance company with whom the mother was insured.

LIABILITY OF THE PROFESSIONAL

It can be seen from Box 17.2 that the professional who takes reasonable care when acting in a professional capacity for treating or advising the parent would not be liable to the child if born disabled. The statute uses the test of the 'then received professional opinion to that particular class of case' which is comparable with the Bolam Test discussed in Chapter 13. However, as in Bolam itself and Maynard's case, the fact that a professional departs from the received opinion is not in itself evidence of negligence. Documentation would have to show clearly the reasons why the professional acted in the way she did and the justification for not following the usual practice.

In February 2001, a girl, then aged 8, received £2.43 million from Buckinghamshire Health Authority for injuries she sustained when she was stabbed in the head with an amniocentesis needle while a fetus of 16 weeks' gestation. She was born profoundly brain damaged and could barely communicate.[6]

EXCLUSIONS TO LIABILITY AND DEFENCES UNDER THE ACT

It must be emphasised that the child's action under the Congenital Disabilities Act is derivative, i.e. it relies upon a negligent act against the mother or father which results in the child being born disabled. If there would be no liability of the defendant to the parent, then there is no liability to the child (the exception to this is the mother's duty to the child when driving a car). The Unfair Contract Terms Act prevents any exclusion of liability for negligence which causes personal injury or death. Voluntary assumption of risk and contributory negligence may however be effective as defences (see Ch. 13).

COMMON LAW AND CIVIL LIABILITY TO THE UNBORN CHILD

Prior to the commencement of the Congenital Disabilities (Civil Liability) Act 1976, it was possible for a child, if born alive, to bring a case at common law (i.e. judge-made law) in respect of pre-birth negligence or illegal activities. This is shown in the case in Box 17.3.[7]

Box 17.3 B v. Islington Health Authority 1991[7]

The facts of this case were that an operation for dilation and curettage was carried out when the plaintiff was an embryo in her mother's womb. She was born disabled with brain damage and asphyxia after a failed forceps delivery. The birth occurred before the Congenital Disabilities (Civil Liability) Act 1976 was passed and therefore the child had to bring a claim at common law. This claim was recognised. A duty of care was therefore recognised as existing towards an unborn child and this becomes actionable at the suit of the child when born alive.

It was held that children with disabilities caused by alleged negligent medical treatment before they were born had a cause of action against the health authorities.

However, under s.4(5) of the Congenital Disabilities (Civil Liability) Act 1976, the common law is replaced in respect of all births after the Act was brought into force on 22 July 1976. The consequence of this is that a child can only sue the mother in respect of prebirth injuries caused by the mother's negligence, if she were negligent while driving a car, i.e. action can only be brought under the 1976 Act.

NO POWER TO MAKE A FETUS A WARD OF COURT

There is no power for the courts to make the baby a ward of court while still *in utero*. The Court of Appeal has held that there is no jurisdiction to make the unborn child of a mentally disturbed woman a ward of court. It rejected the local authority's application that the court should extend wardship jurisdiction where a viable child was at risk (Box 17.4).[8]

Box 17.4 Re F (*in utero*) 1988[8]

In this case, the mother was aged 36 and had suffered from severe mental disturbance since 1977. Throughout 1982, she had led a nomadic existence, wandering around Europe. She had returned in 1983 and had been settled in a flat in south London. Her only means of support was supplementary benefit. The local authority was concerned about the baby expected towards the end of January. Early in January, the mother disappeared. The local authority instituted wardship proceedings. The Court of Appeal were of the opinion that they did not have the power to institute wardship proceedings in relation to a fetus. They pointed to the difficulties of enforcing such an order against the expectant mother.

AN ACTION FOR WRONGFUL LIFE?

What, however, if the child should never have been born, for example if a sterilisation or abortion operation does not proceed correctly? Does the child have a right of action for wrongful life?

Such a case was McKay v. Essex AHA (1982)[9] which is considered in Chapter 16. It was held that a child did not have an action because he or she should not have been born. In this case, the mother was wrongly informed that the baby she was carrying was not disabled and therefore she did not have an abortion.

CONCLUSIONS

The principle that the unborn child has no legal personality has major implications for the law in this area and there are likely to be constant pressures for change in this area from such groups as the Society for the Protection of the Unborn Child. If the European Court of Human Rights were to declare that an unborn child had a legal personality and could therefore claim rights under Article 2, the right to life, this would have major implications for our laws on termination (see Ch. 26) and the rights of the fetus.

QUESTIONS AND EXERCISES

1. Do you consider that the unborn child should have clear rights to be protected from an unacceptable lifestyle of the mother?

2. If you were concerned about an unborn baby because the mother was a drug addict, what action would you take?

3. To what extent does the Congenital Disabilities Act give protection to the midwife against litigation being brought in the name of a brain-damaged baby?

References

1 Human Rights Act 1998 (Amendment) Order 2004 SI 2004 1574.

2 Hamilton v. Fife Health Board. Times Law Report, 28 January 1992.

3 R v. Morgan. The Times, 21 May 1992.

4 A-G's Reference (No 3 1994) [1997] 3 All ER 936.

5 Burton v. Islington Health Authority; De Martell v. Merton and Sutton Health Authority [1992] 10 BMLR 63; [1993] QB 204.

6 News item. The Times, 27 February 2001.

7 B v. Islington Health Authority [1991] 1 All ER 325.

8 Re F (in utero) [1998] 2 All ER 193.

9 McKay v. Essex AHA [1982] 2 All ER 771.

Chapter 18
CRIMINAL LIABILITY

This chapter considers the accountability of the midwife in the criminal courts and looks at the following topics:

- Coroner's jurisdiction

- Murder

- Manslaughter

- The case of R v. Cox[1]

- Infanticide

- Other crimes

- Female Genital Mutilation Act 2003

- Criminal proceedings

- Criminal injury compensation.

In Chapter 1, it was explained that criminal offences may be statutory (e.g. theft) or derived from the common law (e.g. murder). In order to establish that the accused is guilty of the offence with which he or she is charged, the prosecution must prove beyond reasonable doubt that both the actual physical requirements of the offence (i.e. the *actus reus*) and the required mental element (*mens rea*) are present. When a client – mother or baby – dies in the course of being cared for by health professionals, the death could be classified as accidental death, voluntary manslaughter, involuntary manslaughter or murder.

CORONER'S JURISDICTION

The death, unless it has resulted from natural causes and can therefore be certified by the doctor caring for the patient, would be reported to the coroner, who then has the responsibility for deciding whether to request a post-mortem and whether or not an inquest should be held. The coroner will also decide whether or not a jury should be summoned to decide upon the cause of death. The purpose of the inquest is to decide:

- the identity of the deceased

- how, where and when the deceased came by his death, and

– the particulars required by the Registration Acts to be registered concerning his death.

The finding of any person guilty of murder, manslaughter or infanticide is specifically prohibited by the Coroners Act 1988 s.11(6).

Following an unexpected death, there would probably be an inquest carried out by the coroner. If criminal offences are suspected, the coroner has the power to adjourn the hearing. The Director of Public Prosecutions may also ask the coroner to adjourn the hearing. Following the coroner's hearing, the papers in the case may be placed before the Crown Prosecution Service (CPS). The CPS has the right to decide if proceedings should be brought in the criminal courts against the defendant. If a midwife is asked to provide a statement and give evidence at an inquest, she should seek assistance from senior management or the solicitor to the trust (see Ch. 15).

Major reforms to the coroner's jurisdiction and appointments were recommended by the Report following the Inquiry into the Shipman murders.[2]

MURDER

In order to secure a conviction of murder, the prosecution have to prove beyond all reasonable doubt that the defendant must either have intended to cause death or intended to cause grievous bodily harm. Unless a situation comparable with that of the Beverley Allitt case or the Shipman case exists, which is extremely rare (see Ch. 14), it would be very unusual to be able to prove the intent necessary to convict a health professional of the murder of a patient. Following a conviction for murder, a judge at the present time has no discretion over sentencing but must sentence the convicted person to life imprisonment, i.e. a life sentence is mandatory. The judge can indicate the minimum time that must be served. The House of Lords held that the power of the Home Secretary to set tariffs (under s.29 of the Crime (Sentences) Act 1997) was incompatible with Article 6(1) of the European Convention on Human Rights.[3] It made a declaration that s.29 of the 1997 Act was incompatible with the Convention. This was accepted by the Home Secretary, who introduced sentencing principles into the Criminal Justice Act 2003. The Law Commission has recommended that the present mandatory sentence of life imprisonment for murder should be abolished and should be replaced by a range of sanctions depending upon the different circumstances of the death.

INVOLUNTARY MANSLAUGHTER

This may arise where death results from the gross negligence of a health professional, where there is no intention to kill or to cause grievous harm. There will not be a charge of murder. In such cases, there may be a prosecution for involuntary manslaughter or there may be no prosecution at all. It depends upon the circumstances. If, for example, there is gross recklessness leading to the death, then there may be a prosecution for manslaughter. The following two cases illustrate two different situations.

Death by misadventure
In 1991, two junior doctors were each given a 9-month suspended prison sentence for the manslaughter of a 16-year-old with leukaemia. He died after being wrongly injected in the spine with a cytotoxic drug which should have been administered intravenously. The conviction for manslaughter was quashed by the Court of Appeal on the grounds that the jury should have been directed by the judge to decide whether the defendants were guilty of 'gross negligence' and not 'recklessness' and whether there were any mitigating circumstances, such as the lack of supervision from more experienced staff.[4]

Manslaughter
In the second case, Dr Adomako, the person charged, was, during the latter part of an operation, the anaesthetist in charge of the patient, who was undergoing an eye operation. At approximately 11.05 a.m. a disconnection occurred at the endotracheal tube connection. The supply of oxygen to the patient ceased and led to a cardiac arrest at 11.14 a.m. During that period, the defendant failed to notice or remedy the disconnection. He first became aware that something was amiss when an alarm sounded on the Dinamap machine, which monitored the patient's blood pressure. From the evidence it appeared that some 4.5 minutes would have elapsed between the disconnection and the sounding of the alarm. When the alarm sounded, the defendant responded in various ways by checking the equipment and by administering atropine to raise the patient's pulse. But at no stage before the cardiac arrest did he check the integrity of the endotracheal tube connection. The disconnection was not discovered until after resuscitation measures had been commenced.

Dr Adomako accepted at his trial that he had been negligent. The issue was whether his conduct was criminal. He was convicted of involuntary manslaughter but appealed against his conviction. He lost his appeal in the Court of Appeal and then appealed to the House of Lords.[5]

The House of Lords clarified the legal situation.

The stages which the House of Lords suggested should be followed were:

– The ordinary principles of the law of negligence should be applied to ascertain whether or not the defendant had been in breach of a duty of care towards the victim who had died.

– If such a breach of duty was established, the next question was whether that breach of duty caused the death of the victim.

– If so, the jury had to go on to consider whether that breach of duty should be characterised as gross negligence and therefore as a crime. That would depend on

351

the seriousness of the breach of duty committed by the defendant in all the circumstances in which the defendant was placed when it occurred.

– The jury would have to consider whether the extent to which the defendant's conduct departed from the proper standard of care incumbent upon him, involving as it must have done a risk of death to the patient, was such that it should be judged criminal.

The judge was required to give the jury a direction on the meaning of 'gross negligence' as had been given in the present case by the Court of Appeal.

The jury might properly find gross negligence on proof of

– *indifference to an obvious risk of injury to health, or*

– *actual foresight of the risk coupled with either*

  - *a determination nevertheless to run it, or*

  - *an intention to avoid it but involving such a high degree of negligence in the attempted avoidance as the jury considered justified conviction, or*

– *inattention or failure to advert to a serious risk going beyond mere inadvertence in respect of an obvious and important matter which the defendant's duty demanded he should address.'*

The House of Lords held that the Court of Appeal had applied the correct test and his appeal was dismissed.

The judge has full discretion over the sentencing in a case of conviction for involuntary manslaughter.

THE CASE OF R v. DR NIGEL COX[6]

Dr Nigel Cox was convicted when he prescribed potassium chloride to a terminally ill patient, and was sentenced to 1 year's imprisonment which was suspended for 1 year. He also had to appear before disciplinary proceedings of the Regional Health Authority, his employers and before the General Medical Council.

VOLUNTARY MANSLAUGHTER

This term is used to cover the situation where the defendant has caused the death of a person with intent, but owing to special circumstances, a charge or conviction of murder is not appropriate. The term covers:

– death as a result of the provocation of the accused

– death as a result of diminished responsibility of the accused

– killing as a result of a suicide pact.

HOW DOES THIS AFFECT THE MIDWIFE?

If a midwife has been responsible for an action of gross negligence which has led to the death of the mother or baby, she may well face criminal proceedings, in addition to professional conduct proceedings by the NMC (see Ch. 4) and disciplinary proceedings by the employer (see Ch. 22). The criminal procedure which would be followed is considered below.

The midwife might also be involved in a criminal case because of the alleged criminal conduct of a colleague, in which case she may be asked to provide a statement and give evidence in court (see Ch. 15).

ASSISTING IN THE SUICIDE OF ANOTHER

Reference should be made to Chapter 9, where it is pointed out that it is a criminal offence to aid or abet another person in committing suicide. The same chapter discusses the legalities involved in letting a severely disabled child die.

INFANTICIDE

Under s.1(1) of the Infanticide Act 1938, a woman can be found guilty of an offence if she causes the death of a baby under 12 months, but if it is found that the balance of her mind was disturbed by reason of her not having fully recovered from the effect of giving birth or by reason of the effect of lactation, then instead of a murder conviction, she can be found guilty of manslaughter.

This offence was criticised in 1975 in the Butler Report,[7] which recommended the abolition of the offence of infanticide. In 2005, the Court of Appeal stated that the law relating to infanticide is unsatisfactory and outdated, when dismissing the appeal of a woman who was serving life for the murder of her 12-week-old son.[8] The woman had been found guilty of killing her baby by asphyxiation after becoming frustrated with his refusal to breastfeed.

OTHER CRIMES

The chances of the midwife being involved in criminal proceedings for murder or manslaughter are extremely rare. However, she does face the possibility of other criminal charges particularly in relation to property, motor offences or health and safety offences which are prosecuted in the criminal courts (see Ch. 19).

Community midwives are in particular vulnerable to the allegation that they have been guilty of theft of property in a person's house, particularly where they visit on their own. There should be a clear protocol against the receipt of any gifts to the midwife from clients, to protect the midwife against false accusations.

In addition, the community midwife, in driving a car, will have to make arrangements that it is appropriately insured and that driving it at work has been agreed in advance with the insurers. The nature of the work would have to be specified, including whether or not she uses the car to drive clients and equipment. She would be responsible for any breach of the Road Traffic Acts on her own account.

If it is known that the defendant is a registered midwife, any conviction for a criminal offence would automatically be reported to the NMC. The midwife would not have any right to sue the police for breach of confidentiality.[9]

Other offences are discussed in the context of specific chapters, e.g. abortion (Ch. 26), offences against the person (Ch. 17) and offences under the Human Fertilisation and Embryology Act (Ch. 29). Breaches of the Health and Safety at Work Act and the Regulations can result in criminal prosecutions, and these are discussed in Chapter 19.

FEMALE GENITAL MUTILATION ACT 2003

Under the Prohibition of Female Circumcision Act 1985 female circumcision was a criminal offence. There was however evidence that some girls from ethnic minorities were being returned home to be circumcised. Following a parliamentary hearing, the All-Party Parliamentary Group on population development and reproductive health published a report in 2000 recommending that there should be amendments to the Prohibition of Female Circumcision Act 1985 to enable persons who take girls abroad for circumcision to be prosecuted under UK law when they return. This led to the 1985 Act being replaced by the Female Genital Mutilation Act 2003 which strengthens the law against female genital mutilation (FGM).

Under s.1(1) of this Act it is a criminal offence for any person to:

excise, infibulate or otherwise mutilate the whole or any part of a girl's labia majora or labia minora or clitoris.

The word 'girl' includes woman. Section 1(1) is subject to s.1(2), which states no offence is committed by an approved person who performs:

a. a surgical operation on a girl which is necessary for her physical or mental health, or

b. a surgical operation on a girl who is in any stage of labour, or has just given birth, for purposes connected with the labour or birth.

An approved person is defined as:

a. in relation to an operation falling within sub-section 1(2)a, a registered medical practitioner

b. in relation to an operation falling within sub-section 1(2)b, a registered medical practitioner, a registered midwife, or a person undergoing a course of training with a view to becoming such a practitioner or midwife.

There is also no offence if a person performs a surgical operation falling within s.1(2)(a) or (b) outside the UK and exercises functions corresponding to those of an approved person.

Section 1(5) states that for the purpose of determining whether an operation is necessary for the mental health of a girl, it is immaterial whether she or any other person believes that the operation is required as matter of custom or ritual.

Section 2 makes it an offence for a person to aid, abet, counsel or procure a girl to excise, infibulate or otherwise mutilate the whole or any part of her own labia majora, labia minora or clitoris.

Under s.3 it an offence to aid, abet, counsel or procure a person who is not a UK national or permanent in the UK to do a relevant act of female genital mutilation outside the UK. An act is a relevant act of female genital mutilation if it is done in relation to a UK resident and it would constitute an offence under s.1. Similar exceptions in relation to surgical operation and childbirth by approved persons apply. The Act also extends the offences to any act done outside the UK by a UK national or permanent resident.

Midwives may come across information that female circumcision is being carried out illegally in this country. Disclosure of this information to the appropriate authorities would be justified in the public interest and therefore an exception to the duty of confidentiality (see Ch. 10). The RCM has published a revised position paper on female genital mutilation.[10] The British Medical Association has published guidelines about female genital mutilation,[11] recommending that GPs should do all they can to deter families from the practice as soon as they register with a surgery. If a doctor suspects that a girl may be about to undergo circumcision in the UK or be sent 'on holiday', then the GP should inform social services' child protection units. Such advice would also apply to midwives. The NHS pays for at least 200 operations a year to reverse female circumcision.[12] Comfort Momoh considers attitudes to female genital mutilation and emphasises the need to share information with those working at grass root level in other countries and the importance of midwives condemning FGM and identifying and protecting children at risk.[13] Joyce Sihwa and Maurina Baron consider the case of a doctor who was struck off by the GMC for offering to carry out FGM.[14] Baroness Ruth Rendell asked the Attorney General in the House of Lords on 3 March 2005 how many prosecutions there had been under the new legislation and was told that no prosecutions had taken place. Yana Richens and Sarah Creighton discuss the failure of the UK to take action, in spite of the fact that it is estimated that there are 3000–4000 new cases of FGM in the UK every year.[15]

CRIMINAL PROCEEDINGS

For serious crimes known as 'indictable only offences', criminal proceedings would commence with committal proceedings before the magistrates court. In their capacity as examining justices, magistrates have the task of determining whether there is a case to answer. If they agree that there is a case to answer, the case is then committed to the Crown Court for trial before a jury. For less serious crimes, known as summary offences (which can only be heard before the magistrates) or offences which are triable either way (i.e. they can be heard by magistrates or in the Crown Court), the magistrates act as both judge and jury in hearing the case. If they consider that the accused is guilty, then the magistrates sentence the accused. There is power to refer to the Crown Court for sentencing if the magistrates consider the accused should receive a stiffer sentence than they have the power to give.

In a Crown Court hearing, where the accused enters a 'not guilty' plea, the jury is sworn in and the case would begin with an opening speech by the prosecution lawyer. The witnesses for the prosecution give evidence in turn: initially evidence in chief (when they are questioned by the prosecution and leading questions cannot be asked); then they can be cross-examined by the defence and then re-examined by the prosecution. After the end of the prosecution case, the judge could order the jury to bring forward a 'not guilty' verdict if he is satisfied that there is insufficient evidence from the prosecution to justify a conviction. Otherwise, the case proceeds with the evidence of the defence. At present the accused does not have to give evidence, but the prosecution can comment on that fact. After the witnesses for the defence have given evidence, there are closing speeches from the prosecution and defence and the judge then sums up for the jury, directing the jury on the law which applies, the evidence which they have heard and the responsibility upon them. If the jury brings forward a 'guilty' verdict or verdicts, the judge then sentences the accused, but may delay this stage in order to have evidence of the accused's social and financial background.

CRIMINAL INJURY COMPENSATION

A scheme to compensate those who have suffered personal injuries as the result of criminal action has been in existence since 1964. A new scheme for compensation following injuries or death as a result of a crime was established on 1 April 1996 under the Criminal Injuries Compensation Act 1995 based on a statutory scale of awards known as the 'tariff'. This was revised in April 2001 and information is available from the Criminal Injuries Compensation Authority (CICA) headquarters in Glasgow.[16-18]

Claims are processed by the Criminal Injury Compensation Authority (CICA) and claims officers and adjudicators on a panel determine whether a claim can be met. The criminal injury must have been sustained in Great Britain. The assailant does not have to have been convicted of a criminal offence, but the police should have been informed of the incident. There is a discretion to refuse to pay awards where the applicant has unduly delayed in making a claim, failed to cooperate with the police in bringing the assailant to justice, or the applicant's conduct before or after the incident makes it inappropriate that a full or any award should be made, or the applicant's character as shown by his criminal convictions makes it inappropriate for an award to be made. An application must be made within 2 years of the date of the incident giving rise to the injury, though discretion to extend this limit can be exercised where it is reasonable and in the interests of justice to do so.

Payments are made according to a tariff set out in the Scheme. There are 25 levels of compensation: the minimum level 1 is set at £1000 (e.g. blurred vision of eyes lasting 6–13 weeks), level 25 is set at £250 000 (e.g. quadriplegia/tetraplegia or permanent brain damage with no effective control of functions). The death of a viable fetus is set at level 10, £5000. Compensation is paid for loss of earnings as a direct result of the injury after the first 28 weeks of incapacity.

Information relating to the CICA should be available to all NHS staff, who should ensure that, if they are injured at work as a result of a crime, a check is made on their eligibility to receive compensation. It is important that any assaults on staff are reported to the police since information on this would be required by the CICA.

CONCLUSIONS

The Law Commission[19] has recommended that there should be a new law of corporate manslaughter introduced so that senior managers within an organisation can be held criminally liable when persons die as a result of gross negligence by their organisation. The government has still to introduce legislation to implement these proposals. If such legislation were to be enacted then this could have major implications for the functioning of NHS trusts and senior management within them.

QUESTIONS AND EXERCISES

1. The husband of a client attacks a midwife by grabbing her arm. She is contemplating bringing proceedings against him. What is the difference between a civil action and a criminal prosecution in this context? (See also Chs 1 and 13.)

2. A client dies following an unsuccessful caesarean operation. What factors would lead to a prosecution being brought against the staff involved?

3. A community midwife has not insured her car for use in transporting clients. She takes a pregnant woman to hospital in an emergency situation. What are the likely repercussions? (Consider the insurance issues as well as issues of reasonable professional practice.)

4. In what circumstances would a midwife be entitled to receive compensation from the Criminal Injury Compensation Scheme?

References

1 R v. Cox [1993] 2 All ER 19.

2 Shipman Inquiry Third Report. Death and cremation certification, published 14 July 2003. Online. Available: www.the-shipman-inquiry.org.uk/reports.asp

3 R (on the application of Anderson) v. Secretary of State for the Home Department [2002] 4 All ER 1089.

4 R v. Prentice; R. v Adomako; R.v Holloway [1993] 4 All ER 935.

5 R v. Adomako House of Lords. The Times Law Report, 4 July 1994; [1994] 2 All ER 79.

6 R v. Cox. The Times, 22 September 1992; [1992] 12 BMLR 38.

7 Report of the Committee on Mentally Abnormal Offenders (Butler Report) Cmnd 6244 HMSO 1975.

8 News item. R.v Chaha'Oh-Niyol Kai-Whitewind. The Times, 4 May 2005; 4.

9 Woolgar v. Chief Constable of Sussex Police and another [1999] 3 All ER 604 CA.

10 Royal College of Midwives. Position Paper 20: Female genital mutilation (Female circumcision). London: RCM revised 2002 position paper 21 RCM; 1998.

11 British Medical Association. Guidelines on female genital mutilation. London: BMA; 2001.

12 Charter D, Kennedy D. Doctors put on alert for girl butchery. The Times, 21 August 2000.

13 Momoh Comfort. Attitudes to female genital mutilation. Br J Midwifery 2004; 12(10):631–635.

14 Sihwa J, Baron M. Female genital mutilation: cause for concern in the UK. Br J Midwifery 2004; 12(11):717.

15 Richens Y, Creighton S. The question is how many, my lord. Br J Midwifery 2005; 13(4):216.

16 Criminal Injuries Compensation Authority (CICA). Contact: Glasgow (headquarters), Tay House, 300 Bath Street, Glasgow G2 4LN; Tel: 0141 331 2726; Fax: 0141 331 2287.

17 Criminal Injuries Compensation Authority (CICA). Contact: London (headquarters), Morley House, 26–30 Holborn Viaduct, London EC1A 2JQ; Tel: 020 7842 6800; Fax: 020 7436 0804.

18 Criminal Injuries Compensation Scheme. Issue No 1. London: Home Office; 2001.

19 Law Commission Report No 237. Legislating the Criminal Code: Involuntary manslaughter. London: Stationery Office; 1996.

Chapter 19
HEALTH AND SAFETY

This chapter on health and safety is included in the section on accountability since liability for incidents relating to health and safety can lead to hearings in the four main forums which could determine the accountability of the midwife:

1. to the public through the criminal law (see Ch. 18)

2. to the patient/client through the civil law (see Ch. 13)

3. to her employer through the contract of employment (see Ch. 22)

4. to her profession through the NMC fitness to practise proceedings (see Ch. 4).

Box 19.1 shows the areas of law which relate to health and safety.

Box 19.1 Health and safety laws

Employer's duty under the contract of employment

Employee's duty under the contract of employment

Health and Safety at Work Act 1974 and subsequent regulations

Occupier's Liability Acts 1957 and 1984

Consumer Protection Act 1987

Medical Devices Regulations SI 2002 No 618

Control of Substances Hazardous to Health, SI 2002, SI 2002/2677

Reporting of Injuries, Diseases and Dangerous Occurrences Regulations (RIDDOR) 1995/3163

Not all of the areas of law shown in Box 19.1 can be covered in detail here, and the purpose of this chapter is to give the midwife a general understanding of the broad principles which apply so that she can build upon this knowledge with her own research and reading.[1]

The obligations placed by the Acts of Parliament and the common law create similar fields of accountability to those discussed in Chapter 13. This is shown in Box 19.2.[2,3,4]

Box 19.2 Accountability in relation to health and safety

1. Criminal laws

    – Health and Safety at Work Act 1974 and Regulations

    – Offices Shops and Railway Premises Act 1963

    – Factories Act 1961

    – Food Safety Act 1990 and other legislation

    – Environmental Protection Act 1990

    – Medical Devices Regulations SI 2002 No 618

    – Control of Substances Hazardous to Health SI 1999 No 437

2. Civil action

    – Breach of statutory duty

    – Action for negligence

    – Occupier's Liability Act 1957

    – Occupier's Liability Act 1984

    – Consumer Protection Act 1987

3. Employer and contract of employment

    – Laws of contract

    – Statutory Protection provided by the Employment Protection Legislation

    – Rules relating to Employment Tribunals

4. Professional Registration and Codes

– Midwives Rules[2] and Standards[3]

– Code of Professional Conduct: standards for conduct, performance and ethics NMC 2004[4]

CRIMINAL LAWS

The Health and Safety at Work Act 1974 is enforced through the criminal courts by the Health and Safety Inspectorate who have the power to prosecute for offences under the Act and the Regulations and who have also powers of inspection and can issue enforcement or prohibition notices. Since the abolition of the Crown's immunity (by the National Health Service Amendment Act 1986) in relation to the health and safety laws, prosecutions and notices can be brought against the Health Authorities. Trusts do not enjoy any immunity from health and safety legislation.

The basic duty on the employer is set out in Box 19.3.

The Act also places a specific responsibility upon the employee. This is shown in Box 19.4.

Box 19.3 Duty under the Health and Safety at Work Act 1974

Section 2(1) It shall be the duty of every employer to ensure, so far as is reasonably practicable, the health, safety and welfare at work of all his employees.

Section 2(2) of the 1974 Act gives examples of the various duties which must be carried out but these do not detract from the width and comprehensiveness of the general duty.

Box 19.4 Statutory duty of the employee under Section 7 of the Health and Safety at Work Act 1974

1. To take reasonable care for the health and safety of himself and of others who may be affected by his acts or omissions at work.

2. As regards any duty imposed on his employer or any other person, to co-operate with him so far as is reasonable to enable that duty to be performed or complied with.

It is also a criminal offence for an employee to interfere with health and safety measures (Box 19.5).

New regulations came into force on 1 January 1993 as a result of European Directives. These are shown in Box 19.6. Many have subsequently been updated.

Box 19.6 Health and Safety Regulations which came into force on 1 January 1993

1. Management of Health and Safety at Work Regulations 1992 (SI (1992) 2051) (revised 1999 SI 1999 No 3242)

2. Provision and Use of Work Equipment Regulations 1992 (SI (1992) 2932) (revised 1998 SI 1998/2306)

3. Manual Handling Operations Regulations 1992 (SI 1992 2793)

4. Workplace (Health, Safety and Welfare) Regulations 1992 (SI (1992) 3004) (amended by SI 1999/2024)

5. Personal Protective Equipment at Work Regulations 1992 (SI (1992) 2966) (amended by SI 1999/3232)

6. Health and Safety (Display Screen Equipment) Regulations 1992 (SI (1992) 2792)

Box 19.7 shows the areas covered by the Regulations relating to the Management of Health and Safety at Work Act 1999.

The Health and Safety Commission has provided an approved Code of Practice and Guidance along with these Regulations.[5] The legal status of this Code is explained in the introduction:

This Code has been approved by the Health and Safety Commission, with the consent of the Secretary of State. . . If you are prosecuted for breach of health and safety law, and it is proved

Box 19.7 Management of Health and Safety at Work Act Regulations 1999

Regulations cover the following topics:

1 Commencement and interpretation

2 Areas exempt from the rules

3 Risk assessment

4 Principles of prevention to be applied

5 Health and safety arrangements

6 Health surveillance

7 Health and safety assistance

8 Procedures for serious and imminent danger and for danger areas

9 Contacts with external services

10 Information for employees

11 Cooperation and coordination

12 Persons working in host employers' or self-employed persons' undertakings

13 Capabilities and training

14 Employees' duties

15 Temporary workers and other specialist categories

16 Risk assessment in respect of new and expectant mothers

17 Certificate from a registered medical practitioner in respect of new or expectant mothers

18 Notification by new or expectant mothers

19 Protection of young persons

▶

that you did not follow the relevant provisions of the Code, you will need to show that you have complied with the law in some other way or a court will find you at fault. This document also includes other, more general guidance not having this special status . . .

NEW AND EXPECTANT MOTHERS

The new Regulations introduce provisions for the protection of new and expectant mothers and young persons. A 'new and expectant mother' is defined as an employee who is pregnant; who has given birth within the previous 6 months; or who is breastfeeding. Under Regulation 16, employers have a specific duty to carry out an assessment of risk which arises by reason of their condition and if the risk cannot be avoided, then to alter her working conditions or hours of work and if this would not remove the risk, then the employer should suspend the employee as long as is necessary to avoid such a risk.

Regulation 17 states that where a new or expectant mother works at night, and there is a certificate from a registered medical practitioner or registered midwife that she should not work for any period identified in the certificate, then the employer shall suspend her from work as long as it is necessary for her health or safety. The onus is on the woman to notify the employer in writing that she is pregnant (and to provide a certificate of that fact), has given birth within the previous 6 months or is breastfeeding. The suspension would be on full pay.

YOUNG PERSONS

Under Regulation 19, an employer must ensure that any young person employed by him is protected at work from any risks to their health or safety which are a consequence of their lack of experience, or absence of awareness of existing or potential risks, or the fact that young persons have not yet fully matured. In addition, employers are prohibited from employing a young person for work which is beyond his physical or psychological capacity, involves harmful exposure to agents which are toxic, carcinogenic, cause heritable genetic damage or harm the unborn child, or in any other way chronically affect human health; involve harmful exposure to radiation; or where there is a risk to health from extreme cold or heat, noise or vibration.

RISK ASSESSMENT: THE LAW

Not all these regulations can be covered in detail in a book like this, but Regulation 3 on risk assessment is selected to be looked at in detail.

Regulation 3 requires that:

Every employer shall make a suitable and sufficient assessment of

(a) *the risks to the health and safety of his employee to which they are exposed whilst they are at work; and*

(b) *the risks to the health and safety of persons not in his employment arising out of or in connection with the conduct by him of his undertaking,*

for the purpose of identifying the measures he needs to take to comply with the requirements and prohibitions imposed upon him by or under the relevant statutory provisions.

The duty also applies to independent midwives: Regulation 3 Para. (2) requires that:

Every self-employed person . . . make a suitable and sufficient assessment of

(a) *the risks to his own health and safety to which he is exposed while he is at work; and*

(b) *the risks to the health and safety of persons not in his employment arising out of or in connection with the conduct by him of his undertaking,*

for the purposes of identifying the measures he needs to take to comply with the requirements and prohibitions imposed upon him by or under the relevant statutory provisions.

There is a duty under Regulation 3(3) to review the assessment when there is reason to suspect that it is no longer valid or there has been significant change in the matters to which it relates.

Regulation 3(4) requires an employer to make an assessment before employing a young person (a person below 18 years).

RISK ASSESSMENT: THE APPROVED CODE OF PRACTICE (ACOP) AND GUIDANCE

The Approved Code of Practice emphasises that risk assessment must be a systematic general examination of the effect of their undertaking, their work activities and the condition of the premises. There should be a record of the significant findings of that risk assessment.

The definition of risk includes both the likelihood that harm will occur and its severity. The aim of risk assessment is to help the employer or self-employed person to determine what measures should be taken to comply with their statutory obligations laid down under the Health and Safety at Work Act 1974 and its regulations.

Suitable and sufficient is defined in the ACOP as

(a) identifying the risks arising out of work

(b) enabling the employer or the self-employed person to take reasonable steps to help themselves identify risks

(c) being appropriate to the nature of the work and having an identified period for which it is likely to be valid.

HOW IS THE RISK ASSESSMENT TO BE CARRIED OUT?

The ACOP states that there are no fixed rules about how a risk assessment should be carried out, and it will depend upon the nature of the work and the types of hazards and risks. The ACOP sets out some general principles that should be followed and these are summarised in Box 19.8.

Box 19.8 Requirements of valid risk assessment

- Ensure that all relevant risks or hazards are addressed

- Ensure all aspects of the work activity are reviewed

- Take account of non-routine operations

- Take account of the management of incidents

- Be systematic

▶

- Take account of the way in which work is organised

- Take account of risks to the public

- Take account of the need to cover fire risks.

RECORDING

The record should represent an effective statement of hazards and risks which then leads management to take the relevant actions to protect health and safety. It should be in writing unless in computerised form and should be easily retrievable. It should include:

- a record of the preventive and protective measures in place to control risks

- what further action, if any, needs to be taken to reduce risk sufficiently

- proof that a suitable and sufficient assessment has been made.

PREVENTIVE AND PROTECTIVE MEASURES

Schedule 1 of the Regulations specifies the general principles of prevention required by the EEC and in Regulation 4. These include:

- avoiding risks

- evaluating the risks which cannot be avoided

- combating the risks at source

- adapting the work to the individual

- adapting to technical progress

- replacing the dangerous by the non-dangerous or the less dangerous

- developing a coherent overall prevention policy

- giving collective protective measures priority over individual protective measures

- giving appropriate instructions to employees.

How do these regulations relate to the role of the midwife?

For the most part, the midwife would share common health and safety hazards with other hospital or community-based employees and thus models of risk assessment and management which applied to midwifery would also apply to other health professionals. Hazards relating to the safety of equipment, cross-infection risks, safe working practices or violence at work would all apply to midwives, who should be involved in the assessment of risk. The midwife could also apply these same principles of risk assessment to the care of the woman and baby, identifying any particular circumstances which could cause harm and ensuring that reasonable action is taken to prevent such an occurrence. Risk management in midwifery practice is considered by Robina Aslam.[6] It is emphasised that the focus of clinical risk management should not be the reduction of litigation but should be the enhancement of client care. The setting up of a risk management programme in a small, private birth unit is described by Patricia Scott.[7] Among the many benefits resulting from the scheme are:

- early recognition of risk factors

- written care plans

- improved documentation and audit of case notes

- statistics are regularly analysed, e.g. postpartum haemorrhage rates

- study days on CTG traces.

Reference should also be made to the work in clinical risk management of the Clinical Negligence Scheme for Trusts discussed in Chapter 13. The RCM has also published guidance for members on the assessment of risk[8] which looks at the meaning and implications of risk management in relation to midwifery care of pregnant women.

The midwife and violence

Many health professionals, including community midwives, work in fear of violence from strangers in the street as well as abuse from relatives of clients and even clients themselves. If this is a real fear in a particular locality then an assessment should be carried out.

- Is it possible to remove the risk altogether?

  If the answer to this is yes, but only by stopping all home confinements and community visits by midwives, then it could be said not to be a realistic possibility.

- What preventive action or protective measures can be taken?

  The answer to this might include the provision of two-way radios, personal alarms or, in very dangerous areas or on visits to clients who present a threat, midwives going in pairs or accompanied by another person, who may be the police. Are attacks due to the view that midwives carry drugs? Could this be prevented by necessary medication being obtained by the patients on prescription and kept at the home, so that midwives do not have to carry them?

- Review the situation to ascertain if the nature of the risk has changed (e.g. the district is more violent than it was formerly assessed to be) and the extent of the success of the measures taken to prevent harm to midwives. Are any further measures necessary?

This type of analysis will not relate only to community midwives – it could be part of a wider assessment of all community health professionals into which the community midwife could have an input. Clearly, the risk assessment is dependent upon having accurate feedback from employees and others about incidents and threatening situations.

Guidance is available from the Health and Safety Commission.[9] This gives practical advice for reducing the risk of violence in a variety of settings and emphasises the importance of commitment from the highest levels of management. An appendix includes a checklist for home visiting. The RCM has also provided advice on safety in maternity units[10] and for midwives working in the community.[11] Because of the growing concerns about violence to health staff, some general practitioners in Bristol[12] have decided that violent patients will only be attended to in the police station, not in the surgery. It is unlikely that such a rule could apply to midwives attending pregnant women, but in exceptional circumstances, police could be brought into antenatal clinics or onto the wards. The Secretary of State announced in November 2001[13] the publication of new national guidelines on withholding treatment from violent and abusive patients. (This does not apply to patients with severe mental health problems or suffering life-threatening conditions, and is seen as a last resort.) In 2003 the National Audit Office reported that reports of violence against NHS staff had risen by 13% in 2 years, costing the service at least £69 million annually.[14] The report estimated that about 40% of incidents were not being reported. The BMA reported in October 2003 that one in ten doctors is assaulted every year.[15] Those most likely to be assaulted were those working in A&E Departments, in psychiatric services and in General Practice.

The zero tolerance site[16] provides a list of issues which should be included in any local policy. These include:

– a pledge to protect staff at work

– the definition of violence

– details of the employers' legal requirements

– details of managers' and employees' responsibilities

– information on risk assessment measures

– details of local prevention and reduction plans and local emergency procedures

– an explanation of staff training and local reporting procedures.

Examples are given of successful prosecutions brought against individuals assaulting NHS staff.

In June 2004, the Court ordered the banning of a man from every hospital and doctor's surgery in England and Wales.[17] Norman Hutchins was prohibited from entering or making contact with any NHS or private medical centre. He was also barred from seeking medical clothing or equipment. He had been accused of upsetting staff on 47 occasions since November 2003 in his endeavours to obtain medical clothing and equipment. The South West London and St George's Mental Health NHS Trust was fined £28 000 and ordered to pay £14 000 prosecution costs for systematic failures which led to a nurse being battered to death by a patient at Springfield Hospital.[18]

The NHS Security Management Service (NHS SMS) launched a poster campaign to explain how staff can protect themselves against violence in the NHS. The Government zero tolerance campaign against violence is reviewed by Maggie Rew and Terry Ferns.[19] The Health and Safety Executive commenced in 2000 a 3-year programme to help employers tackle work-related violence and further details of its work are available on its website.[20]

Domestic violence against pregnant women

Concern is growing at the numbers of pregnant women who are subjected to domestic violence.[21] Midwives may be told of the violence in confidence. However, reporting such information may be a justifiable exception to the duty of confidentiality, since it would be in the public interest (see Ch. 10) to ensure that a woman with learning disabilities and children at risk received protection. The Home Office published a consultation paper[22] in June 2003 on ways to prevent and follow-up domestic violence. It looked at three areas: prevention, protection and justice and support for victims. The Domestic Violence, Crime and Victims Act 2004 Part 1 covers the topics shown below:

- Breach of non-molestation order to be a criminal offence
- Additional considerations if parties are cohabitants or former cohabitants
- Cohabitants in Part 4 of the Family Law Act 1996 to include same-sex couples
- Extension of Part 4 of the Family Law Act 1996 to non-cohabiting couples
- Causing or allowing the death of a child or vulnerable adult to be an offence
- Establishment and conduct of domestic homicide reviews.

Under Part 2 of the Act common assault becomes an arrestable offence for the purposes of the Police and Criminal Evidence Act 1984, thereby increasing the powers of the police and citizens in relation to such an offence.

The provisions under Part 3 of the Act relating to victims should also benefit those suffering from domestic violence. A Victim's Code of Practice is to be issued by the Secretary of State to cover the services to be provided to a victim of criminal conduct. Failure to comply with the Code, while not an offence in itself, could be used in evidence in civil and criminal proceedings.

Midwives can play a significant role in the detection and support of women who are exposed to domestic violence[23,24] and midwives should have access to a local policy on domestic violence and good links with any local organisation aimed at protecting partners and children against such violence. A study by the University of the West of England has introduced and evaluated the introduction of the Bristol Pregnancy and Domestic Violence Programme in the North Bristol NHS trust, which was aimed at equipping community midwives with the knowledge and confidence to enquire effectively about their clients' experiences of domestic violence.[25] Sally Price and others have evaluated the training provided in Bristol for midwives to make routine enquiries at antenatal clinics.[26] The prevalence and nature of domestic abuse in an early pregnancy unit was explored in another study[27] which concluded that there was a significant association between the age of the woman and the prevalence of domestic abuse and the majority of women felt that questions about possible abuse were appropriate. Current developments and the necessary training for midwives are reviewed by Jane Morgan.[28]

A domestic violence website has been set up for midwives.[29] Midwives should have the training and confidence to be able to ask women about domestic abuse.[27] A comprehensive book on midwifery practice which includes chapters on domestic violence in pregnancy and the role of the midwife;[30] women's response to screening for domestic violence in a healthcare setting;[31] and addressing domestic violence through maternity services: policy and practice[32] is provided in a volume edited by Wickham.[33] See also Shipway's handbook on domestic violence[34] and Mander's book 'Men and Maternity', which includes a chapter on childbearing and domestic vio-lence.[35] In a survey of the prevalence of domestic violence in pregnancy, Bacchus and colleagues found that routine enquiry for domestic violence increased the rate of detection in maternity settings.[36]

Risk assessment and midwife-managed units
Other assessments of risk could apply to midwifery activity. For example, it may be that the NHS trust is considering setting up a midwife-managed unit. In the planning of this unit it would be necessary to assess which mothers should not be admitted to such a unit but should be delivered with the facilities of a district general hospital. Such an assessment would require the identification of which tests were required during the antenatal stages to identify contraindications. An analysis would then be necessary of those risks in childbirth which could occur and the measures necessary either to prevent them occurring or to reduce their seriousness. Should the unit have storage facilities for blood? What additional procedures should the midwife receive training in, in case certain risks materialised (e.g. resuscitation of the newborn)? Working parties could plan procedures for coping with emergencies and the neces-sary cooperation with paramedical ambulance staff and staff in the operating theatres of nearby general hospitals.[37,38] Reference could also be made to the RCM Stewards Briefings and newsletters prepared by the Royal College of Midwives for health and safety representatives.[39]

Conclusions on risk assessment and management
The emphasis in the guidance from the Health and Safety Commission is on the assessment of significant risks. There is a realism therefore about the Regulations

which may have been lacking in health and safety audits carried out in the past. The midwives are central to the assessment process, since they have first-hand knowledge of the dangers which they face.

MANUAL HANDLING REGULATIONS

Back injuries have been recognised as a major reason for sickness and staff retiring early on grounds of ill health. The Royal College of Midwives has provided guidance on manual handling.[40] The Royal College of Midwives in its handbook[41] for health and safety representatives states that back injury is the commonest single hazard for nurses and midwives:

> Nurses and midwives take almost twice as much sick leave due to back pain as the rest of the working population. 16% of all NHS sickness absence is due to back pain. One out of six nurses or midwives is said to suffer back pain or injury each year, costing an estimated 1.5 million lost working days each year. Nearly half of all working age adults experience some low back pain in any 6-week period.

The handbook also quotes a Health and Safety Executive survey in 1982 which showed that 25% of midwives had at one time been off sick from work because of back injury, and this is about the average figure for nurses, midwives and health visitors generally. The handbook points out that community midwives are more likely to have sustained a back injury.

> There is also some evidence to suggest that back injury is even more likely among part-time, bank or agency staff, maybe because they may be older ... Risk also correlates with length of service, partly because back troubles can accumulate. The longer in midwifery, the greater the chances of back injury.

Regulations have been enacted under the Health and Safety Act 1974 and are published with guidance by the Health and Safety Executive.[42] The guidelines are not themselves the law and the booklet advises that the guidelines set out in Appendix 1 'should not be regarded as precise recommendations. They should be applied with caution. Where doubt remains, a more detailed assessment should be made'.

A Working Group set up by the Health and Safety Commission has produced a booklet of guidance on manual handling of loads in the health services.[43] This document is described as 'an authoritative document which will be used by health and safety inspectors in describing reliable and fully acceptable methods of achieving health and safety in the workplace'. Part of this health services specific guidance material relates to staff working in the community.

CONTENT OF THE REGULATIONS

The duty under the regulations can be summed up as follows:

– If possible, avoid the hazardous manual handling.

– Make a suitable and sufficient assessment of any hazardous manual handling which cannot be avoided.

– Reduce the risk of injury from this handling so far as is reasonably practicable.

– Provide information about the load and centre of weight.

– Review the assessment.

Avoiding the risk

Regulation 4(1) Each employer shall:

(a) so far as is reasonably practicable, avoid the need for his employees to undertake any manual handling operations at work which involve a risk of their being injured.

The guidance asks the question, as an example of this, 'Can a treatment be brought to a patient rather than taking the patient to the treatment?' It may be that in the case of midwifery, it would be very difficult to remove the risk of injury entirely without reducing patient choice to unacceptable levels. For example, water births or births in alternative positions may be considered to cause unacceptable risks to the health of the midwife. In such situations, it is necessary to balance the risk of harm against the freedom of choice for the mother.

Carrying out the assessment

Regulation 4(1) Each employer shall:

(b) where it is not reasonably practicable to avoid the need for his employees to undertake any manual handling operations at work which involve a risk of their being injured –

   (i) make a suitable and sufficient assessment of all such manual handling operations to be undertaken by them, having regard to the factors which are specified in column 1 of Schedule 1 to these Regulations and considering the questions which are specified in the corresponding entry in column 2 of that Schedule.

Schedule 1 is set out as shown in Box 19.9.

Application of the schedule to midwifery

The Royal College of Midwives has identified the following areas as particularly relevant to midwives:

Box 19.9 Schedule 1 of Manual Handling Regulations 1992

Factors to which the employer must have regard and questions he must consider when making an assessment of manual handling operations.

Questions	Factors
1. The tasks	e.g. do they involve holding or manipulating loads at a distance from trunk, etc.?
2. The loads	e.g. are they heavy, bulky or unwieldy, etc.?
3. The working environment	e.g. are there space constraints preventing good posture, uneven, slippery or unstable floors, etc.?
4. Individual capability	Does the job require unusual strength, height, etc.?
5. Other factors	Is movement or posture hindered by personal protective equipment or by clothing?

- helping clients to breastfeed
- delivery, particularly in water births and alternative positions
- clients with epidurals
- clients who have had lower segment caesarean sections
- baby bathing
- transfer between ward or theatre
- handicapped mothers
- lifting of equipment, in hospital, home or car.

The assessment should take into account the mother's choice of place of confinement. It may be for example that following an assessment, the mother is advised that the accommodation is unsuitable to ensure the health and safety of the mother and baby and also of the midwife during the confinement.

Management checklist

Appendix 2 of the Regulations gives an example of an assessment checklist: Section A covering the preliminary stages, Section B the more detailed assessment where necessary and Section C identifying the remedial action which should be taken.

Taking appropriate steps to reduce the risk
Regulation 4(1)

Each employer shall

(b) where it is not reasonably practicable to avoid the need for his employees to undertake any manual handling operations at work which involve a risk of their being injured

   (ii) take appropriate steps to reduce the risk of injury to those employees arising out of their undertaking any such manual handling operations to the lowest level reasonably practicable.

For example, in carrying out the assessment of risk and deciding how to minimise the risk, it might be concluded that hoists should be installed. This may include the possibility of installing a hoist for a domiciliary confinement, even though temporarily.

Employer's duty to inform employees, so far as is reasonably practicable, about the weight
Regulation 4(1)(b)(iii) requires the employer to provide the employee with information about the weight of each load and the heaviest side of any load whose centre of gravity is not positioned centrally.

Review
Regulation 4(2) requires the employer to review the assessment

(a) if there is reason to suspect that it is no longer valid; or

(b) if there has been a significant change in the manual handling operations to which it relates

and where as a result of any such review changes to an assessment are required, the relevant employer shall make them.

It is in the interests of all midwives in whatever capacity they are employed and whatever their hours per week to ensure that the employer is reminded when a review becomes necessary under the above provisions.

Agency and bank midwives and independent midwives
The duty which is owed by the employer is owed not only to employees but also to temporary staff such as agency or bank midwives who are called in to assist. All such employees are entitled to be included in the risk assessment process, since as has been seen, the assessment must take into account the individual characteristics of each employee.

Midwives who are unusually small in height or not so strong as the average might require special provisions in relation to manual handling. Independent midwives are not employees and as self-employed persons would be responsible for carrying out the assessments and taking the necessary precautions for themselves and any staff whom they employ. Where they work alongside employed midwives in maternity delivery units, they should ensure that the NHS trust takes into account hazards to their health and safety and that the agreement which they have with the NHS trust reflects this duty.

What action can be taken if the employer ignores these regulations?

The Regulations are part of the health and safety provisions which form part of the criminal law. Infringement of the Regulations can lead to prosecution by the Health and Safety Inspectorate. The Inspectorate has the power to issue enforcement or prohibition notices against any corporate body or individual.

A Health Authority no longer enjoys the immunity from the criminal sanctions which it once did as a Crown Authority and therefore these enforcement provisions are available against it. Similarly, an NHS trust and its employees are subject to the full force of the criminal law.

What remedies exist for compensation?

Section 47 of the Health and Safety at Work Act 1974 prevents breach of a duty under ss. 2–8 of the Act being used as the basis for a claim in the civil courts. Breach of the Regulations can however be the basis of a civil claim for compensation unless the Regulations provide to the contrary. Even where what is alleged is a breach of the basic duties, a midwife who suffered harm, as a result of the failure of the employer to take reasonable steps to safeguard her health and safety, could sue in the civil courts on the basis of the employer's duty at common law.

Employer's duty at common law and manual handling

The statutory duty to ensure the Act is implemented is paralleled by a duty at common law placed upon the employer to take reasonable steps to ensure the employee's health and safety. Contracts of employment should state clearly the duty upon the employer to take reasonable care of the employee's safety and also the employee's duty to cooperate with the employer in carrying out health and safety duties under the Act and at common law. It is of course in the long-term interest of the employer to prevent back injuries, thereby avoiding payment of substantial compensation to his injured employees and also reducing the incidence of sickness and absenteeism. Considerable sums of compensation have been awarded by the civil courts in recent years in situations where the employer is in breach of the duty to take reasonable care of the health and safety of the employee in manual handling.

Wiles v. Bedfordshire CC[44]

The County Court held that there was a breach of the Manual Handling Regulations 1992 Regulation 4.1(a) when W, a residential social worker, sustained an injury when taking M, a disabled girl, to the lavatory. W lifted the girl out of her wheelchair, propping her against the wall while she bent down to remove her underclothes but the girl, whose upper limbs were prone to occasional involuntary spasms, threw out her hands and fell backwards onto W, who suffered a back injury. W claimed that two persons should have carried out that activity. Following the incident, staff were instructed to use a hoist and two staff when taking M to the lavatory. The judge held that even though at the precise time, W was not actually carrying out a manual handling operation, the whole task of taking M to the lavatory should be considered a manual handling operation. The employers were in breach of the Regulations by failing to avoid the need for manual handling and for failing to carry out a proper assessment or taking steps to reduce the risk of injury.

Training
This is essential to ensure that staff have the understanding to carry out the assessments and to advise on lifting and the appropriate equipment. Regular monitoring should take place to ensure that the training is effective and the policies for ensuring the safety of midwives are being implemented.

Record keeping
The guidance emphasises the importance of recording significant findings of the assessment and that the record should be kept, readily accessible, as long as it remains relevant. In addition, the Royal College of Midwives has emphasised the importance of the HA (or NHS trust) keeping adequate statistics. It recommends that the following are kept:

– numbers and incident rate of injuries

– type of injuries

– handling methods involved

– numbers of staff involved

– age and training of the injured parties

– location and time of the accident

– the cause of the accident

– the related costs, e.g. time lost.

There is a statutory duty under Health and Safety Regulations for certain accidents to be notified to the appropriate authority, usually the Health and Safety Inspectorate.

In keeping records of accidents at work, the principles set out in the guidance by the NMC[45] should be followed.

It is in the interest of every practising midwife to ensure that the regulations on manual handling are implemented comprehensively. It should be the aim of every midwife to ensure that the level of injuries is reduced. She, her employer, her colleagues and her clients stand to gain.

Lifting Operations and Lifting Equipment Regulations 1998 (LOLER 1998)[46]

These regulations came into force for all lifting equipment on 5 December 1998, as a result of the lifting provisions of the Amending Directive to the Use of Work Equipment Directive (AUWED 95/63/EC). They are to be read in conjunction with the Provision and Use of Work Equipment Regulations 1998 (PUWER).[47] Further information on these Regulations can be found in Dimond (2004).[1]

In August 2003, the Health and Safety Executive published a manual handling assessment chart (MAC) and also set up a website[48] which can be used by employers, employees, safety representatives and others to obtain information about Musculoskeletal Disorders (MSD), case studies, guidance and research on MSD.

Manual handling and human rights (A and B against East Sussex County Council[49])

In a manual handling case in East Sussex, two severely disabled women claimed that they had a human right not to be manually handled. The judge accepted that both A and B and also their carers had rights under Article 8 of the European Convention on Human Rights to dignity. He stated it was highly questionable to state that manual handling is dignified whereas mechanical handling is undignified and said that:

one must guard against jumping too readily to the conclusion that manual handling is necessarily more dignified than the use of equipment . . . Hoisting is not inherently undignified, let alone inherently inhuman or degrading. I agree . . . that certain forms of manual lift, for example the drag lift, may in certain circumstances be less dignified than hoisting. Hoisting can facilitate dignity, comfort, safety and independence. It all depends on the context.

The judge went on to consider a framework for decision making, setting out the principles which should apply and considering the factors which should be taken into account in determining how to assess reasonable practicability. These factors included:

– The possible methods

– The context

– The risks to the employee

– The impact upon the disabled person which would necessitate an analysis of her physical and mental personality; their wishes and feelings; effect upon the person's dignity and rights.

Following this assessment, there then had to be a balancing exercise between the assessment of the carer and of the disabled person. Once the balance has been struck, if it comes down in favour of manual handling, then the employer must make appropriate assessments and take all appropriate steps to minimise the risks that exist. The assessment must be properly documented and lead to clear protocols which cover *all* situations, including foreseeable emergencies and, in the case of patients such as A and B, events such as spasm and distress which might arise. The outcome of the case was that the judge required East Sussex to carry out the necessary assessments for each activity for A and B, taking into account the considerations and factors which he had set out.

Only reasonable precautions need be taken to prevent risk of injury from manual handling

The Court of Appeal[50] found against an ambulance man who had been injured while carrying a heavy man in a chairlift down stairs. It held that the employers were not in breach of the directive or regulations on manual handling. There was nothing to suggest that calling the fire brigade would have been appropriate in the case. The ambulance service owed the same duty of care to its employees as did any other employer. However, the question of what was reasonable for it to do might have to be judged in the light of its duties to the public and the resources available to it when performing those duties.

MEDICAL DEVICES REGULATIONS 1994 (REVISED 2002)

The Medical Devices Agency (MDA) was established in September 1994 to promote the safe and effective use of devices. In particular, its role is to ensure that whenever a medical device is used, it is:

- suitable for its intended purpose

- properly understood by the professional user, and

- maintained in a safe and reliable condition.

In April 2003 the MDA, together with the Medicines Control Agency, were incorporated into the Medicines and Healthcare Products Regulatory Agency.

What is a medical device?

The definition used by the MDA is based upon the European Directive definition.[51]

Any instrument, apparatus, material or other article, whether used alone or in combination, including the software necessary for its proper application, intended by the manufacturer to be used for human beings for the purpose of:

- diagnosis, prevention, monitoring, treatment or alleviation of disease

- diagnosis, monitoring, treatment, alleviation of or compensation for an injury or handicap

– investigation, replacement or modification of the anatomy or of a physiological process

– control of contraception

and which does not achieve its principal intended action in or on the human body by pharmacological, immunological or metabolic means, but which may be assisted in its function by such means.

Annex B to Safety Notice 9801 from the MDA gives examples of medical devices. It covers the following:

– equipment used in the diagnosis or treatment of disease, monitoring of patients, e.g. syringes and needles, dressings, catheters, beds, mattresses and covers and other equipment

– equipment used in life support, e.g. ventilators, defibrillators

– *in vitro* diagnostic medical devices and their accessories, e.g. blood gas analysers

– equipment used in the care of disabled people, e.g. orthotic and prosthetic appliances, wheelchairs and special support seating, patient hoists, walking aids, pressure sore prevention equipment

– aids to daily living, e.g. commodes, hearing aids, urine drainage systems, domiciliary oxygen therapy systems, incontinence pads, prescribable footwear

– equipment used by ambulance services (but not the vehicles themselves), e.g. stretchers and trolleys, resuscitators.

Other examples of medical devices include condoms, contact lenses and care products, intrauterine devices.

From these examples, it can be seen that almost all the equipment which a midwife would use during the care of a pregnant woman would come under the definition of a medical device.

Regulations[52] require that from 14 June 1998 all medical devices placed on the market (made available for use or distribution even if no charge is made) must conform to 'the essential requirements' including safety required by law, and bear a CE marking as a sign of that conformity. Although most of the obligations contained in the Regulations fall on manufacturers, purchasers who are positioned further down the supply chain may also be liable, for example, 'for supplying equipment which does not bear a CE marking or which carries a marking liable to mislead people'.[53] This is the requirement of the EC Directive on medical devices.[54] The manufacturer who can demonstrate conformity with the Regulations is entitled to apply the CE marking to a medical device.

The essential requirements include the general principle that, 'A device must not harm patients or users, and any risks must be outweighed by benefits'. Design and construction must be inherently safe, and if there are residual risks, users must be informed about them. Devices must perform as claimed, and not fail due to the stresses of normal use. Transport and storage must not have adverse effects. Essential requirements also include prerequisites in relation to the design and construction, infection and microbial contamination, mechanical construction, measuring devices, exposure to radiation, built-in computer systems, electrical and electronic design, mechanical design, devices which deliver fluids to a patient, and the function of controls and indicators.

In January 1998, the MDA issued a device bulletin[55] giving guidance to organisations on implementing the regulations. The MDA has powers under the Consumer Protection Act 1987 to issue warnings or remove devices from the market.

Devices are divided into three classes according to possible hazards, class 2 being further subdivided. Thus class 1 with a low risk, e.g. a bandage; class 2a medium risk, e.g. a simple breast pump; class 2b medium risk, e.g. a ventilator; class 3 high risk, e.g. an intraortic balloon.

Any warning about equipment issued by the MDA should be acted upon immediately. Notices from the Agency are sent to Regional General Managers, Chief Executives of HAs and NHS trusts, directors of social services, managers of independent health-care units and rehabilitation service managers. Failure to ensure that these notices are obtained and acted upon could be used as evidence of failure to provide a reasonable standard of care.

Adverse incident reporting procedures
In 1998 the MDA issued a safety notice[52] requiring healthcare managers, healthcare and social care professionals and other users of medical devices to establish a system to encourage the prompt reporting of adverse incidents relating to medical devices to the MDA. The procedures should be regularly reviewed, updated as necessary, and should ensure that adverse incident reports are submitted to MDA in accordance with the notice.

REPORTING OF INJURIES, DISEASES AND DANGEROUS OCCURRENCES REGULATIONS 1995 (RIDDOR 1995)

Regulations were introduced in 1985 to govern the reporting of injuries, diseases and dangerous occurrences. They were replaced by new Regulations (dated 1995), which came into force on 1 April 1996. There is now one set of regulations in place of the four sets under the 1985 Regulations. The list of reportable diseases has been updated, as has the list of dangerous occurrences. It will be legally possible for reports to be made by telephone. A pilot scheme was tested out in Scotland.

Following the successful HSE pilot scheme in Scotland, in February 2000 it was announced that funding was to be made available to the HSE to set up a centralised national workplace accident and incident reporting system instead of the 500 different addresses which have to be used at present. Reports can be made in the following ways:

– By phone: 0845 300 9923

– By Fax: 0845 300 9924

– By internet: www.riddor.gov.uk

– By e-mail: riddor@natbrit.com

– By post: Incident Contact Centre: Caerphilly Business Park, Caerphilly CF83 3GG.

National Patient Safety Agency

In April 2001 the Department of Health published its proposals for establishing a National Patient Safety Agency (NPSA) which would run the mandatory reporting system for logging all failures, mistakes, errors and near misses across the health services. The Department of Health's publication, 'Building a Safer NHS for Patients', sets out details of the scheme together with recommendations for an improved system for handling investigations and inquiries across the NHS. The NPSA is an independent body which has the following statutory functions:

– Collecting and analysing information on adverse events from local NHS organisations, NHS staff and patients and carers

– Assimilating other safety-related information from a variety of existing reporting systems and other sources in this country and abroad

– Learning lessons and ensuring that they are fed back into practice, service organisation and delivery

– Producing solutions to prevent harm where risks are identified, and setting out national goals and establishing ways of tracking progress towards these goals.

The aim of this new national reporting system is to ensure that adverse events, including specified near misses, will be identified, recorded, analysed, reported, and lessons learnt will be shared to effect change at local and national levels.

The NPSA coordinates its work with other reporting systems (e.g. RIDDOR and Medicines and Healthcare Products Regulatory Agency) on adverse reactions to medicines.

The first patient alert from the NPSA was on the risks associated with the administration of potassium chloride concentrate solutions. Subsequent alerts include a standardisation for crash call numbers to 2222; risks associated with oral methotrexate and steps to ensure that surgery was on the correct site. An alert in February 2005 related to the misplacing of nasal gastric tubes.[56] It was aware of 11 deaths and one case of serious harm as a result of misplacement. Further information on this and all the other alerts, its other work and copies of the NPSA annual reports can be obtained from its website.[57]

On 1 October 2003, the NPSA appointed a midwife to its team to advise on improving patient safety in midwifery. The appointment is a combined post with the Royal College of Midwives. Isobelle Madden and Frank Milligan apply the concept of patient safety incidents and near miss events to maternity care and show how an enhanced focus on patient safety led to significant improvements in maternity care.[58]

CONTROL OF SUBSTANCES HAZARDOUS TO HEALTH (COSHH)

All health workers have responsibilities under the Regulations Relating to the Control of Substances Hazardous to Health. The Regulations were first introduced in 1988 but have subsequently been updated, the current regulations dating from 2002.[59]

Where the Regulations have not been followed, there can be a prosecution in the criminal courts against the offender. In addition, any person who has been injured as a result of a failure to ensure reasonable care was taken by the employer would have a right of civil action to claim compensation. The HSE[60] has issued guidance on the implementation of the new regulations providing both a 'COSHH in a hurry publication', as well as more detailed guidance on preventing or controlling exposure to hazardous substances at work. The HSE guidance covers: the current legal base, legal developments, key message, the hazardous substances covered by COSHH, the COSHH requirements, assessing risk, preventing or controlling exposure, ensuring that control measures are used and maintained, monitoring exposure, health surveillance, planning for accidents, incidents and emergencies and ensuring that employees are properly informed, trained and supervised. It recommends an eight-stage assessment. These eight stages are shown in Box 19.10.

Box 19.10 Guidance in carrying out an 8-step COSHH assessment

1. Work out what hazardous substances are used in your workplace and find out the risks from using these substances to people's health.

2. Decide what precautions are needed before starting work with hazardous substances.

3. Prevent people being exposed to hazardous substances, but where this is not reasonably practicable, control the exposure.

4. Make sure control measures are used and maintained properly and that safety procedures are followed.

▶

▶

5. If required, monitor exposure of employees to hazardous substances.

6. Carry out health surveillance where your assessment has shown that this is necessary or where COSHH makes specific requirements.

7. If required, prepare plans and procedures to deal with accidents, incidents and emergencies.

8. Make sure employees are properly informed, trained and supervised.

CIVIL LAW

BREACH OF STATUTORY DUTY

The injured person can bring a civil claim for breach of the statutory duty in certain cases. However, breach of the general duties under the Health and Safety at Work Act 1974 does not give rise to a civil action of breach of statutory duty, but breach of the Regulations may give rise to such an action (see above).

ACTION FOR NEGLIGENCE

The person injured is more likely to bring a claim under the law of negligence (see Ch. 13) by establishing that a duty of care which is owed has been breached and that as a reasonably foreseeable consequence, harm has been caused. Where an employee has been injured by alleged failures of the employer, the employee can sue for breach of contract of an implied term in the contract of employment (see below).

OCCUPIER'S LIABILITY ACTS 1957 AND 1984

These Acts are enforceable in the civil courts where harm has occurred to a visitor (1957 Act) or to a trespasser (1984 Act). Under the 1957 Act, the duty of care owed by the occupier (of whom there may be several) is what is reasonable in the circumstances to ensure that the visitor will be safe for the purposes for which he is permitted to be on the premises. Extra care is required of the occupier when a child is the visitor.

CONSUMER PROTECTION ACT 1987

This enables a claim to be brought where harm has occurred as a result of a defect in a product. It is a form of strict liability in that negligence by the supplier or manufacturer does not have to be established. The claimant will however have to show that there was a defect. The supplier can rely upon a defence colloquially known as 'state of the art', i.e. that the state of scientific and technical knowledge at the time the goods were supplied was not such that the producer of products of that kind might be expected to have discovered the defect.

There have been few examples of actions being brought under the Consumer Protection Act 1987 in healthcare cases. One reported in March 1993[61] led to Simon Garratt being awarded £1400 against the manufacturers of a pair of surgical scissors which broke during an operation on his knee, with the blade being left embedded. A second operation was required to remove it. Had he relied upon the law of negligence to obtain compensation he would have had to show that the manufacturers were in breach of the duty of care which they owed to him. Under the Consumer Protection Act 1987, he had to show the harm, the defect and the fact that the equipment was produced by the defendant.

The Consumer Protection Act 1987 is significant for the midwife in that she should ensure that she keeps records of the supplier of any goods (both equipment and drugs) which she provides for the client. If she is unable to cite the name and address of the supplier, she, or her employer, may become the supplier of the goods for the purposes of the Consumer Protection Act 1987 and therefore have to defend an action alleging that there was a defect in the goods which caused harm. Harm includes both personal injury and death, and loss or damage of property.

In a recent case,[62] it was held that patients who had contracted hepatitis C from blood and blood products used in blood transfusions were able to bring a claim under the Consumer Protection Act 1987. This decision may well lead to greater use of the Consumer Protection Act 1987, where personal injuries are caused as a result of defective products, since negligence does not have to be established under the Consumer Protection Act 1987, only that there was a defect in the product which has caused the harm.

The Blood Safety and Quality regulations[63] introduce new safety and quality requirements on human blood collection and storage, thereby implementing an EC Directive.[64]

EMPLOYER AND CONTRACT OF EMPLOYMENT

Under the contract of employment, both employer and employee have duties in relation to health and safety. It is the employer's duty to take reasonable care for the health and safety of the employee. It is the employee's duty to obey reasonable orders (which could include instructions in relation to health and safety) and to act with reasonable care and skill. These duties are enforced on the employer's part by disciplinary procedures and ultimately dismissal and on the employee's part by an action for breach of contract or an allegation of constructive dismissal which, if the employee has the requisite length of continuous service, may result in a hearing before an employment tribunal.

Under the contract of employment, the employee must obey the express terms on the contract of employment. In addition, there are implied terms binding on the employee and employer.

The employee:

– must obey the reasonable instructions of the employer

– must act with all reasonable care and skill in the performance of his duties

– must respect confidential information obtained during the course of employment.

The employer must take all reasonable care for the employee's safety in:

– employing competent staff

– ensuring a safe system of work

– providing safe plant, premises and equipment.

Failure on the employer's part could lead to an action for constructive dismissal, breach of contract or an action for negligence if harm occurs.

Stress
An example of the employer's duty under the contract to take reasonable care of the employee's health and safety is the legal situation relating to stress. The following facts would have to be proved by the employee:

– The employee is under considerable pressure which is causing unacceptable stress

– The employer is aware of that fact

– There is reasonable action which the employer could take but has failed to take

– As a reasonably foreseeable result of the employer's failure,

– the employee has suffered severe mental illness.

The case in Box 19.11[65] illustrates these factors.

In a more recent case it was reported[66] that a former social worker was awarded £140 000 after stress forced her to give up her job as head of a care home. It was

Box 19.11 Walker v. Northumberland County Council[65]

A social worker obtained compensation when his employer failed to provide the necessary support in a stressful work situation when he returned to work following an earlier absence due to stress. The employer was not liable for the initial absence, but that put the employer on notice that the employee was vulnerable and its failure to provide the assistance he needed was a breach of its duty to provide reasonable care for his health and safety as required under the contract of employment.

alleged that Worcestershire County Council had refused to accept that she was unqualified for the position and unable to cope. In contrast, a case brought by a teacher of children with special educational needs, claiming compensation for stress and psychiatric injury, failed on the grounds that the court held that she had not provided any evidence that the head teacher was aware that she was likely to suffer any psychiatric injury as a result of her employment. Breach of the duty of care had not been established.[67]

The Court of Appeal[68] recently overruled three decisions where awards ranging from £7000 to £101 041 had been made on grounds of stress. The Court of Appeal stated that where an employee is bringing a claim against the employer for breach of its contractual duty to take reasonable care of the health and safety of the employee, the employee had to show that it was reasonably foreseeable to the employer that the employee was suffering from stress which was work related, and that it was reasonable for the employer to take action, and that the employer's failure to take action had caused the harm. The employer was entitled to assume that the employee could withstand the normal pressures of the job unless he knew of some particular problem or vulnerability. Relevant factors could include the nature and extent of the work done by the employee and the signs from the employee of impending harm to health. The size and scope of the employer's operation were relevant, including the redistribution of duties to other employees and the need to treat them fairly. The Court of Appeal also stated that an employer who offered a confidential counselling or treatment service was unlikely to be in breach of duty. The assessment of compensation would take account of any pre-existing disorder or vulnerability.

One of the claimants succeeded in an appeal before the House of Lords which overruled the Court of Appeal decision.[69]

Mr Barber, the head of the Maths Department at East Bridgwater Community School, was involved in a restructuring of staffing at the school following which he became 'mathematical area of experience co-ordinator' and in order to maintain his salary level he had also taken on the post of project manager for public and media relations. In order to discharge all his responsibilities he was working between 61 and 70 hours/

week. Stress took its toll and in the summer term of 1996 he was off sick for 3 weeks with sick notes showing 'overstressed/depression' and 'stress'. On his return to work, he had filled in the council's form of sickness declaration stating his troubles as 'overstressed/depression'. He initiated a meeting with the headmistress, but found that she treated him unsympathetically by telling him that all the staff were under stress. Similarly, meetings with the two deputy heads, though more sympathetic, resulted in no steps being taken to improve or consider the situation beyond urging him to prioritise his work. In the autumn, he found himself with the same or even possibly a slightly heavier workload. In November, he lost control of himself and found himself shaking a pupil. He left school that day and never returned. Since then he had been unable to work as a teacher or do any work other than undemanding part-time work. He took early retirement in March 1997, aged 52 years.

The House of Lords held that the guidance issued by the Court of Appeal that unless the employer knows of some particular problem or vulnerability, he is usually entitled to assume that his employee is up to the normal pressures of the job, was only guidance and not a rule of law. Every case had to be decided on its own facts. The House of Lords quoted the principle established in an earlier case (Stokes v. Guest 1968[70]):

> The overall test is still the conduct of the reasonable and prudent employer taking positive thought for the safety of his workers in the light of what he knows or ought to know.

The House of Lords held (in a majority decision) that on the facts there it had not been a flagrant breach of duty by the employer, but nor was it an obviously hopeless claim. It decided that there was insufficient reason for the Court of Appeal to set aside the decision of the High Court. At the very least, the school's senior management team should have taken the initiative in making sympathetic inquiries about him when he returned to work in June 1996 and in making some reduction to his workload to ease his return. Even a small reduction in workload, coupled with the feeling that the team was on his side, might have made a difference. In any event, his condition should have been monitored and if it did not improve some more drastic action should have been taken.

The Barber case was followed in a case where a teacher claimed compensation for a severe clinical depression on two occasions as a result of pressures at work.[71] The court held that her two bouts of depression were not caused by any breach of duty on the part of the defendants.

Stress and the midwife

There is evidence that a high proportion of midwives consider that they are stressed in their work. In one study, 78% of midwives in a labour ward reported having insufficient time to perform their duties, causing high degrees of stress.[72] The same authors concluded in another article that poor communications between doctors and midwives also caused stress.[73] Work in a neonatal unit can be particularly stressful, especially in dealing with dying babies.[74] A staffing survey by the RCM in 2004 showed that stress and heavy workloads were the first and second most important reason given for recruitment and retention problems.[75]

If a midwife considers that she is suffering from unacceptable stress, then she must ensure that she makes senior management aware of this so that reasonable action can be taken to support her. Conversely, a midwife manager should ensure that she identifies when midwives would appear to be under stress and that reasonable action is taken to support them and that this is documented (see Ch. 24 and the role of the midwife manager). Some trusts have counselling services for staff and similar services are available from the Royal College of Midwives.[76] A useful guide for managers on stress among healthcare professionals is provided in a work edited by Firth-Cozens and Payne (1999).[77]

Bullying

The duty owed by the employer to the employee to take reasonable care of the health and safety of the employee would also include the duty to protect the employee against bullying. In one case, £100 000 was accepted in an out-of-court settlement by a teacher who alleged that he had been bullied by the head teacher and other staff, when he was teaching in a school in Pembrokeshire.[78] The Andrea Adams Trust, a support organisation that helps health service employees, has provided a fact sheet on workplace bullying.[79] Bullying may be associated with racial or other harassment. For example in 2004, a black nurse was awarded £20 000 because she was prevented from looking after a white baby.[80] The employment tribunal held that her employers, the Southampton University Hospitals NHS Trust, was effectively silent and complicit in the racist demands made by the woman (see Ch. 22 for racial and other harassment). An overview of workplace bullying in midwifery departments and how it may be addressed is provided by Ruth Hadikin.[81] She provides an action checklist for targets of workplace bullying. Records are of course essential. In November 2001 it was reported that two senior midwives in Portsmouth were dismissed following allegations of harassment and bullying.[82] Research carried out by Professor Mavis Kirkham shows that bullying and harassment are part of the culture of maternity services in England and Wales.[83] This is supported by research carried out by Leivers (2004).[84] The liabilities of the employer for workplace bullying are considered by the author.[85] Bullying in midwifery is reviewed by Rosemary Mander, who shows its damaging effects on both the midwife victim and the pregnant women.[86]

Smoking

Health and safety duties would include the protection of the employee against working in a dangerous smoke-filled environment. Most hospitals and clinics these days follow a no-smoking policy, only allowing smoking in certain designated (and hopefully well-ventilated) areas. However, a complete ban on smoking by patients can cause difficulties and potential dangers for long-term patients who are addicted, as is discussed in an article by the author.[87] The Government initiated smoking cessation services in Health Action Zones in 1999/2000 following the White Paper 'Smoking Kills', December 1998. There were three key targets: young people, adult smoking and pregnant women. The results of the first monitoring of these services were published in February 2002.[88]

Cross-infection
The problems, dangers and duties which arise from cross-infection are considered in Chapter 29.

PROTECTION OF EMPLOYEE WITH HEALTH AND SAFETY CONCERNS

Changes to the law have boosted the protection of the employee in the event of disputes over health and safety matters. The law provides a right not to suffer detriment in health and safety cases so that an employee who is concerned about a health and safety danger can, if the appropriate procedure is followed, be protected from any victimisation such as dismissal. The criteria for judging the appropriateness of the employee's actions are 'all the circumstances including, in particular, his knowledge and the facilities and advice available to him at the time'. There is also provision for the protection of health and safety representatives carrying out their duties.

A defence is available to the employer if the employee's actions were so negligent that a reasonable employer might have treated him as the employer did.[89]

The Public Interest Disclosure Act 1998 has extended this provision to protect the whistle-blower from victimisation (see Ch. 22).

PROFESSIONAL ACCOUNTABILITY BEFORE THE NMC

The Midwives Rules[2] contain several provisions in relation to health and safety.

Rule 6 on responsibility and sphere of practice emphasises that except in an emergency, she must not provide any care, or undertake any treatment, which she has not been trained to give (see Ch. 5).

Rule 7 limits her role in relation to the administration of medicines and other forms of pain relief (see Ch. 20).

Rule 10 requires her to give her supervisor, the LSA and the Council every reasonable facility to inspect her methods of practice, records, equipment and premises (see Ch. 3).

In addition, the standards and guidance provided by the NMC[90] give further advice on these rules.

The Rules, standards and guidance by the NMC are enforceable through the Fitness to Practise proceedings of the NMC (see Ch. 4).

CONCLUSION

While the areas of accountability and liability have been considered separately it is of course possible that there could be criminal proceedings, civil proceedings, disciplinary proceedings and fitness to practise proceedings resulting from the same health and safety incident, especially where someone has died. Most NHS organisations employ health and safety officers who provide training, guidance and information for employees and can be contacted for updates on health and safety publications. However, it remains the personal and professional responsibility of the individual midwife to ensure that health and safety laws are implemented and that this implementation is regularly monitored. A survey by the Health Foundation, an independent charity, found that health and safety was not considered to be a top priority by NHS chief executives.[91] A lack of commitment from senior management will make the task of the individual midwife in implementing health and safety laws and good practice extremely challenging.

Legal issues relating to cross-infection are considered in Chapter 29.

QUESTIONS AND EXERCISES

1. Following the risk assessment regulations, identify the risks in your practice and consider the action which should be taken to prevent them or reduce them.

2. Your trust wishes to protect clients against the possibility of babies being abducted. Carry out a risk assessment on your unit and decide what action it would be reasonably practicable to take.

3. Look carefully at your working practices over a week and identify any dangers to you in relation to manual handling. What changes, if any, should be made?

4. A colleague asks you for advice because she has been injured by the relative of a client and wants to obtain compensation. What form of legal action may she have?

5. You are aware that a senior midwife has a reputation for bullying junior staff. What action would you take if you were (a) a student midwife, (b) a junior midwife.

References

1 Dimond B. Legal aspects of health and safety. Dinton, Wiltshire: Quay Publications; 2004.
2 Nursing and Midwifery Council. (Midwives) Rules Order of Council 2004, Statutory Instrument 2004 1764.
3 Nurses, Midwives and Health Visitors. (Midwives Amendment) Rules Approval Order, SI 1998 No 2649.

4 Nursing and Midwifery Council. Code of professional conduct: standards for conduct, performance and ethics. NMC; 2004.

5 Health and Safety Commission. Management of health and safety at work: Approved Code of Practice and Guidance. London: HMSO; 2000.

6 Aslam R. Risk management in midwifery practice. Br J Midwifery 1999; 7(1):41–44.

7 Scott P. Setting up a risk management programme in a small, private birth unit. Practising Midwife 1998; 1(10):15–17.

8 Royal College of Midwives. Reassessing risk: a midwifery perspective. London: RCM; 2000.

9 Health and Safety Commission. Violence and aggression to staff in health services. London: HSE Books; 1997.

10 Royal College of Midwives. Safety in maternity units. London: RCM; 2000.

11 Royal College of Midwives. Safety for midwives working in the community. London: RCM; 1996.

12 News report. BBC1 West, 24 July 2001.

13 Department of Health. Violent patients can now be denied NHS treatment. Press release 2001/0509, 2001.

14 National Audit Office. A Safer Place to Work: protecting NHS Hospital and Ambulance Staff from Violence and Aggression. Report of the Comptroller and Auditor General HC 527 Session 2002–2003, 27 March 2003.

15 British Medical Association. Violence at work: the experience of UK doctors. BMA; 2003.

16 NHS Responseline. Contact: 0541 555455 or www.nhs.uk/zerotolerance.

17 Lister S. Court to ban fetishist from health units. The Times, 2 June 2004.

18 News item. The Times, 6 May 2005.

19 Rew M, Ferns T. A balanced approach to dealing with violence and aggression at work. Br J Nurs 2005; 14(4):227–232.

20 The Health and Safety Executive. Online. Available: www.hse.gov.uk

21 Hunt SC, Martin AM. Pregnant women: Violent men. MIDIRS; 2000.

22 Home Office Safety and Justice: the Government's Proposals on Domestic Violence. Home Office; June 2003. Online. Available: http://www.domesticviolence.gov.uk

23 Dimond B. Domestic violence and the midwife: Can you report it? Br J Midwifery 2003; 11(8):557–561.

24 Johnstone J. Domestic violence – midwives can make a difference. MIDIRS Midwifery Digest 2003; 13(3):311–315.

25 Salmon D, Baird K, Price S, et al. An Evaluation of the Bristol Pregnancy and Domestic Violence Programme to promote the introduction of routine antenatal enquiry for domestic violence at North Bristol NHS trust. University of the West of England; March 2004.

26 Price S, Baird K, Salmon D. Asking the question: antenatal domestic violence. Practising Midwife 2005; 8(3):21–25.

27 Keeling J, Birch L. Asking pregnant women about domestic abuse. Br J Midwifery 2004; 12(12):746–749.

28 Morgan J. Tackling domestic violence during pregnancy. Br J Midwifery 2005 13(3):176–181.

29 NHS. Online. Available: www.northbristol.nhs.uk/midwives/domesticviolence

30 Price S, Baird K. Domestic violence in pregnancy. How can midwives make a difference? In: Wickham S, ed. Midwifery: Best Practice 2. Edinburgh: Books for Midwives; 2004:46–49.

31 Webster J, Stratigos SM, Grimes KM. Women's response to screening for domestic violence in a healthcare setting. In: Wickham S, ed. Midwifery: best practice 2. Edinburgh: Books for Midwives; 2004:59–65.

32 Marchant S, Davidson LL, Garcia J, et al. Addressing domestic violence through maternity services: policy and practice. In: Wickham S, ed. Midwifery: best practice 2. Edinburgh: Books for Midwives; 2004:52–58.

33 Wickham S, ed. Midwifery: best practice 2. Edinburgh: Books for Midwives; 2004.

34 Shipway L. Domestic violence: a handbook for health professionals. London: Routledge; 2004.

35 Mander R. Childbearing and domestic violence. In Mander R, ed. Men and maternity. London: Routledge; 2004:118–138.

36 Bacchus L, Mezey G, Bewley S, Haworth A. Prevalence of domestic violence when midwives routinely enquire in pregnancy. MIDIRS Midwifery Digest 2004; 14(3):339–342.

37 Dimond B. Risk management and the midwife. Modern Midwife 1994; 4(4):36–67

38 Dimond B. Midwife managed units. Modern Midwife 1994; 4(6):31–33.

39 Royal College of Midwives. Stewards Briefings, on-going.

40 Royal College of Midwives. Handle with care: a midwife's guide to preventing back injury, 2nd edn. London: RCM; 1999.

41 Royal College of Midwives. Handbook for health and safety representatives. London: RCM; 1992.

42 Health and Safety Executive. Manual handling: Guidance on regulations. London: HMSO; 1992.

43 Health and Safety Commission. Guidance on manual handling of loads in the health services. London: HMSO; 1992.

44 Wiles v. Bedfordshire CC CLR 365 June 2001.

45 NMC. Guidelines for records and record keeping. London: NMC; 2004.

46 Lifting Operations and Lifting Equipment Regulations (LOLER)1998, SI1998/2307.

47 Provision and Use of Work Equipment Regulations (PUWER) 1992, SI 1992/2932, revised 1998, SI 1998/2306.

48 The Health and Safety Executive. Online. Available: www.hse.gov.uk/msd/mac

49 A and B v. East Sussex County Council (The Disability Rights Commission an interested party) [2003] EWHC 167 (Admin).

50 King v. Sussex Ambulance NHS Trust [2002] EWCA 953; Current law, August 2002:408.

51 European Union Directive 93/42/EEC.

52 Medical Devices Agency. SN 9801: reporting adverse incidents relating to medical devices. London: MDA; 1998.

53 SI 1994/3017 Medical Devices Regulations 1994 came into force 1 January 1995, mandatory from 14 June 1998. Directive 93/42/EEC.

54 93/42/EEC Directive concerning medical devices.

55 Medical Devices Agency. DB 9801: Medical device and equipment management for hospital and community based organisations. London: MDA; 1998.

56 National Patient Safety Agency Advice to NHS on reducing harm caused by the misplacement of nasogastric feeding tubes. 22 February 2005.

57 National Patient Safety Agency. Online. Available: www.npsa.org.uk

58 Madden I, Milligan F. Enhancing patient safety and reporting near misses. Br J Midwifery 2004; 12(10):643–647.

59 Control of Substances Hazardous to Health 2002, SI 2002/2677.

60 HSE Preventing or controlling exposure to hazardous substances at work. HSE; 2002. Online. Available: www.hse.gov.uk/hthdir/noframes/coshh/coshh9a.htm; www.hse.gov.uk/coshh/index.htm

61 Dimond B. Protecting the consumer. Nurs Stand 1993; 7(24):18–19.

62 A and others v. National Blood Authority and another. Times Law Report, 4 April 2001; Lloyd's Law Rep Med [2001] 187.

63 Blood Safety and Quality Regulations 2005, SI 2005 No 50.

64 EC Directive 2002/98 [2003] OJL33/30.

65 Walker v. Northumberland County Council. Times Law Report, 24 November 1994 QBD.

66 News item. Care Chief's £140 000 stress award. The Times, 5 September 2001.

67 Salisbury v. Kirklees MBC 21 June 2001. Current Law Digest 392, October 2001.

68 Hatton v. Sutherland, Barber v. Somerset County Council, Jones v. Sandwell Metropolitan Borough Council, Baker v. Baker Refractories Ltd (2002) The Times Law Report, 12 February; [2002] EWCA 76 [2002] 2 All ER 1.

69 Barber v. Somerset County Council 2004. The Times Law Report, 5 April 2004 HL; [2002] EWCA Cuv 76; [2002] 2 All ER 1.

70 Stokes v. Guest, Keen and Nettlefold (Bolts and Nuts) Ltd [1968] 1 WLR 1776.

71 Vahidi v. Fairstead House School Trust LTD [2004] EWHC 2102; [2005] PIQR P9.

72 Mackin P, Sinclair M. Midwives' experience of stress on the labour ward. Br J Midwifery 2004; 7(5):323–326.

73 Mackin P, Sinclair M. Labour ward midwives' perceptions of stress. J Adv Nurs 1998; 27:986–991.

74 Raeside L. Caring for dying babies: perceptions of neonatal nurses. J Neonat Nurs 2000; 6(3):93–99.

75 Royal College of Midwives. Staffing survey 2004. RCM; 2004.

76 RCM. Service always available to members and their families. Contact: Tel 0846 605 0044.

77 Firth-Cozens J, Payne RL, eds. Stress in health professionals: psychological and organisational causes and interventions. Chichester: Wiley; 1999.

78 Fletcher V. Teacher 'bullied by staff' wins £100,000. The Times, 17 July 1998.

79 Andrea Adams Trust. Factsheet on workplace bullying. 2000. Contact: Andrea Adams Trust, Maritime House, Basin Road, North Portslade, Brighton BN41 1WA. Tel/fax: 01273 704 900; e-mail: aat@btinternet.com

80 Purves R. Racist abuse ruined my life. Nursing Times, 10 August 2004; 100(32):24–25.

81 Hadikin R. MIDIRS Midwifery Digest 2001; 11(3):308–311.

82 News item. Practising Midwife 2001; 4(10):6.

83 Kirkham M, ed. Informed choice in maternity care. Basingstoke: Palgrave Macmillan; 2004.

84 Leivers G. Harassment by staff in the workplace: the experiences of midwives. MIDIRS Midwifery Digest 2002; 14(1):19–24.

85 Dimond B. Workplace stress and bullying: liabilities of the employer. Br J Nurs 2002; 11(10):699–710.

86 Mander R. The B-word in Midwifery. MIDIRS Midwifery Digest 2004; 14(3):320–322.

87 Dimond B. Smoking mothers' rights and the maternity department. Modern Midwife 1996; 6(6):10–11.

88 Department of Health. Press release 2002/0075.

89 Trade Union Reform and Employment Rights Act 1993, Para. 3(3), Schedule 5.

90 Nursing and Midwifery Council. Midwives Rules and Standards. August 2004.

91 The Health Foundation. Healthcare Leaders Panel Survey 1: Patient Safety Report and Table of Results. London: The Health Foundation and YouGov; 2004.

Chapter 20
MEDICATION

The midwife has extended powers in relation to the prescribing and administration of medicines compared with the nurse/health visitor practitioner. These powers have been further expanded as midwives are one of the designated practitioners with additional powers of prescribing under changes to the statutory provisions for prescribing. Amendments have been made by s.63 of the Health and Social Care Act 2001 to the Medicines Act 1968, expanding the health practitioners who will be eligible to prescribe following the recommendations of the Final Crown Report[1] (see below). This chapter looks at the specific powers of the midwife in relation to the statutory provisions dealing with medicines and the legal issues which are likely to arise.[2]

The NMC has provided guidance on the administration of medicines[3] in addition to the Standards it has set on the Midwives Rules (see below). All practising midwives should have an up-to-date copy of the British National Formulary (BNF), which is published jointly by the British Medical Association and the Royal Pharmaceutical Society of Great Britain. Updates on the most recent edition of the BNF can be obtained from its website.[4] At the front of the BNF there is a very useful introductory section which gives guidance on prescribing for different categories of drugs and different groups of patients. In addition a directory is published annually on over-the-counter medicinal products.[5] Reference should also be made to the Appendix on Further Reading.

THE STATUTORY FRAMEWORK

The two main Acts of Parliament controlling the administration and use of medicines are the Medicines Act 1968 and the Misuse of Drugs Act 1971.

THE MEDICINES ACT 1968

This Act set up an administrative and licensing system to control the sale and supply of medicines to the public, retail pharmacies and the packing and labelling of medicinal products. It classifies medicines in the categories shown in Box 20.1.

Box 20.1 Classification of medicines under the Medicines Act 1968

1. Pharmacy only products. These can only be sold or supplied retail by someone conducting a retail pharmacy when the product must be sold for a registered pharmacy by, or under the supervision of, a registered pharmacist.

2. General sales list. These are medicinal products which may be sold other than from a retail pharmacy so long as the provisions relating to s.53 of the Medicines Act are complied with. This means that the place of sale must be the premises where the business is carried out; they must be capable of excluding the public; the medicines must have been made up elsewhere and the contents must not have been opened since make-up.

3. Prescription-only list. The medicines are only available on a practitioner's prescription. Schedule I of the Regulations lists the prescription-only products and Part II of the Schedule lists the prescription-only products which are covered by the Misuse of Drugs Act 1971. Special provisions apply to prescriptions in hospitals.

THE MISUSE OF DRUGS ACT 1971

This Act and subsequent legislation makes provision for the classification of Controlled Drugs and their possession, supply and manufacture.

The Act makes it a criminal offence to carry on the manufacture, supply and possession of Controlled Drugs contrary to the Regulations. Controlled drugs are divided into three categories:

Class A includes, among others: cocaine, diamorphine, morphine, opium, pethidine and class B substances when prepared for injection.

Class B includes, among others: oral amphetamines, barbiturates, cannabis, codeine.

Class C includes, among others: most benzodiazepines, meprobamate.

(The classification of cannabis was changed from a class B drug to a class C drug in January 2004.)

THE MISUSE OF DRUGS REGULATIONS 2001[6]

The Misuse of Drugs Regulations 2001 divides Controlled Drugs into 5 Schedules, each specifying the requirements governing activities such as import, export, production, supply, possession, prescribing and record keeping. These schedules are shown in Box 20.2.

Box 20.2 Schedules under the Misuse of Drugs Regulations 2001

Schedule 1, e.g. cannabis, lysergide. Possession and supply prohibited except in accordance with Home Office authority given in a licence. They cannot be used for medicinal purposes and their production and possession is limited to research or other specified purposes. Rules cover the documentation, keeping of records, preservation of records, supply on prescription, marking of containers and procedure for destruction.

Schedule 2, e.g. diamorphine, morphine, pethidine, glutethimide, amphetamine – are subject to full Controlled Drug requirements relating to prescriptions, safe custody, the need to keep registers. These drugs may only be administered to a patient by a doctor or dentist or any person acting in accordance with the directions of a doctor or dentist.

Schedule 3, e.g. barbiturates, diethylpropion, mazindol – subject to similar controls as Schedule 2 such as the special prescription requirements but they may be manufactured by persons authorised in writing by the Secretary of State. There is a difference in the classes of person who may possess and supply them, entries in the register of Controlled Drugs need not be made in respect of these drugs, but invoices or similar records must be kept for at least 2 years.

Schedule 4, Part 1 includes lorazepam and diazepam.

Part 2, drugs which are subject to less control. In particular, Controlled Drug prescription requirements do NOT apply and they are NOT subject to safe custody requirements.

Schedule 5, preparations which because of their strength are exempt from most Controlled Drug requirements, other than retention of invoices for two years.

MIDWIVES AND SUPPLY OF MEDICINES

By Statutory Instrument[7] the midwife can supply:

– All medicines that are not Prescription Only Medicines (POM)

– Prescription Only Medicines containing any of the following substances but no other Prescription Only Medicine:

- Chloral hydrate

- Ergometrine maleate (only when contained in a medicinal product which is not for parenteral administration)

- Pentazocine hydrochloride

- Phytomenadione[8]

- Triclofos sodium

– The midwife can also administer parenterally in the course of professional practice Prescription Only Medicines containing any of the following substances:[7]

- Ergometrine maleate

- Lignocaine

- Lignocaine hydrochloride

- Naloxone hydrochloride

- Oxytocin, natural and synthetic

- Pentazocine lactate

- Pethidine hydrochloride

- Phytomenadione

- Promazine hydrochloride.

Lignocaine, Lignocaine hydrochloride and Promazine hydrochloride may only be administered by a midwife while attending a woman in childbirth.

MIDWIFE AND CONTROLLED DRUGS

A registered midwife who has notified the local supervising authority of her intention to practise may, as far as is necessary for the practice of her profession or employment as a midwife, possess and administer any Controlled Drug which the Medicines Act 1968 permits her to administer (Regulation 11 of the Misuse of Drugs Regulations 2001).[6] Supplies may only be made to her or possessed by her, on the authority of a midwife's supply order. This supply order must specify the name and occupation of the midwife, the purpose for which it is required and the total quantity to be obtained. The supply order must be signed:

– by a doctor who is authorised by the local supervising authority for the region or area in which the Controlled Drug was, or is to be, obtained or

– by the Supervisor of Midwives appointed by the local supervising authority for that area.

The Regulation defines a midwife's supply order as 'an order in writing specifying the name and occupation of the midwife obtaining the drug, the purpose for which it is required and the total quantity to be obtained'.

Diamorphine and morphine were added to the list of exemptions for midwives[9] as noted in an NMC Circular,[10] which provides an updated list of the midwives' exemption drugs. The list that the midwives can also supply as well as administer can be obtained from the Statutory Instrument[11] which is available from the HMSO website.[12]

DISPOSAL OF UNWANTED STOCKS OF CONTROLLED DRUGS

A midwife may surrender any stocks of Controlled Drugs in her possession which she no longer requires to the doctor as identified above (Reg. 11) or any doctor, or pharmacist (Reg. 6).

DOCUMENTATION OF CONTROLLED DRUGS

The midwife must keep a Controlled Drug book in which she must record the following:

– the date

– the name and address of the person from whom the drug was obtained

– the amount obtained and

– the form in which it was obtained

– the name and address of the patient to whom the drug was administered

– the amount administered and

– the form in which it was administered.

When the midwife receives the Controlled Drug from the pharmacist, she must sign the pharmacist's Controlled Drugs register and the pharmacist must keep the midwife's supply order for 2 years.

NON-POM MEDICINES

The NMC emphasised that midwives can supply and administer all non-prescription only medicines (non-POMs) and general sales list medicines in the course of their professional practice.[13] The NMC was concerned that the supply and administration of some non-prescription medicines such as nitrous oxide and oxygen have been wrongly written into Patient Group Directions. In its guidance for employers and registered midwives, it emphasises that under Statutory Instrument 1980 No 1924[14] a registered midwife can supply and administer all non-prescription only medicines, including pharmacy and general sale list medicines. A student midwife, during the course of her programme of education, can administer those medicines under the guidance of a practising midwife, for which the registered midwife remains accountable. The NMC feared that including medicines unnecessarily in Patient Group Directions would have implications for student midwives gaining experience in the administration of nitrous oxide and oxygen to women in the course of their education.

THE MIDWIVES RULES

Rule 7 of the Midwives Rules[15] details further legally binding regulations in relation to the administration of medicines by midwives. For convenience these are set out in Box 20.3.

Box 20.3 Rule 7 Administration of medicines

A practising midwife shall only administer those medicines, including analgesics, in respect of which she has received the appropriate training as to use, dosage and methods of administration.

In its standards on Rule 7, the NMC states that:

- A midwife must abide by the regulations relating to the destruction of Controlled Drugs.

- A midwife must respect the right of individuals to self-administer substances of their choice.

The NMC guidance on Rule 7 replaces the guidance originally contained in the Midwives Code of Practice. It states that:

You are able to supply and administer all non-prescription medicines, which include all pharmacy and general sales list medicines without a prescription. The list of medicines are all those in the British National Formulary that are not prescription medicines. These medicines do not need to be in a Patient Group Direction for you to be able to supply and/or administer them as part of your professional practice.

Local policies, sometimes referred to as 'standing orders', have frequently been developed to supplement the legislation on medicines that practising midwives may supply and/or administer. There is no legal requirement to replace these with Patient Group Directions.

You should expect your Supervisor of Midwives to audit your records relating to drug administration from time to time.

Some medicines, which are normally only available on a prescription issued by a medical practitioner, may be supplied by you for use in your practice either from a retail or hospital pharmacy. Further details can be found on page 37 of the NMC guidance document[16] under supplementary information and legislation.

You should advise a woman who has not used a Controlled Drug, which has been prescribed by her GP, to destroy it and suggest that she does so in your presence. Alternatively, you can advise the woman to return the unused controlled drug to the pharmacist from where it was obtained. You must not do this for her.

The NMC guidance on homeopathic and herbal medicines is set out and discussed in Chapter 34.

RECORDS

The Midwives Rule 9 requires the midwife to keep records in relation to medicines. Record keeping is considered in Chapter 15 of this book.

PRESCRIPTION ONLY AND OTHER MEDICINES USED BY MIDWIVES

Nurse/midwife prescribing

Following the first Crown Report,[17] the provisions of the Medicinal Products: Prescription by Nurses Act 1992, introducing nurse prescribing, came into force in October 1994 when pilot schemes for prescribing by community nurses and health visitors commenced. Nurses and health visitors who have recorded their prescribing qualification on the NMC Register can prescribe against the Nurse Prescriber's Formulary. Subsequently, a further Crown Report[18] recommended the recognition of Patient Group Directions (group protocols), whereby registered nurses, midwives and other registered health practitioners could prescribe in accordance with a protocol containing the information specified in the Regulations.[19] These provide for 'Patient Group Directions' to be drawn up to make provision for the sale or supply of a prescription only medicine in hospitals in accordance with the written direction of a doctor or dentist. To be lawful, the Patient Group Direction must cover the particulars which are set out in Part 1 of Schedule 7 of the Statutory Instrument, shown in Box 20.4.

As noted in the NMC guidance above, Patient Group Directions are only required for drugs which cannot otherwise be prescribed and administered by midwives, i.e. they are not necessary for non-prescription and general sales medicines.

Box 20.4 Particulars for Patient Group Direction

a. the period during which the Direction shall have effect

b. the description or class of prescription only medicines to which the Direction relates

c. whether there are any restrictions on the quantity of medicine which may be supplied on any one occasion, and if so, what restrictions

d. the clinical situations which prescription only medicines of that description or class may be used to treat

e. the clinical criteria under which a person shall be eligible for treatment

f. whether any class of person is excluded from treatment under the Direction, and if so, what class of person

g. whether there are circumstances in which further advice should be sought from a doctor or dentist and, if so, what circumstances

h. the pharmaceutical form or forms in which prescription only medicines of that description or class are to be administered

i. the strength, or maximum strength, at which prescription only medicines of that description or class are to be administered

j. the applicable dosage or maximum dosage

k. the route of administration

l. the frequency of administration

m. any minimum or maximum period of administration applicable to prescription only medicines of that description or class

n. whether there are any relevant warnings to note, and if so, what warnings

o. whether there is any follow-up action to be taken in any circumstances, and if so, what action and in what circumstances

p. arrangements for referral for medical advice

q. details of the records to be kept of the supply or the administration of medicines under the Direction.

The final report of the Crown Review was published in March 1999.[1] One of its most significant recommendations was that the legal authority in the UK to prescribe should be extended beyond currently authorised prescribers and two types of prescribers should be recognised: the independent prescriber and the dependent prescriber (now known as the supplementary prescriber). In addition a UK-wide advisory body, provisionally entitled the 'New Prescribers Advisory Committee' should be established, under s.4 of the Medicines Act, to assess submissions from professional organisations seeking powers for suitably trained members to become independent or dependent prescribers.

An 'independent prescriber' is a clinician who is responsible for the assessment of patients with undiagnosed conditions and for the decisions about the clinical management required, including prescriptions.

A 'dependent (or supplementary) prescriber' is a clinician who takes over the continuing care of a patient which may include prescribing, after initial assessment by an independent prescriber.

A 'clinician' is a healthcare professional who is engaged in the direct examination, treatment and care of patients.

On 25 October 2000, the Department of Health issued a consultation paper to extend nurse prescribing. This was followed by legislation enacted in the Health and Social Care Act 2001 to extend prescribing powers. Section 63 amends s.58 of the Medicines Act 1968 to enable additional persons to be eligible to prescribe, including persons registered by a board established under the Professions Supplementary to Medicine Act 1960, persons who are pharmacists and also persons who are registered in any register established, continued or maintained under an Order in Council under s.60(1) of the Health Act 1999. The latter would include midwives registered under the Nursing and Midwifery Council. In other words, the possibility of all registered health professionals having powers to prescribe is envisaged by the amendments to the Medicines Act 1968. However, who actually in practice is able to prescribe depends upon the detailed regulations to be enacted by the Secretary of State. The Secretary of State has the power to draw up orders which set the conditions for prescribing and administering specified medicines. Anyone failing to obey these conditions would be guilty of a criminal offence.

Regulations were passed in 2003 covering supplementary prescribing.[20] Under these regulations, where a doctor employs a supplementary prescriber, the conditions under which she/he can prescribe prescription only medicines, can administer a prescription only medicine for parenteral administration, or give directions for the administration of a prescription only medicine for parenteral administration are that:

(a) The person satisfies the applicable conditions set out in Article 3B(3) of the POM order (prescribing and administration by supplementary prescribers)[21] unless those conditions do not apply by virtue of any of the exemptions set out in the subsequent provisions of that Order.

(b) The medicine is not a Controlled Drug within the meaning of the Misuse of Drugs Act 1971.

(c) The medicine is not specified in Schedule 10 to the Medical Regulations (drugs and other substances not to be prescribed for supply under pharmaceutical services).[22]

(d) The medicine is not specified in an entry in column 1 of Schedule 11 to the Medical Regulations (drugs to be prescribed under pharmaceutical services only in certain circumstances).

Where a doctor employs a supplementary prescriber, the conditions on which he or she can give a prescription for an appliance or a medicine which is not a prescription only medicine include:

(a) that he acts in accordance with a clinical management plan (which may be amended from time to time) which is in effect at the time he acts, which has been agreed by the patient to whom the plan relates, the doctor or dentist who is a party to the plan and any supplementary prescriber who is to prescribe, give directions for the administration or administer under the plan and which contains the following particulars:

   i   the name of the patient to whom the plan relates

   ii   the illness or conditions which may be treated by the supplementary prescriber

   iii the date on which the plan is to take effect, and when it is to be reviewed by the doctor or dentist who is a party to the plan

   iv   reference to the class or description of medicines or types of appliances which may be prescribed or administered under the plan

   v   any restrictions or limitations as to the strength or dose of any medicine which may be prescribed or administered under the plan, any period of administration or use of any medicine or appliance which may be prescribed or administered under the plan

   vi   relevant warnings about known sensitivities of the patient to, or known difficulties of the patient with, particular medicines or appliances

   vii the arrangements for the notification of suspected or known adverse reactions; incidents occurring with the appliance which might lead to the death or serious deterioration of the patient and

   viii the circumstances in which the supplementary prescriber should refer to, or seek the advice of, the doctor or dentist who is a party to the plan.

(b) that he has access to the health records of the patient to whom the plan relates which are used by any doctor or dentist who is a party to the plan

(c) if it is a prescription for a medicine, the medicine is not a Controlled Drug within the meaning of the Misuse of Drugs Act 1971

(d) if it is a prescription for a medicine, the medicine is not specified in Schedule 10 to the Medical Regulations (drugs and other substances not to be prescribed for supply under pharmaceutical services).

NMC STANDARDS ON EXTENDED INDEPENDENT NURSE PRESCRIBING AND SUPPLEMENTARY PRESCRIBING

In November 2002 the NMC published a copy of new NMC standards for the extension of independent prescribing by nurses, midwives and health visitors and supplementary prescribing.[23] Successful completion of a course meeting these standards can lead to an entry on the register which will enable the practitioners to prescribe independently or as supplementary prescribers. The NMC requirements cover:

– The standard of programme

– The kind of programme

– The content of the programme.

The NMC identified the principal areas, knowledge and competencies required to underpin the practice of prescribing.

MORE RECENT CHANGES

Under Statutory Instrument in 2004[9] further changes were made including changes in the permitted use or route of administration for specified substances when prescribed or administered by an extended formulary nurse prescriber. For example erythromycin is to include oral use. The Statutory Instrument also added diamorphine and morphine to the list of substances that may be parenterally administered by registered nurses and midwives (see above).

PRESCRIBING IN PREGNANCY

There is evidence that the use of over-the-counter medication by pregnant women is common.[24] In another research study on pregnant women and medication, it was found that only 17% of mothers did not take any conventional medicine throughout pregnancy.[25] In response to this study, the British National Formulary (BNF) has issued new advice on medication use during pregnancy.[26] The BNF guidance emphasises that women need to take special care about their entire lifestyle during pregnancy: this means taking care with eating, drinking, exercising and, indeed, taking medicines. Women should consult their doctor or pharmacist before embarking on any treatment with medicines or herbal remedies during pregnancy. The BNF advises that medicines should be avoided during pregnancy as far as possible. Drugs which have been extensively used in pregnancy and appear to be usually safe should be prescribed in preference to new or untried drugs; and the smallest effective dose should be used. The BNF advises caution and not overstating the potential for harm. It suggests that:

Before we get too concerned about the level of medicine taking during pregnancy, we need to have a clearer idea of whether the clinical outcome of the pregnancy in women who have taken medicines is statistically different from those who have not.

The BNF lists the drugs which are to be avoided or used with caution in pregnancy.

Occasionally a heroic story is told of a sacrifice of a mother for the unborn baby. One such is that of Michelle Doyle who, it is reported,[27] gave birth to a healthy boy after being told soon after she became pregnant that she was suffering from ovarian cancer. She refused cytotoxic drugs knowing that they would have harmed the baby. After the birth of the baby she had surgery for the cancer but it was too late to save her life.

Such sacrifices cannot be insisted upon and as the law stands at present, the mother can take medications which are necessary to save her life, even if they are likely to be harmful to the child. Only if she takes the drugs intending to cause a miscarriage to the baby would she be acting illegally under the criminal law (see Chs 17, 25 and 26).

PRESCRIBING AND BREASTFEEDING

Similar precautions about medications taken by the pregnant woman should also be taken by the breastfeeding mother. The BNF has published a Breastfeeding Network Newsletter[28] which considers an overview of the safety of antibiotics during breastfeeding. A study from the Netherlands provides an insight into drug use during breastfeeding.[29]

ROUTINE ANTENATAL ANTI-D PROPHYLAXIS FOR RHD-NEGATIVE WOMEN

A position statement issued by the UKCC on 11 February 1999 was withdrawn by the NMC in March 2003.[30] It followed guidance from the National Institute for Clinical Excellence (NICE).[31] NICE has recommended that pregnant rhesus negative women should be offered Anti-D prophylaxis as preventative treatment (to haemolytic disease in the newborn) routinely, unless they already have antibodies to the D antigen in their blood. NICE also recommended that healthcare professionals should explain the options available to rhesus negative mothers, so they can make an informed choice about treatment.

CONTROLLED DRUGS: THE FOURTH SHIPMAN REPORT

Following the conviction of Harold Shipman for murdering 15 patients (see Ch. 14), an Inquiry was established under the chairmanship of Dame Janet Smith. The Fourth Report[32] from the Inquiry was concerned with the regulation of Controlled Drugs. There were three major groups of recommendations:

1. The setting up of an integrated and multidisciplinary inspectorate to monitor and audit the prescription, storage, distribution and disposal of Controlled Drugs.

2. A number of restrictions on the prescribing of Controlled Drugs to discourage or prevent health professionals from prescribing in circumstances in which it could be considered to be unsafe or unwise for them to do so. The unsafe circumstances include: prescribing for their own use, prescribing by professionals convicted of Controlled Drug Offences.

3. A series of measures should be introduced to tighten up the handling and safe-keeping of Controlled Drugs along each part of the supply chain from supplier to the patient's home and to provide a complete 'audit trail' to account for the movement of Controlled Drugs at each stage, both in the NHS and in the private sector.

The Department of Health is discussing these recommendations with relevant organisations including the Advisory Council on the Misuse of Drugs (ACMD). The Department of Health emphasised the finding in the Fourth Shipman Report that no system for the regulation of Controlled Drugs can offer complete security against abuse from minds as devious as Shipman's, while allowing for their legitimate use by health professionals to ease suffering, but much can still be done to deter and detect improper use.

MANAGEMENT OF ERRORS OR INCIDENTS IN THE ADMINISTRATION OF MEDICINES

Guidelines provided by the NMC[33] suggest a sensitive management of any incidents relating to the administration of medicines and require the registered practitioner to report the error or incident immediately to the line manager or employer. In addition the NMC recommends that:

If a practising midwife makes or identifies a drug error or incident, she should also inform her Supervisor of Midwives as soon as possible after the event.

The NMC published an advice note on medicines management[34] as a consequence of the large number of calls received by its professional advice team. This advice covers the principles for prescribing and also administering medicines. Where complex drug calculations are required it suggests that it may be necessary for a second practitioner to check the calculation to minimise the risk of error.

DRUG ADDICTS

What action does a midwife take if she discovers that one of the mothers referred to her is a drug addict? In the past, particulars of persons addicted to specific drugs had to be notified to the Chief Medical Officer or Home Office by the doctor within 7 days of his considering or having reasonable grounds to believe the addiction (Misuse of Drugs (Notification of and Supply to Addicts) Regulations 1973). However, this requirement was revoked by the Misuse of Drugs (Supply to Addicts) Regulations SI 1997 No 1001. Doctors are now expected to report on a standard form a case of drug misuse to their local Drug Misuse Database (DMD). The BNF states:

A report (notification) to the Drug Misuse Database (DMD) should be made when a patient first presents with a drug problem or re-presents after a gap of six months or more. All types of problem drug misuse should be reported including opioid, benzodiazepine and CNS stimulant.

The NMC has provided guidance[16] on a situation where the midwife suspects that a woman is taking illegal substances:

If you are aware that a woman is self-administering illegal substances you should discuss the health implications for her and her baby with her. You should also assist her by liaison with others in the multi-professional team to gain further support or access to detoxification programmes.

If a midwife suspects that one of her clients is addicted she should ensure that a medical practitioner is informed, who would send the requisite details to the DMD. Apart from the criminal offences relating to the possession and supply of illegal drugs, there are no laws in this country which enable action to be taken against a mother to prevent the fetus being harmed by drugs. Nor can the fetus be made a ward of court before it is born, as the case Re F (*in utero*) 1988[35] illustrates (this case is discussed in Ch. 17). However, the midwife would have responsibilities to ensure that appropriate care is taken of a vulnerable adult. It may be that the mother refuses all assistance offered by the midwife. If there are concerns that the mother lacks the mental capacity to make her own decisions, then action can be taken in her best interests (see Ch. 7). Close contact with social services will be essential to ensure that action is taken in the best interests of the child once born. A report by the Audit Commission in February 2002[36] recommended fundamental reforms of the drug treatment services in England and Wales. At present they provided little value for the £234 million spent on helping addicts and mis-users. As a consequence of this audit, midwives might find that a new strategy for drug treatment services may be planned and implemented which would assist them in their work. The Drugs Act 2005 introduces a new offence of aggravated supply of controlled drugs, to cover the situation where drugs are supplied in the vicinity of school premises. Police powers in relation to searches for controlled drugs are also increased.

LIABILITY AND MEDICINAL PRODUCTS

There are unfortunately many cases where litigation arises as a result of breaches of the duty of care in relation to the prescribing or administration of medicinal products.

In examples of contested cases, £119 302 was ordered to be paid to a man who had suffered permanent brain damage because of a badly written prescription.[37] The doctor had written a prescription for Amoxil, but this was read by the pharmacist as Daonil. The doctor was held 25% liable and the employers of the pharmacist 75% liable.

In another case,[38] the doctor prescribed Migril but failed to heed the manufacturer's warnings and instead of limiting the dose to not more that 12 tablets in the course of 1 week and not more than 1 every 4 hours, prescribed 60 tablets to be taken at 2 tablets every 4 hours. The pharmacist did not spot the error. The patient's condition deteriorated and the mistake was not noticed by another doctor in the practice who visited the patient. In the High Court, compensation of £100 000 was agreed, 45% payable by the prescribing doctor, 40% by the pharmacist and the remaining 15% by the second doctor who visited. On appeal, the second doctor was found not liable and his 15% contribution was accepted by the pharmacist.

In one case, bad handwriting on a prescription for a top-up epidural resulted in a junior doctor administering to a woman following a hysterectomy operation 30 mg of epidural diamorphine in 10 ml of saline instead of 3 mg.[39] A woman of 53 had entered the Princess Grace private hospital in London for a routine hysterectomy. As a result of the drug administration error (it was also only the second time the junior doctor had added drugs to an epidural) and the fact that the junior doctor had not been trained to use the resuscitation equipment, the patient died a few days later.

Other examples of errors in medication and prescribing are described in the Journal of the Medical Defence Union and reports are to be found regularly in newspapers and professional journals. The Royal Pharmaceutical Society of Great Britain has published leaflets on legal and ethical issues in medicines which include a leaflet on dealing with dispensing errors.[40]

At the heart of the issue of negligence is the question of whether the accepted standard of the reasonable professional has been followed. This is known as the Bolam Test[41] and is discussed in Chapter 13. If midwives are to have extended powers of prescribing as a result of the new legislation, standards will have to be defined, protocols drawn up and procedures agreed to ensure that there are recognised standards for professional practice.[42] However, the public should not expect a lower standard of care because midwives have the role of prescribing.

The Consumer Protection Act 1987 can be used by those who have suffered harm as a result of a defect in medication, without having to establish that there was negligence on the part of the manufacturers or suppliers (the Act is discussed in Ch. 19).

INFLUENCE OF THE NATIONAL INSTITUTE FOR HEALTH AND CLINICAL EXCELLENCE (NICE)

The establishment of NICE is discussed in Chapter 21. One of its main functions is to consider research relating to medicinal products and to identify effective products. Its recommendations are not binding upon the NHS, but in practice any Health Authority or NHS trust which ignored its guidelines that a specific medication was effective would probably face an action for judicial review if it prevented the medication from being made available on the NHS within its own catchment area. In May 2000, NICE issued guidance on the use of Taxanes in the treatment of ovarian cancer. It recommended that the drug paclitaxel (Taxol) should be used to treat women who have previously received it and whose cancer has recurred or been resistant to other forms of treatment.[43] While the guidelines of NICE are not law in the sense that patients have the right to insist that they are followed, they may well become absorbed into any definition of what is reasonable professional practice according to the Bolam Test (see Ch. 13), thus creating a presumption that they are followed. Midwives should ensure that they receive information about NICE publications and guidelines and also, if possible, have an input into the thinking behind NICE's publications.

CLINICAL TRIALS

Rule 8 of the Midwives Rules states:

A practising midwife may only participate in clinical trials if there is a protocol approved by a relevant ethics committee.

Ethics committee is defined in the rules. As a result of an EC Directive[44] strict rules relating to the conduct of clinical trials on medicinal products have been implemented. (For further information on ethics committees and the EC Directive see Ch. 31.)

CONCLUSION

Recent changes in prescribing powers are supporting a radical development in the traditional demarcation boundaries of health professional activities. There are now great opportunities for professional development. However, any such widening of the scope of professional practice must ensure that midwives work within their competence and they obtain the training and necessary practice under supervision (see Ch. 5). It is illegal for any health professional other than a midwife or doctor to attend a woman in childbirth. Errors and negligent practice will be followed by litigation, disciplinary and fitness to practise proceedings and, in situations where there has been gross negligence, criminal prosecution. The regulation of complementary and alternative medicines is considered in Chapter 34. Under regulations (The Medicines (Advisor Bodies) Regulations, SI 2005 No 1094) which came into force in October 2005, the Medicines Commission is replaced by the Commission on Human Medicines which appoints sub-committees known as expert advisory groups, which must include the following:

– The Biological Expert Advisory Group

– The Chemistry, Pharmacy and Standards Expert Advisory Group

– The Pharmacovigilance Expert Advisory Group and such other groups as it considers appropriate.

The Committee for the Safety of Medicines is replaced.

QUESTIONS AND EXERCISES

1. Prepare a policy in relation to the supply and administration of Controlled Drugs in the community.

2. In what ways would you consider that the powers of the midwife could be enhanced by the changes in prescribing legislation?

3. A client is a drug addict. What action do you take?

References

1 Department of Health. Final report on the prescribing, supply and administration of medicines. Chaired by Dr June Crown. London: HMSO; 1999.

2 Dimond B. The legal aspects of medicines. Dinton, Wilts: Quay Books; 2005.

3 NMC. 2004 Guidelines for the administration of medicines. London, replacing UKCC. 2000 guidance.

4 British National Formulary. Online. Available: www.bnf.org.uk

5 Proprietary Association of Great Britain. OTC Directory. London: Proprietary Association of Great Britain; annual.

6 Misuse of Drugs Regulations SI 2001 No 3998 amending and re-enacting the Misuse of Drugs Regulations SI 1985 2066.

7 Statutory Instrument 1997 No 1830.

8 Statutory instrument 1998 No 2081.

9 The Prescription only Medicines (Human Use) Amendment Order 2004 No 2.

10 Nursing and Midwifery Council. NMC Circular 10/2004.

11 The Prescription only Medicines (Human Use) Order 1997 SI 1997 No 1830.

12 HMSO. Online. Available: www.hmso.gov.uk

13 Nursing and Midwifery Council. Circular 8/2003 31 March 2003.

14 Medicines (Pharmacy and General Sale Exemption) Order 1980 Article 4 Statutory Instrument 1980 No 1924.

15 Nursing and Midwifery Council. (Midwives) Rules Order of Council 2004 Statutory Instrument 2004/1764 as contained in the Nursing and Midwifery Council Midwives Rules and Standards. London: NMC; August 2004.

16 Nursing and Midwifery Council. Midwives Rules and Standards. London: NMC; August 2004.

17 Department of Health. Report on the nurse prescribing and supply. Advisory Group chaired by Dr June Crown. London: HMSO; 1989.

18 Department of Health. Review of prescribing, supply and administration of medicines: a Report on the supply and administration of medicines under Group Protocols. London: HMSO; 1998.

19 Prescription only Medicines (Human Use) Amendment Order 2000 SI 2000 No 1917.

20 The National Health Service (Amendments Relating to Prescribing by Nurses and Pharmacists etc.) (England) Regulations 2003 SI 2003 No 699.

21 Prescription only Medicines (Human Use) Order 1997 SI 1997 No 1830 (amended by SI 2002/549 and 2003/696.

22 SI 1992/635 as amended by AI 1992/2412; SI 1993/2421; 1994/2620; 1995/3093; 1997/981; 1998/682and 2838; 1999/326 ad 1627; 2000/1645; 2001/1178, 3386 and 37742; 2002/554, 881, 1768, 1920 and 2469; and 2003/26.

23 Nursing and Midwifery Council. NMC Circular 25/2002 Extended independent nurse prescribing and supplementary prescribing. NMC; November 2002.

24 Tillett J, Kostich LM, VandeVusse L. Use of over-the-counter medications during pregnancy. J Perinat Neonat Nurs 2003; 17(1):3–18.

25 Nursing and Midwifery Council. NMC News, 8 October 2004, reporting research by Headley J, Northstone K, Simmons H, et al. Medication use during pregnancy: data from the Avon longitudinal Study of Parents and Children. Eur J Clin Pharmacol 2004.

26 British National Formulary Extra: News, 6 October 2004. Online. Available: www.bnf.uk

27 News item. The Times, 19 March 1994.

28 BNF. Breastfeeding Network Newsletter 2004; 24:9–10.

29 Schirm E, Schwagermann MP, Toi H, et al. Drug use during breastfeeding. A survey from the Netherlands. Eur J Clin Nutr 2004; 58(2):386–390.

30 Nursing and Midwifery Council. Routine antenatal anti-D prophylaxis for RhD-negative women. NMC Circular 5/2003.

31 National Institute for Clinical Excellence. Guidance for rhesus negative women during pregnancy 2002/024. Online. Available: www.nice.org.uk

32 Shipman Inquiry Fourth Report. The Regulation of Controlled Drugs in the Community, published 15 July 2004. Online. Available: www.the-shipman-inquiry.org.uk/reports.asp

33 Nursing and Midwifery Council. Guidelines for the administration of medicines 2004, reprint of UKCC 2000.

34 Nursing and Midwifery Council News 2004; October:9.

35 Re F (*in utero*) [1988] 2 All ER 193.

36 Audit Commission. Acute hospital portfolio: Medicines management. 2002. Online. Available: www.auditcommission

37 Prendergast v. Sam & Dee and others. Independent, 17 March 1988.

38 Dwyer v. Roderick and others. The Times, 12 November 1983 (1983) 127 SI 805.

39 Kennedy D. Hospital blamed in report on overdose death. The Times, 3 July 1996.

40 Royal Pharmaceutical Society of Great Britain law and ethics facts sheet. Dealing with dispensing errors. November 2004. Online. Available: www.rpsgb.org.uk

41 Bolam v. Friern Hospital Management Committee. QBD [1957] 2 All ER 118.

42 Dimond B. Legal aspects of medicines. Dinton, Wilts: Quay Books; 2005.

43 NICE. Online. Available: www.nice.org.uk/appraisals/taxguide.htm

44 EC Directive 2001/20/EC. On the implementation of good clinical practice in the conduct of clinical trials on medicinal products for human use.

SECTION D
MANAGEMENT ISSUES

This Section of the book considers the management issues in relation to the provision of maternity services. Chapter 21 will consider the statutory authorities and the regulations relating to the provision of medical maternity services by general practitioners. Subsequent chapters look at employment law, the position of the independent midwife and the laws relating to the registration of private maternity hospitals and the role of the midwifery manager.

Chapter 21

THE STRUCTURE OF THE NHS AND THE PROVISION OF HOSPITAL, COMMUNITY AND PRIMARY CARE SERVICES

In this chapter we consider the statutory framework of the National Health Service in the light of the changes which have been made under the NHS and Community Care Act 1990, the Primary Care Act 1997, the Health Act 1999, the Health and Social Care Act 2001, NHS Reform and Healthcare Professions Act 2002, the Health and Social Care (Community Health and Standards) Act 2003 and the provision of maternity medical services by General Practitioners.

Over the past 10 years there have been constant changes to the NHS structure and some midwives may have found that their contracts of employment have been transferred several times between different health organisations.

The Secretary of State has the responsibility for providing NHS services within the UK and appoints the statutory bodies which have the tasks of commissioning and providing care. The Secretary of State is under a general duty[1] to:

continue the promotion in England and Wales of a comprehensive health service designed to secure improvement

(a) in the physical and mental health of the people of those countries, and

(b) in the prevention, diagnosis and treatment of illness, and for that purpose to provide or secure the effective provision of services in accordance with this Act.

Section 3(1) of the NHS Act 1977 requires the Secretary of State to provide throughout England and Wales, to such extent as he considers necessary to meet all reasonable requirements:

(a) hospital accommodation

(b) other accommodation for the purpose of any service provided under this Act

(c) medical, dental, nursing and ambulance services

(d) such other facilities for the care of the expectant and nursing mothers and young children as he considers are appropriate as part of the health service.

The discretionary nature of this power should be recognised. The phrases 'to such extent as he considers necessary' 'to meet all reasonable requirements' qualify the duty and have meant that actions for failure to provide services brought against statutory authorities have usually failed in the context of healthcare.[2–4] However, a recent decision of the High Court held the NHS should pay for a patient to have treatment abroad, if the patient had waited a significantly long time for NHS treatment.[5]

The Secretary of State fulfils the task of providing a comprehensive health service by delegating the work to statutory authorities.

STRATEGIC HEALTH AUTHORITIES

These are statutory bodies which are appointed to carry out the functions of the Secretary of State in ensuring the provision of health services. As part of their functions they undertake an assessment of needs for healthcare and services in relation to public health. Strategic Health Authorities arrange for the provision of primary care services through Primary Care Trusts (in Wales Local Health Boards) (see below). Hospital and some community services are provided by NHS trusts, which receive their funding from the Strategic Health Authorities. A reorganisation of the boundaries and number of Health Authorities took place following publication of the Department of Health's paper 'Shifting the Balance of Power within the NHS',[6] which was designed to strengthen the strategic role of Health Authorities.

The NHS and Community Care Act 1990 introduced into the law relating to healthcare the concept of the internal market, and led to the establishment of NHS trusts from whom the Health Authorities purchased services. The White Paper of 1997[7] recommended the abolition of the internal market and the GP fundholding arrangements. Following the implementation of the Health Act 1999, GP fundholders were abolished, Primary Care Groups (which became trusts) were established and new institutions such as the Commission for Health Improvement (now the Healthcare Commission) were established. At the same time, the National Institute for Clinical Excellence was set up (re-named as the National Institute for Health and Clinical Excellence following its joining with the Health Development Agency in April 2005).

NHS TRUSTS

Section 5 of the NHS and Community Care Act 1990 enabled NHS trusts to be established. These are statutory bodies appointed by the Secretary of State which are responsible for the provision of NHS services. The NHS trust can make long-term arrangements with Strategic Health Authorities and Primary Care Trusts for the provision of health services in their area.

NHS FOUNDATION TRUSTS

After considerable controversy, the Health and Social Care (Community Health and Standards) Act was passed in 2003 and Foundation Hospitals were set up in April 2004. The Act defines an NHS foundation trust as:

a public benefit corporation which is authorised to provide goods and services for the purposes of the health service in England.

It is a body corporate and rules relating to its constitution are set out in Schedule 1 of the Act. A body corporate known as the Independent Regulator of NHS Foundation Trusts (called the regulator)[8] is set up under s.2 of the Act, with additional provisions relating to membership, tenure of office, general and specific powers, finance and reports set out in Schedule 2. The regulator has a duty to exercise its functions in a manner that is consistent with the performance by the Secretary of State of the duties under ss.1, 3 and 51 of the NHS Act 1977 (Duty as to health service and services generally and as to university clinical teaching and research). NHS Trusts can apply to the regulator for authorisation to become an NHS foundation trust. The application must describe the goods and services it intends to provide together with a copy of the proposed constitution of the trust. The regulator must maintain a register of NHS foundation trusts together with a copy of its constitution, latest annual report and accounts and any notice relating to its being a failing NHS foundation trust. Once an NHS foundation is established, it ceases to be regarded as the servant or agent of the Crown or as enjoying any status, immunity or privilege of the Crown.

The main differences between an NHS foundation trust and an NHS trust are as follows:

– An NHS foundation trust is an independent public benefit corporation, not under the direct control of the Secretary of State.

– An NHS foundation trust comes under the control of an Independent Regulator which gives an authorisation for the establishment of the NHS foundation trust and must secure that the principal purpose of the trust is the provision of goods and services for the purposes of the health service in England. (These include education and training, accommodation and other facilities and carrying out research.) An authorisation can restrict the provision of private health care by the NHS foundation trust.

– The NHS foundation trust has a general duty to exercise its functions effectively, efficiently and economically (s.39 HSC(CHS) Act).

– Ownership and accountability for the NHS foundation trust is in the hands of the local community rather than the Secretary of State.

– NHS foundation trusts will be able to raise capital (s.13) within overall limits and according to a prudential borrowing code (PBC – s.12) and retain any operating surplus. (The PBC is to be drawn by the Regulator and placed before Parliament[9]).

– NHS foundation trusts are able to recruit and employ their own staff.

– NHS foundation trusts will be expected to comply with national standards and targets, but will not be subject to directions from the Secretary of State or performance management by strategic health authorities and the Department of Health. (They will however be subject to inspections and inquiries carried out by CHAI (i.e. the Healthcare Commission) who must report to the Regulator.)

– Individuals with an interest in the development and wellbeing of an NHS foundation trust can register as members. These members become responsible as owners of the trust.

– Each NHS foundation trust will establish a Board of Governors who will ensure that the local community is directly involved in the governance of the trust. Regulations may make provision for the conduct of elections for membership of the board of governors.

– PCT Patient Forums for any PCT area served by an NHS foundation trust will have the right to inspect the NHS foundation trust's services, commission independent advocacy in relation to services provided by the NHS foundation trust, promote the involvement of members of the public in consultations, decisions and policy development by the NHS foundation trust, advise the trust on encouraging public involvement and monitor its success in achieving public involvement.

– An NHS foundation trust may do anything which appears to it to be necessary or desirable for the purpose of or in connection with its functions (s.18(1)) including the acquiring and disposing of property, entering into contracts, accepting gifts of property.

– The authorisation must require an NHS foundation trust to disclose such information as the Secretary of State specifies to the regulator and may require an NHS foundation trust to allow the regulator to enter and inspect premises owned or controlled by the trust.

– Sections 27 and 28 provide for the mergers of NHS foundation trusts with NHS foundation trusts and/or NHS trusts.

Bill Moyes was appointed in December 2003 as chair of the Independent Regulator of NHS Foundation Trusts. He has the responsibility of authorising, monitoring and regulating NHS Foundation Trusts and works with a Board of up to five members including the chair and a deputy chair.

The RCM has provided a guide for midwives on NHS Foundation Trusts.[10]

FAILING NHS FOUNDATION TRUSTS

If the independent regulator is satisfied that an NHS foundation trust is contravening or failing to comply with the terms of its authorisation then it may serve a notice on the trust that the Board of Governors is required to do a specified thing, or that all of the directors or the members of the board of governors are removed and replaced with interim directors or members or suspended. The directors can be required to take steps to obtain a moratorium or propose a voluntary arrangement under insolvency legislation. Ultimately the regulator can make an order (after following a specified procedure) providing for the dissolution of the trust and the transfer of its property or liabilities to another NHS foundation trust, a PCT, an NHS trust or the Secretary of State.

PRIMARY CARE TRUSTS

Primary Care Trusts evolved from the primary care groups, established to provide or arrange for the provision of primary care services. Midwifery services are sometimes included in Primary Care Trusts, but there is no uniformity: in some areas only community maternity services are transferred to the Primary Care Trust; in others the hospital and community midwifery services are transferred (Ealing is an example of the latter). Under the Health and Social Care Act 2001 powers are given to enable Care Trusts to be set up which can provide both Local Authority and health services. The thinking behind the provision is that by combining both NHS responsibilities and Local Authority responsibilities under single management, care trusts increase continuity of care and simplify administration. Further information on the regulations relating to care trusts and guidance on estate and facilities management and on governance is available on the DH website.

Children Trusts have also been created so that all health and local services relating to children are coordinated in a single agency. It is too early to assess the effectiveness of either Care Trusts or Children Trusts.

HOW DOES THIS AFFECT THE MIDWIFE AND MIDWIFERY SERVICES?

Many midwives may now find that they are employed by a Primary Care Trust and the employment implications of this are considered in Chapter 22. Initially their contracts are likely to be as they were under Whitley Council arrangements but since trusts have the power to make local agreements for terms and conditions of service this might eventually change. Regulations relating to the transfer to a Primary Care Trust are set out in the Health Act 1999 (Schedule 1).

GENERAL PRACTITIONERS

There are about 30 000 GPs in England with on average 2000 patients per GP. About 10% of all GPs work without partners. The majority however work in group practices which may be attached to a health centre. The NHS and Community Care Act 1990 saw the introduction of some GPs receiving approval as fundholders working in fundholding practices. However, fundholding was abolished under the Health Act 1999. Under the NHS (Primary Care) Act 1977, pilot schemes were introduced to enable General Practitioners and dentists to provide personal medical and dental services outside the framework of the Health Authorities. Primary Care Trusts have powers to take over the administration of personal medical services. New contracts came into place in April 2004.

General Practitioners working within the NHS agree contracts with primary care trusts over the services which they provide according to the new contractual arrangements which came into force in 2004[11-14] and were amended in 2005.[15] (Transitional arrangements covered the interim period).[16] The Regulations set the terms on which Primary Care Trusts can contract for services with general medical practitioners.

The regulations enable contracts to be agreed with GPs for the provision of essential services throughout the core hours. Essential services include:

Services required for the management of registered patients and temporary residents who are or believe themselves to be:

a. ill, with conditions from which recovery is generally expected

b. terminally ill or

c. suffering from chronic disease.

The core hours are defined as the period beginning at 8.00 a.m. and ending at 6.30 p.m. on any day from Monday to Friday, except Good Friday, Christmas Day or bank holidays.

A contractor must provide primary medical services required in core hours for the immediately necessary treatment of any person to whom the contractor had been requested to provide treatment owing to an accident or emergency at any place in the practice area (Regulation 15(6)).

ADDITIONAL SERVICES

The Regulations identify the following as additional services which the contractor may provide:

- Cervical screening services

- Contraceptive services

- Vaccination and immunisations

- Childhood vaccinations and immunisations

- Child health surveillance services

- Maternity medical services and

- Minor surgery.

The Regulations also cover the provision of out of hours services, which the primary care trust can negotiate with contractors (Regulation 30).

MATERNITY MEDICAL SERVICES

Schedule 2(7) sets out the requirements in relation to the provision of the additional service of maternity medical services. A contractor whose contract includes the provision of maternity services shall:

a. provide to female patients who have been diagnosed as pregnant all necessary maternity medical services throughout the antenatal period

b. provide to female patients and their babies all necessary maternity medical services throughout the postnatal period other than neonatal checks

c. provide all necessary maternity medical services to female patients whose pregnancy has terminated as a result of miscarriage or abortion or, where the contractor has a conscientious objection to the termination of pregnancy, prompt referral to another provider of primary medical services who does not have such conscientious objection.

Antenatal means the period from the start of the pregnancy to the onset of labour.

Maternity medical services is defined as:

a. in relation to female patients (other than babies) all primary medical services relating to pregnancy, excluding intrapartum care, and

b. in relation to babies, any primary medical services necessary in their first 14 days of life.

Postnatal period means the period starting from the conclusion of delivery of the baby or the patient's discharge from secondary care services, whichever is the later and ending on the 14(th) day after the birth.

There is no longer a list of GPs who provide intrapartum care (i.e. an obstetric list which used to be held by the FHSA and then health authorities). It is open to an individual PCT (in Wales an LHB) to agree with a local general practitioner that he or she would provide intrapartum services. There are no national arrangements for such provision.

QUALITY ASSURANCE MECHANISM

The White Paper on the NHS envisaged new institutions and strategies for raising standards within the NHS.[17] These included the concept of Clinical Governance, the Commission for Health Improvement (subsequently replaced by the Commission for Healthcare Audit and Inspection, now known as the Healthcare Commission), the National Institute for Clinical Excellence, National Service Frameworks and new arrangements for professional registration and concerning misconduct.

THE INTRODUCTION OF CLINICAL GOVERNANCE

The White Paper on the NHS introduced the concept of Clinical Governance. It is defined as:

A framework through which NHS organisations are accountable for continuously improving the quality of their services.[18]

The idea of Clinical Governance is basically simple. In the past, the trust board and its Chief Executive have been responsible for the financial probity of the organisation; there has been no statutory responsibility of the trust for the overall quality of the organisation. Under the concept of Clinical Governance, the board and its Chief Executive are responsible for the quality of clinical services provided by the organisation. In theory this could mean that a board is removed or a Chief Executive dismissed if a baby suffers brain damage at birth or a mother dies in childbirth as a result of negligence.

The concept of Clinical Governance is based on the statutory duty of quality set out under s.18 of the Health Act 1999 and as subsequently amended in the Health and Social Care (Community Health and Standards) Act 2003 and shown in Box 21.1.

> ## Box 21.1 Section 45 Health and Social Care (Community Health and Standards) Act 2003
>
> It is the duty of each NHS body to put and keep in place arrangements for the purpose of monitoring and improving the quality of health care provided by and for that body.

'Healthcare' means the services provided to individuals for or in connection with the prevention, diagnosis or treatment of illness and the promotion and protection of public health.

The duty falls primarily upon the Chief Executive of each Health Authority and NHS trust to implement. In practice, each Chief Executive designates officers to be responsible for quality or Clinical Governance in specified areas of clinical practice. Government guidance was published in March 1999.[18] This follows from the original consultation document, A First Class Service: Quality in the new NHS.[19] The aim to develop quality within the NHS is to be secured in three ways:

– setting clear national quality standards

– ensuring local delivery of high quality clinical services, and

– effective systems for monitoring the quality of services.

The UKCC published a position paper for NHS employers in 2001[20] identifying the major issues in strengthening and supporting the midwifery contribution to maternity care for women and their families which link with the concept of Clinical Governance. These major issues include clinical issues such as variations in practice and care, the management of emergencies, the absence of or failure to use the guidelines and protocols and poor quality of record keeping; issues associated with women's experience of care, such as informed choice and communication; and organisational issues such as effective use of resources, effective leadership, communication and collaboration, lack of consensus on the midwife's role and organisational constraints on providing optimum maternity care. The UKCC suggested that 'using the Clinical Governance and supervisory frameworks together in a proactive way can lead to major benefits for the organisation overall but more particularly will improve outcomes for women . . .'.

THE HEALTHCARE COMMISSION (OTHERWISE KNOWN AS THE COMMISSION FOR HEALTHCARE AUDIT AND INSPECTION, FORMERLY THE COMMISSION FOR HEALTH IMPROVEMENT (CHI))

The Commission for Health Improvement replaced the Clinical Standards Advisory Group (CSAG) but had much wider functions and powers. Sections 19–24 of the

Health Act 1999 establish the Commission for Health Improvement and set out its functions and powers. It is a body corporate, i.e. it can sue and be sued on its own account. The functions are listed in Box 21.2.

Box 21.2 Functions of the Commission for Health Audit and Inspection (known as the Healthcare Commission)

a. Provide advice or information with respect to arrangements by Primary Care Trusts or NHS trusts for the purpose of monitoring and improving the quality of healthcare for which they have responsibility.

b. Conducting reviews of, and making reports on, arrangements by Primary Care Trusts or NHS trusts for the purpose of monitoring and improving the quality of healthcare for which they have responsibility.

c. Carrying out investigations into, and making reports on, the management, provision or quality of healthcare for which Health Authorities, Primary Care Trusts or NHS trusts have responsibility.

d. Conducting reviews of, and making reports on, the quality of data obtained by others relating to the management, provision or quality of, or access to, or availability of healthcare, for which NHS bodies or service providers have responsibility, the validity of conclusions drawn from such data, and the methods used in their collection and analysis.

e. Registering and inspecting private hospitals.

f. Providing an independent investigation of complaints.

g. Other functions as may be prescribed relating to the management, provision or quality of, or access to or availability of, healthcare for which prescribed NHS bodies or prescribed service providers have responsibility.

Section 19(2) of the Health Act 1999 gives powers to the Secretary of State to make regulations covering:

– the times at which, the cases in which, the manner in which, the persons in relation to which or matters with respect to which any functions of the Commission are to be exercised

– the matters to be considered or taken into account in connection with the exercise of any functions of the Commission

– the persons to whom any advice, information or reports are to be given or made

– the publication of reports and summaries of reports

– the recovery from prescribed persons of amounts in respect of expenditure incurred by the Commission in the exercise of any of its functions, and

– the exercise of functions of the Commission in conjunction with the exercise of statutory functions of other persons.

Activities of the CHI

One of the earliest tasks undertaken by the CHI on the day it was established was to visit Garlands Hospital in Carlisle, run by the North Lakeland Healthcare NHS Trust, in Cumbria. An independent investigation[21] had found that staff had physically and mentally abused patients. The Chairman of the NHS trust was dismissed by the Secretary of State. The Secretary of State ordered CHI to visit the hospital.

A spokesman for the Commission stated that its programme for scrutinising NHS trusts could include questions about the resuscitation of older people, following complaints that some hospital doctors were ignoring guidelines.[22] CHI had a programme of inspections so that over 5 years, all NHS trusts would be visited and a report published. The powers of CHI were wide: to ask for the production of documents, require people to be interviewed by them and make strong recommendations to the Secretary of State. The NHS Health and Social Care (Community Health and Standards) Act 2003 replaced CHI with the Commission for Health Audit and Inspection which has subsequently become known as the Healthcare Commission. It has extensive powers and is a principal tool in the Government's aim to raise standards within the NHS. It has also taken on the role of the independent investigation of NHS complaints (see Ch. 11).

In April 2005 the Healthcare Commission carried out an unannounced inspection of Northwick Park Hospital in Northwest London where ten deaths had occurred in the maternity unit over three years.[23] Its visit showed that there were serious system failures, and it demanded that the Health Secretary took urgent action to protect the safety of patients, by putting special measures in place, including daily supervision through a clinical partnership, support from the National Clinical Governance support team and a new acting chief executive and a new medical director. It was also revealed that the workload had doubled at the hospital after a neighbouring facility was closed.[24]

PERFORMANCE STANDARDS

Another initiative envisaged in the NHS Plan is the establishment of nationwide assessment of performance in the NHS. Performance ratings were established and for the first year of assessment were based on waiting times and hospital cleanliness. Hospitals were awarded stars according to their performance and the best trusts were permitted to spend their share of the £155m Performance Fund. In addition the best performing trusts were given 10 key freedoms including: less frequent monitoring from the centre, fewer and better coordinated inspections, development of their own investment programmes without receiving prior approval, extra cash and resources and opportunities for their Chief Executives to provide direct advice to Ministers and to join the learning set which will consider additional freedoms for their organisations. The Healthcare Commission assists in refining the criteria for assessing performance. Four failing trusts which were given a zero star rating in the CHI assessment and failed to make improvements had their management franchised to other NHS organisations. New Chief Executives were appointed. The Government announced its intention of establishing a Register of Experts who would act as 'public service entrepreneurs' (DoH Press release 2002/0069). The best performing trusts were able to apply for NHS foundation trust status (see above).

AUDIT COMMISSION

The Audit Commission is a non-departmental public body sponsored by the Office of the Deputy Prime Minister with the Department of Health and the National Assembly for Wales. It is responsible for ensuring that public money is used economically, efficiently and effectively. Its reports are available from its website.[25] An Audit Commission Report in 1997[26] made significant recommendations for all aspects of maternity services including the care of women in pregnancy, labour and birth and the care of women after childbirth and the care of newborn babies (see Ch. 6 on standards of care).

NATIONAL INSTITUTE FOR HEALTH AND CLINICAL EXCELLENCE (NICE)

This statutory body was established on 1 April 1999 to promote clinical- and cost-effectiveness. (In 2005 it became known as the National Institute for Health and Clinical Excellence.) The then Secretary of State stated that its task would be to abolish postcode variation in the country, so that there would be national standards for the provision of healthcare such as medicines. There had been a lack of uniformity in the decisions of Health Authorities over the provision of services, particularly of medicines. One of the functions of NICE is to issue clinical guidelines and clinical audit methodologies and information on good practice. The National Institute for Health and Clinical Excellence has a major role to play in the setting of standards of practice, by disseminating the results of research of what is proved to be clinically effective, research-based practice. NICE guidelines on caesarean sections which were commissioned from the National Collaborating Centre for Women's and Children's Health were published in April 2004 (see Ch. 6 for further discussion on these).

In May 2001, NICE published clinical guidelines on the use of electronic fetal monitoring: the use and interpretation of cardiography in intrapartum fetal surveillance,[27,28] which are discussed in the RCM Journal[29] and MIDIRS.[30] Other guidelines published by NICE and relevant to the midwife include: Induction of labour;[31] Guidance on the use of routine antenatal anti-D prophylaxis for RhD-negative women,[32] considered by MacKenzie[33] and Jarvis;[34] Antenatal care guidelines,[35] commented on in a letter to MIDIRS;[36] Fertility: assessment and treatment for people with fertility problems[37] (see Ch. 27). The NICE antenatal care guidelines were developed by an expert group under the auspices of the charity Action on Pre-eclampsia[38] and are available on its website.[39] Locally devised guidelines for pre-eclampsia are considered by Jankowicz and Tufnell.[40]

On 1 April 2005, NICE joined with the Health Development Agency to become the new National Institute for Health and Clinical Excellence (also to be known as NICE). NICE announced that it was to establish social value judgements guidelines in addition to the scientific value judgements (which interpret the significance and relevance of the totality of the available scientific, technical and clinical data) it already undertakes. These social value judgements will take account of societal aspirations, preferences and ethical principles that ought to underpin the manner and extent of the care provided to NHS patients.[41] (The legal significance of NICE guidelines is considered in Ch. 13.)

The difficulties faced by midwives in attempting to use evidence-based practice are illustrated by Helen Hindle in a case study concerned with group B Streptococcus in breast milk.[42]

SETTING UP OF NATIONAL SERVICE FRAMEWORKS (NSFs)

The White Paper envisaged that there would be evidence-based National Service Frameworks (NSFs), which set out what patients can expect to receive from the NHS in major care areas or disease groups. One of the first NSFs to be published was that for Mental Health[43] (see Ch. 33).

An NSF for children and maternity services was published in 2004 and is considered in Chapter 6 (maternity services), Chapter 12 (teenage pregnancies) and Chapter 32 (children). Eventually NSFs will cover most of the main sphere of clinical practice. They will doubtless assist managers and clinicians in obtaining the resources to ensure a reasonable standard of care for the patients. Inevitably however they are also likely to support litigation where patients who have suffered personal injuries are able to compare local facilities unfavourably with the norm laid down in the NSF. Mandy Renton provides a constructive comment on how effective the NSF is likely to be.[44]

NHS DIRECT

The White Paper on the NHS[45] proposed the establishment of NHS Direct. The Government's aim was that by the end of the year 2000, the whole country would be covered by a 24-hour telephone advice line staffed by nurses. NHS Direct in Wales became operational in January 2000, with separate funding and organisation from England's. The service aims to provide both clinical advice to support self-care and appropriate self-referral to NHS services as well as access to more general advice and information. In June 2001, the Department of Health announced that as part of a £5 million pilot programme, people with digital television sets will be able to get on-screen consultations with NHS Direct nurses.[46] Patients in the pilot scheme will be able to book appointments with their GPs, get general and local health information and speak to NHS Direct nurses on screen. Clearly any NHS Direct nurse responding to a call would have to question whether the caller is pregnant and ensure that she does not give advice which is outside the limits of her competence. In certain call centres it may be possible to ensure that the woman speaks to a midwife. The caller would be advised to contact her own midwife and doctor and inform them of her contact with NHS Direct.

NATIONAL PLAN FOR THE NHS

On 22 March 2000 the Prime Minister announced to the House of Commons that there were five challenges to be faced in the NHS. These are shown in Box 21.3.

Box 21.3 Challenges for the NHS

– Partnership: making all parts of the health and social care system work better together and ensuring the right emphasis at each level of care

– Performance: improving both clinical performance and health service productivity

– Professions: increasing flexibility in training and working practices and removing demarcations, in the context of major expansion of the healthcare workforce

– Patient care: which has two components: ensuring fast and convenient access to services and empowering and informing patients so that they can be more involved in their own care

– Prevention: tackling inequalities and focussing the health system on its contribution to tackling the causes of avoidable ill health.

Following the Prime Minister's announcement, the Secretary for Health announced that he was setting up discussions with key professionals in the NHS to develop a National Plan based on these five challenges. He intended to establish six modernisation action teams with a specific remit to address variations in performance and standards across the care system.

The NHS Plan was published in July 2000[47] and set out significant proposals for the reform of the NHS, envisaging significant increase in resources and numbers of professional staff, changes in the professional registration, and controls of professional standards. The significant changes in the representation of patients which have taken place are considered in Chapters 6 and 11 of this book. Changes are envisaged in the relationships between the NHS and social services and the NHS and private sector. A modernisation agency has been set up to spread best practice, which is to be combined with the NHS University, the NHS leadership centre, in a new NHS Institute by July 2005. At the time of writing, work is under way with most of the recommendations contained in the NHS Plan. Additional funding has been allocated, targeted on maternity units. The first tranche was announced in May 2001, to support maternity services and bereavement. In October 2001 it was announced[48] a further £100m would be made available for major refurbishment, new facilities for fathers and families and the modernisation of antenatal units. A list of how the money was to be allocated accompanied the press release. Some 2000 extra midwives were to be recruited over the following 3 years and national standards would be set for maternity services. The Maternity and Neonatal Workforce Group (chaired by the Deputy Chief Medical Officer of Health, Dr Sheila Adams, and including representatives of the RCM, RCOG and Health Authorities) was established to examine the best way to provide high quality maternity services and make recommendations to Ministers (see Ch. 6 and Models of staffing in Ch. 24).

THE BRISTOL INQUIRY

Such were the wide, sweeping recommendations in the Report of the Inquiry chaired by Professor Ian Kennedy into children's heart surgery at the Bristol Royal Infirmary[49] that one commentator suggested that in future the NHS would be talked about in terms of 'Before Bristol' and 'After Bristol'. Concerns at the high death rates among the children receiving heart surgery in Bristol were expressed increasingly from the late 1980s onwards. Subsequently, complaints were made to the General Medical Council and in 1998 two cardiac surgeons and the Chief Executive of the trust were found guilty of serious professional misconduct: one cardiac surgeon and the chief executive were struck off from the Register and the other cardiac surgeon's registration was made conditional for 3 years that he did not operate on children. A public inquiry was appointed in June 1998 which reported in 2001. Significant recommendations were made across several areas, shown in Box 21.4.

Box 21.4 Subjects covered by recommendations of the Bristol Inquiry

1. Respect and honesty

2. A health service which is well led

3. Competent healthcare professionals

4. The safety of care

5. Care of an appropriate standard

6. Public involvement through empowerment

7. The care of children

8. Healthcare services and the treatment for children with congenital heart disease.

Many of the recommendations, such as the greater respect given to the rights of the patient, the National Patient Safety Agency, and the changes to control over professional standards exercised by the Registration bodies, had already been included in the NHS Plan. In its introduction to its recommendations the Inquiry makes some extremely salient points:

– There are no right answers; just, perhaps, less wrong answers.

– Cultural and institutional change takes time and can be slow, requiring patience and forbearance.

– Nothing can be achieved on the cheap.

– There are no quick fixes, but progress is possible and can be achieved.

– Change can only be brought about with the willing and active participation of those involved in healthcare; the public, patients, healthcare professionals, trusts and Health Authorities and government.

The Inquiry outlined specific principles which it wished the Report to give effect to. These are summarised in Box 21.5.

Box 21.5 Principles recognised by the Inquiry

- The patient must be at the centre of everything the NHS does.

- The commitment and dedication of staff in the NHS must be valued and acknowledged; those caring for patients must themselves be supported and cared for.

- There must be openness and transparency in everything the NHS does.

- The impact of the way in which services are organised on the quality of care which patients receive must be recognised: the quality of care depends on systems and on facilities, as well as on individual healthcare professionals.

- All those involved in healthcare ... must recognise and acknowledge the contribution of the others in the service of patients.

- The safety of patients must be the foundation of the NHS's commitment to the quality of its services.

- Sentinel events, that is, errors, other adverse events, and near misses, which occur during the care of patients, must be seen as opportunities to learn, not just as reasons to blame.

- There must be clear and understood systems of responsibility and accountability: a culture of blame is no substitute for such systems.

- The quality of healthcare must be guided by agreed standards, compliance with which is regularly monitored.

- The role of central government in relation to the NHS should be:

  a. to act as its HQ in terms of management, and

  b. to create independent mechanisms for regulating the quality of healthcare and the competence of healthcare professionals.

- The various independent bodies must themselves be coordinated so as to avoid the fragmentation of responsibility which arose in the past.

The next few years are likely to see the working through of the recommendations contained in the Bristol Inquiry Report.

CONCLUSION

Major changes have taken place in the organisation and structure of the NHS in recent years. The establishment of Primary Care Trusts should put the emphasis on primary care services and thus have a significant impact on the delivery of maternity services and the role of the General Practitioner. In addition, the institutions of NICE, Healthcare Commission, the National Service Frameworks and the strategy set out in the NHS Plan have an important impact on the setting and the monitoring of standards within midwifery and obstetric practice. Of great significance is the Report of the Bristol Inquiry. Its comprehensive and far-reaching proposals affect all aspects of patient care and professional practice (see especially Ch. 6). The NSF on maternity and children, if supported by the necessary resources, should result in the establishment of a minimum standard of care in maternity services. Major concerns still remain, particularly the problem of the recruitment and retention of midwives (see Ch. 24), which currently are thwarting attempts to create a woman-led service.

QUESTIONS AND EXERCISES

1. What are the advantages of the concept of Clinical Governance in the provision of maternity services?

2. Ask your primary care trust for details of General Practitioners who you know provide medical maternity services.

3. What services does the Local Authority provide for the care of the pregnant woman, before, during and after confinement?

4. What do you consider would be the best administrative arrangement for the provision of hospital, community health and social services for the pregnant woman and her family?

5. Obtain a copy of the NSF on maternity and children's services and consider the extent to which the department within which you work meets these standards. What action, if any, is necessary to bring the department into compliance with the NSF standards?

6. Obtain a copy of the Report of the Bristol Inquiry and discuss with colleagues the action necessary to ensure the implementation of its recommendations in your department.

References

1 Section 1 of the National Health Service Act 1977.
2 R. v. Secretary of State for Social Services *ex parte* Hincks and others. Solicitors' J 29 June 1979 436.

3 In Re Walker's application, The Times 26 November 1987.

4 R. v. Cambridge Health Authority *ex parte* B (a minor) (1995) 23 BMLR 1 CA; [1995] 2 All ER 129.

5 R.(Watts) v. Bedford Primary Care Trust and another. The Times Law Report, 3 October 2003; Lloyd's Rep Med [2004] 113.

6 Department of Health. Shifting the balance of power within the NHS. London: HMSO; 2001.

7 Department of Health. The New NHS: Modern, dependable. London: HMSO; 1997.

8 Department of Health. Online. Available: www.doh.gov.uk/nhsfoundationtrusts/independentregulator.htm

9 Department of Health. Online. Available: www.doh.gov.uk/nhsfoundationtrusts/finance.htm

10 Royal College of Midwives. NHS Foundation Trusts: A guide for Midwives and Physiotherapists. RCM; October 2004.

11 The National Health Service (General Medical Service Contracts) Regulations 2004 SI 2004 No 291.

12 National Health Service (Primary Medical Services Agreements) Regulations 2004 SI 2004 No 627.

13 National Health Service (Performers Lists) Regulations 2004 SI 2004 No 585.

14 National Health Service (Primary Medical Services (Miscellaneous Amendment)) Regulations 2004 SI 2004 No 2694.

15 National Health Service (Primary Medical Services (Miscellaneous Amendment)) Regulations 2005 SI 2005 No 893.

16 General Medical Services Transitional and Consequential Provisions Order 2004 SI 2004 No 865.

17 Department of Health. A first class service: Quality in the new NHS. London: HMSO; 1998.

18 NHS Executive. Health Service Circular 1999/065. Clinical Governance: Quality in the new NHS. NHS;1999.

19 NHS Executive. Health Service Circular 1998/113 A First Class Service: Quality in the new NHS. NHS; 1998

20 UKCC. Strengthening and supporting the midwifery contribution to maternity care for women and their families. Registrar's Letter 22/2001.

21 North Lakeland Healthcare NHS Trust. Report of Independent Inquiry into Garlands Hospital. 2000.

22 Healthcare Parliamentary Monitor 2000; 250:3.

23 Lister S. Task force ordered in after ten deaths at maternity unit. The Times, 22 April 2005.

24 Lister S. Workload doubled at hospital where ten mothers died. The Times, 2 May 2005.

25 Audit Commission. Online. Available: www.audit-commission.gov.uk/aboutus/index.asp

26 Audit Commission. First class delivery: Improving maternity services in England and Wales. London: HMSO; 1997.

27 NICE. The use of electronic fetal monitoring: Inherited clinical guideline C. London: NICE; 2001.

28 NICE. Online. Available: website www.nice.org.uk

29 Harvey B. Use of CTG monitoring: are recommendations suitable? RCM Midwives 2004; 7(12):518–520.

30 Costello J, Munro J. An audit of the NICE guidelines for the use of electronic fetal monitoring in labour. MIDIRS Midwifery Digest 2003; 13(1):66–68.

31 NICE. Induction of labour: Inherited clinical guideline D. London: NICE; 2001. Online. Available: www.nice.org.uk

32 NICE. Guidance on the use of routine antenatal anti-D prophylaxis for RhD-negative women. London: NICE; 2002.

33 MacKenzie I. Antenatal anti-D prophylaxis: one dose or two? Br J Midwifery 2004; 12(1):13–14, 16–19.

34 Jarvis S. Routine anti-D prophylaxis for RhD negative pregnant women. Br J Midwifery 2003; 11(1):13–15.

35 NICE. Antenatal care: routine care for the healthy pregnant woman. London: NICE; 2003.

36 Jeffery A, Wilkin I. NICE guidelines for routine antenatal care. MIDIRS Midwifery Digest 2004; 14(2):201–202.

37 NICE. Fertility: assessment and treatment for people with fertility problems. London: NICE; 2004.

38 News item. Pre-eclampsia guideline for community midwives. The Practising Midwife 2005; 8(4):9.

39 Action on Pre-eclampsia. Online. Available: www.apec.org.uk

40 Jankowicz D, Tufnell D. Managing pre-eclampsia 1: establishing guidelines. Br J Midwifery 2004; 12(11):687–691.

41 NICE. Social value judgement guidelines, 4 April 2005 DH.

42 Hindle H. The clinical application of evidence-based practice. Br J Midwifery 2001; 9(11):672–675.

43 Department of Health. National Service Framework for mental health services. London: HMSO; 1999.

44 Renton M. The NSF – use it or lose it. The Practising Midwife 2004; 7(11):4–5.

45 Department of Health. White Paper on the NHS: Modern, dependable. London: HMSO; 1997.

46 Department of Health. Switch to Health Care on your TV. Press release 2001/0289.

47 Department of Health. The NHS Plan: A plan for investment, a plan for reform. London: HMSO; 2000.

48 Department of Health. Maternity units receive £100 million to modernise and improve facilities. Press release 2001/0470.

49 Bristol Royal Infirmary. Learning from Bristol: the report of the public inquiry into children's heart surgery at the Bristol Royal Infirmary 1984–1995. 2001. Command Paper CM 5207. Online. Available: www.bristol-inquiry.org.uk

Chapter 22
EMPLOYMENT LAW

It is important for midwives to have a good understanding of the law relating to employment, whether they are employees or independent midwives. Some may be managers who are responsible for other employees and need to know the situation from both the employer's and the employee's perspective. It is impossible in a work of this nature to go fully into the complexities of employment law. The aim is to provide an introduction and understanding of the basic principles so that when necessary the subject can be supplemented with more specialist works listed in the list of Further Reading.

The areas to be considered are shown in Box 22.1.

Box 22.1 Topics considered in this chapter

– Human Rights

– The contract of employment: formation and content

– Changing the contract

– Performance of the contract

– Breach of contract

– Termination of contract

– Sex, race and disability discrimination

– Male midwives

– Rights of part-time staff

– Maternity benefits

– The Working Time Directive

– Whistle-blowing

HUMAN RIGHTS

The human rights set out in Schedule 1 of the Human Rights Act 1998 (see Appendix 1 of this book) apply to employees within the public sector or those working for organisations which exercise functions of a public nature. Employees are able to argue a breach of Article 3 if they are subjected to inhuman or degrading treatment or punishment, or a breach of Article 6 if in the determination of their civil rights and obligations (which of course include rights under a contract of employment) they are not given a fair hearing, or a breach of Article 8 and their right to a private and family life, home and correspondence, or a breach of Article 14 if they suffer discrimination in the recognition of their human rights. Most practising midwives would therefore be able to bring an action in the courts of this country if their human rights as set out in Schedule 1 to the Human Rights Act 1998 are violated (see Ch. 6).

CONTRACT OF EMPLOYMENT

At the heart of the employment relationship is a contract. It may not always be evidenced in writing but it exists as soon as there is agreement by one person to work for another in payment of consideration. The basic principles of contract law apply and in addition there are many Acts of Parliament giving employees rights through employment and regulating the powers of employers and also the rights of workers to combine to withdraw labour. Some of the more significant Statutes are shown in Box 22.2. European Directives have led to changes in employees' rights, and new maternity rights were implemented in October 2002[1] as a result of an EC directive.[2]

Box 22.2 Acts of Parliament covering employment law

Disability Discrimination Act 1995

Employment Acts 1980, 1982, 1988, 1989, 1990, 2002, 2004

Employers Liability (Compulsory Insurance) Act 1969

Employers Liability (Defective Equipment) Act 1969

Employment Protection (Consolidation) Act 1978

Employment Rights (Dispute Resolution) Act 1998

Employment Rights Act 1996

Employment Relations Act 1999

Employment Tribunals Act 1996

Equal Pay Act 1970

Health and Safety at Work Act 1974

Human Rights Act 1998

Industrial Relations Act 1971

National Minimum Wage Act 1998

Race Relations Act 1976

Race Relations (Amendment) Act 2000

Rehabilitation of Offenders Act 1974

Sex Discrimination Acts 1975, 1986

Trade Union Act 1984

Trade Union and Labour Relations (Consolidation) Act 1992

Trade Union Reform and Employment Rights Act 1993

Wages Act 1986

The essential elements of a contract are:

– agreement

– consideration

– intention to be legally binding.

The law recognises that a legally enforceable contract has come into existence when an offer is accepted and the main terms are agreed. In the employment situation, the advertisement and initial applications and interviews would be regarded as preliminary negotiations, part of the invitation to treat. However, statements made then may become part of the terms of the eventual agreement. It is not until an offer is made, usually by the employer to the prospective employee, and this is accepted, that the contract comes into existence. The contract may be conditional, e.g. subject to satisfactory medical examination or subject to the receipt of satisfactory references. Should the medical examination and/or the references not be satisfactory, then the relationship will end or not come into existence.

Many employers fail to put the terms of the contract into writing and thus some employees assume that they have no contract. This is not so. A contract exists in law if there has been this offer and acceptance and if there is no reason, e.g. that it is contrary to public policy, for the contract to be unlawful. There is however a statutory duty for written particulars of the contract to be given to all employees within two months of commencing work. The necessary details are shown in Box 22.3 taken from s.1 of the Employment Rights Act 1996.

Box 22.3 Written statement of the terms must include

- identity of the parties*

- date on which the employment began*

- date when the employee's period of continuous employment began*

- remuneration*

- intervals at which paid*

- holidays*

- sick pay

- pensions

- notice or reference to the law on minimum periods of notice or any collective agreements

- title of job or brief description of the work for which the employee is employed*

- any terms and conditions on hours of work and holidays*

- any disciplinary rules or access to a document setting them out (unless fewer than 20 employees)

- person to whom employee can apply if dissatisfied with any disciplinary decision and how such application should be made

▶

▶ - in case of non-permanent employment, the period for which it is expected to continue

- either the place of work, or, where the employee is required or permitted to work at various places, an indication of that fact and the address of the employer*

- any collective agreement which directly affects the terms and conditions of the employment including, where the employer is not a party, the persons by whom they were made

- details if the employee is required to work outside the UK.

All the items with an asterisk (*) must be included in a single document given to the employee (s.2(4) Employment Rights Act 1996). Those items without an asterisk may be contained in some other document which the employee has reasonable opportunities of reading in the course of her employment or which is made reasonably accessible to her in some other way. The particulars must be provided within 2 months of the beginning of the employment.

Changes to the particulars must be given not later than:

- 1 month after the change, or

- where the change arises from the requirement to work outside the UK for more than 1 month, the time when the employee leaves the UK.

Under the Employment Act 2002, the written statement must include the details of the new minimum statutory disciplinary and dismissal procedures (see below) and this duty is binding on employers of not less than 20 employees. Particulars included in a copy of the contract of employment or letter of engagement can form part of the written statement and an employment tribunal is given power to award compensation to an employee where the lack, incompleteness or inaccuracy of the written statement becomes evident when a claim is made.

The statement is not the contract, which includes other terms.

CONTENT OF THE CONTRACT

Not all terms are agreed at the time the offer is accepted. Box 22.4 shows the variety of terms of which the contract is made.

Box 22.4 Content of contract of employment

– Express terms agreed between the parties at the time the contract is formed.

– Express terms agreed through collective bargaining for that type of post.

– Terms implied by the law imposing duties on both employer and employee.

– Statutory rights given to employer and employee through Acts of Parliament, Regulations and European Directives.

If a midwife applies for a post with an NHS trust, she may be offered employment.

– She will agree with the employer the starting date, the grade and the location and her duties.

– She will be offered commencement at a specific point either on the Whitley Council grade with all the terms and conditions which have been agreed over the years, or she will be offered the terms which the trust has negotiated through local bargaining.

– As an employee she will be expected to recognise the implied duties imposed upon her by law and set out in Box 22.5. She will also have the benefit of the implied duties placed upon her employer by law and set out in Box 22.6.

– As an employee she will be entitled to specific statutory rights which are set out in Box 22.7.

IMPLIED TERMS

The common law (i.e. judge-made law) implies into a contract of employment, however long or short it is, certain duties on both employer and employee (see Box 22.5 and Box 22.6). No specific mention need be made of these during the negotiations leading up to the appointment or in the documents. Yet they are enforceable through the courts of law. If the employer is in breach of any of the implied terms, this, depending upon the circumstances, may be regarded as a fundamental breach such that the employee is entitled to see the contract as at an end (see below). If the employee is in breach of any of the implied terms, disciplinary action may be taken.

Box 22.5 Duties implied by the law and imposed upon employees

– The employee is expected to obey the reasonable orders of the employer.

– The employee owes a duty of cooperation and loyalty to his employer:

442

a. the duty to account

b. to disclose misdeeds

c. not to disclose confidential information

d. to work with care and skill.

Box 22.6 Duties implied by the law and imposed upon employers

– To cooperate with the employees (e.g. not to criticise employees in front of subordinates, not to use foul language, to show proper respect for senior employees).

– To take reasonable care for the safety of his employees.

Legislation has added to the rights of the employees, and a list of some of the statutory rights is shown in Box 22.7.

Box 22.7 Statutory rights

– Written statement of particulars

– Itemised statement of pay

– Maternity benefits

– Payment and limitations on deductions

– Time off work:

  a. to take part in Trade Union activities (unpaid)

  b. if a Trade Union official, to undertake Trade Union duties and training (paid)

  c. reasonable time off to search for work in a redundancy situation (pay for at least 2 days)

  d. to work as member of Local Authority, JP, statutory tribunal, Health Authority or school governor (unpaid)

▶
- Holidays (Bank Holidays)

- Patents

- Guarantee payments

- Unemployment benefit

- Redundancy

- Medical suspension payment.

CHANGING THE CONTRACT

It is a rule of law that a contract cannot be changed unilaterally, i.e. if changes are to be made, they must be agreed either expressly or impliedly by both parties to the contract. If, therefore, a midwife is employed as a community midwife and this is a term of her contract of employment, and she is asked to work in a hospital as a midwife or gynaecology nurse, she is entitled to refuse the change in her contract. Should the employer attempt to force this through, it would be a fundamental breach on his part. Should she agree to the change, then the contract can be amended to reflect the agreement of both parties.

What about the transfer from an NHS trust to a Primary Care Trust?

An employee who is required to transfer from one NHS trust to a Primary Care Trust has protection under the Health Act 1999. In addition, protection in relation to the original terms of contract is given under the Transfer of Undertaking Regulations which ensures that the new employer is bound to accept the contractual conditions which the employees who are now transferred originally enjoyed.

Thus, the same contract provisions will apply initially. The new employer is however entitled to require a change of terms if promotion is being offered. In addition, any new employee can be asked to agree terms which are different from those of the transferred employees.

What if the midwife is forced to agree changes against her will?

The midwife is legally entitled to refuse to accept any changes which were not agreed. Should the employer attempt to force them upon her, she could claim that he is in fundamental breach of the contract and claim an unfair constructive dismissal. However, she needs to look at the situation carefully: is it a redundancy situation, which means that the offer of alternative work and conditions is the choice instead of redundancy? Is the employer's request a reasonable one and has he given reasonable notice of it? The answers to these questions would determine whether or not she would win an unfair dismissal case.

PERFORMANCE OF THE CONTRACT

Both the express and implied terms anticipate that both parties will perform their share of the contract's responsibilities. Failure to perform would be regarded as a breach unless justified by the other party's conduct.

Working to rule has been regarded by the courts as a failure to fulfil the contract even though those working to rule would regard it as technically following the contract exactly. The Court of Appeal[3] has held that withdrawal of cooperation in the form of working to rule can amount to a breach of contract. Similarly, going on strike, i.e. withdrawing labour, is a breach of contract by employees. They are however given certain protection. Should the employer dismiss some of the strikers but not all, that is an unfair dismissal for those who are dismissed. Should the employer dismiss all the strikers and then re-employ some of them, that would be an unfair dismissal of those not re-employed. The employer could sue strikers for damages but since the aim is usually to obtain a return to work this is not a preferred option and the amount of damages would be difficult to calculate. Pay would normally be withheld during a strike. Certain protection is given to trade unions which take industrial action. These are known as 'immunities'. Section 219 of the Trade Union and Labour Relations (Consolidation) Act 1992 provides as follows:

An act done in contemplation or furtherance of a trade dispute shall not be actionable in tort on the ground only that

– *it induces a breach of contract,*

– *that it interferes with a contract,*

– *that it induces any other person to interfere with its performance,*

– *that it constitutes a threat of breach, inducement, or interference, or*

– *that it constitutes a conspiracy to do any of these things.*

There is no immunity in respect of breaches of contract or crime. The words 'trade dispute' are strictly defined and secondary action where employees of firms not involved in the trade dispute are encouraged to take part is not covered by the immunity. Reference should be made to works in the Appendix on further reading for more information relating to the legal position of trade unions and the rights of officials and members.

BREACH OF CONTRACT

Failure to comply with the terms and conditions of contract by either party is a *prima facie* breach of contract.

WHERE THE EMPLOYEE IS IN BREACH

Where the employee is in breach, the employer would be entitled to take disciplinary action which may include dismissal. Statutory requirements in relation to an employer with 20 or more employees include the setting out in the written statement of terms, any disciplinary rules or a reasonably accessible document containing details. The employee must also be notified of a person to whom he can apply if he is dissatisfied with any disciplinary decision and how the application is to be made. Most trusts should have in place a disciplinary procedure and the midwife should ensure that she is familiar with its contents, particularly where she has a managerial function.

Counselling an employee following misconduct or unauthorised absenteeism is not usually regarded as part of the disciplinary procedure. The stages which most procedures recognise are:

– oral warning

– first written warning

– second written warning

– final warning

– suspension and/or dismissal.

Not all these stages have to be followed consecutively and in cases of serious misconduct, instant suspension or a final written warning may be justified.

Unfair dismissal
At common law (i.e. judge-made law), it would be lawful for an employer to give an employee the requisite period of notice and terminate the contract of employment without any specific reason. This would not be unlawful but could clearly be unjust. Statutory provision has therefore been made for the employee to be protected against dismissal which would be regarded as unfair.

The statute recognises that certain reasons will make the dismissal automatically fair. Other reasons may make the dismissal unfair and in certain cases, the dismissal will be automatically unfair. These three categories are shown in Box 22.8.

Definition of dismissal
The definition of dismissal covers the three situations shown in Box 22.9.

Box 22.8 Statutory reasons for fair or unfair dismissal

a. National security

b. Dismissal during a strike or lockout.

Statutory reasons which may make the dismissal fair:

a. Capability and qualifications

b. Misconduct

c. Redundancy

d. Illegality for the employee to continue

e. Some other substantial reason.

Automatically unfair reasons:

a. Dismissal on the grounds of pregnancy or childbirth

b. Dismissal on transfer of undertaking

c. Dismissal in relation to Trade Union membership or activities

d. Dismissal for assertion of a statutory right.

Box 22.9 Definition of dismissal

1. When a contract of employment is terminated by the employer with or without notice.

2. When the contract of employment is for a fixed term and this expires without renewal of the contract.

3. When the employee terminates the contract, with or without notice, in circumstances such that he is entitled to terminate it without notice by reason of the employer's conduct. (This is known as 'constructive dismissal'.)

In addition, leaving early when under notice, taking a new job for a trial period, lay-off and short time working, and implied termination will all count as dismissal for the purposes of statutory protection of the employee against unfair dismissal.

The first situation is the usual form of dismissal. The second situation rarely results in an unfair dismissal claim, since most short-term, fixed-term contracts would have a clause which removed the employee's right to make an application for unfair dismissal if the contract is not renewed.

The third situation in Box 22.9 is commonly known as 'constructive dismissal' and entitles the employee, if she has the requisite continuous service requirement, to claim unfair dismissal. This is discussed below.

Dispute resolution

A statutory dispute resolution is set out in Schedule 2 to the Employment Act 2002. There are two forms: a standard three-step procedure and a modified two-step procedure. There are separate procedures for dealing with grievance issues and for disciplinary matters.

Schedule 2 Part 1 sets out the dismissal and disciplinary procedures.

The standard procedure for dismissal and discipline covers the following three steps:

Step 1: Statement of grounds for action and invitation to meeting

i.   The employer must set out in writing the employee's alleged conduct or characteristics, or other circumstances, which lead him to contemplate dismissing or taking disciplinary action against the employee.

ii. The employer must send the statement or a copy of it to the employee and invite the employee to attend a meeting to discuss the matter.

Step 2: Meeting

i.   The meeting must take place before action is taken, except in the case where the disciplinary action consists of suspension.

ii. The meeting must not take place unless:

  a. the employer has informed the employee what the basis was for including in the statement under Para. 1(1) the ground or grounds given in it and

  b. the employee has had a reasonable opportunity to consider his response to that information

iii. The employee must take all reasonable steps to attend the meeting.

iv. After the meeting, the employer must inform the employee of his decision and notify him of the right to appeal against the decision if he is not satisfied with it.

Step 3 Appeal

i.   If the employee does wish to appeal, he must inform the employer.

ii.   If the employee informs the employer of his wish to appeal, the employer must invite him to attend a further meeting.

iii. The employee must take all reasonable steps to attend the hearing.

iv.   The appeal meeting need not take place before the dismissal or disciplinary action takes effect.

v.   After the appeal meeting, the employer must inform the employee of his final decision.

The modified procedure for dismissal and discipline has two steps:

Step 1: Statement of grounds for action

The employer must:

i.   Set out in writing:

    a. The employee's alleged misconduct which has led to the dismissal

    b. What the basis was for thinking at the time of the dismissal that the employee was guilty of the alleged misconduct, and

    c. The employee's right to appeal against dismissal, and

ii.   Send the statement or a copy of it to the employee.

Step 2: Appeal

i.   If the employee does wish to appeal, he must inform the employer.

ii.   If the employee informs the employer of his wish to appeal, the employer must invite him to attend a meeting.

iii. The employee must take all reasonable steps to attend the hearing.

iv.   After the appeal meeting, the employer must inform the employee of his final decision.

Procedure for grievances

Schedule 2 Part 2 sets out the procedure for grievances.

The standard procedure for grievances has three steps:

Step 1: Statement of grievance

The employee must set out the grievance in writing and send the statement or a copy of it to the employer.

Step 2: Meeting

1. The employer must invite the employee to attend a meeting to discuss the grievance.

2. The meeting must not take place unless:

   a. the employee has informed the employer what the basis for the grievance was when he made the statement under the above paragraph.

   b. The employer has had a reasonable opportunity to consider his response to that information.

3. The employee must take all reasonable steps to attend the meeting.

4. After the meeting, the employer must inform the employee of his decisions as to his response to the grievance and notify him of the right to appeal against the decision if he is not satisfied with it.

Step 3: Appeal

1. If the employee does not wish to appeal, he must inform the employer.

2. If the employee informs the employer of his wish to appeal, the employer must invite him to attend a further meeting.

3. The employee must take all reasonable steps to attend the meeting.

4. After the appeal meeting, the employer must inform the employee of the final decision.

Modified procedure for grievances in two stages
Step 1: Statement of grievance

1. The employee must:

   a. set out in writing:

      i. the grievance and

      ii. the basis for it and

   b. send the statement or a copy of it to the employer.

Step 2: The response

The employer must set out his response in writing and send the statement or a copy of it to the employee.

General requirements
In addition to the new procedures for disciplinary and grievance matters, Schedule 2 to the Act sets out general requirements which must be followed by the parties. These are shown in Box 22.10.

Box 22.10 General requirements of the procedures

- Each step and action under the procedure must be taken without unreasonable delay.

- Timing and location of meetings must be reasonable.

- Meetings must be conducted in a manner that enables both employer and employee to explain their cases.

- In the case of appeal meetings which are not the first meeting, the employer should, as far as is reasonably practicable, be represented by a more senior manager than attended the first meeting (unless the most senior manager attended that meeting).

- The employee has a right to be accompanied to these meetings (s.10 of the Employment Relations Act 1999).

The aim of these procedural requirements is to facilitate agreement between the parties. Because it is recognised that where former employees are involved and a case of constructive dismissal is being brought, it would not be appropriate to expect the former employee to return to the work place for discussions with the employer, the modified procedures are available and matters can be considered by correspondence if that would be preferable. The modified procedure would apply in disciplinary cases, where there has been a situation of summary dismissal on the basis of gross misconduct.

To illustrate the importance attached to these new dispute resolutions, under s.30 of the Employment Act 2002, it is a statutory requirement that a contract of employment shall require every employee and employer to comply with the new statutory procedure for dispute resolution. Furthermore, s.31 enables an employment tribunal to take into account the failure of either party to comply with the dispute procedure by varying the award which it makes.

Unfair dismissal: the procedures

If an employee alleges that there has been an unfair dismissal and she has worked for at least 1 year, she has the right to apply to an employment tribunal for unfair dismissal. If the dismissal is in the circumstances listed in the third category shown in Box 22.8, no continuous service requirement is necessary.

New procedures have been introduced whereby the Advisory, Conciliation and Arbitration Service (ACAS) will attempt to secure a reconciliation between the parties. In 2001, ACAS issued a guide to the scheme to resolve unfair dismissal disputes. This new scheme is an alternative to a hearing before an employment tribunal and is set up under the Employment Rights (Dispute Resolution) Act 1998 and the statutory instrument.[4] Further details are available from ACAS.[5]

The employer must show:

a. What was the reason for the dismissal. The onus is on the employer to establish the reason.

b. Where the reason is potentially fair (rather than automatically fair), the tribunal has to decide if the employer acted reasonably in all the circumstances in treating the reason as justifying the dismissal.

The circumstances taken into account in deciding the reasonableness of the employer's actions include:

– whether the employer followed an agreed procedure (this may include the giving of a warning)

– whether the principles of natural justice were followed, e.g. the employee was allowed to speak in her own defence

– whether the employer has been consistent in his dealings with employees.

If the employee's claim for unfair dismissal is upheld, the following remedies are available:

– reinstatement

– re-engagement

– compensation.

The basic award of compensation is calculated on the number of years of continuous service of the employee.

In addition, a compensatory award provides what is just and equitable as compensation having regard to the loss suffered as a result of the dismissal.

Both the basic award and the compensatory award can be reduced owing to failure of the employee to mitigate (reduce or offset) the loss or on account of the contributory fault of the employee. If the employee is found to have contributed to the dismissal, the award of compensation may be reduced by as much as 100%.

WHERE THE EMPLOYER IS IN BREACH OF CONTRACT

Where it is the employer who is in breach of contract, the employee has the option of continuing with the contract and seeking damages for the breach or of deciding that the breach by the employer has brought the contract to an end and that therefore she is entitled to see the contract as terminated. This is the constructive dismissal situation shown in Box 22.9. If the employee has the necessary continuous service requirements, where this is required, she can pursue an action in the employment tribunal for unfair dismissal.

TERMINATION OF CONTRACT

A contract of employment can end in the ways shown in Box 22.11.

Box 22.11 Ways of ending a contract of employment

- Notice

- Performance

- Termination by agreement

- Breach of contract

- Frustration

NOTICE GIVEN BY EITHER PARTY

The employer must give:

- 1 week's notice to an employee who has served him for between 1 month and 2 years
- 1 week for each year served up to a maximum of 12 weeks for 12 years.

The employee must give:

- at least 1 week's notice if employed for more than 1 month (Employment Rights Act 1996 ss.86 and 87).

It is open to the parties to agree different lengths of notice than those specified by statute. Where the parties fail to provide for notice lengths, the common law will imply a reasonable length depending upon the seniority of the post and the intervals of payment.

Sometimes, rather than provide the notice time, an employer might prefer to give the employee pay in lieu of notice.

PERFORMANCE

Where the contract is for a fixed term then the expiry of that fixed term will bring the contract to an end. However, as we have seen, failure to renew the contract counts as a dismissal.

TERMINATION BY AGREEMENT

It is possible for the parties to agree together that the contract can be ended without the set notice periods running. In this situation, there would be no dismissal.

BREACH OF CONTRACT

If either party is in fundamental breach of contract, this entitles the other party to see the contract as at an end. The employer might dismiss the employee (subject of course to the employee's statutory right to claim unfair dismissal); the employee might consider himself released from his contractual obligations and claim that he has been constructively dismissed.

FRUSTRATION

This is a concept in law which covers the situation where the intention of the parties when the contract was first arranged has been made impossible to perform and the contract thus comes to an end by operation of law. No notice is required, nor dismissal. A lengthy prison term, which makes it impossible for the employee to perform his job, would be a frustrating event. In one case[6] an employee was suspended from medical practice and his name temporarily removed from the Register; this was considered to be a frustrating event so as to bring the contract of employment to an end by operation of law.

Where the contract is terminated through frustration, the employer does not have to dismiss the employee and the employee has no claim for unfair dismissal. Because it is not always clear if the event would actually constitute frustration in law, it is wiser for an employer to assume that the contract is continuing and regard the event as potential grounds for fair dismissal and act reasonably in all the circumstances of the case. Because of the injustices of this situation, certain remedies are available under the Law Reform (Frustrated Contracts) Act 1943.

SEX, RACE AND DISABILITY DISCRIMINATION

Statutory rights to be protected against unlawful discrimination on the grounds of sex or race are given by the Sex Discrimination Acts 1975 and 1986 and the Race

Relations Act 1976. The Acts prevent direct discrimination, indirect discrimination and victimisation. However, there are many exceptions to unlawful discrimination. For example, discrimination is justified on grounds of sex and race where a genuine occupational qualification requires a specific sex or race. A European Council Directive[7] sets out the definition of indirect discrimination for the purposes of the principle of equal treatment and requires each Member State to take such measures as are necessary to ensure that in complaints of sex discrimination before a court or other competent authority, the burden is on the complainant initially to establish facts from which the court or competent authority may presume there has been direct or indirect discrimination. Thereafter the burden of proof shifts to the person who has allegedly discriminated against the complainant to prove that there has been no such discrimination. The Directive has been followed by statutory regulations.[8]

Under The Race Relations (Amendment) Act 2000 a 'General Statutory Duty' is placed upon the organisations which are listed in Schedule 1A of the Act. Under this duty, public authorities are required to have due regard to the need:

1. to eliminate unlawful racial discrimination and

2. to promote equality of opportunity and good relations between persons of different racial groups.

Each public authority is required to publish a Race Equality Scheme in accordance with the general and specific duties set out in the legislation.

Under Article 13 of the Treaty of Amsterdam, the European Council can take action to combat discrimination based on sex, racial or ethnic origin, religion or belief, disability, age or sexual orientation. In 2000, the EC issued an Employment Directive and a Race Directive[9] which require member states to introduce, if not already in existence, measures to combat discrimination.

Midwives who care for ethnic minorities should ensure that as far as possible their specific needs should be taken into account in the provision of services for them. However, there is no legal requirement that the midwife should be of a specific race. A midwife was awarded £41 720 compensation for persistent racial discrimination. Her complaints of racial discrimination were not taken seriously by her employers, who failed to carry out an investigation.[10] In 2004, a black nurse was awarded £20 000 because she was prevented from looking after a white baby[11] (see Ch. 19 for further details of this case).

Reference should be made to Further Reading for further information relating to the statutory provisions on discrimination and equal pay. The RCM has published a position paper on racism and maternity services[12] and the rights of employees.[13] The Department of Health set targets for the ending of racial harassment as part of a national strategy.[14,15]

THE DISABILITY DISCRIMINATION ACT 1995

The Disability Discrimination Act 1995 protects disabled people from discrimination in the areas of:

– access to goods, facilities and services

– buying or renting land and property, and

– employment.

It has been brought into force in several stages and came completely into force in October 2004.

A person is disabled if they have a physical or mental impairment which has a substantial and long-term adverse effect on their ability to carry out normal day-to-day activities. Long-term means 'lasting' or likely to last at least 12 months. There must be an effect on at least one of the following aspects:

– Mobility

– Manual dexterity

– Physical coordination

– Continence

– Ability to lift, carry or otherwise move everyday objects

– Speech

– Hearing or eyesight

– Memory or ability to concentrate, learn or understand

– Perception of the risk of physical danger.

Discrimination occurs if a disabled person is treated less favourably than a person without a disability. A National Disability Council was established which, following consultation, advised the Secretary of State on relevant matters as requested, and prepared Codes of Practice. It was replaced in April 2000 by the Disability Rights Commission. The Commission can sue any company that denied equal treatment to disabled people. In March 2001 the Disability Rights Commission published details of a new service to settle discrimination disputes called the Disability Conciliation Service.[16]

NEW COMMISSION FOR EQUALITY AND HUMAN RIGHTS

The Joint Committee on Human Rights in its sixth report[17] recommended that human rights and equalities functions should be integrated within one body. Following these recommendations and the feedback from its consultation document

'Equality and Diversity: Making in Happen',[18] the Government announced in October 2003 that it was preparing a White Paper on the establishment of a new Commission for Equality and Human Rights. The White Paper 'Fairness For All'[19] was published in May 2004 and envisaged the replacement of the Equal Opportunities Commission, the Commission for Racial Harassment and the Disability Rights Commission, by new Commission in 2006.

MALE MIDWIVES

Under the Sex Discrimination Act 1975 s.20, the employment, training, promotion and transfer of men as midwives were restricted. These restrictions were brought to an end by Statutory Instrument in 1983[20] and implemented from 1 January 1984.[21] Health Authorities were notified that in implementing these changes they should make appropriate arrangements to ensure that women have freedom of choice to be attended by a female midwife and that where male midwives are employed, provision is made for them to be chaperoned as necessary. In the statistics for 2003–2004 (see Ch. 2), the number of midwives with an effective registration was: women: 33 578 and men: 108 (not recorded: 1).

RIGHTS OF PART-TIME STAFF

On 1 July 2000, regulations came into force to prevent part-time workers being treated less favourably than full-time workers,[22] implementing the European Directive.[23] Paragraph 5 of these regulations gives the part-time worker:

the right not to be treated by his employer less favourably than the employer treats a comparable full-time worker

– *as regards the terms of his contract, or*

– *by being subjected to any other detriment by any act, or deliberate failure to act of his employer.*

Any worker who considers that his rights have been infringed can present a complaint to an employment tribunal within 3 months of the day of less favourable treatment or detriment taking place. This is subject to the right of the tribunal to consider out-of-time cases, if in all the circumstances it is just and equitable to do so.

MATERNITY RIGHTS AND BENEFITS

In addition to any contractual rights that an employee has, they may also be entitled to many statutory provisions for the pregnant employee. These include:

- Time off for antenatal care

- Protection against detriment or dismissal on grounds of pregnancy or childbirth

- Maternity leave

- Maternity benefit

- Return to work after maternity leave

- Entitlements on redundancy during maternity leave

- Special provisions on health and safety while pregnant or breast feeding

- Protection against sex discrimination.

Each benefit is subject to qualifications and conditions and further details on each is available from the DTI website.[24] Further amendments have been made to the current maternity benefits by 2005 Regulations which provide for continuity of employment where a person is dismissed and following the statutory dispute resolution procedure is reinstated or re-engaged.[25]

In addition to these employee-related benefits, maternity benefits are available from Social Security. The Maternity Alliance provides update information on these.[26]

THE EUROPEAN WORKING TIME DIRECTIVE (EWTD)

A Directive had been adopted by the member states of the European Community on 23 November 1996, but implementation in the UK was delayed until 1 October 1998, when the Working Time Regulations[27] came into force.[28,29] The fundamental provision is that a worker's working time, including overtime, should not exceed an average of 48 hours for each period of 7 days over a specified period of 17 weeks. Regulations also specify provisions for rest breaks and annual leave. Night work should not normally exceed an average of 8 hours for each 24 hours. There is an entitlement of annual leave of 4 weeks' paid leave in each holiday year.

Doctors in training, and civil protection services (ambulance) were initially specifically excluded from the Regulations. NMC practitioners are not specifically excluded. However, they come within the definition of the group:

where the worker's activities involve the need for continuity of service or production, as the case may be, in relation to:

- *services relating to the reception, treatment or care provided by hospitals or similar establishments, residential institutions and prisons.*

The effect of this is that the Regulations on night work, daily rest, weekly rest period, and rest breaks do not apply to NMC practitioners where there is a need for continuity of service. However, Regulation 24 requires that where a worker is required to work during a period which would otherwise be a rest period or rest break, the employer shall wherever possible allow her to take an equivalent period of compensatory rest and in exceptional cases, where this is not possible, the employer shall afford her such protection as may be appropriate in order to safeguard the worker's health and safety.

The meaning of rest break was considered by the Court of Appeal[30] where it was held that a rest break was an uninterrupted period of at least 20 min that was neither a rest period nor working time, both of which were defined at Regulation 2(1).

The General Whitley Council (GWC) has agreed the implementation of the Regulations for non-medical staff.[31] Section 44 of the GWC Handbook sets out the new provisions which apply to all non-medical staff.

Individual employees can, if they wish, agree to work more than the average of 48 hours a week. However, this must be an individual decision.

The Working Time Directive was applied to junior doctors from August 2004. The British Medical Association issued a press release about the implications of its implementation.[32] Guidance on working patterns for junior doctors was issued by the Department of Health.[33] Resources were allocated to Strategic health authorities in respect of the Working Time Directive strategic change fund.[34]

INFORMATION AND CONSULTATION WITH EMPLOYEES

New Regulations[35] came into force on 6 April 2005, which establish a general framework for improving information and consultation rights of employees in the EC. From 6 April 2005, employers with 150 or more employees will have a right to be informed and consulted on a regular basis about issues in the organisation they work for. From April 2007 this will cover organisations with 100 or more employees and from April 2009 those with 50 or more employees. Further information is available from the Department of Trade and Industry website.[24]

WHISTLE-BLOWING

This is the term which refers to a person (usually an employee) who draws attention to concerns which have health and safety implications. Because of a fear that persons, many of whom had a professional duty to draw attention to dangers and hazards, would be victimised as a result of their actions, the Department of Health issued a circular recommending that each trust and Authority should set up a procedure whereby an individual employee could draw these concerns to the management internally without being victimised and thus not needing to bring in the media or other external bodies.

The need to establish statutory protection for employees who raised concerns led to the passing of the Public Interest Disclosure Act 1998.

PUBLIC INTEREST DISCLOSURE ACT 1998

The Public Interest Disclosure Act received the royal assent on 2 July 1998 and came into force on 2 July 1999. It introduces amendments to the Employment Rights Act 1996. The explanatory memorandum envisages that the Act will protect workers who disclose information about certain types of matters from being dismissed or penalised by their employers as a result. The Act applies to specific disclosures:

– that a criminal offence has been committed, is being committed or is likely to be committed

– that a person has failed, is failing or is likely to fail to comply with any legal obligation to which he is subject

– that a miscarriage of justice has occurred, is occurring or is likely to occur

– that the health or safety of any individual has been, is being or is likely to be endangered

– that the environment has been, is being or is likely to be damaged, or

– that information tending to show any matter falling within any one of the preceding paragraphs has been, is being or is likely to be deliberately concealed.

To qualify for protection, the worker making the disclosure must:

– Make the disclosure to his employer or to another person to whom the failure relates or who has legal responsibility

– Be acting in good faith.

Protected disclosures include:

– Disclosures made to obtain legal advice

– Disclosures to a Minister of the Crown if the employee's employer is appointed by the Crown.

Any provision in an agreement between employer and worker is void if it purports to preclude the worker from making a protected disclosure.

Guidance has been issued by the Department of Health,[36] which requires every NHS trust and Health Authority to have in place local policies and procedures which comply with the provisions of the Act.

In one of the first cases to be reported after the coming into force of the Act, compensation of more than £250 000 was awarded.

Box 22.12 Compensation for a whistle-blower[37]

An accountant who was dismissed after blowing the whistle on his managing director's expenses claims was awarded compensation of £293 441 by an employment tribunal. The Tribunal held that he was victimised by his employers for raising genuine concerns.

CONCLUSIONS

Like many other areas of law, employment law is constantly changing as new Statutes, Directives and Regulations are introduced as a result of changes to the law in the European Community, and the courts then determine how these statutory provisions are to be interpreted. In addition, the incorporation of the European Convention on Human Rights into the laws of the UK has enabled employees to bring actions against their public authority employers if there is an alleged violation of their human rights. Changes may follow reports by the Equal Opportunities Commission that employers are not giving pregnant employees their entitlements, partly because of the ignorance of pregnant employees.[38] The EOC has suggested that a written statement of maternity rights and responsibilities should be given to every pregnant woman at her first antenatal visit with a tear-off copy to hand to her employer. Clearly, midwives will have a significant role in ensuring that this is implemented. At the time of writing, 'Agenda for Change' is being implemented across the NHS and each midwife is personally involved in assessing the scope and level of responsibility of her post.

QUESTIONS AND EXERCISES

1. Examine the written particulars of your contract and compare them with the list shown in Box 22.3. Are there any other terms which you consider should be included?

2. The trust has decided that in view of future uncertainties, midwives will be placed on fixed-term contracts. What are your rights in this situation?

3. A colleague is facing disciplinary action as a result of pointing out the need for improved staffing levels. Advise her on the legal situation. Refer also to Chapter 19 on health and safety.

References

1 Maternity and Parental Leave (Amendment) Regulations 2002 SI 2002 No 2789.

2 EC Directive 96/34 [1996] OJL 1451/14.

3 Secretary of State for Employment v. ASLEF (No. 2) [1972] 2 All ER 949.

4 ACAS Arbitration Scheme (England and Wales) Order 2001 SI 2001 No 1185.

5 ACAS. The ACAS arbitration scheme for the resolution of unfair dismissal disputes: a guide to the scheme. 2001. Online. Available: www.acas.org.uk/arbitration.htm

6 Tarnesby v. Kensington and Chelsea AHA [1981] IRLR 369.

7 Council Directive 97/80 [1998] OJL 14/6.

8 Sex Discrimination (Indirect Discrimination and the Burden of Proof) Regulations 2001 SI 2660.

9 EC Directive 2000/43 EC 29 June 2000.

10 Royal College of Midwives. Race case midwife awarded substantial compensation. London: RCM; 1997.

11 Purves R. Racist abuse ruined my life. Nursing Times 2004; 100(32):24–25.

12 Royal College of Midwives. Racism and the maternity services. London: RCM; 2000.

13 Royal College of Midwives. Know your rights 4: Racial harassment. RCM Midwives J 2001; 4(5):146–147.

14 Department of Health. New plan to end racial harassment in the NHS. London: DoH; 1998.

15 Department of Health. Tough action to tackle racism. London: DoH; 1999.

16 Disability Rights Commission. Press release: New Service to settle discrimination disputes launched by the DRC; 2001.

17 Joint Committee on Human Rights Sixth Report, March 2003.

18 Department of Trade and Industry. Equality and diversity: Making it happen. DTI; 2003.

19 Department of Trade and Industry and Department of Constitutional Affairs. Fairness for all: A new Commission for Equality and Human Rights. DTI/DCA; 2004.

20 Statutory Instrument 1983 No. 1202.

21 Statutory Instrument 1983 No. 1841.

22 The Part-time Workers (Prevention of Less Favourable Treatment) Regulations 2000, SI No 1551 and SI 2001 No 1107.

23 Directive 97/81/EC; Part-time Work Directive as extended to the UK by Directive 98/23/EC.

24 Department of Trade and Industry. Online. Available: www.dti.gov.uk

25 Statutory Maternity Pay (General) and the Statutory Paternity Pay and the Statutory Adoption Pay (General) (Amendment) Regulations 2005, SI 2005 No 358.

26 Maternity Alliance. Contact: 45 Beech Street, London EC2P 2LX; Tel: 020 7588 8583; Fax: 020 7588 8584; e-mail: ma@mail.pro-net.co.uk

27 Working Time Regulations 1998, SI 1998 No 1833.

28 NHS Executive. Working Time Regulations: Implementation in the NHS. Health Service 1998; Circular (98)204.

29 Department of Trade and Industry. A Guide to the Working Time Regulations. URN 1998/894. Online. Available: www.dti.gov.uk

30 Gallagher v. Alpha Catering Services Ltd [2004] EWCA Civ 1559; [2005] I.R.L.R. 102.

31 NHS Advance letter (GC) 3/98, 18 November 1998; see DoH website (www.dh.gov.uk) for further information on the EWTD.

32 British Medical Association. Still time to meet Euro hours law, trusts told. Press release, June 2004.

33 Department of Health. Guidance on working patterns for junior doctors. DoH; November 2002.

34 Department of Health. Resource and cash limit adjustment in respect of the working time directive strategic change fund. DoH; June 2004.

35 Information and Consultation of Employees Regulations 2004, SI 2004 No 3426.

36 Department of Health. Public Interest Disclosure Act. Health Service Circular (99)198.

37 Booth J. Man who shopped boss wins £290 000. The Times, 11 July 2000.

38 Equal Opportunity Commission. Great Expectations. Final report on pregnancy discrimination. EOC; June 2005.

Chapter 23

THE INDEPENDENT MIDWIFE AND PRIVATE MATERNITY HOSPITALS

This chapter explores the legal issues relating to the independent midwife. It also considers the legal situation of private maternity hospitals in which many midwives are employed.

INDEPENDENT MIDWIVES

In Chapter 22, we looked at the situation of employed midwives and the terms of the contract of employment. The vast majority of midwives are employed. As can be seen from Chapter 2, out of a total number of 33 687 practising midwives in the UK only 44 are identified as working in private practice and 468 working in a private institution.

The employed midwives (whether working for the NHS or for a private employer) enjoy not only the contractual and statutory rights which are given to them by virtue of their employment, they also enjoy the indemnity of the employer who on the basis of his vicarious liability for the employee will pay out to those harmed by the negligence of the employee the compensation due (see Ch. 13). Here we look at the situation of the independent midwife.[1]

The independent midwife is self-employed. She has no employer and is comparable with a small business person. This section on independent midwives will look at those issues set out in Box 23.1.

Box 23.1 Legal issues and the private practitioner

Contract for services: not contract of employment

- No vicarious liability

- No indemnity by employer

▶

▶

- Contracts with trusts

- No employee rights

- Personal liability for health and safety of self and others

- Liable for breach of contract.

In addition, since the independent midwife is a self-employed contractor, she must ensure that she has an understanding of the topics set out in Box 23.2.

It is impossible in a work of this kind to look in detail at all the topics listed in Box 23.2. Advice on running a business is provided[2] and the independent midwife should refer to specialist books on the different areas. Helpful guidance on setting up in independent practice with details of the equipment she would require, money matters, marketing and other concerns is provided by the independent midwife Lesley Hobbs.[3] The independent midwife should also remember that like any employed midwife she is bound by the Midwives Rules, standards and guidance from the NMC and by the rules, standards and guidance relating to supervision. She should also be aware that if she employs others, then as an employer she has statutory and contractual duties under health and safety legislation.

Box 23.2 The independent midwife and business law

- Inland revenue and VAT

- National insurance: self and employees

- Insurance and indemnity

- Health and safety regulations – personal accident cover

- Contracts for supplies and services

- Training and development

- Employment law

- Data protection regulations

- Pensions and sickness

▶

▶

– Formation of business

  - Type: Sole trader

        Partnership

        Limited company

        Cooperative

  - Name

  - Protection through patents

– Registering designs

– Premises

  - Planning permission

  - Building regulations

  - The lease

– Special trades

  - Trading laws

– Sale of goods and services

  - Trade descriptions acts

– Unfair Contract Terms Act

– UKCC advisory paper on advertising

– Taxation and starting up

– Capital allowances

– Deciding on the tax year.

EMPLOYEES AND VICARIOUS LIABILITY

All employees are covered for indemnity payments by their employers provided that the unlawful or negligent acts which lead to compensation being payable take place during the 'course of employment'. This is discussed in full in Chapter 13.

Midwives who are employed by an NHS trust, whether acute or community, or by a Primary Care Trust, or who work in a private hospital, are covered by the vicarious liability of the employer. Even if a midwife is personally sued, it would be the usual procedure for the employer to accept liability if it can be established that the negligent person was an employee acting in the course of employment. The employer could of course dispute that the act was carried out in the course of employment, but recent case law has made this more difficult[4] (see Ch. 13).

INDEPENDENT MIDWIVES

Independent midwives are self-employed. Even though they have to have a Supervisor of Midwives (or often supervisors), who may be a midwife manager in a nearby hospital, the fact of supervision does not make the supervisor liable for the negligence of the midwife, nor does it make the supervisor's employer vicariously liable for the negligence of the independent midwife.

Independent midwives therefore have to ensure that they have adequate insurance cover to protect them against the claims and which would cover not only their legal expenses but also the compensation payable. Such indemnity cover must be sufficient to cover the greatest sum likely to be awarded and be upgraded each year to cover any inflationary rises.

In August 1993 the RCM was advised that higher insurance premiums would be payable in respect of independent midwives who had previously enjoyed the same insurance cover as their employed colleagues via the RCM. An additional cost of almost £500 000 was requested but it was made clear this would not be required if self-employed midwives were excluded from protection. After the failure of attempts to renegotiate the insurance cover, the RCM notified the self-employed midwives that their cover via the RCM would terminate on 31 March 1994. As a consequence independent midwives were required to pay £4950 per annum premium for indemnity insurance.[5] In 1997, £10 000 premium was required by the MDU to provide insurance for an independent midwife. This led to many midwives giving up independent practice. Obtaining reasonable insurance cover for independent midwives to practise is still an on-going concern.

The NMC has amended its Code of Professional Conduct to include a recommendation that registered practitioners should obtain professional indemnity cover. Clause 9 was added to the Code and took effect from August 2004. It states:

9.1 The NMC recommends that a registered nurse, midwife or specialist community public health nurse, in advising, treating and caring for patients/clients, has professional indemnity insurance. This is in the interests of clients, patients and registrants in the event of claims of professional negligence.

9.2 Some employers accept vicarious liability for the negligent acts and/or omissions of their employees. Such cover does not normally extend to activities undertaken outside the registrant's employment. Independent practice would not normally be covered by vicarious liability, while agency work may not. It is the individual registrant's responsibility to establish their insurance status and take appropriate action.

9.3 In situations where employers do not accept vicarious liability, the NMC recommends that registrants obtain adequate professional indemnity insurance. If unable to secure professional indemnity insurance, a registrant will need to demonstrate that all their clients/patients are fully informed of this fact and the implications this might have in the event of a claim for professional negligence.[6]

The Clause is considered in Chapter 13 in respect of employed midwives. The last paragraph considers the situation where registrants are unable to secure professional indemnity insurance. It does not cover the situation, often encountered by independent midwives, where insurance cover can be obtained, but at such a high premium (over £10 000/year) that it is unaffordable. If the independent midwife decides that she cannot afford this cover, the NMC would clearly expect her to notify the client and advise her that in the event of any alleged incident, there is no cover to pay compensation.

Insurance cover is also essential for the car, for any equipment used, for negligence by any employees employed by the independent midwife and for personal injuries. Insurance cover for any legal expenses is also useful.

EXCLUDING LIABILITY

Could the independent midwife ask the mother to agree to use her services on the understanding that the mother would accept all the risks and in the event of negligence occurring would not sue her?

Such an arrangement could constitute either an exclusion of liability by the midwife or a voluntary assumption of risk by the mother. The former is prohibited by the Unfair Contract Terms Act 1977 which prevents a person excluding herself from liability in the event of her negligence causing personal injury or death. The latter would only be valid if it can be shown that the person voluntarily assuming all the risks of negligence had all these risks spelt out and agreed not to sue in respect of these risks. Clearly, if the kind of negligence which arose had not been contemplated

469

by the parties, it would be outside the agreement and the mother could bring a claim. Such a defence as voluntary assumption of risk would be fraught with difficulties in these circumstances and there may well be a view that it is not professionally acceptable for the midwife to reach such an agreement since it deprives the mother of a legitimate claim for compensation.

If the independent midwife were to take the risk and not pay for insurance cover and was sued successfully by a claimant, she would find that any assets which she owned (e.g. house, car and other property) could be taken by bailiffs in satisfaction of any debt, subject to the exclusion of certain statutory necessities (e.g. bed and tools of her trade).

CONTRACTS WITH TRUSTS

When an independent midwife works in a hospital to take part in the delivery of her own patient, it is often customary to provide an honorary contract. An example of the content which might be included is shown in Box 23.3.

Box 23.3 Contents of an honorary contract

Names of parties

Duration of the contract

Duty of the midwife to take out indemnity insurance cover

Duty of midwife in arranging admission of patient

Procedure on arrival in hospital

Provisions for the subsequent care of the patient, covering such issues as:

- relationship between the independent midwife and the hospital midwives

- any procedures which the independent midwife may not perform in the hospital

- record keeping and documentation

- drugs

- equipment

– procedure following delivery

– subsequent care.

HONORARY CONTRACTS AND THE LAW

Honorary contracts have not, to the author's knowledge, been the subject of any court decision on their legality.

Contractual requirement of consideration

The honorary contract would not be considered valid as an agreement with binding contractual force unless there was an element of reciprocity. If the agreement simply said 'the independent midwife can use our facilities', what has the midwife done in return for this undertaking? An agreement where there is no consideration (i.e. some act/payment/token) is not a valid contract in law. To be binding, a promise to do/give/ perform etc. where there is no consideration must be made under seal. Thus, if a wealthy grandfather were to sign a deed promising to pay money to his grandchild and it was made under seal then the grandchild could enforce the payment. Alternatively, the grandfather could promise to give money to his grandson provided 'he wore my tartan shirt once a week'. This element of reciprocity would then count as considera- tion and the promise could be enforced even though it were not under seal.

If it can be shown that the midwife does indeed perform some service for the trust, the honorary contract to permit her to use the premises and facilities might then be enforceable.

Accountability of the independent midwife remains

The honorary contract usually makes it clear that the independent midwife remains personally and professionally accountable for her care of the patient. However, there could be considerable difficulties in determining liability.

Disputes over liability

What if the contract requires the independent midwife to use the equipment pro- vided by the hospital, and the midwife alleges that harm occurred because this was defective? Such a claim is likely to be disputed by the hospital who might claim that any harm to the patient was entirely caused by the midwife. In addition, the inde- pendent midwife will be working with a team of hospital midwives and doctors in the delivery suite and when harm occurs it is not always easy to pinpoint which person in the team caused the harm. The courts do not accept any principle of team liability and each and every member of the team is personally and professionally accountable for his/her actions.

If harm occurs, where does the claimant stand?

If a mother or baby is harmed following delivery by an independent midwife in an NHS hospital working alongside NHS employees and there then follows a dispute over liability between the independent midwife and the others on the team who are employed by the trust, it is likely that the patient would bring a claim against the trust. The latter could then bring in the independent midwife as a third party and if found liable could claim an indemnity against the independent midwife. At the heart of the dispute would be the issue of causation and which of the many persons involved caused the harm and were in breach of their duty of care.

What if the independent midwife is injured?

The honorary contract should not affect the duty of care owed to the independent midwife as a visitor to the hospital. If she is injured on the premises, the same obligations would be owed to her under the Occupier's Liability Act 1957 as are owed to any other visitor. The occupier would be the NHS trust or the Primary Care Trust. It might even be an independent contractor if the harm has occurred because of the negligence of one of its employees on site (see Ch. 19).

Would the independent midwife be regarded as an employee for the purposes of the employer's duty to care for the health and safety of his employees?

While not an employee, the independent midwife is comparable with a volunteer coming onto the premises to assist in the working of the organisation. There are guidelines which suggest that volunteers should be the recipients of the same duty of care that the employer owes to his employees. Thus if the independent midwife is infected as a result of the negligence of an employee of the trust or Health Authority, she should be compensated by the employer. A duty of care would be owed to her in the law of negligence and she might be able to sue the NHS organisation for its direct responsibility in failing to take reasonable care of her safety or for its vicarious liability for the negligence of an employee. In addition, under s.3 of the Health and Safety at Work Act 1974 (see Ch. 19), an employer has a general duty to ensure the reasonable health and safety of the public at large, which would include the independent midwife working in a hospital.

NO EMPLOYEE RIGHTS

The independent midwife cannot benefit from the statutory rights which the law gives to the employee (see Ch. 22). However, if she herself employs staff, she will have to ensure that she enables them to have the rights to which they are entitled.

PERSONAL LIABILITY FOR THE HEALTH AND SAFETY OF HERSELF AND OTHERS

In Chapter 19, the laws on health and safety were considered. Most of the duties under the Health and Safety at Work Act 1974 and the Regulations under it are binding on the self-employed person who employs others. The independent midwife is therefore required to ensure that she observes the Regulations. Ignorance of the law is no defence to a prosecution for breach of the regulations.

LIABILITY FOR BREACH OF CONTRACT

Box 23.4 shows some of the different parties with whom the independent midwife may contract.

Box 23.4 Contracting parties for the independent midwife

- Private patients

- NHS Trusts

- Primary Care Trusts

- Care Trusts

- General Practitioners

- Private hospitals

- Agencies

- Charities and voluntary bodies

When the independent midwife agrees a contract with a client, that agreement would be subject to the same laws which bind any contract for the sale of goods and services. Should the midwife be in breach of that contract the client may be able to sue her for compensation.

If as a result of negligence, the midwife causes harm to the client, unlike the NHS patient, the private patient has a remedy, not only in negligence (as the NHS patient has) but also has a remedy for breach of contract. This may not be of any significance since the contract is likely to require the same duty of care as required under the laws of negligence; however, it depends upon the nature of the alleged breach of contract.

Where a private practitioner or organisation has a contract with an NHS trust for the provision of health services the agreement for the provision of and payment for midwifery services would be enforceable in a court of law.

SUSPENSION FROM PRACTICE

Like any employed midwife, the independent midwife could face suspension from practice by the Local Supervising Authority. Suspension from practice for the independent midwife means that she will immediately cease to be able to obtain income from her practice within the geographical area of that Local Supervising Authority. Where an employed midwife is suspended from practice, this would not necessarily mean that she is suspended from her contract of employment, and she may continue to receive her full pay even though she is unable to work within the geographical area of the LSA which has suspended her. The new Midwives Rules require the Practice Committee of the NMC, when notified of a suspension by the LSA, to consider whether or not to make an interim suspension order or interim conditions of practice order in respect of the midwife concerned.[7] If the Practice Committee decides not to make an interim suspension order, or having made one, revokes it, the LSA must revoke the suspension. Where the NMC makes an interim suspension order, the midwife cannot of course practise as a registered midwife.

CONCLUSION ON INDEPENDENT MIDWIFERY

Independent midwifery is fraught with financial and contractual problems, but it does provide, for those women who can afford it, an alternative service which may meet their needs in a way in which the NHS is failing. The financial problems in obtaining reasonable insurance cover for the ever increasing value of claims following brain damage at birth is the biggest deterrent to midwives being prepared to undertake independent practice. Many have suggested that independent midwives should be able to contract with the NHS so that care to individual women and their families can be more responsive.[8,9] Alice Coyle, an independent midwife interviewed in The Practising Midwife,[10] recommended a central fund so that women could 'choose their care, a bit like the dreaded voucher system. This would enable women to vote with their feet, and services which weren't meeting their needs would be under-used and hopefully scrapped with popular services built on and funded properly such as caseload practices with realistic caseloads'. It is clear that if such schemes are not set up, the days of independent midwifery are coming to an end because of the financial problems of indemnity insurance.

The NSF for Maternity and Children's Services (see Chs 6, 12 and 32) suggests the support and positive promotion of women's choice and states:

Women are able to choose the most appropriate place to give birth from a range of local options including home birth and delivery in midwife-led units, with the facility for women delivering in the community to be transferred to hospital rapidly if complications arise.

It does not specifically include the choice of being able to choose an independent midwife.

The Independent Midwives Association has set up a database to collect on-going details of low-intervention midwifery practice in the home setting, which is being undertaken by self-employed midwives. The project is intended to run until the end of 2005 and should provide some interesting data.[11]

PRIVATE MATERNITY HOSPITALS

CARE STANDARDS ACT 2000

Many wealthy celebrities opt for obstetric and midwifery care outside the NHS. It has been estimated that £25 000 would in August 2001 cover the cost of a birth in a private hospital such as the Portland Hospital in London, a maternity nurse for 6 weeks, a *doula* for 5 hours a day for the next 3 months and a night nanny for 5 nights a week for 5 months.[12] (*Doula* comes from the Greek word for the most important female servant in the house. They are trained to provide practical and emotional support. A birth *doula* would attend labour, providing support and encouragement. A post-birth *doula* provides general support and help for the mother.)

Private maternity homes have, in the past, come under the provisions of the Registered Homes Act 1984. This Act has now been repealed by the Care Standards Act 2000, which established a new central registration body, known as the National Care Standards Commission (NCSC), which was a new, independent regulatory body for social care and private and voluntary healthcare services. (The National Assembly for Wales has established a department/unit to be the regulatory body for such services in Wales.) The NCSC was subsequently replaced by the Commission for Health Audit and Inspection (now known as the Healthcare Commission) and the Commission for Social Care Inspection. The Healthcare Commission is the registration body for private hospitals and the Commission for Social Care Inspection is the registration body for care homes (formerly residential and nursing homes). The legislation follows a government report on the regulation of private and voluntary healthcare.[13–17] Under the Registered Homes Act 1984, individual Health Authorities had been the registration authorities for nursing homes and Local Authorities for residential care homes within their catchment areas. The emphasis is now on national standards set out by the Secretary of State and the National Assembly of Wales which have powers under the Act to make regulations and issue national minimum standards.

MIDWIVES IN AN INDEPENDENT HOSPITAL

The midwife may be employed to work in an independent hospital which is used in connection with maternity services so she needs to have an understanding of the registration provisions and how these affect the environment and standard of care. Of those registered in 2003–2004 as practising midwives, 468 work for a private institution (44 are identified as working in private practice, 511 work for an agency,

105 for a family practitioner; 1529 work in a midwifery bank). (Midwives may of course operate in more than one of these fields.)

Box 23.5 shows the definition of independent hospital for the purposes of the Care Standards Act 2000.

Box 23.5 Section 2 Care Standards Act 2000

(2) A hospital which is not a health service hospital is an independent hospital.

(3) 'Hospital' (except in the expression health service hospital) means

  a. an establishment

    i. the main purpose of which is to provide medical or psychiatric treatment for illness or mental disorder or palliative care; or

    ii. in which (whether or not other services are also provided) any of the listed services are provided;

  b. any other establishment in which treatment or nursing (or both) are provided for persons liable to be detained under the Mental Health Act 1983.

(4) 'Independent clinic' means an establishment of a prescribed kind (not being a hospital) in which services are provided by medical practitioners (whether or nor any services are also provided for the purposes of the establishment elsewhere).

But an establishment in which, or for the purposes of which, services are provided by medical practitioners in pursuance of the NHS Act 1977 is not an independent clinic.

(5) 'Independent medical agency' . . .

(6) . . .

(7) In this section 'listed services' means:

  a. Medical treatment under anaesthesia or sedation

  b. Dental treatment under general anaesthesia

  c. Obstetric services and in connection with childbirth, medical services

▶

d. Termination of pregnancies

e. Cosmetic surgery

f. Treatment using prescribed techniques or prescribed technology.

These independent hospitals are regulated under the Care Standards Act 2000.

Care homes are defined as establishments providing accommodation, together with nursing or personal care, for people who are or have been ill, persons who have or have had a mental disorder, persons who are disabled or infirm, persons who are or have been dependent on alcohol or drugs. However, an establishment is not a care home if it is a hospital, an independent clinic or a children's home (s.3(3)). The old distinction in the Registered Homes Act 1984 between nursing and residential care home is thus abolished.

Most midwives working outside the NHS would be providing services in an independent hospital, but there may be some establishments providing post-convalescent nursing and personal care which would come under the definition of care home.

Box 23.6 shows a summary of the provisions of Part 2 of the Care Standards Act in so far as they are likely to affect midwifery.

Box 23.6 Provisions of Part 2 of the Care Standards Act 2000

Section 11 Requirements to register

Section 12 Application for registration

Section 13 Grant or refusal of registration

Section 14 Cancellation of registration

Section 15 Application by registered persons

Section 16 Regulations about registration

Section 17 Notice of proposals

Section 18 Right to make representations

Section 19 Notice of decisions

► Section 20 Urgent procedure for cancellation

Section 21 Appeals to the tribunal

Section 22 Regulations of establishments and agencies

Section 23 National minimum standards

Section 24 Offence of failure to comply with conditions

Section 25 Offence of contravention of regulations

Section 26 Offence of false descriptions of establishments and agencies

Section 27 Offence of false statements in applications

Section 28 Offence of failure to display certificate of registration

Section 29 Proceedings for offences

Section 30 Offences by bodies corporate

Section 31 Inspections by persons authorised by registration authority

Section 32 Inspections supplementary

Section 33 Annual returns

It is not the intention to go through each of these sections in detail but rather to give to the midwife who works in this area an understanding of the basic provisions and a knowledge of where she can seek further information.

It is an offence to carry on an unregistered independent hospital. Any independent hospital offering abortion facilities must obtain the prior approval of the Secretary of State under s.1(3) of the Abortion Act 1967 (see Ch. 26).

Section 16 enables regulations to be made relating to registration. Section 22 enables the Secretary of State to make regulations which impose specific requirements on the establishment in relation to the persons who are fit to carry on or manage the establishment, the fitness of the premises, the numbers of persons working there.[18] Under s.23, national minimum standards can be prepared and published by the Minister.[19] Regulations under s.22 will give effect to these standards.

General rules relating to the regulation of independent hospitals cover the following topics:

The provision of a statement of purpose (Clause 6)

The provision of a patients' guide (Clause 7)

Review of statement of purpose and patients' guide (Clause 8)

Preparation and implementation of policies and procedures covering specified areas such as arrangements for admission, discharge and transfer of patients, arrangements for assessment, diagnosis and treatment of patients, creation, management, handling and storage of records and other information (Clause 9)

Quality of service provision (Part III Clauses 15–32) covering areas such as care and welfare of patients, staffing, fitness of workers, records, staff views as to conduct of establishment or agency, complaints, research, fitness of premises, management including financial position and notices to be given to the Regulator

Specific provisions are laid down for independent hospitals which provide obstetric services. Under Clause 39, a Head of Midwifery Services must be appointed who is responsible for managing the provisions of midwifery services, and in addition a Head of Obstetric Services (unless services are provided primarily by midwives). The healthcare professional providing services must be a midwife, or an appropriately qualified medical practitioner. Where midwives primarily provide the obstetric services, the registered person must ensure that the services of a medical practitioner who is competent to deal with obstetric emergencies are available at all times. In addition there must be available at all times a healthcare professional who is competent to undertake resuscitation of a newborn baby and that his skills are regularly reviewed and if necessary updated.

Additional requirements relating to obstetric services are laid down under Clause 40. These include:

– Reporting the death of a patient during or as a result of pregnancy or childbirth, and of any stillbirth or neonatal death, to any person undertaking an enquiry into such deaths

– Ensuring facilities are available within the hospital to provide adequate treatment to patients who have undergone a delivery requiring surgical intervention or the use of forceps and care by an appropriately experienced midwife

– Ensuring that appropriate arrangements are in place for the immediate transfer, where necessary, of a patient and her newborn baby to critical care facilities within the hospital or elsewhere in the near vicinity

– Ensuring that appropriate arrangements are in place for the treatment and, if necessary, transfer to a specialist care facility, of a very sick person or new born child

– Ensuring a maternity record is maintained for each patient receiving obstetric services and each child born in the hospital (see Boxes 23.7 and 23.8).

Essential information required under the Regulations about the birth of a child[20] is shown in Box 23.7.

Box 23.7 Particulars of child born (Part 2 Schedule 4 Private and Voluntary Health (England) Regulations 2001)

1. Details of the weight and condition of the child at birth

2. A daily statement of the child's health

3. If any paediatric examination is carried out involving any of the following procedures:

   a. examination for congenital abnormalities including congenital dislocation of the hip

   b. measurement of the circumference of the head of the child

   c. measurement of the length of the child

   d. screening for phenylketonuria

   details of each such examination and the result.

Essential information required under the Regulations about the patient receiving obstetric services[20] is shown in Box 23.8.

Box 23.8 Particulars of patient receiving obstetric services (Part 1 Schedule 4 Private and Voluntary Health (England) Regulations 2001)

1. The date and time of delivery of each patient, the number of children born to the patient, the sex of each child and whether the birth was a live birth or a still birth

2. The name and qualification of the person who delivered the patient

3. The date and time of any miscarriage occurring in the hospital

4. The date on which any child born to a patient left the hospital

5. If any child born to a patient died in the hospital, the date and time of death.

Under Clause 40(5) of the Regulations, these records must be retained for a period of not less than 25 years beginning on the date of the last entry.

NATIONAL MINIMUM STANDARDS FOR INDEPENDENT HEALTHCARE

The 2001 Regulations have been strengthened by the setting of national minimum standards by the Department of Health, using powers given by s.23(1) of the Care Standards Act 2000.[19] These can be obtained from the Department of Health website (www.dh.gov.uk). Core standards cover the following topics:

– Information provision

– Quality of treatment and care

– Management and personnel

– Complaints management

– Premises, facilities and equipment

– Risk management procedures

– Records and information management

– Research

In addition, there are service-specific standards. Those of maternity hospitals cover:

– Human resources

– Infection control

– Records management

– Antenatal care

– Additional standards for midwife-led units

– Childbirth

– Maternal death or stillbirth

– Care of the newborn baby

Each standard has a specified outcome and identifies the criteria for securing that standard. The standards are enforced through the inspections of the Healthcare Commission and a report is published following each inspection visit.

Midwives who work in the NHS might find these standards relevant and useful for their own departments.

BIRTH CENTRES

An example of a privately run birth centre is that of the Wessex Maternity Centre of which the parent company is Independent Maternity Centres Ltd (IMC Ltd). Kate Walmsley[21] described how it started as a pilot scheme, employing five midwives who work as autonomous practitioners in a non-hierarchical setting. It takes referrals from GPs who feel that particular women would benefit from the individualised care the midwives give. The centre provides indemnity cover for the midwives. The author, who is also a director of IMC Ltd, considers that this model of a midwifery service is one which would work well within the primary care sector.

Jilly Rosser and Tricia Anderson launched a project to encourage the establishment of small, community-based birth centres with the emphasis on normal birth.[22] Such centres could either be provided within the NHS (see Bristol,[23] Watford[24] St Thomas's[25] and Southern Derbyshire[26] experience) or they could be part of the private sector but receive NHS funding like the Wessex Maternity Centre described above. The Royal College of Midwives published a position statement on birth centres in May 2004[27] and the National Childbirth Trust has reviewed maternity care in birth centres, providing an analysis of the outcomes of birth centre care compared with hospital care[28] (see also Kirkham (2003)[29] and Ch. 24).

CONCLUSION

Any midwife who works in an independent hospital or care home should make herself aware of the conditions for registration including the numbers of persons permitted to be cared for. She should ensure that she brings to the manager or the proprietor any conditions which would appear to be unacceptable in relation to both the registration of the hospital or home and also under the Code of Professional Conduct: standards for conduct, performance and ethics of the NMC.

QUESTIONS AND EXERCISES

1. If you are an employed midwife, consider the advantages and disadvantages of becoming independent from the point of view of the client and from the point of view of the midwife.

2. What are the main legal differences between the situation of the employed midwife and that of the independent midwife?

3. What do you consider should be the minimum requirements of an agreement between a trust and an independent midwife for the latter to be able to deliver her clients in the trust hospital when necessary?

4. Make enquiries to ascertain the number and type of private maternity hospitals in your area and if possible obtain details of the registration provisions.

5. A client asks you for details of the differences between maternity hospitals provided within the NHS and those provided privately. Obtain the answers for her.

6. Obtain from the National Care Standards Commission (or the Welsh equivalent) a copy of the national minimum standards for private maternity homes and assess the extent to which you consider that they are in place in the organisation in which you work.

References

1 Hobbs L. The independent midwife, 2nd edn. Hale: Books for Midwives Press; 2000.

2 How to make your independent midwifery practice more business-like: key tips for lifting performance. Communique 2000; 8:37–38.

3 Hobbs L. Going independent. Nursing Times 1993; 89(20): 68–69.

4 L. and Others v. Hesley Hall Ltd. Times Law Reports, May 10 2001 HL; [2001] UKHL 22; [2001] 2 WLR 1311.

5 Independent Midwives Association. Women lose their right to choose as midwives lose indemnity insurance cover. Botley: Independent Midwives Association; 1995.

6 NMC. New NMC register: Addendum to the Code of Professional Conduct 22/2004 NMC Circular; 28 July 2004.

7 Nursing and Midwifery Council. Midwives Rules and Standards, Rule 5. NMC; August 2004.

8 Page L. The independent midwife. Br J Midwifery 2004; 12(6):360.

9 Independent Midwives Association. IMA proposes new model of care. Practising Midwife 2004; 7(6):13.

10 Coyle A. Pleased to meet you. Practising Midwife 1999; 2(4): 42.

11 Milan M. The Independent Midwives Association Database project. MIDIRS Midwifery Digest 2004; 14(4):548–554.

12 O'Driscoll E. Putting mothers and children first. The Daily Telegraph, 17 August 2001.

13 Department of Health. Regulating private and voluntary healthcare: a Consultation Document. London: HMSO; 1999.

14 Welsh Office. Regulation and inspection of social and healthcare services in Wales – A Commission for Care Standards in Wales. Cardiff: Welsh Office; 1999.

15 Welsh Office. Regulating private and voluntary healthcare in Wales. Cardiff: Welsh Office; 1999.

16 Department of Health. Regulating private and voluntary healthcare: The way forward. London: HMSO; 2000.

17 Department of Health. Regulating private and voluntary healthcare: Developing the way forward. London: HMSO; 2001.

18 The Private and Voluntary Health (England) Regulations 2001, SI 2001 No 3968.

19 Department of Health. Independent Health Care National Minimum Standards Regulations. London: The Stationery Office; 2002.

20 Private and Voluntary Health (England) Regulations 2001, Schedule 4 Part 2, SI 2001 No 3968.

21 Walmsley K. The Wessex Maternity Centre. Practising Midwife 1999; 2(8):12–13.

22 Rosser J, Anderson T. What next? Taking normal birth out of the labour ward. Practising Midwife 2000; 3(4):4–5.

23 Paterson S. Campaigning for a birth centre within the NHS. Midwifery Matters 2004; 103:13–14.

24 Harlev-Lam B, Lucey N. An integrated midwifery led birthing centre – creating a successful birth centre within a hospital. MIDIRS Midwifery Digest 2004; 14:S20–S22.

25 Ackerman B. Home from home. Practising Midwife 2005; 8(4):15–16.

26 Cotton L. Evidence to the House of Commons Select Committee meeting. Midwifery Matters 2004; 101:3.

27 Royal College of Midwives. Position Statement No 7, birth centres. RCM; May 2004.

28 Walsh D. NCT evidence based briefing. Maternity care in birth centres. New Digest 2005; 2918–21.

29 Kirkham M., ed. Birth Centres: a social model for maternity care. Edinburgh: Elsevier Science Ltd; 2003.

Chapter 24
MIDWIFERY MANAGEMENT

The management of a maternity department in a hospital, or a midwife-managed unit, or a community midwifery service, or a combination of all three, requires a high standard of management practice and a clear understanding of the laws which apply. The challenges for midwife managers are evident. The twenty-first staffing survey carried out by the RCM[1] showed that there are still very high vacancy rates in most regions and where recruitment and retention of midwives is becoming harder, then the main reasons appear to be stress and heavy workloads, placing considerable strains on the midwife manager.

In this chapter some of the specific laws which relate to management will be considered with references to chapters where some of the topics are discussed in more detail.

The topics set out below will be considered:

– Expanded role

– Delegation and supervision

– Difference between supervision as a Supervisor of Midwives (see Ch. 2) and line management supervision

– Standards of care

– Staffing levels and resource issues

– Audit and quality assurance

– Record keeping

– Employment and health and safety issues

– Primary Care Trusts and transfer of employment contracts

– Consultant midwives

– Midwife-managed units.

EXPANDED ROLE OF THE MIDWIFE

Professional development within midwifery knows no bounds: where necessary legislative changes can be made to expand the midwife's role (as in independent and supplementary prescribing). While there is no formal document on advanced midwifery practice issued by the NMC (see Ch. 2), midwives continue to develop their skills beyond those achieved at initial registration.

AREAS OF PRACTICE WHICH NOT ALL MIDWIVES AT PRESENT PRACTISE INCLUDE:

– examination[2] and resuscitation of the newborn[3]

– resuscitation in pregnancy[4]

– suturing

– transfusion of blood

– i.v. administration of antibiotics and other medications not presently normally covered by the midwives' powers of prescribing and medication, see Rule 7 (see Ch. 20)

– epidurals (midwives now top up epidurals in conjunction with medical staff but it may be that they can develop the skills for the complete administration of an epidural)

– forceps (this has been an activity in the past which was carried out only by medical staff)

– vacuum extraction

– acting as first assistant in theatre[5] (see Box 5.4)

– undertaking various complementary therapies such as acupuncture (see Ch. 34)

– advice: on fertility; gynaecology; adolescent health; child protection and infant feeding.[6]

The training and development of the midwife ventouse practitioner in community maternity units is considered by Tinsley.[7] She emphasises that any expansion of the midwife's role cannot be undertaken lightly and considers the extensive preparation and training, supervised practice, clear protocols, on-going clinical audit and appropriate equipment which must be made available, together with support from management, GPs and obstetricians. This would apply to every other area of potential role expansion which midwives might consider. An evaluation of a course for ventouse practitioners has been carried out.[8]

A consultant midwife described her role in public health which covered advice on domestic violence, rape and sexual assault, traumatic childbirth, mental ill health and maternal request for caesarean section.[9]

All these expansions in the role of the midwife have significant implications for the midwife manager.[10] The basic principles formerly set out by the UKCC in its scope of professional practice, which are now incorporated in the NMC Code of Professional Conduct[11] to ensure that they have the necessary professional competence to develop their practice safely, include the following basic principles.

The registered nurse, midwife or health visitor:

1. must be satisfied that each aspect of practice is directed to meeting the needs and serving the interests of the patient or client

2. must endeavour always to achieve, maintain and develop knowledge, skill and competence to respond to those needs and interests

3. must honestly acknowledge any limits of personal knowledge and skill and take steps to remedy any relevant deficits in order effectively and appropriately to meet the needs of patients and clients

4. must ensure that any enlargement or adjustment of the scope of personal professional practice must be achieved without compromising or fragmenting existing aspects of professional practice and care and that requirements of the Council's Code of Professional Conduct are satisfied throughout the whole area of practice

5. must recognise and honour the direct or indirect personal accountability borne for all aspects of professional practice and

6. must, in serving the interests of patients and clients and the wider interests of society, avoid any inappropriate delegation to others which compromises those interests.

Where a midwife undertakes an expanded role activity for which she is not competent then she could face disciplinary action, fitness to practise proceedings and be a witness in civil action brought by anyone harmed as a consequence of her negligence against her employer because of its vicarious liability for her negligence. The Modernisation Agency and the Department of Health issued a consultation document on 24 March 2005 which would allow nurses (and this would include midwives) to train for work as assistants in surgery. If these proposals are implemented, midwives may well have the opportunity to assist in caesarean sections.

DELEGATION AND SUPERVISION

The NMC standard set for Rule 6 Responsibility and sphere of practice[12] states that:

A midwife cannot arrange for anyone to act as a substitute, other than another practising midwife or a registered medical practitioner.

The NMC cites Article 45 of the Nursing and Midwifery Order 2001[13] as the source for this standard. The Article is headed: 'Attendance by unqualified persons at childbirth'.

This states that:

Article 45

(1) *A person other than a registered midwife or a registered medical practitioner shall not attend a woman in childbirth.*

(2) *Paragraph (1) does not apply –*

(a) *where the attention is given in a case of sudden or urgent necessity; or*

(b) *in the case of a person who, while undergoing training with a view to becoming a medical practitioner or to becoming a midwife, attends a woman in childbirth as part of a course of practical instruction in midwifery recognised by the Council or by the General Medical Council.*

(3) *A person who contravenes paragraph (1) shall be liable on summary conviction to a fine not exceeding level 5 on the standard scale.*

Article 45 refers to 'attendance at childbirth'; however, the NMC standard refers to all activities of the midwife, since the definition of childbirth in the new rules states that '"childbirth" includes the antenatal, intranatal and postnatal periods'. A strict interpretation of this would therefore appear to imply that no activities carried out by a midwife in connection with the antenatal, intranatal and postnatal stages of pregnancy can be delegated by a midwife other than to another midwife or doctor.

That this is not the intention of the NMC is clear from their guidance in the NMC circular on delegation of midwifery care to others.[14] This circular emphasises that there is no such person as a non-practising midwife who can be legally involved in antenatal or intrapartum or postnatal care. The NMC also states that:

It is for the midwife to decide whether delegation of tasks is appropriate in the care of a woman or her baby.

The midwife remains responsible for the care provided.

It follows therefore that specific activities of a midwife, except that of attendance at childbirth, can be delegated to a person who has the training competence and experience to undertake the activity to the required standard. It is the midwife's personal responsibility to decide on that delegation and to ensure that the appropriate level of supervision is provided.

It is the midwife manager's responsibility to ensure that appropriate delegation and supervision is taking place in her department. A woman/baby is entitled to the reasonable standard of care, whoever has provided that care. It is no defence to a woman to argue that harm occurred because a person of a lower grade or less experience undertook a particular activity. This means that where activities are being delegated to non-registered staff (Note: attendance at a confinement cannot be so delegated), the delegator must ensure that the knowledge, experience and training of the person who is to carry out that activity is sufficient to ensure that the patient/client will receive a reasonable standard of care. The person delegating must also decide the level of supervision required. Initially probably a high level of close supervision will be required, but this could be reduced as confidence in the abilities of the person undertaking the activities grows. The situation should be constantly reviewed and monitored.

Where activities are safely and appropriately delegated and supervised, the manager would not be responsible if the person undertaking the activities acts negligently. Nor is there a concept of vicarious liability for the delegation of a senior to a junior. However, where the delegator has delegated or supervised negligently, then there would be personal liability of the delegator, though in practice, the employer would be sued for its vicarious liability for the negligent employee.

The NHS Plan[15] envisages greater use of support staff to alleviate the chronic shortage of registered professionals across many different areas including midwifery. The use of support workers in maternity care is considered by Doug Charlton[16] who discusses the many concerns which arise including the vexed question of the supervision of support workers in the community, when they may not be under the direct supervision of the registered midwife, the education of support workers and the dangers of breaking the law relating to the attendance at childbirth of only the registered midwife, doctor or student of either. He suggests that:

the way ahead looks rocky and untried. Many of the issues raised in this article will need further debate before the profession launches headlong into accepting healthcare support workers as equal partners in maternity care.

Pat Lindsay and Susan Burvill consider the role that maternity care assistants (MCA) can play in home births[17] and emphasise that with appropriate preparation and supervision the MCA appears to be a safe and workable proposition. A new pilot training scheme for MCAs is considered by Pat Lindsay.[18]

SUPERVISION AND LINE MANAGEMENT

There is a clear distinction between the role of the Supervisor of Midwives, which is based on the statutory provisions, and the role of a manager who as part of her management responsibilities has a line management supervision responsibility. To add to the confusion, sometimes the same person might hold both roles in relation to the midwife being supervised. The role of the Supervisor of Midwives is considered in Chapter 3. As a line manager, a midwife would have responsibilities to ensure that clear instructions were given over the delegation of responsibilities, that records were audited, that the employer's responsibilities to the midwife were carried out (e.g. in the management of stress, see below) and in being accessible to any concerns which the midwife wishes to raise.

STANDARDS OF CARE

While each individual practitioner is personally and professionally accountable for her own practice, a manager has an overall responsibility in ensuring that the unit she manages is meeting the reasonable standards of care to which the patient is entitled. Guidance published by the National Institute for Health and Clinical Excellence, reports from the Audit Commission or from the Healthcare Commission, any relevant National Service Frameworks, criteria published by the Clinical Negligence Scheme for Trusts and any other information from registration bodies or professional associations should, where appropriate, be incorporated within the standards of the department/unit (see Ch. 13). Guidance is provided by the NHS Executive on the role of the ward sister which would also apply to the midwife who is responsible for running a ward or maternity unit.[19] This guidance envisages that under the NHS Plan (see Ch. 21) senior nurses or charge nurses will have the authority and support they need to get the basics of care right. By April 2002, NHS Trusts and Primary Care Trusts with wards were required to have identified matrons, each accountable for a group of wards. Supporting policies for these roles include:

- tackling standards of cleanliness

- improving the quality of hospital food

- introducing ward housekeepers

- patient forums and the Patient Advocacy and Liaison Service (PALS) (see Ch. 11 on Complaints)

- ward environment budgets

- benchmarking the fundamental and essential aspects of care

- prevention and control of hospital acquired infection

- clinical leadership development

- the Chief Nursing Officer's ten key roles for nurses.

The implementation of the policy of hospital matrons required the review of job descriptions and organisational structures, ensuring that adequate support is given to the ward sisters, reviewing staff establishments and skill mix, ensuring that Clinical Governance (see Ch. 21) is in place and ensuring that leadership development exists and there is investment in education and training.

STAFFING LEVELS AND RESOURCE ISSUES

The manager should be in constant dialogue with senior management to ensure that the resources necessary to implement the identified standards are available. In addition the manager would have the responsibility of advising the trust board or employer if the level of staffing resources is such that a safe system of work cannot be guaranteed for mothers and babies. In some circumstances, the scope of the service might have to be curtailed to ensure that priority was given to clinical need; in others arrangements may have to be agreed with neighbouring trusts to share workloads and staff. Failure to take such reasonable measures might if a mother or baby were harmed lead to a successful action either because of breach of the direct duty of care owed to the patient by the trust or because of its vicarious liability for negligence by an employee. (See discussion in Chapter 6 on home births and situations where employers have had to curtail a home birth service.)

CASE LOAD

Midwives frequently ask, 'What does the law say about the workload that any midwife should be undertaking?' Unfortunately laws, whether statute or case (common) law, are rarely so precise as to give an answer to the question of 'for how many clients should any midwife be responsible?' The circumstances are of course extremely wide. To compare the case load of a community midwife working in a rural area of the West Country with that of a midwife in an obstetric unit in a district hospital would be very difficult. Travelling time would not feature in the latter's working hours; it may be a significant feature in the former's. There are other differences depending upon whether the midwife in the obstetric unit would be working on the labour or antenatal wards. However, even though there is no stated figure on workloads given by law, there must be an attempt at formulating what would or would not be reasonable. The mother may have to show, if she is seeking compensation for a brain-damaged baby, that there was not a reasonable number of staff allocated to her care; the midwives need to have clear evidence to place before managers if they are alleging that the lack of sufficient staff is placing patients at risk, and therefore they are in danger of breaking the Code of Professional Conduct: standards for conduct, performance and ethics. Particularly at this time, when there is a national shortage of midwifery staff, managers need to know what are recommended figures for staffing levels so that they can inform the trust board of the significance of the current situation.

The law requires the NHS Trust, its managers and staff to provide a reasonable standard of care for pregnant women. The National Health Service Act 1977 places a statutory duty upon the Secretary of State to provide a comprehensive service to such extent as he considers necessary to meet all reasonable requirements. The stipulated services include hospital and medical and nursing services and 'such other facilities for the care of expectant and nursing mothers and young children as he considers are appropriate as part of the health service' (see Ch. 21).

There is also a duty recognised in common law or case law for the staff of the hospital to act with reasonable care according to the standards of competent professional practice (i.e. the Bolam Test; see Ch. 13). It is therefore no defence for a midwife to claim that she acted in error in caring for a mother because she was so pressured as a result of shortage of staff.

It could therefore be said that both statute and common law require a reasonable standard of care to be provided for the care of expectant women and their children. In addition the NMC will hold any registered midwife accountable if it can be shown that she is responsible for management failures resulting in patient harm. Thus it was reported that three midwives were cautioned by the UKCC (the predecessor of the NMC) when a baby died 10 days after birth, partly as a result of inadequate staffing levels.[20]

REASONABLE WORKLOADS

How can the demands of a reasonable standard of care be translated into a reasonable workload for the midwife? Research has been undertaken in this area by Marie Washbrook and Jean Ball whose earlier research into assessing midwifery staffing requirements[21,22] for the Nuffield Centre for Health Services Studies and Trent Region Midwifery Manpower Project led to their textbook on the subject.[23] The book provides guidance to managers in assessing staffing required for antenatal clinic, delivery suite, hospital-based postnatal care and community care.

The Royal College of Obstetricians and Gynaecologists established a working party to identify minimum standards of care in labour.[24] The report sets out the basic standards of care required to provide a safe and pleasant childbirth experience and provides an assessment of staffing, facility and equipment levels in relation to the number and kind of deliveries. Various models for measuring workload in midwifery services have been applied including the GRASP systems workload methodology used by Hurley and Dickson in identifying staffing needs based on patient dependency levels on a labour ward.[25] The Clinical Negligence Scheme for Trusts has also given guidance on staffing figures (see Ch. 13). In addition Appendix C of the Report of the Maternity and Neonatal Workforce Group (MNWG) set up under the Chairmanship of Dr Sheila Adam, the Deputy Chief Medical Officer of Health which reported to the Department of Health in January 2003[26] set workforce models for maternity services for a range of facilities, which it recommended should be explored further by the Department of Health and Royal Colleges.

Constant updating of such figures is essential to take account of new technologies,[27] new systems of working such as team midwifery,[28] how midwives work with nurses and GP[29] and the actual work that midwives undertake as shown by their diaries[30] or observation and what are predictors of obstetric intervention.[31] Sandra Walsh provides an overview of a new Government strategy to deal with midwifery staffing issues.[32] Annie Lester makes a strong argument for case load midwifery and using the Albany Midwifery Practice model suggests an individual case load of 36 women as primary midwife and a further 36 as the second midwife.[33]

The legal issues arising from inadequate staffing are considered in Dimond (1998).[34]

PERSONAL RESPONSIBILITY OF THE MIDWIFE

A midwife who believes that she is under too much pressure to provide a safe service is required by the Code of Professional Conduct: standards for conduct, performance and ethics to ensure that she brings this to the attention of the appropriate person. If this is not an isolated situation, then there are clear management failings in not providing a safe environment. There can be legal liability if managers, knowing that staff are suffering from stress to such extent that it amounts to a serious illness, fail to take reasonable steps to remedy the situation.[35] There would also be a duty on the manager to prevent any bullying (see Ch. 19).

AUDIT AND QUALITY ASSURANCE

The concept of Clinical Governance derives from s.45 of the Health and Social Care (Community Health and Standards) Act 2003 which imposes a duty of quality upon NMS bodies (re-enacting s.18 of the Health Act 1999; see Ch. 21). This statutory duty requires the establishment of quality standards and their regular monitoring. In practice the trust board would delegate these responsibilities to the directorate managers and in turn to the departmental managers. Any manager would therefore have responsibilities in defining reasonable standards of practice and ensuring that arrangements were in place for their regular monitoring. Records should be kept of both the standards and the dates and results of the monitoring.

RECORD KEEPING

One of the main ways of ensuring that standards of records and record keeping are maintained is by carrying out regular internal audit. This could be undertaken in a non-confrontational, constructive manner within each department or ward, when a set of records are taken and then reviewed to identify the errors, omissions, ambiguities etc. (see Ch. 15) and to assess the extent to which they would be robust in defending professional practice in 10 years' time in a court of law. A record could be made of the main ways in which standards could be improved and a similar audit carried out a few weeks later to see if improvements had been maintained.

EMPLOYMENT AND HEALTH AND SAFETY ISSUES

A manager has a responsibility for ensuring that the duties in the health and safety laws and employment rights are implemented on behalf of the employer. For example, if an employee is being subjected to unreasonable stress and reasonable action is not taken by the manager to secure the reasonable health and safety of the employee, then the employee may have grounds for suing for compensation (see Ch. 19). Many of the statutory duties placed upon the employer would in practice be delegated to the manager to ensure that they are implemented and that the processes are in place to ensure they are regularly monitored. Records maintained by the manager on health and safety audit, training, disciplinary action, counselling, complaints by staff would all be relevant in the event of any dispute arising. The manager would also have responsibility for ensuring that complaints were correctly recorded and the proper procedure followed in their investigation (see Ch. 11). In addition, the manager would have to ensure that the procedure drawn up by the trust under the Public Interest Disclosure Act 1998 ('whistle blowing charter'; see Ch. 22) is made known to the staff and is operating effectively.

IMPROVING WORKING LIVES (IWL)

The Department of Health in 2005 published a guide for midwife managers.[36] This sets out several ways in which midwifery managers can improve levels of flexibility. Units will be audited to identify the extent to which they comply with the principles of the guide. Employers are required to:

– recognise that modern health services require modern employment services

– understand that staff work best when they can strike a balance between work and home life

– jointly develop with staff a variety of working arrangements that balance the needs of the service and staff

– value support staff according to the contribution they make to patient care and service needs

– provide personal and professional development and training opportunities that are accessible to all staff

– have a range of policies and practices that enable staff to manage a healthy balance between work and their commitments outside work.

PRIMARY CARE TRUSTS AND TRANSFER OF EMPLOYMENT CONTRACTS

The transfer of employment contracts to new Primary Care Trusts or Care Trusts raised concerns about employment rights and the conditions of employment. The manager has a major responsibility to ensure that arrangements are made for staff to receive the appropriate advice and counselling.

CONSULTANT MIDWIVES

One of the recommendations of 'Making a Difference',[37] a report from the Department of Health published in 1999 with the aim of improving recruitment, strengthening education, improving working lives and enhancing the quality of care, was that Consultant nurses and midwives should be appointed. The key features of the Consultant midwife, as envisaged in 'Making a Difference',[38] are shown in Box 24.1.

Box 24.1 Key features of the Consultant midwife

– Expert practice

– Professional leadership and consultancy

– Education and development

– Practice and service development linked to research and evaluation.

It was envisaged that Consultant midwives would spend at least 50% of their time on clinical work with career opportunities. NHS trusts were required to agree the posts with regional offices of the DoH. It is perhaps too early to determine the effectiveness of the role of the Consultant midwife and the likely impact of this role on advanced midwifery practice (see Ch 2).

SPECIALIST MIDWIVES

The delegation of some midwifery activities (excluding attendance at birth) may facilitate the development of specialist midwives. Such areas as teenage pregnancy, alcohol and substance misuse, ethnic minority women and parent education and practice support could be covered by midwives specialising in those topics.[39] Such developments may assist in raising the morale of the midwife as well as providing a more expert service for women. Clearly, the midwifery manager has a significant role to play in such developments.

MIDWIFE-MANAGED UNITS

On the basis of what we have heard, this Committee must draw the conclusion that the policy of encouraging all women to give birth in hospitals cannot be justified on grounds of safety.

These are the words of the Health Committee of the House of Commons,[40] which recommended that maternity services should be provided which gave women a greater choice in the maternity care which they received. At present the choice of home births or birth in small maternity units appear to be options which have been substantially withdrawn. For most women, there is no choice. This does not appear to be in accordance with their wishes. In Chapter 6, we considered the implications of the House of Commons report on maternity services[40] and the Expert Committee report Changing Childbirth[41] in relation to the choices that women should have. The UKCC position statement on supporting women to have a home birth is discussed in Chapter 6. An analysis of a risk assessment carried out by midwives who were planning a midwifery managed unit was documented by the author.[42,43] Concerns of the midwives about the new unit included:

- risks of harm to mother and baby

- difficulties of transfers from the unit to the District General Hospital

- refusals by clients to accept the unit's criteria

- indemnity/litigation/protection by management and

- prescribing, training and updating.

These concerns were discussed in a workshop and appropriate protocols and training set in place, together with collaboration with other groups such as consultant obstetricians, pharmacists and ambulance paramedics (see discussion in Ch. 19 on Risk management and the midwife).

BIRTH CENTRES

Another variant of the midwife-managed unit which is becoming increasingly popular is a birth centre which is managed, staffed and run by midwives. They may be outside the NHS or contract with the NHS for the provision of their services (see Ch. 23), or they may be run within the NHS by an NHS trust or Primary Care Group. Details of the Edgware Birth Centre were given by Jane Walker to the All-Party Parliamentary Group on Maternity at its meeting on 18 July 2001 as an example of a midwife-managed unit run by midwives and midwifery assistants funded by the NHS.[44] A comparison of its results since it opened in 1997 showed a significantly lower rate of inductions, interventions in labour, planned caesarean sections, episiotomies and pharmacological analgesia than births in the local hospital. In the previous 2 years, 50% of women at the Centre birthed in water, compared with 2% in the UK, and 85% breast-fed.

Clearly the midwife manager of such a unit would require specific training in the necessary management skills and would also have responsibility for clarifying and enforcing the criteria for admission to ensure that only those women suitable for delivery in such a unit were admitted.[45–47]

CONCLUSIONS

It cannot be assumed that a midwife can become a manager without additional training. The management activities described in this chapter have serious implications for the professional accountability of the midwife manager. As in all other areas of midwifery practice, the midwife manager should ensure that she has the training, competence and experience to carry out her management functions satisfactorily. Recent initiatives have presented considerable challenges for the midwife manager. These include the NHS Plan (see Ch. 21), the implementation of Clinical Governance (see Ch. 21), the National Service Frameworks for midwifery services and children (see Ch. 6), the recommendations of NICE (see Ch. 21) and of the NPSA (see Ch. 19). In addition the midwife manager faces complex problems of recruiting and retaining midwifery staff and ensuring adequate staffing and skill mix to ensure a reasonable standard of care is provided. It is the personal responsibility of the midwifery manager to ensure that she keeps up to date with publications from many different organisations and quangos and that the recommended standards are secured in her unit. The Report of the Inquiry of the Healthcare Commission into the management of the maternity unit at Northwick Park Hospital in 2004[48] would be invaluable reading for many midwifery managers. A task force was sent in to manage the unit as a consequence of the recommendations of the Healthcare Commission. In the light of three inquiries into maternity departments (Northwick Park London, New Cross Hospital Wolverhampton and Ashford St Peters Hospital in Chertsey), the Chairman of the Healthcare Commission called for improvements into maternity services. He wished to see boards of NHS Trusts put in place immediately measures whereby they can assess their maternity services.[49] The midwife manager will have a crucial role to play in raising and maintaining standards.

QUESTIONS AND EXERCISES

1. Your NHS trust has suggested that you might like to apply for a senior midwifery management post and that you might like to write a job description for the post. How would you set about responding to this invitation? What would you put in the job description and what training would you consider was essential for such a position?

2. A midwife-managed unit is to be set up in your locality. Examine the factors which should be taken into account to ensure that risks to the mother and child are reduced to a minimum.

3. Discuss the suggestion that a specialist body of trained midwives should be capable of carrying out caesarean operations.

4. Prepare a leaflet giving information to a client about a new midwife-managed unit which is to be established.

5. How would you distinguish between the roles of the Supervisor of Midwives (see Ch. 3) and the midwifery line manager?

References

1 Royal College of Midwives. Staffing survey 2004. RCM; 2004

2 Lomax A. Expanding the midwife's role in examining the new-born. Br J Midwifery 2001; 9(2):100–102.

3 Jevon P. Resuscitation of the newborn – a practical approach. London: Butterworth Heinemann; 2000.

4 Jevon P. Resuscitation in pregnancy – a practical approach. London: Butterworth Heinemann; 2002.

5 Jackson-Baker A. Changing roles and responsibilities: the midwife's challenge. RCM Midwives J 2000; 3:177.

6 Barrell M. Midwives need to make a difference. Practising Midwife 2000; 3(6):4–5.

7 Tinsley V. Rethinking the role of the midwife: midwife ventouse practitioners in community maternity units. Midwifery Matters 2001; 90:19–23.

8 Anderson T, Cunningham S. An evaluation by focus group and survey of a course for midwifery ventouse practitioners. Midwifery 2002; 18(2):165–172.

9 Dunkley-Bent J. A consultant midwife's community clinic. Br J Midwifery 2004; 12(3):144–150.

10 Andrews S. Managerial implications of expanding practice. Br J Midwifery 2004; 12(2):114–119.

11 Nursing and Midwifery Council. Code of Professional Conduct: standards for performance, conduct and ethics, 2004.

12 Nursing and Midwifery Council. (Midwives) Rules Order of Council 2004, Statutory Instrument 2004/1764; Nursing and Midwifery Council Midwives Rules and Standards, August 2004.

13 The Nursing and Midwifery Order 2001, Statutory Instrument 2002 No 253.

14 Nursing and Midwifery Council. NMC Circular 1/2004.

15 Department of Health. NHS Plan: A plan for investment, a plan for reform. London: HMSO; 2000.

16 Charlton D. Support workers in maternity care. MIDIRS Midwifery Digest 2001; 11(3):405–406.

17 Pat L, Burvill S. An extra pair of hands. The Practising Midwife 2005; 8(4):22–24.

18 Pat L. Introduction of maternity care assistants. Br J Midwifery 2004; 12(10):650–653.

19 NHS Executive. Implementing the NHS Plan: Modern Matrons. Health Service Circular 2001/010.

20 News item. UKCC cautions midwives. Nursing Times 1998; 94(22):11.

21 Ball JA. Birthrate: using clinical indicators to assess case mix, workload outcomes and staffing needs in intrapartum care and for predicting postnatal bed needs. Oxford: Nuffield; 1992.

22 Centre for Health Care Studies, Washbrook M. Assessing midwifery staffing requirements. Nursing Standard 1992; 6(25):39.

23 Ball JA, Washbrook M. Birthrate plus: a framework for workforce planning and decision making for midwifery services. Oxford: Books for Midwives Press; 1996.

24 Royal College of Obstetricians and Gynaecologists. Minimum standards of care in labour. London: RCOG; 1994.

25 Hurley J, Dickson K. Assessing midwifery workload on a labour ward. Br J Midwifery 1998; 6(7): 444–449.

26 Department of Health. Report to the DH Children's taskforce from the Maternity and Neonatal workforce group. London: DoH; 2003.

27 Mugford MA. Review of the economics of care for sick newborn infants. Comm Med 1998; 10(2):99–111.

28 Stock J. Continuity of care in maternity services – the implications for midwives. Health Manpower Management 1994; 20(3):30–36.

29 Young D, Lees A, Twaddle S. The costs to the NHS of maternity care: midwife managed vs shared. Br J Midwifery1997; 5(8):465–471.

30 McCourt C. Working patterns of caseload midwives: a diary analysis. Br J Midwifery 1998; 6(9):580–585.

31 Joyce R, Webb R, Peacock J. Predictors of obstetric intervention rates: case-mix, staffing levels and organisational factors of hospital of birth. J Obstet Gynaecol 2002; 22(6):618–625.

32 Walsh S. Tackling midwives' recruitment, retention and return. Practising Midwife 2003; 6(9):34–36.

33 Lester A. The argument for caseload midwifery. MIDIRS Midwifery Digest 2004; 15(1):27–30, reprinted from Midwifery Matters 2004; 103:9–12.

34 Dimond B. Crisis in midwifery staffing: The legal aspects. Br J Midwifery 1998; 6(12):755–759.

35 Dimond B. Legal aspects of health and safety. Dinton, Wiltshire: Quay Books; 2004.

36 Department of Health. Improving Working Lives: a guide for midwives and managers. London: DoH; 2005.

37 Department of Health. Making a Difference: strengthening the nursing, midwifery and health visiting contribution to healthcare. London: HMSO; 1999.

38 Department of Health. Making a Difference: The new NHS. London: HMSO; 1999.

39 Herve J. Specialist posts for specialist needs. The Practising Midwife 2005; 8(4):30–32.

40 House of Commons report on maternity services 1993. Second Report Session 1991–1992. London: HMSO; 1993.

41 Department of Health. Changing Childbirth: Report of the Expert Maternity Group. London: HMSO; 1993.

42 Dimond B. Risk management and the midwife. Modern Midwife 1994; 4(4):36–67.

43 Dimond B. Midwife managed units. Modern Midwife 1994; 4(6):31–33.

44 National Childbirth Trust. For report of the meeting (and other meetings) contact: Catherine Eden at the National Childbirth Trust, Tel: 020 8992 2616; e-mail: c_eden@national-childbirth-trust.co.uk

45 Rosser J. Birth centres: the key to modernising the maternity services. MIDIRS Midwifery Digest 2001; 11(Suppl. 2):S22–S26, 43.

46 Nursing and Midwifery Council. (Midwives) Rules Order of Council 2004, Statutory Instrument 2004/1764.

47 Nursing and Midwifery Council. Midwives Rules and Standards, August 2004.

48 Healthcare Commission. Online. Available: www.healthcarecommission.org.uk

49 Healthcare Commission. Press release, 18 July 2005.

SECTION E

STATUTORY PROVISIONS AND CHILDBIRTH

This Section considers certain statutory provisions which impact upon the work of the midwife. Chapter 25 sets out the legal duties placed upon midwives and others in relation to the confinement, the notification and registration of birth and the registration of death including stillbirths. Laws relating to the termination of pregnancy are then considered. Chapter 26 looks at the statutory provisions covering human fertilisation and embryology, followed by the provisions relating to vaccine damage compensation, infectious disease notification and the midwife's situation in relation to AIDS/HIV.

Chapter 25
CRIMINAL LAW
AND CONFINEMENTS

ATTENDANCE AT A CHILDBIRTH

Article 45 of the Nursing and Midwifery Order 2001[1] (re-enacting s.16 of the Nurses, Midwives and Health Visitors Act 1997, which itself re-enacted the Midwives Act 1951, s.9 and the Nurses, Midwives and Health Visitors Act 1979), made it a criminal offence for a person other than a registered midwife or a registered medical practitioner to attend at a childbirth. Article 45 of the Nursing and Midwifery Order is set out in full in Box 25.1.

Box 25.1 Criminal offence for unauthorised persons to attend at childbirth

Article 45 of the Nursing and Midwifery Order

(1) A person other than a registered midwife or registered medical practitioner shall not attend a woman in childbirth.

(2) Paragraph 1 does not apply:

a. where the attention is given in a case of sudden or urgent necessity; or

b. in the case of a person who, while undergoing training with a view to becoming a medical practitioner or to becoming a midwife, attends a woman in childbirth as part of a course of practical instruction in midwifery recognised by the Council or by the General Medical Council.

(3) A person who contravenes Paragraph 1 shall be liable on summary conviction to a fine not exceeding level 5 on the standard scale.

The fact that an authorised person can be prosecuted for attending a woman in childbirth gives the midwife some powers in the situation where a husband or co-habitee or the mother herself is anxious that a midwife should not be present at the birth but that the partner should be in control. The midwife can make it clear that failure to summon the midwife in order that the partner can attend would be a criminal offence. She should report any such possibility to her Supervisor. If there are records that a written warning has been given to the couple, it is less likely that a defence under Para. 2 would succeed.

There have been several convictions under this section. Brian Radley from Wolverhampton was charged with attending a woman in childbirth otherwise than under the direction and personal supervision of a duly qualified practitioner and was fined £100 (August 1983). If the charge were defended, the midwife would of course be a key witness for the prosecution and her records would come under close scrutiny.

In October 2000 the UKCC reported that a nurse who delivered a baby despite having no midwifery qualification was found guilty of professional misconduct and removed from the UK Register. The offence took place in April 1999 when the registered nurse delivered a baby at a home in North London. It was said that she was a member of a religious group which banned members from attending hospitals or seeing mid-wives when they give birth. The UKCC Director of Professional Conduct stated that registered practitioners were entitled to hold strong religious beliefs and convictions. However, the nurse was not entitled to use these beliefs as a justification for breaking the law and endangering women and babies. Her belief that her religious views put her above the law meant that removing her from the Register was the only appropri-ate penalty to ensure the protection of the public.

REGISTRATION AND NOTIFICATION OF BIRTHS

Certain duties are placed upon the registered midwife in connection with the regis-tration of births and stillbirths and she should therefore have a good understanding of her statutory duties in this respect. In addition, she may be asked by the clients about the duties of registration, about changing the registered names or about the situation in relation to an illegitimate child. Full details are therefore given for refer-ence. The statutory provisions governing this area are shown in Box 25.2.

Box 25.2 Statutory provisions for birth and death

Births and Deaths Registration Act 1953

Regulations of the Births, Deaths and Marriages Regulations, Statutory Instrument 1968 No 2049

Stillbirth Definition Act 1992

National Health Service Act 1977 s.124

◀

National Health Service (Notification of Births and Deaths) Regulations Statutory Instrument 1982 No. 286

Some of the main provisions of the 1953 Act are shown in Box 25.3.

Box 25.3 Births and Deaths Registration Act 1953

1. (1) the birth of every child born in England and Wales shall be registered by the registrar of births and deaths . . . by entering in a register kept for that sub-district such particulars concerning the birth as may be prescribed . . .

   (2) The following person shall be qualified to give information concerning a birth . . .

   a. the father and mother of the child

   b. the occupier of the house in which the child was to the knowledge of that occupier born

   c. any person present at the birth

   d. any person having charge of the child

   e. in the case of a stillborn child found exposed, the person who found the child. (Added by Children Act 1975 Schedule 3 Para. 13(2).)

2. In the case of every birth it shall be the duty

   a. of the father and mother of the child; and

   b. in the case of the death or inability of the father and mother, of each other qualified informant,

   to give to the registrar, before the expiration of a period of 42 days from the date of the birth, information of the particulars required to be registered concerning the birth, and in the presence of the registrar to sign the register:

   Provided that

   1. the giving of information and the signing of the register by any one qualified informant shall act as a discharge of any duty under this section of every other informant

▶

2. this section shall cease to apply if, before the expiration of the said period and before the birth has been registered, an inquest is held at which the child is found to have been stillborn

3. where any stillborn child is found exposed, it shall be the duty of the person finding the child . . . to give to the best of his knowledge and belief to the registrar, before the expiration of 42 days from the date on which the child was found, such information of the particulars required to be registered concerning the birth of the child as the informant possesses, and in the presence of the registrar to sign the register.

3A. (1) Where the place and date of birth of a child who was abandoned are unknown to, and cannot be ascertained by, the person who has charge of the child, that person may apply to the Registrar General for the child's birth to be registered under this section.

The Registrar General's duties are detailed in the Act, but he shall not register a child's birth if he is satisfied that the child was not born in England or Wales, or has been adopted, or the birth is known to have been previously registered under this Act.

NOTIFICATION OF BIRTHS

There is a statutory duty on the midwife or doctor attending the woman in childbirth to give notification to the prescribed medical officer (the District Medical Officer) of the birth or stillbirth within 36 hours (s.124 National Health Service Act 1977). The duty applies whether the birth is at home or in hospital.

REGISTRATION

There is a statutory duty placed upon certain informants for the birth to be registered with the registrar for births, marriages and deaths. Details of the duty are shown in Box 25.4.

Box 25.4 Duties of informants

Under the Births and Deaths Registration Act 1953 it is the duty of the mother or father to give information to the Registrar within 42 days of the birth or stillbirth and to sign the register. If either of them cannot, then there is a duty to do so on the occupier of the house, or any person present at the birth, or any person having charge of the child.

'House' is defined as including a public institution, which covers a prison, lock-up or hospital, and such other public or charitable institution as may be prescribed. The occupier is defined in relation to a public institution as including a governor, keeper, master, matron, superintendent or other chief resident officer. The unit general manager or other person nominated by him would therefore have the responsibility for registering the birth. The nominated person might well be the midwife.

Powers of enforcement

If there is a failure to register within 42 days, the Registrar can compel any qualified informant to attend to give information and sign the register. The Registrar must give 7 days notice in writing (s.4 of 1953 Act). If the birth is registered within 3 months of the date of the birth, no registration fee is required.

There are additional powers if there is no registration after that date (s.6). After 12 months since the date of the birth, the birth can only be registered with the written authority of the Registrar General. This does not apply to a stillbirth (s.7(3)).

The Registrar shall if required by the informant give to the informant a certificate that he has registered the birth (s.12).

Registration of the name of the child or alteration of the name (s.13)

Where before the expiration of 12 months from the date of the birth of any child, the name by which it was registered is altered, or, if it was registered without a name, a name is given to the child, the registrar or superintendent registrar having custody of the register in which the birth was registered, upon delivery to him at any time of a certificate in the prescribed form signed:

a. if the name was altered or given in baptism, either by the person who performed the rite of baptism or by the person who has custody of the register, if any, in which the baptism is recorded, or

b. if a name has not been given to the child in baptism, by the father, mother or guardian of the child or other person procuring the name of the child to be altered or given . . .

shall without any erasure of the original entry, forthwith enter in the register the name mentioned in the certificate as having been given to the child, and, after stating upon the certificate the fact that the entry has been made, shall forthwith send the certificate to the Registrar General together with a certified copy of the entry of the birth with the name added under this subsection.

ILLEGITIMATE CHILDREN

Under s.10, in the case of a child whose father and mother were not married to each other at the time of his birth, no person shall as father of the child be required to give information concerning the birth of the child, and the registrar shall not enter in the register the name of any person as father of the child unless certain specified exceptions apply. These exceptions include the joint request of the mother and the person acknowledging himself to be the father of the child (in which case that person shall sign the register together with the mother), or at the request of the mother or the putative father on production of specified declarations.

Since December 2003, it has been possible for an unmarried couple to register the birth of the baby together, in which case the unmarried father acquires parental responsibilities in relation to the child, which he would not otherwise have.

Under s.10A, where the birth of a child whose parents were not married at the time of its birth has been registered under this Act, but no person has been registered as the child's father, the registrar shall re-register the birth so as to show a person as the father at the joint request of the mother and that person; or at the request of the mother or of the putative father on production of specified documentation.

Re-registration of births of legitimated persons

Section 14 enables the Registrar General (subject to certain conditions) at any time to authorise the re-registration of a person's birth on the production of evidence which appears to him to be satisfactory that the person has become a legitimated person. Both parents must furnish the information for the re-registration.

REGISTRATION OF GENDER

Originally, the gender recorded on the birth certificate could not be changed at the request of a person who wished to change their sex. The Court of Appeal held that even where a person had undergone gender re-assignment surgery, the registration of the person at birth as male remained as such. This meant that the transsexual could not validly marry a man, since she was in law still male.[2]

However, as a result of the Gender Recognition Act 2004 which came into force on 4 April 2005 a person can apply for a gender recognition certificate on the basis of:

– living in the other gender or

– having changed gender under the law of a country or territory outside the UK.

The application is put before a panel who must grant the application if satisfied that the applicant:

– has or has had gender dysphoria

– has lived in the acquired gender throughout the period of 2 years ending with the date on which the application is made

– intends to continue to live in the acquired gender until death and

– complies with the requirements imposed by s.3. (This covers the evidence to be provided by the applicant.)

An interim certificate can be issued if the applicant is married, a full certificate if the applicant is not married. The interim certificate can be followed by a full certificate once the marriage is dissolved or annulled or the spouse dies. There is a procedure for appeals where an applicant can appeal against the ruling of the panel to the High Court or Court of Session on a point of law.

The effect of the issue of a full gender recognition certificate is that the person's gender becomes for all purposes the acquired gender. The Registrar General is required to maintain a Gender Recognition Register, which is not open to public inspection or search.

An interesting provision of the Act is that for the purposes of sport, the organisers can prohibit or restrict the participation in a gender-affected sport of a person with an acquired gender if necessary for fair competition or the safety of competitors. Supplementary provisions make it an offence for information about an application for acquired gender to be disclosed by a person in an official capacity. There are specific defences to this offence, including disclosure with the consent of the person. Schedule 1 sets out provisions relating to the setting-up of gender recognition panels of persons with legal or medical qualifications.

REGISTRATION OF DEATH

If the baby is born alive and then dies, there must be a registration of both the birth and the death.

MATERNAL DEATH

In the rare event of a maternal death, the midwife should be conversant with the legal requirements for the certification and registration of the death and the requirements when the family request a cremation rather than a burial. She should also ensure that she is familiar with specific ethnic and religious requirements when appropriate.

STILLBIRTH

A stillbirth is defined as

Where a child issues forth from its mother after the 24th week of pregnancy, and which did not at any time after being completely expelled from its mother breathe or show any signs of life

(s.41 of the 1953 Act as amended by s.1 of the Stillbirth Act 1992)

The stillbirth has to be registered as such and the informant has to deliver to the Registrar a written certificate that the child was not born alive. This must be signed by the registered medical practitioner or the registered midwife who was in attendance at the birth or who has examined the body. The certificate must state to the best of the knowledge and the belief of the person signing it, the cause of death and the estimated duration of the pregnancy (s.11(1)(a)). Where the midwife is in sole attendance at the confinement, whether in a home or in a hospital, she must complete the certificate.

Alternatively a declaration in the prescribed form giving the reasons for the absence of a certificate and that the child was not born alive could be made (s.11(1)(b)).

A stillbirth should be disposed of by burial in a burial ground or churchyard or by cremation at an authorised crematorium.

Under the supplementary information and legislation placed by the NMC at the end of its publication on the Midwives Rules and Standards,[3] the NMC sets out the provisions of the Births and Deaths Registration Act and outlines the duties of the midwife. The guidance contained in the earlier Midwives Code of Practice[4] Para. 39 is that the midwife must inform the Supervisor of Midwives of any maternal death, stillbirth or neonatal death occurring when she is the midwife responsible for the care of that mother and her baby. However, the need for this communication would be implied from the relationship of the midwife and Supervisor as set out in the NMC guidance.

A Health Authority should not dispose of a stillbirth without the consent of the parents. In October 1993 the manager at the Bishop Auckland General Hospital, Co. Durham, admitted causing distress to Tracey Turner for burying her stillborn baby without her permission. It was stated that there would be an investigation into how the mistake occurred[5] (see below on the disposal of fetus and organs after post-mortems).

Fetus of less than 24 weeks

If the fetus was delivered without any signs of life, then no registration is necessary. The fetus may be disposed of without formality in any way which does not constitute a nuisance or an affront to public decency. If the fetus shows signs of life and then dies, it would have to be treated as both a birth and a death.

Midwives should be sensitive to the fact that parents may suffer the same feelings of bereavement whatever the period of gestation and should therefore arrange for counselling and support as they would if the baby were full term.

The Human Fertilisation and Embryology Act 1990 s.37 changed the law relating to abortion. It substituted a new section for the Abortion Act 1967 and apart from some exceptional circumstances, the rule now is that the pregnancy must not have exceeded its 24th week and that the continuance of the pregnancy would involve a risk greater than if the pregnancy were terminated to the physical or mental health of the pregnant woman or any existing children of her family (see Ch. 26). However, a stillbirth was defined as one where the pregnancy had lasted 28 weeks or more. This anomaly was redressed by the Stillbirth (Definition) Act 1992.

Live birth followed by death
A fetus of 24 weeks or more gestation which is born alive, but subsequently dies, is not a stillbirth but must be registered as a birth and a death.

An abortion after 24 weeks
What happens in the very exceptional circumstances when an abortion takes place after 24 weeks' gestation?

This is possible (under the amendments to the Abortion Act 1967 by the Human Fertilisation and Embryology Act 1990) in the circumstances set out in Chapter 26.

How is the length of gestation determined?
The midwife or doctor have to use their professional judgement in determining whether the fetus comes within the provisions of the stillbirth regulations. If the fetus is considered to be less than 24 weeks the parents could still arrange a ceremony and formal disposal of the body if they so wish.

Should the fetus survive a termination, every reasonable care should be taken of him/her (see Ch. 17).

Other implications of the Act
The change of time for the definition of stillbirth also affects the right of the mother to maternity allowances. The meaning of confinement for the purposes of benefits under the Social Security and Benefits Act 1992 will cover confinements of 24 or more weeks, rather than 28 weeks.

OFFENCES UNDER THE 1953 ACT

Sections 35–38 create certain offences in relation to registration. These are shown in Box 25.5.

Box 25.5 Offences in relation to registration

Section 35: Offences in relation to failure by the registrar to register or in carelessly losing or injuring the register

Section 36: Penalties for failure to give information

▶
Section 37: Penalty for forging or falsifying any certificate, declaration or order under the Act or knowingly using or giving, sending as genuine any false or forged certificate, document etc.

Section 38: Gives the power to the superintendent registrar to prosecute any person for an offence under this Act.

POST-MORTEMS AND INQUESTS

POST-MORTEM REQUESTED BY THE HOSPITAL

Post-mortem consent forms have to be signed by one of the parents where a post-mortem has been requested. They have the right of refusal and the post-mortem cannot be carried out against their wishes unless the case has been referred to the coroner who has the right to order a post-mortem.

A post-mortem must be carried out by or under the instructions of a fully registered medical practitioner and must have the authority of the person lawfully in possession of the body.

CORONER'S POST-MORTEM AND INQUEST

Relatives cannot refuse to give consent where the coroner requires a post-mortem to be carried out in order to fulfil his/her statutory provisions.

The Coroner's Rules require material removed from the body to be preserved for such a period as the coroner thinks fit.[6]

Significant changes to the coroner's office and jurisdiction are recommended in the Third Report of the Shipman Inquiry.[7]

Where death occurs in a hospital in circumstances where the patient is suffering from a condition which could lead to death if monitoring and treatment is omitted, then the coroner is required to hold an inquest unless he/she can say there are no grounds for suspecting that the omission was an effective cause of death. This was the ruling in a case[8] where a woman gave birth to twins by caesarean section at 10.25 p.m. on 6 February 1999. Her blood pressure was normal post-delivery but was not monitored between that time and 1.35 a.m. on 7 February 1999. It was then checked and discovered to be raised and treatment began. She suffered a left-sided intracerebral haemorrhage at 5.15 a.m. and died on 15 February 1999. The coroner accepted that the failure to monitor her blood pressure post-delivery was wholly inadequate but held that it was not a case in which the defects and human fault complained of rendered the death unnatural, and refused to hold an inquest. The High Court held that an inquest should be held unless there are no grounds for suspecting that the omission of monitoring and treatment was an effective cause of death. The Court of Appeal dismissed the coroner's appeal, since there was material evidence available to the coroner upon which he could not properly decide otherwise than that there was reasonable cause to suspect that her death was

a. at the least contributed to by neglect, and was thus

b. unnatural.

Stillbirth and the coroner

If it is found that the body was that of a stillborn child there can be no complete inquest since there has been no independent life and therefore no subsequent death. Accordingly, in such cases the inquisition should be marked 'stillbirth' and not completed. It is usual for the coroner to fill in Part Three of the certificate for disposal after an inquest which relates to a stillbirth.

REMOVAL, RETENTION AND STORAGE OF ORGANS, BODY PARTS AND TISSUE

The Human Tissue Act 2004 (see below) now regulates the removal and retention of tissues and, apart from specified exceptions, requires the 'appropriate consent' as defined in the Act.

The Department of Health and Social Security provided a 'Post-Mortem Declaration Form' to ensure that inquiries of relatives were made not only as to any relevant objection to the post-mortem examination itself, but also to the removal and retention of tissue.[9] The Royal College of Pathologists has issued a consensus statement on the use of human tissue in research, education and quality control[10] and also guidelines for the retention of tissues and organs at post-mortem examination.[11] In October 2000 the British Medical Association issued advice to its members that relatives should give informed consent to the retention of organs. It should also be made clear that relatives can refuse consent to a post-mortem examination, unless it has been ordered by a coroner.[12] In the 6th Annual Report of CESDI,[13] Appendix 4 gives guidance on fetal and infant post-mortems.

REFORMS POST-ALDER HEY AND OTHER CENTRES

Following an outcry by parents about organs from their dead children having been removed and retained without their explicit consent, an Inquiry was set up to look at the removal, retention and storage of body parts at Alder Hey Children's Hospital. The Report of the Royal Liverpool Children's Inquiry (chaired by Michael Redfern QC)[14] on the retention of organs and body parts was published on 30 January 2001. Its publication coincided with three other publications:

– A report of a Census of Organs and Tissues Retained by Pathology Services in England carried out by the Chief Medical Officer[15]

– The Removal, Retention and use of Human Organs and Tissue from Post-Mortem Examination Advice from the Chief Medical Officer[16]

– Consent to Organ and Tissue Retention at Post-Mortem Examination and Disposal of Human Materials.[17]

The Inquiry found that thousands of children's body parts had been collected at the hospital, some going back to before 1973. Most however were retained after 1988 when Professor Richard Van Velzen was appointed to the Department of Pathology and there was a huge increase in the number of organs removed and retained. Between 1988 and the end of 1995, it was the practice to remove every organ from every child in a post-mortem.

RETAINED ORGANS COMMISSION

In response to the Redfern Report, the Secretary of State set up a Retained Organs Commission under the Chairmanship of Professor Margaret Brazier. It was a special Health Authority with the following functions:

– Oversee the return of tissues and organs from collections around the country

– Ensure that collections are accurately catalogued

– Provide information on collections throughout the country

– Ensure that suitable counselling is available

– Act as an advocate for parents if problems arise

– Advise on good practice in this area

– Handle inquiries from families and the public.

In addition it advised Ministers, provided guidance to the NHS and universities, and monitored trusts to ensure that they deal properly with organ returns. It also provided a national help-line initially via NHS Direct for parents and relatives. It ceased to function in March 2004.

LEGAL ACTION BY PARENTS

Legal action by parents who had suffered as a result of the removal and retention of organs from their dead children in a group litigation action was initiated and the court agreed that the legal costs would be capped at £506 500.[18] On 26 March 2004 the High Court ruled, in respect of three test cases, that doctors could owe a duty of care to a mother after the death of her baby, therefore the practice of not warning parents that a post-mortem examination might involve the removal and retention of an organ could not be justified in all cases. Parents could claim damages if they had suffered psychological injury as a consequence.[19] Damages of £2750 were awarded in one of the test cases; the other two lost.

THE HUMAN TISSUE ACT 2004

The Human Tissue Act 2004 was passed as a result of the concerns resulting from the Alder Hey and other hospital scandals on organ removal retention and storage and in the light of the feedback from the consultation document 'Human Bodies Human Choices', which was published in July 2002.[20] Proposals for new legislation on human organs and tissue were published in September 2003[21] and the Human Tissue Act 2004 was enacted as a consequence. A Human Tissue Authority was appointed in April 2005 and will be responsible for the implementation of the Act in April 2006. The Act makes provisions for:

– Removal, storage and use of human organs and other tissue for scheduled purposes

– Regulation of activities involving human tissue

– Establishment of the Human Tissue Authority

– Preservation for transplantation

– Non-consensual analysis of DNA

– Powers of inspection, entry, search and seizures

– Offences by bodies corporate and prosecutions.

The storage of a body or body parts or removal and use are lawful if done with appropriate consent for one of the purposes listed in Schedule 1 which sets out the following:

– Anatomical examination (after the registration of death)

– Determining the cause of death

– Establishing after a person's death the efficacy of any drug or other treatment administered to him

– Obtaining scientific or medical information about a living or deceased person which may be relevant to any other person (including a future person)

– Public display

– Transplantation

– Clinical audit

- Education in training relating to human health

- Performance assessment

- Public health monitoring

- Quality assurance.

Special provisions apply to the use of body material for research, where it must be ethically approved under Regulations made by the Secretary of State.

Appropriate consent for a child means consent by the child, or if he is not competent to deal with the issue of consent, the consent of a person with parental responsibility. Where the child has died, appropriate consent means either the consent in writing by the child and the consent is for public display or anatomical examination (of non-excepted material), or the consent of the person who had parental responsibility before the death.

Appropriate consent for an adult means either the consent of the person, or his consent in writing before his death. This must have been signed by the person in the presence of at least one witness or signed at the direction of the person concerned, in his presence and in the presence of at least one witness, or have been contained in a will. For purposes other than public display or anatomical examination (of non-excepted material) appropriate consent means consent before death, consent by a person appointed (under s.4) or the consent of a person who stood in a qualifying relationship to him immediately before he died. Section 4 enables a person to appoint one or more persons to represent him after his death in relation to consent for the purposes of s.1.

Excepted material means material which has come from the body of a living person or has come from the body of a deceased person otherwise than in the course of use of the body for the purposes of anatomical examination.

The Human Tissue Authority has considerable duties in providing information and monitoring developments in relation to the removal from a human body of material, the storage of the body or relevant material, the disposal of the body or relevant material. It issues licences for specified activities and failure to obtain a licence is a criminal offence. The Human Tissue Authority also has responsibility for preparing and issuing codes of practice. Section 45 creates an offence of attempting or taking an analysis of DNA without appropriate consent. The necessary consent with specified exceptions are defined in Schedule 4.

A criminal offence occurs if a person, without the appropriate consent, does one of the following activities unless he reasonably believes that he has the appropriate consent or that the activity is not one covered by this offence. The specified activities are:

– Storage of a body for use for a purpose specified in Schedule 1 other than anatomical examination

– The use of a body for a purpose specified in Schedule 1 other than anatomical examination

– The removal from the body for use for a purpose specified in Schedule 1 of any relevant material of which the body consists or which it contains.

Regulations are to be drawn up to cover the situation where activities involve taking material from adults who lack capacity to consent.

Nothing in Part 1 of the Act applies to the powers of the coroner.

The Human Tissue Act 2004 replaces the Human Tissue Act 1961, the Anatomy Act 1984 and the Human Organ Transplants Act 1989.

Disposal of fetal material following a termination is considered in Chapter 26.

CONCLUSION

The midwife should find that within the medical records department or general office of the trust, expertise is available to assist her on the forms which have to be completed and the notifications which must be carried out on a stillbirth, birth or death. She must ensure that the guidance is followed relating to obtaining consent from parents before a hospital (as opposed to a coroner's) post-mortem is carried out and that the parents are notified and agree to any retention and storage of organs and that the provisions of the Human Tissue Act 2004 are followed.

QUESTIONS AND EXERCISES

1. You are asked to prepare a booklet for your clients on information which they would require to have in the event of a stillbirth. What topics would you include?

2. A client who has a miscarriage at 15 weeks has asked you if she could have a service and burial. What is the legal situation?

3. You are involved in caring for a client, when the child is born alive but dies within minutes of delivery. What is the legal situation?

4. A pathologist in your hospital is undertaking research into neonatal deaths and has asked you to obtain the consent of the relevant mothers for a post-mortem to be undertaken. What laws apply and what procedures should be followed?

References

1 Nursing and Midwifery Order 2001, Statutory Instrument 2002 No 253.

2 B v. B (validity for marriage: transsexual) [2001] EWCA Civ 1140; The Times, August 15 2001.

3 Nursing and Midwifery Council. Midwives Rules and Standards. NMC; August 2004.

4 UKCC. Midwives Rules and Code of Practice. London: UKCC; 1998.

5 News item. The Times, 11 October 1993.

6 Coroners Rules 1984, SI 1984 No 552 Rule 9.

7 Shipman Inquiry Third Report. Death and Cremation Certification, published 14 July 2003. Online. Available: www.the-shipman-inquiry.org.uk/reports.asp

8 Her Majesty's Coroner for Inner London North *ex parte* Peter Francis v. Touche. Lloyds Rep Med [2001] 327.

9 Department of Health. Post-Mortem Declaration Forms. Health Service Circular 77:28.

10 Royal College of Pathologists, Institute of Bio-Medical Science. Consensus statement of recommended policies for uses of human tissue in research, education and quality control. With notes reflecting UK law and practices prepared by a working party of the Royal College of Pathologists and the Institute of Bio-Medical Science. London: RCPath; 1999.

11 Royal College of Pathologists. Guidelines for the retention of tissues and organs at post-mortem examination. London: RCPath; 2000.

12 British Medical Association. Consent to organ retention. London: BMA; 2000.

13 Confidential Enquiry into Stillbirths and Deaths in Infancy. 6th Annual Report 1996–1997. London: Maternal and Child Health Research Consortium; 1999.

14 Department of Health. The Royal Liverpool Children's Inquiry Report. London: HMSO; 2001.

15 Chief Medical Officer. A report of a Census of Organs and Tissues Retained by Pathology Services in England. London: HMSO; 2001.

16 Department of Health. The removal, retention and use of human organs and tissue from post-mortem examination: Advice from the Chief Medical Officer. London: HMSO; 2001.

17 Department of Health. Consent to organ and tissue retention at post-mortem examination and disposal of human materials. London: HMSO; 2001.

18 AB and others v. Leeds Teaching Hospitals NHS Trust and in the Matter of the Nationwide Organ Group Litigation. Lloyd's Rep Med 7[2003] 355.

19 AB and Others v. Leeds Teaching Hospital NHS Trust and Another. The Times Law Report, 12 April 2004; [2004] Lloyd's Rep Med 1.

20 Department of Health and Welsh Assembly Government. Human Bodies, Human Choices. A Consultation Report, July 2002.

21 Department of Health and Welsh Assembly Government. Proposals for new legislation on human organs and tissue, September 2003. Online. Available: www.doh.gov.uk/tissue

Chapter 26

TERMINATION OF PREGNANCY

In 2003 abortions were at an all time high reaching 18.6 per 1000 of all women. The total number of all ages having a termination of pregnancy was 190 700.[1] Some 80% of these were funded by the NHS. There were 34 200 abortions among girls aged 16–19 years. The number of women aged between 30 and 34 having abortions doubled between 1976 and 2003, to 14 600. A total of 1229 terminations were carried out on fetuses between 22 and 24 weeks; one-fifth of these were due to a risk that the baby would be born with a serious disability.[2]

ABORTION AND THE CRIMINAL LAW

The Abortion Act 1967, as amended by the Human Fertilisation and Embryology Act 1990 (see Box 26.1) provides a statutory defence to certain offences under the Offences Against The Person Act 1861 and the Infant Life Preservation Act 1929. To bring about the death of a fetus, either intentionally or as a result of gross negligence, is unlawful under ss.58 and 59 of the Offences Against The Person Act 1861, unless the Abortion Act applies. The Infant Life Preservation Act 1929 makes it a criminal offence to destroy the life of a child capable of being born alive (see below). However, the Abortion Act 1967 s.5(1) makes it clear that 'no offence under the Infant Life (Preservation) Act shall be committed by a registered medical practitioner who terminates a pregnancy in accordance with the provisions of this Act'. (For further discussion on the rights of the fetus see Ch. 17.)

To avail oneself of the defence under the Abortion Act 1967 it must be shown that the requirements set out in s.1 were present (Box 26.1). It would be a question of fact and evidence as to whether this situation existed.

Box 26.1 Abortion Act 1967 (as amended by the Human Fertilisation and Embryology Act 1990)

1(1) Subject to the provisions of this section, a person shall not be guilty of an offence under the law relating to abortion when a pregnancy is terminated by a registered medical practitioner, if two registered medical practitioners are of the opinion formed in good faith:

a. that the pregnancy has not exceeded its twenty-fourth week and that the continuance of the pregnancy would involve risk, greater than if the pregnancy were terminated, of injury to the physical or mental health of the pregnant woman or any existing children of her family; or

b. that the termination is necessary to prevent grave permanent injury to the physical or mental health of the pregnant woman; or

c. that the continuance of the pregnancy would involve risk to the life of the pregnant woman, greater than if the pregnancy were terminated; or

d. that there is substantial risk that if the child were born it would suffer from such physical or mental abnormalities as to be seriously handicapped.

1(2) In determining whether the continuance of a pregnancy would involve such risk of injury to health as is mentioned in para. (a) or (b) of sub-section (1) of this section, account may be taken of the pregnant woman's actual or reasonably foreseeable environment.

1(3) Except as provided by sub-section (4) of this section, any treatment for the termination of pregnancy must be carried out in a hospital vested in the Minister of Health or the Secretary of State under the National Health Service Acts (NHS Trust or NHS Foundation Trust), or in a place for the time being approved for the purposes of this section by the said Minister or the Secretary of State.

a. The power under sub-section (3) of this section to approve a place includes power, in relation to treatment consisting primarily in the use of such medicines as may be specified in the approval and carried out in such manner as may be so specified, to approve a class of places.

1(4) Sub-section (3) of this section, and so much of subsection (1) as relates to the opinion of two registered medical practitioners, shall not apply to the termination of a pregnancy by a registered medical practitioner in a case where he is of the opinion, formed in good faith, that the termination is immediately necessary to save the life or to prevent grave permanent injury to the physical or mental health of the pregnant woman.

The Human Fertilisation and Embryology Act 1990 added a further amendment to the Abortion Act 1967 to cover the situation where one or more fetus(es) in a multiple pregnancy is terminated. The termination may be justified either to protect the health or life of the mother or where there is a substantial risk that if the child were born it would suffer from such physical or mental abnormalities as to be seriously handicapped (i.e. s.1(1)(d)).

SUCH PHYSICAL OR MENTAL ABNORMALITIES AS TO BE SERIOUSLY HANDICAPPED

There is no definition in the Act of the meaning of seriously handicapped and the issue was recently raised when a woman curate challenged the fact that a fetus with a cleft palate had been aborted. Joanna Jepson,[3] a curate at St Michael's Church Chester, was herself born with a congenital jaw defect and has a brother with Down's syndrome, but claims that following surgery, her life has not been unbearable as a consequence of that defect and therefore it should not be grounds for a termination of pregnancy. She brought a legal action in December 2003 and won the right of judicial review from the High Court to challenge the failure of West Mercia Police to investigate the late abortion. The case was due to commence on 24 May 2004 but has been delayed indefinitely under pressure from West Mercia Police who have re-opened a criminal investigation into the case. The termination in question was performed on a 28-week-old fetus with a bilateral cleft lip and palate. The procedure was carried out at Hereford County Hospital in December 2001, 4 weeks after the time limit set out in s.1(1)(a), as shown in Box 26.1. Had it been claimed that 'the continuance of the pregnancy would involve risk, greater than if the pregnancy were terminated, of injury to the physical or mental health of the pregnant woman or any existing children of her family' and the fetus was less than 24 weeks' gestation, then the termination could have been carried out without any reference to the defect. At the time of writing, it is reported that West Mercia police have sent a file to the Crown Prosecution Service.[4]

If the case goes ahead, the court will be required to define 'seriously handicapped' for the purposes of Para. (1)d. of the Abortion Act 1967 (as amended).

EMERGENCY SITUATION

In an emergency situation s.1(1) does not apply, where a registered medical practitioner is of the opinion, formed in good faith, that the termination is immediately necessary to save the life or to prevent grave permanent injury to the physical or mental health of the pregnant woman (s.1(4)) (see Box 26.1). Where an emergency situation as defined in this Section exists, the termination would not have to take place in an NHS hospital or one approved for the purposes of the Act by the Secretary of State. (See ss.1(3) and 1(4). Section 1(4) could also cover the situation where a surgeon who had no reasonable cause to believe that a woman was pregnant had no option but to continue with an operation even though this might result in a termination of pregnancy if the life of the mother was to be saved.)

CAPABLE OF BEING BORN ALIVE AND THE INFANT LIFE PRESERVATION ACT 1929

Prior to the amendments to the Abortion Act 1967 (which came into force on 1 April 1991), it was an offence to terminate a pregnancy where the fetus was capable of being born alive. In the case of C v. S[5] it was argued by the father, who was trying to stop the termination taking place, that a doctor who attempted to terminate a pregnancy of 18 weeks would be committing an offence under the Infant Life Preservation Act 1929, since the fetus was capable of being born alive. The Court of Appeal held that there was no evidence that the fetus was capable of breathing and so was not a child capable of being born alive. The termination would not therefore be an offence under the 1929 Act. In a case in 1991[6] a claim was made against the Health Authority by a woman who had a spina bifida baby on the grounds that the defect could have been found on a scan and therefore she could have had a termination. The claim was lost because the defendants claimed that at 26 weeks the fetus was capable of being born alive and therefore termination would have been an offence under the 1929 Act. The law has now been changed.

The amendments to the Abortion Act 1967 (effected by the Human Fertilisation and Embryology Act) make it clear that:

no offence under the Infant Life (Preservation) Act shall be committed by a registered medical practitioner who terminates a pregnancy in accordance with the provisions of this Act. (s.5(1) Abortion Act 1967 as amended)

Viability of the fetus and the capacity to be born alive are not now concerns in the lawful termination of a pregnancy. It became an public issue prior to the general election of 2005 that the 24-week limit should be lowered to 20 weeks. Much of the discussion appeared to ignore the fact that under the present law, ss.1(1) (b), (c) and (d) did not require any time limit. The Health Secretary announced on 22 March 2005 that he expected time to be made for an Abortion Bill after the election.[7]

ABORTION RESULTING IN A LIVE BIRTH

As can be seen from Box 26.1, there can be an abortion after 24 weeks where the conditions set out in s.1(1)b, c and d are present. Section 5(1) enables an abortion to be carried out at a later stage of pregnancy even though the child is capable of being born alive, providing that the conditions set out in s.1 are met. However, if following a lawful abortion the child were to be born alive, there is no right to kill the child. If the child were to be considerably disabled with a very poor prognosis, there is no duty to keep the child alive against all the odds (see Ch. 9). However, where the child is capable of surviving with a reasonable quality of life, there would be a duty of care to ensure that every reasonable means were taken to do so.

There are now very few abortions which take place after 24 weeks' gestation. Figures from the Department of Health published in July 2005 show that 42 women had terminations at 28 weeks or more gestation in 2004 compared with 49 the year before. There were 18 cases that involved pregnancies of 32 weeks or more, compared with 22 in 2003.

TERMINATION BY A REGISTERED MEDICAL PRACTITIONER

The Act requires a termination of pregnancy to be carried out by a registered medical practitioner.

The Royal College of Nursing challenged the lawfulness of the use of prostaglandins to terminate a pregnancy, since the patient was cared for by nursing staff and therefore the termination was not being carried out by a registered medical practitioner. In a majority decision, the House of Lords[8] held that when prostaglandins are used to terminate a pregnancy, the termination is lawful provided that it is under the control of a registered medical practitioner. Lord Diplock stated the position as follows:

In the context of the Act, what was required was that a registered medical practitioner – a doctor – should accept responsibility for all stages of the treatment for the termination of the pregnancy. The particular method to be used should be decided by the doctor in charge of that treatment; he should carry out any physical acts, forming part of the treatment, that in accordance with accepted medical practice were done only by qualified medical practitioners, and should give specific instructions as to the carrying out of such parts of the treatment as in accordance with accepted medical practice were carried out by nurses or other hospital staff without medical qualifications. To each of them the doctor or his substitute should be available to be consulted or called in for assistance from beginning to end of the treatment. In other words, the doctor need not do everything with his own hands; the subsection's requirements were satisfied when the treatment was one prescribed by a registered medical practitioner carried out in accordance with his directions and of which he remained in charge throughout.

Midwives might sometimes be asked to take part in prostaglandins abortions but they would be entitled to rely upon the right of conscientious refusal (see below).

PROVISIONS RELATING TO NOTIFICATION

The Secretary of State in respect of England and Wales, and the Scottish Executive, are empowered to make regulations to provide:

a. for requiring any such opinion as is referred to in s.1 of this Act to be certified by the practitioners or practitioner concerned in such form and at such time as may be prescribed by the regulations, and for requiring the preservation and disposal of certificates made for the purposes of the regulations

b. for requiring any registered medical practitioner who terminates a pregnancy to give notice of the termination and such other information relating to the termination as may be so prescribed

c. for prohibiting the disclosure, except to such persons or for such purposes as may be so prescribed, of notices given or information furnished pursuant to the regulations.

2(2) The information furnished in pursuance of regulations made by virtue of para. (b) of sub-section (1) of this section shall be notified solely to the Chief Medical Officer of the Department of Health, or of the Welsh Office, or of the Scottish Executive.

2(3) Any person who wilfully contravenes or wilfully fails to comply with require-ments of regulations under sub-section (1) of this section shall be liable on summary conviction to a fine not exceeding level 5 on the standard scale.

2(4) Any statutory instrument made by virtue of this section shall be subject to annulment in pursuance of a resolution of either House of Parliament.

The Abortion Regulations 1991[9] cover

– the Certificate of Opinion
– the Notice of Termination of Pregnancy and information relating to the termination
– restrictions on disclosure of information.

Changes were made to the abortion notification form HSA4 in April 2002.[10] These re-designed the form to allow for scanning in of the document and optical character reading of its contents; encouraged use of patient identification numbers and post-codes, rather than full name and address, so as to improve confidentiality; collection of self-reported ethnicity data where known and collection of data on whether Chlamydia screening was offered.

CONSCIENTIOUS OBJECTION TO ABORTIONS

A statutory defence is given by the law to a person who refuses to take part in abortions under s.4 of the Abortion Act. Section 4(1) of the Abortion Act 1967 permits conscientious objection to participation in treatment and is set out in Box 26.2.

Box 26.2 Section 4 Abortion Act 1967

4(1) Subject to sub-section (2) of this section, no person shall be under any duty, whether by contract or by any statutory or other legal requirement, to par-ticipate in any treatment authorised by this Act to which he has a conscien-tious objection;

– Provided that in any legal proceedings the burden of proof of conscientious objection shall rest on the person claiming to rely on it.

4(2) Nothing in sub-section (1) of this section shall effect any duty to participate in treatment which is necessary to save the life or to prevent grave permanent injury to the physical or mental health of a pregnant woman.

Midwifery is about preparation for, and care during and after, birth. It is not surprising therefore that some midwives should consider that they have no part to play in the termination of pregnancy. However, methods of termination such as the use of prostaglandins rely on the discharge of the fetus through the birth canal as in normal labour. Midwives may therefore sometimes be asked to assist or even take responsibility for the abortion under the supervision of the registered medical practitioner. (A conscientious objection provision similar to s.4 of the Abortion Act is provided by s.38 of the Human Fertilisation and Embryology Act 1990, which is discussed in Ch. 27.)

MEANING AND EVIDENCE OF CONSCIENTIOUS OBJECTION

It can be seen from Box 26.2 that the burden would be on the midwife to prove that she had a conscientious objection. How does she do that? What is the meaning of conscientious objection? There is no statutory definition. Sub-section 4(3) provides that in Scotland it is sufficient for a person to make a statement on oath, that she has a conscientious objection to participating in any treatment under the Act and that is then sufficient evidence to discharge the burden of proof. That sub-section does not apply however in England and Wales.

It would clearly have to be a settled view based perhaps on religious grounds or some other evidence of a belief against abortion. There has been no judicial decision on the definition of the objection but there has on the extent of the defence.

Extent of the defence of conscientious objection

In the case of Janaway v. Salford AHA,[11] Mrs Janaway was a devout Roman Catholic who was a secretary employed by the Health Authority. She refused to type abortion referral letters and was dismissed. She applied to the Industrial Tribunal claiming the dismissal was unfair in that she was protected from having to participate in such activities by reason of her conscientious objection and the defence under s.4(1) of the Abortion Act 1967. The House of Lords held that she was fairly dismissed since the protection of s.4(1) did not extend to typing letters. 'Participate' actually meant taking part in treatment designed to terminate a pregnancy.

This means that while the midwife would be protected by s.4(1) in her refusal to take part in the abortion treatment, she could not refuse to give advice to clients about abortion facilities, amniocentesis and other information which may lead to an abortion taking place.

This clearly places the midwife who has a conscientious objection to abortion in a difficult position. If during antenatal care, for example, a mother became aware of a possible genetical abnormality in her child and the appropriate advice would be to inform her about the possibility and need for an amniocentesis, a midwife would have a duty of care to ensure that the mother received this information, which might result in an abortion taking place, even though the midwife conscientiously objected to abortions for whatever reason.

The implications are two-fold:

– either the midwife refuses to give the advice in which case she faces the possibility of being disciplined and even dismissed. The midwife's refusal may also be contrary to the human rights of the woman as set out in the European Convention on Human Rights and enacted in the Human Rights Act 1998 (see Ch. 6 and Appendix 1 of this book); or

– the midwife gives the client the information, against her own principles and beliefs.

A possible compromise solution is for another midwife to take over the responsibility for the antenatal care at that stage, but this would be contrary to the philosophy of the Cumberlege Report, Changing Childbirth,[12] and the continuity of care provided by the named midwife. In addition it is recognised by the European Community Midwives Direction that included within the activities of a midwife are those shown in Box 26.3.

Box 26.3 Definition of a midwife in European Directive[13] (see Ch. 2)

Member states shall ensure that midwives are at least entitled to take up and pursue the following activities:

To provide sound family planning information and advice.

The activity shown in Box 26.3 might include advice on contraception, including the post-coital pill, and the midwife could not claim protection from carrying out that task. It must not of course be assumed that because the midwife had a strongly held personal view against abortion, she would not be capable of giving impartial, sound, comprehensive advice. Unpublished research has shown that there was no difference in the uptake of serum screening for risk estimation of Down's Syndrome of women in the second trimester, between patients counselled by midwives who held a conscientious objection to abortions and those counselled by midwives who did not object to abortions, provided that there was adherence to a protocol (pers. comm., 1992).

CONSCIENTIOUS OBJECTIONS AND AN EMERGENCY SITUATION

The right to refuse to participate given by s.4(1) does not apply in the circumstances set out in s.4(2) which are shown in Box 26.4.

Box 26.4 Section 4 (2) Abortion Act 1967

Nothing in sub-section (1) of this section shall effect any duty to participate in treatment which is necessary to save the life or to prevent grave permanent injury to the physical or mental health of a pregnant woman.

Where life is at stake or the possibility of grave permanent injury is present, the duty of care to the mother takes precedence over any conscientious objection held by the midwife.

CONSCIENTIOUS OBJECTION AND THE NMC CODE OF PROFESSIONAL CONDUCT: STANDARDS FOR CONDUCT, PERFORMANCE AND ETHICS

Clause 2.5 of the Code of Professional Conduct: standards for conduct, performance and ethics[14] is set out in Box 26.5.

Box 26.5 Clause 2.5 Code of Professional Conduct: standards for conduct, performance and ethics

You must report to a relevant person or authority, at the earliest possible time, any conscientious objection that may be relevant to your professional practice. You must continue to provide care to the best of your ability until alternative arrangements are implemented.

To comply with the requirement shown in Box 26.5 the midwife would have to declare her conscientious objections at the time of the interview for a post. She may therefore face discrimination against her appointment, because of the possibility of the midwife having to give advice during the antenatal stage as discussed above. In this controversial area where the midwife might not wish to be involved in abortions, whether through the actual activity or in giving advice, there are two rights which have to be balanced:

– on the one hand, the right of the woman to make available to herself the opportunities provided within the law to have an abortion and the necessary information;

– on the other hand, the right of the midwife to be entitled to work within her principles and beliefs.

Section 4(1) provides a compromise but inevitably it will not always satisfy both sides.

Should the midwife be asked for advice about procuring an abortion, she should make sure that the questioner is referred to the correct authority and should be very careful about giving any advice which could assist a person in carrying out an unlawful termination of pregnancy. To do so would be a criminal offence under the Offences Against The Person Act 1861.

HUMAN RIGHTS AND ABORTION

Since a fetus is not recognised as having a legal personality, it does not acquire legal rights until it is born (see Ch. 17 and the Congenital Disabilities Act). This means that probably no action can be taken on behalf of a fetus which is aborted under the Human Rights Act 1998 and Article 2 and the right to life, though the Strasbourg court has not ruled on the issue.[15] (In the case of Paton v BPAS[16] the European Commission on Human Rights ruled that the father had no right to be consulted – his Article 8 rights were subject under para. 2 to the rights of another person, i.e. the mother). The legal situation is different in Ireland, where the Irish Bill of Rights recognises the right to life of the unborn child. The human rights of the mother may become engaged, if it is alleged that a woman was unjustly refused an abortion and her Article 3 or 8 or 14 Rights were therefore violated (see case of an NHS Trust v. D, below).

POST-COITAL PILL AND THE INTRAUTERINE DEVICE

There has been some controversy over whether the above forms of family planning are properly regarded as contraception or abortion. They both aim at preventing the fertilised egg being implanted in the womb. In the case of R v. Price[17] a doctor was charged and convicted under s.58 of the Offences Against The Person Act 1861 after fitting a woman with an intrauterine device. His conviction was quashed in the Court of Appeal. Crucial to his defence was the fact that he believed the woman not to be pregnant at the time, i.e. he was preventing an implantation not assisting a termination. The Medical Protection Society[18] cited four cases in 1983 which were referred to the Director of Public Prosecutions to consider criminal proceedings (two were referred by LIFE) on grounds that the post-coital pill is procuring a miscarriage and that the requirements of the Abortion Act 1967 were not met and therefore there should be a prosecution under the Offences Against The Person Act 1861. In a written Parliamentary Reply, the Attorney General announced that no proceedings would be taken.[19] The provisions of the Offences Against The Person Act 1861 s.58 make it an offence for any woman being with child to unlawfully administer to herself any poison or noxious thing with intent to procure her miscarriage. Section 59 covers the situation of the supply or procurement whether or not she be with child. The Attorney General took the view that the word 'miscarriage' in its ordinary meaning is not apt to describe a failure to implant, whether spontaneous or not, and that it refers to a later stage of antenatal development than implantation and also that the phrase 'procure a miscarriage' cannot be construed to include the prevention of implantation.

In a more recent case,[20] an anti-abortion group won an application to the High Court to proceed with a case to stop the supply of over-the-counter sales of the morning-after pill to women over 16 years. The drug Levonelle-2 had formerly only been available on prescription, but in January 2001 its classification was changed to enable it to be sold by pharmacists. The barrister representing the Council for the Society for the Protection of Unborn Children argued that the change of classification per-mitted the commission of a criminal offence – the administration or supply of poisons or instruments with the intent to procure a miscarriage under the Offences Against The Person Act 1861. The judge decided that an important issue of public policy arose, which should be heard in the civil courts.

Securing a miscarriage through the use of menstrual extraction either mechanically or by induction through a drug such as mifepristone would have to be performed in compliance with the requirements of the Abortion Act 1967. Section 1(3) of the Abortion Act 1967 was amended by the Human Fertilisation and Embryology Act 1990 to give the Secretary of State power to approve centres where such treatment may be carried out (s.1(3A)) (see Box 26.1).

OPPOSITION TO ABORTIONS

In the case C v. S discussed above, the father was not married to the mother. In an earlier case a husband, Mr Paton, tried to prevent his wife obtaining a termination.[21] He failed on the grounds that provided the requirements of the Abortion Act 1967 were satisfied the termination was lawful and the husband had no *locus standi* to bring an action to prevent a lawful termination proceeding.

Mr Paton then took the case to the European Commission of Human Rights in Strasbourg[22] claiming that as a result of Article 8 of the European Convention on Human Rights, which gave a right to respect for family life (see Ch. 6 and Appendix 1 of this book) he had a right to stop the termination going ahead. He lost on the grounds that the Commissioner held the rights of the mother were protected under Para. 2 of Article 8.

In a more recent Scottish case, a father, separated from his wife, attempted to prevent an abortion taking place in the name of the child.[23] The court held that there was in law no justification for recognising the rights of the unborn child against the mother's right to lawfully terminate the pregnancy. The legal status of the unborn child is considered in Chapter 17. In cases where the mother is refusing a caesarean section which is vital to the survival of the fetus, the Court of Appeal has refused to accept the view that the unborn child has rights which are enforceable against the mother[24] (see Ch. 7).

In the Case Re P 1982,[25] parents opposed the abortion wanted by their daughter and offered to bring up the child. The judge decided that the abortion was in the best interests of the girl. (For further discussion of this case see Ch. 7.)

In May 2004, considerable media coverage was given to a situation where a mother discovered by chance that her daughter of 14 years was having an abortion (the situation is discussed in Ch. 12).

APPROVED PLACE

Section 1(3) (see above) requires the termination to take place in an NHS establishment or a place approved for the purposes of this section by the Minister or the Secretary of State (except in an emergency situation). Under the Care Standards Act 2000 regulations have been drawn up for the registration and inspection of independent hospitals and clinics.[26] As well as being subject to the general regulations, there are specific provisions for independent hospitals in which termination of pregnancies take place. Under Regulation 41:

(2) The registered person shall ensure that no patient is admitted to the hospital for a termination of pregnancy, and that no fee is demanded or accepted from a patient in respect of a termination, unless two certificates of opinion have been received in respect of the patient.

(3) The registered person shall ensure that a certificate of opinion in respect of a patient undergoing a termination of a pregnancy is completed and included with the patient's record within the meaning of Regulation 21 (which sets standards on record keeping).

(4) The registered person shall ensure that no termination of a pregnancy is undertaken after the 20(th) week of gestation, unless:

(a) the patient is treated by persons who are suitably qualified, skilled and experienced in the late termination of pregnancy; and

(b) the appropriate procedures are in place to deal with any medical emergency which occurs during or as a result of the termination.

(5) The registered person shall ensure that no termination of a pregnancy is undertaken after the 24(th) week of gestation.

(6) The registered person shall ensure that a register of patients undergoing termination of pregnancy in the hospital is maintained, which is

(a) separate from the register of patients which is to be maintained under para. 1 of Schedule 3;

(b) completed in respect of each patient at the time the termination is undertaken and

(c) retained for a period of not less that 3 years beginning on the date of the last entry.

(7) The registered person shall ensure that a record is maintained of the total numbers of terminations undertaken in the hospital and the requirements of Regulation 21(3) shall apply to that record (i.e. kept up to date, available for inspection at all times and retained for at least 3 years beginning on the date of the last entry).

(8) The registered person shall ensure that notice in writing is sent to the Chief Medical Officer of the DoH of each termination of pregnancy which takes place in the hospital.

(9) If the registered person

(a) receives information concerning the death of a patient who has undergone termination of pregnancy in the hospital during the period of 12 months ending on the date on which the information is received; and

(b) has reason to believe that the patient's death may be associated with the termination he shall give notice in writing to the Commission of that information, within the period of 14 days beginning on the day on which the information is received.

(10) The registered person shall prepare and implement appropriate procedures in the hospital to ensure that fetal tissue is treated with respect.

(11) Certificate of opinion means a certificate required by the regulations made under s.2(1) of the Abortion Act 1967.

The registration authority for an independent hospital is the Commission for Health Audit and Inspection (known as the Healthcare Commission; see Ch. 23 on private hospitals).

The Regulations have been supplemented by national minimum standards drawn up by the Department of Health.[27] As well as the core standards covering such areas as information provision and quality of care and treatment (see Ch. 23), service-specific standards are set for termination of pregnancy establishments. These cover:

– Quality of treatment and care

– Information for patients

– Privacy and confidentiality for patients

– Respect for fetal tissue

– Emergency procedures.

RIGHT TO SECURE A TERMINATION

There appears to be considerable variation across the country in the availability of NHS facilities for termination of pregnancy. An audit carried out by the Royal College of Obstetricians and Gynaecologists in 2001 found that 34% of abortion services failed to meet minimum targets for acceptable waiting periods. The RCOG guidelines suggest that a woman seeking a termination should see a gynaecologist within 5 days and that the procedure should take place within 1 week. The conclusion of the report was that some parts of the country appear to be providing a good service, although not always within the NHS.[28]

TERMINATION AND MENTAL INCAPACITY

In the following case, the court had to decide whether to issue a declaration that a termination could be lawfully carried out.

An NHS Trust v. D[29]

An NHS Trust sought guidance on when it was necessary to obtain a court declaration prior to terminating the pregnancy of a mentally incapacitated person suffering from severe schizophrenia. The court gave a declaration that it was lawful to terminate D's pregnancy following evidence of her incapacity and to the effect that termination was in her best interests. The Trust and Official Solicitor then sought more general guidance at a second hearing in relation to Article 8 of the European Convention on Human Rights. The court set out the following guidance:

– An application to the court was not necessary where issues of capacity and best interests were beyond doubt

– An application should be made promptly when there was any doubt as to either issue

– Applications should ordinarily be made where:

   i. there was a realistic prospect of the patient regaining capacity during or shortly after the pregnancy

   ii. there was a disagreement between medical professionals as to the patient's best interests or the patient or her family or the father expressed views inconsistent with termination

   iii. the procedures under the Abortion Act 1967 had not been followed or

   iv. there was some other exceptional circumstance, such as the pregnancy being the patient's last chance to bear a child.

– A termination in accordance with the Abortion Act 1967 in the best interests of an incapacitated patient was a legitimate and proportionate interference with rights protected by Article 8(1) and 8(2).

DISPOSAL OF PRODUCTS OF ABORTION FOLLOWING TERMINATION

Department of Health guidance was issued on the disposal following pregnancy loss before 24 weeks' gestation.[30] Stillbirths and neonatal deaths do not come under this guidance. Any woman or couple can make their own arrangements for disposal if they so wish. All fetal tissue should be stored in accordance with earlier Department of Health advice.[31] Fetal tissue can be buried, cremated or incinerated by an NHS trust provided the consent has been obtained from the woman or couple. Further guidance on this has been issued by the Department of Health.[32] Guidance has been issued by the Royal College of Nursing.[33] The Independent sector is required to comply with these arrangements as part of its registration rules (see Ch. 23) and NHS Trusts may wish to discuss issues relating to the disposal of fetal tissue with the independent sector clinic carrying out abortions on their behalf. NHS Trust policies should be developed and can take into account gestational age and the nature of the fetal tissue.

ORGAN REMOVAL, RETENTION AND STORAGE

An Inquiry was held into organ removal, retention and storage at Alder Hey Hospital.[34] Following the report, the government set up a Retained Organ Commission under the chairmanship of Professor Margaret Brazier and made recommendations on improving standards in relation to obtaining the informed consent of parents to the removal and use of organs and other body parts and tissue. These recommendations should improve practice in relation to consent for the disposal or use of aborted fetuses. Many of the recommendations have been given statutory force in the Human Tissue Act 2004 (see Ch. 25 on organ removal, retention and storage).

CONFIDENTIALITY OF ABORTION

Information relating to an abortion must be reported on the specific forms to the Department of Health. Otherwise the usual rules of confidentiality apply, subject to exceptions where disclosure is justified (see Ch. 10). In Chapter 12, the situation of the girl of 14 whose mother did not know that she was having an abortion is considered.

The question of confidentiality arose in a criminal case over the disclosure of documents relating to abortions.[35] The defendants jointly organised and participated in a protest outside a clinic run by the British Pregnancy Advice Service at which abortions were regularly performed. The protesters prevented patients and staff from leaving the clinic and failed to comply with police requests to leave the scene. Some 26 people were arrested and charged under s.5(1)(a) of the Public Order Act 1986, which makes it an offence to use threatening, abusive, or insulting words or behaviour . . . within the hearing or sight of a person likely to be caused harassment, alarm or distress thereby.

They were convicted and in their appeal claimed, among other points, that the Crown Court had erred in setting aside a witness summons served on an officer of the British Pregnancy Advice Centre, which would have required him to produce all records relating to abortions which had taken place or were to have taken place at the clinic on the day of the protest. They also claimed that they believed illegal abortions were about to be performed at the clinic on the day of the protest and therefore they were protected by the Criminal Law Act 1967, in that they were using such force as is reasonable in the prevention of a crime. Neither of these grounds of appeal succeeded.

The Court of Appeal referred to the specific provisions of the Abortion Act 1967 and the 1968 Regulations which ensured the maintenance of a high degree of confidentiality in respect of documents relating to abortions carried out under the Act. The documents were not relevant to the defence raised by the defendants. The 1991 regulations, though they came into effect after the case, continued to emphasise the confidentiality of the records.

Nor did the defendants come within the protection of the Criminal Law Act 1967, since their actions were aggressive and prevented other people from exercising their legal rights and did not distinguish between legal and illegal abortions.

FAILED ABORTION

It was reported in April 2005[36] that a mother is suing Tayside University Hospitals NHS Trust, seeking compensation and damages for the financial burden of raising her daughter following an abortion which removed only one pregnancy, leaving her with one fetus. Other similar cases for failed sterilisations are considered in Chapter 16.

CONCLUSIONS

The changes effected in the Abortion Act 1967 by the Human Fertilisation and Embryology Act 1990 have enabled terminations of pregnancies to take place at a much later date than the previous laws, since the time limit of 24 weeks only applies to the first condition for termination under s.1(1)(a). However, in practice, there are very few terminations after 24 weeks. In practice too, the method of ending a late gestation usually ensures the death of the fetus in the womb so that a living child is not the result of the termination. There will always be continual pressure for legislative change in this emotive area since the pro-life groups will continue to press for the criminalising of termination of pregnancy. There are also likely to be concerns over the availability of terminations within the NHS and guidance may be issued by NICE over the provision and availability of termination services.

QUESTIONS AND EXERCISES

1. A mother with four children (the last one only 12 months old) tells you that she is pregnant and probably over 24 weeks. She is anxious to obtain an abortion. What is the legal position?

2. You have been asked to assist in the gynaecology ward in the termination of pregnancies. You are not happy taking part in this work, since you wished to work only as a midwife. What is your legal position and what assistance does the law and the Code of Professional Conduct: standards for conduct, performance and ethics give you?

3. A client tells you that her 14-year-old daughter is pregnant but wants to have an abortion. The client wishes to bring up the child herself and prevent the daughter having a termination. What is the legal position? (See Chs 7 and 12.)

References

1 Office of National Statistics. Online. Available: www.statistics.gov.uk

2 Templeton S-K. Toll of babies aborted with chance of life hits 1,000 a year. Sunday Times, 17 April 2005.

3 Gledhill R. Congregations keep faith with women priests. The Times, 17 May 2004.

4 The Times News Report, 23 September 2004.

5 C v. S [1988] 1 All ER 1230.

6 Rance v. Mid-Downs HA [1991] 1 All ER 801.

7 News item. Abortion Bill. The Times, 23 March 2005.

8 Royal College of Nursing of the UK v. Department of Health and Social Security [1981] AC 800; [1981] 1 All ER 545.

9 The Abortion Regulations 1991, Statutory Instrument 1991 No 499.

10 Abortion (Amendment) (England) Regulations 2002, SI 2002 No 887.

11 Janaway v. Salford [1988] 3 All ER 1051.

12 Department of Health. Changing Childbirth: Report of Expert Maternity Group. London: HMSO; 1993.

13 European Community Midwives Directive 80/155 EEC Article 4, quoted in the Midwives Rules and Standards; 2004:36–37.

14 Nursing and Midwifery. Code of Professional Conduct: standards for conduct, performance and ethics. London: NMC; 2004.

15 Paton v. UK (1981) 3 EHRR 408.

16 Paton v. BPAS [1978] 2 All ER 987.

17 R v. Price [1969] 1 QB 541.

18 Medical Protection Society. Annual Report. Medical Protection Society; 1983:18.

19 House of Commons, May 1983 42 Parl Deb HC 238.

20 Gibb F. High Court Challenge to morning-after pill. The Times, 3 May 2001.

21 Paton v. Trustees of the British Pregnancy Advisory Service [1978] 2 All ER 987.

22 Paton v. United Kingdom [1980] 3 EHRR 408 (EcomHR).

23 Kelly v. Kelly [1997] SLT 896.

24 St George's Healthcare NHS trust v. S; R. v. Collins *ex parte* S [1998] 44 BLMR 160.

25 Re P (a minor) [1982] 80 Local Government Reports 301.

26 The Private and Voluntary Health (England) Regulations 2001, SI 2001 No 3968.

27 Department of Health Independent Health Care National Minimum Standards Regulations London: The Stationery Office; 2002.

28 Templeton A. Audit of abortion services. London: Royal College of Obstetricians and Gynaecologists; 2001.

29 An NHS Trust v. D; sub nom D. v. An NHS Trust (Medical Treatment: Consent: Termination) [2003] EWHC 2793; [2004] 1 FLR 1110; Lloyd's Rep Med [2004] 107.

30 Department of Health. Q and A on disposal following pregnancy loss before 24 weeks gestation. London: DoH; August 2004.

31 Department of Health. Health Service Guidelines – Disposal of fetal tissue. HSG (92)19, 12 November 1991.

32 Department of Health. Code of Practice Families and Post mortems. DoH, April 2003.

33 Royal College of Nursing Sensitive Disposal of All Fetal Remains. RCN; 2001.

34 Department of Health. The Royal Liverpool Children's Inquiry Report. London: HMSO; 2001.

35 Morrow and others v. Director of Public Prosecutions High Court of Justice QBD [1993] 14 BMLR 54 (reported in Medical Law Review 1994 99).

36 Lister D. Mother sues NHS after twin survives abortion. The Times, 25 April 2005.

Chapter 27

LEGAL ISSUES RELATING TO FERTILISATION, EMBRYOLOGY AND GENETICS

Estimates are given that at least one in ten couples are affected at some stage in their lives by infertility problems. The midwife is therefore quite likely to have clients who as a result of problems in conception and fertility may be involved with *in vitro* fertilisation (IVF) and/or surrogacy. This chapter considers the legal issues which arise and the framework which has been established by statute. It also considers recent developments in genetics and the legal implications. The Human Tissue Act 2004 is discussed in Chapter 25. An embryo outside the human body does not come within the provisions of that Act. The Human Tissue Act repeals Paras 8 and 9 of Schedule 4 of the Human Fertilisation and Embryology Act 1990, which relate to organ transplants.

HUMAN EMBRYOS AND *IN VITRO* FERTILISATION

The present law dates from the Warnock report which was published in 1984.[1] Many of its recommendations were subsequently incorporated into the Human Fertilisation and Embryology Act 1990. The Act covers the topics shown in Box 27.1.

Box 27.1 The Human Fertilisation and Embryology Act 1990

1. Establishes a statutory authority

2. Prohibits specific activities in connection with embryos and gametes

3. Enables licences to be issued by the authority

4. Defines mother and father

5. Regulates disclosure of information and confidentiality

6. Amends the Surrogacy Arrangements Act 1985

7. Amends the Abortion Act 1967 (see Ch. 26)

8. Provides a defence of a conscientious objection

9. Gives powers of enforcement and creates offences

10. Makes provision in relation to the giving and withdrawal of consent.

HUMAN FERTILISATION AND EMBRYOLOGY AUTHORITY (HFEA)

This Authority is appointed by the Secretary of State as a statutory non-crown body. The Secretary of State also appoints the chairman and deputy chairman. Registered medical practitioners, those concerned with the keeping or using of gametes or embryos outside the body and any person concerned with commissioning or funding research are ineligible to be appointed as chairman or deputy chairman.

The functions of the HFEA are shown in Box 27.2.

Box 27.2 Functions of HFEA

1. Keep under review information about embryos and advise the Secretary of State

2. Publicise the services provided to the public by the Authority

3. Provide advice and information for persons to whom licences apply or who are receiving treatment

4. Grant, vary, suspend and revoke licences through licence committees

5. Issue directions either generally or specifically

6. Maintain a code of practice giving guidance about the conduct of activities and treatment services

7. Maintain a register containing specified information.

UNAUTHORISED ACTIVITIES

The Act regulates activities in respect of embryos (i.e. a live human embryo where fertilisation is complete and an egg in the process of fertilisation) outside the human body and gametes (eggs or sperm). The activities shown in Box 27.3 and Box 27.4 are regulated: some completely prohibited, others can be undertaken but only under a licence.

Box 27.3 Prohibited activities in relation to embryos

S.3(1) No person shall

    a. bring about the creation of an embryo, or

    b. keep or use an embryo, except in pursuance of a licence.

S.3(2) No person shall place in a woman

    a. a live embryo other than a human embryo, or

    b. any live gametes other than human gametes.

S.3(3) A licence cannot authorise

    a. keeping or using an embryo after the appearance of the primitive streak (i.e. not later than the end of 14 days beginning with the day when the gametes are mixed)

    b. placing an embryo in any animal

    c. keeping or using an embryo in any circumstances in which regulations prohibit its keeping or use, or

    d. replacing a nucleus of a cell of an embryo with a nucleus taken from a cell of any person, embryo or subsequent development of an embryo.

Box 27.4 Prohibited activities in relation to gametes

S.4(1) No person shall

    a. store any gametes, or

    b. during treatment services, use the sperm of any man unless the services are being provided for the woman and the man together, or use the eggs of any other woman, or

▶
c. mix gametes with the live gametes of any animal, except in pursuance of a licence.

S.4(2) A licence cannot authorise storing or using gametes in any circumstances in which regulations prohibit their storage or use.

S.4(3) No person shall place sperm and eggs in a woman in any circumstances specified in the regulations except in pursuance of a licence.

The court has held that the criminal liability for offences in relation to an embryo otherwise than in accordance with a licence contrary to s.3(1) and 41(2)(a) of the 1990 Act did not extend to the person responsible for the supervision of the activities at the clinic where the alleged offences had taken place.[2]

In 1994, an amendment[3] was made to the 1990 Act which came into force on 10 April 1995. This added s.3A to the Act:

No person shall, for the purpose of providing fertility services for any woman, use female germ cells taken or derived from an embryo or a fetus or use embryos created by using such cells.

As a result of this Section, it is a criminal offence to use fetal eggs or embryos derived therefrom in medically assisted reproduction. The statutory definition of female germ cells is 'cells of the female germ line and includes such cells at any stage of maturity including eggs'.

GRANTING OF LICENCES

The Authority can grant licences

– authorising activities in the course of providing treatment services

– authorising the storage of gametes and embryos

– authorising activities for the purpose of a project of research.

Conditions for the giving of licences are laid down in ss.12, 13, 14 and 15 and Schedule 2. Sections 16–22 cover the granting, revocation and suspension of licences.

DEFINITION OF MOTHER AND FATHER

The definition of mother for the purposes of the Act is shown in Box 27.5 and the definition of father in Box 27.6.

CHAPTER 27 | LEGAL ISSUES RELATING TO FERTILISATION, EMBRYOLOGY AND GENETICS

Box 27.5 Definition of mother

S.27(1) The woman who is carrying or has carried a child as a result of the placing in her of an embryo or of sperm and eggs, and no other woman, is to be treated as the mother of the child.

(This does not apply to adoption but applies whether the woman was in the UK or elsewhere at the time of the placing in her of an embryo or the sperm and eggs.)

Box 27.6 Definition of father

S.28(1) Where a child is being or has been carried by a woman as the result of the placing in her of any embryo or of sperm and eggs or her artificial insemination; if

   a. at the time of the placing in her of the embryo or the sperm and eggs or of her insemination, the woman was a party to a marriage, and

   b. the creation of the embryo carried by her was not brought about with the sperm of the other party to the marriage

the other party to the marriage shall be treated as the father of the child unless it is shown that he did not consent to the placing in her of the embryo or the sperm and eggs or to her insemination.

If the treatment services were provided for her and a man together, by a person to whom a licence applies, then he shall be treated as the father of the child.

Where the sperm of a man is given for the treatment of others under Para. 5 of Schedule 3, or the sperm of a man or any embryo created from his sperm is used after his death, he is not to be treated as the father of the child (see Human Fertilisation and Embryology (Deceased Fathers) Act 2003 and the Diane Blood case below).

Under s.30, the courts can make orders providing for a child to be treated in law as the child of the parties to the marriage in certain circumstances. Regulations under this Section apply certain provisions of the Adoption Act 1976 to parental orders under s.30 of the 1990 Act.[4]

DISCLOSURE OF INFORMATION AND CONFIDENTIALITY

Section 33 prohibits any member or employee of a licensing authority disclosing information which is contained in the register so that an individual can be identified. However, the consent of the person(s) protected by these confidentiality provisions can release the person from the prohibition.

The Human Fertilisation and Embryology (Disclosure of Information) Act 1992 was passed to enable additional exceptions to the duty of confidentiality to be recognised. The bar on a doctor passing information direct to the patient's GP has ended. The 1992 Act enables the patient to give consent to disclosure to a specified person or to give general consent to disclosure within a wider circle of people where disclosure is necessary in connection with medical treatment, clinical audit or accounts audit. Before consent is given, reasonable steps must be taken to explain the implications of giving consent to the patient. Disclosure of information is also permissible in an emergency where the person disclosing is satisfied that the disclosure is necessary to avert imminent danger to the health of the patient and at the time, it is not reasonably practicable to obtain the patient's consent. The clinician can also disclose information to his legal adviser where necessary for the purposes preliminary to or in connection with legal proceedings. The 1992 Act allows access to records of treatment to be given to personal representatives and those bringing litigation on behalf of the incapacitated patient.

Power is given for new regulations relating to additional exceptions to the principle of confidentiality to be made if necessary.

Disclosure in the interests of justice can be made under s.34 in proceedings before a court when the question of whether a person is or is not the parent of the child by virtue of the act falls to be determined.

Under the Congenital Disabilities (Civil Liability) Act 1976, the court can make an application to the Authority authorising it to disclose information kept in the register and relevant to the issue of parentage (see Ch. 17, on the 1976 Act).

MISTAKE IN FERTILISING EGGS

During IVF treatment in Leeds, there was a mix up in the creation of embryos, and sperm from one man was wrongly injected into the eggs of the woman of another couple receiving IVF treatment. The error came to light at the birth of the children since one couple were both white and gave birth to twins of mixed race. In the subsequent court hearing to determine who should be treated as parents of the children, the judge held that the mistake in the mixing of Mr B's sperm with Mrs A's egg went to the root of the whole process and vitiated the whole concept of treatment together. Mr A had not given a consent to this fertilisation. Mr B was the biological and the legal father of the twins. An adoption order could safeguard the rights of the twins.[5]

DISCLOSURE OF SPERM AND EGG DONORS

As a result of regulations which came into force in April 2005[6] children born from donated sperm and egg have a right to trace their biological parents when they turn 18 years. The new laws only apply to sperm and egg donated after April 2005. In advance of the loss of anonymity, a campaign was commenced in January 2005 to raise public awareness about the need for egg and sperm donation.[7] The campaign sought to reassure potential donors that they would have no financial or legal responsibilities to any related offspring either now or in 18 years. However, there was evidence that fears of the loss of anonymity had already led to a reduction in those willing to be sperm donors and to couples looking on the internet or going overseas to obtain the services of donors.[8]

SURROGACY

The Surrogacy Arrangements Act 1985 is amended and a new s.1A provided (see below).

ABORTION ACT 1967

Major amendments are made to the Abortion Act 1967 and these are discussed in Chapter 26.

CONSCIENTIOUS OBJECTION

Section 38 provides a similar provision to that contained in the Abortion Act 1967 to protect any person who has a conscientious objection to working in the field. Its provision is shown in Box 27.7. There is no statutory definition of what constitutes a conscientious objection and a similar interpretation of the section in the Abortion Act 1967 can be expected. This did not protect a secretary who refused to type correspondence relating to abortions (see Ch. 26). Unlike the conscientious objection in a termination of pregnancy, there is no exception for emergencies.

Box 27.7 Conscientious objection: Section 38

S.38(1) No person who has a conscientious objection to participating in any activity governed by this Act shall be under any duty, however arising, to do so.

S.38(2) In any legal proceedings the burden of proof of conscientious objection shall rest on the person claiming to rely on it.

ENFORCEMENT PROVISIONS AND OFFENCES

Any member or employee of the Authority on entering and inspecting premises has the right to:

- take possession of anything which he has reasonable grounds to believe may be required
- take steps to preserve anything or prevent interference with anything, and
- can obtain from a JP, if there are reasonable grounds for suspecting that an offence under this Act is being (or has been) committed, a warrant to enter premises, using such force as is necessary and to search premises.

Offences include:

- undertaking activities prohibited by ss.3(2) or 4(1)(c) without a licence or doing anything which cannot be authorised by a licence
- Providing false or misleading information for the purposes of a licence
- Disclosing information in contravention of the Act.

The consent of the Director of Public Prosecutions is required before proceedings can be commenced.

CONSENT TO TREATMENT

The principles of law relating to the giving of consent are covered in Chapter 7. The 1990 Act makes very detailed provisions relating to the giving and use of gametes and embryos and the Act requires counselling to be given before consent is obtained.

Schedule 3 covers the consent to the use of gametes or embryos. Consent has to be given in writing and effective consent means consent which has not been withdrawn.

The provisions of the Schedule are set out in Box 27.8.

Box 27.8 Consent provisions

A. Consent to the use of an embryo must specify one or more of the following purposes:

  i. use in providing treatment services to the person giving consent, or that person and another specified person together

---

ii. use in providing treatment services to persons not including the person giving consent, or

iii. use for the purposes of any project of research,

and may specify conditions subject to which the embryo may be so used.

B. A consent to the storage of any gametes or embryos must:

i. specify the maximum period of storage (if less than the statutory storage period), and

ii. state what is to be done with the gametes or embryo if the person who gave the consent dies or is unable because of incapacity to vary the terms of the consent or to revoke it, and may specify conditions subject to which the gametes or embryo may remain in storage.

C. Other matters to be included in the consent can be specified by the Authority.

D. Procedure for giving consent:

Before a person gives consent under this Schedule

i. he must be given a suitable opportunity to receive proper counselling about the implications of taking the proposed steps, and

ii. he must be provided with such relevant information as is proper

iii. he must be informed of his right to withdraw consent or vary it at any time by notice given by the person who gave the consent to the person keeping the gametes or embryo to which the consent is relevant.

The terms of any consent to the use of any embryo cannot be varied, and such consent cannot be withdrawn, once the embryo has been used:

– in providing treatment services, or

– for the purposes of any project of research.

Use of gametes for the treatment of others

A person's gametes must not be used for the purposes of treatment services unless there is an effective consent by that person to their being so used and they are used in accordance with the terms of the consent.

A person's gametes must not be received for use for those purposes unless there is an effective consent by that person to their being so used. This does not apply to the use of a person's gametes for that person, or that person and another together, receiving treatment services.

In vitro fertilisation and subsequent use of embryo

A person's gametes must not be used to bring about creation of any embryo *in vitro* unless there is an effective consent by that person to any embryo, the creation of which may be brought about with the use of those gametes, being used for one or more of the purposes mentioned in para.2(1) above.

Each person whose gametes were used for IVF must give an effective consent before the embryo can be received (see the case of Diane Blood below).

The House of Lords has held[9] that a former unmarried partner cannot be the legal father of an IVF baby, since the embryo must be placed in the mother at a time when treatment services are being provided for the woman and the man together. In this case, the couple had separated before the successful implantation.

Embryos obtained by lavage

An embryo taken from a woman must not be used for any purpose unless there is an effective consent by her to the use of the embryo for that purpose and it is used in accordance with that consent.

Storage of gametes and embryos

There must be an effective consent by the person whose gametes are to be stored and storage must be in accordance with their consent.

The case of Diane Blood[10] illustrates how tight the rules on consent to the use of gametes are.

Box 27.9 No written consent: The use of sperm from a dead husband

Mr and Mrs Blood had been married for 3 years and were intending to start a family when Mr Blood contracted meningitis and went into a coma. Mrs Blood asked for sperm to be taken from her husband and he died shortly afterwards. She then applied to the Human Fertilisation and Embryology Authority for the sperm to be used for her artificial insemination. The Authority refused on the grounds that the written consent of the donor was required under s.4(1) and Schedule 3 of the Act. Her application to the High Court for judicial review failed and she appealed to the Court of Appeal. It held that the Act clearly required the written consent of the donor to storage of the sperm and the court could not give consent to her being treated. It held however that HFEA has not lawfully exercised

▶

its discretion under ss.23 and 24 to allow export and Mrs Blood would be able to seek treatment abroad.

It was subsequently made known that she had given birth to a child following successful insemination with her husband's sperm abroad. In 2002 it was reported that she was expecting a second child conceived by using her dead husband's sperm.

In a more recent case a couple wished to have children but the husband had had a vasectomy. They agreed to surgical retrieval of the husband's sperm and consent forms regarding the storage and disposal of the sperm were signed. The sperm was retrieved and stored. Subsequently, the husband agreed to sign an amendment to the form which allowed the embryos and sperm to perish after death or incapacitation. There was one attempt at pregnancy which failed and then the husband died unexpectedly. The Centre sought a ruling on the storage and use of the stored sperm and the High Court held that Mr U gave a valid consent to the destruction of his sperm after his death and so the sperm could be destroyed.[11] Mrs U's appeal against this decision was dismissed by the Court of Appeal,[12] which held that Mr U's amendment to the initial consent was not obtained by undue influence and there was no effective consent for the Centre to continue to store or use the sperm following his death.

Following the Blood case, the government set up a review of the law under the Chairmanship of Professor Sheila McLean and a report was published in 1998.[13] The report recommended that in exceptional circumstances the removal of gametes from an unconscious person, if that were in the best interests of that person, should be permitted. It also suggested that the 1990 Act should be amended to remove the need for written consent from the donor for storage. In August 2000, the government published its response to the McLean Report.[14] It accepted all the recommendations of the report and went further, suggesting a retrospective effect:

– The father's name should be allowed to appear on birth certificates where his sperm has been used after his death.

– The legal position on consent and removal of gametes should remain unchanged: gametes can be taken from an incapacitated person who is likely to recover, if the removal of gametes is in their best interests.

– The HFEA should have the power to permit the storage of gametes where consent has not been given, so long as the gametes have been lawfully removed. This will also benefit children who are about to undergo treatment which will affect their future fertility. (Legislation will be required to implement this.)

– Families will be able to make these birth certificate changes retrospectively.

– The best practice is for written consent to be obtained, since this most clearly constitutes effective consent. Where there is doubt over whether an effective consent has been obtained, this should be a matter for the courts.

Subsequently Diane Blood won her claim to have her late husband legally recognised as the father of her two sons, when the Department of Health dropped its opposition.[15] The judge accepted that her inability to name her deceased husband as the father of her children was contrary to her human rights and he ordered the Department of Health to pay Mrs Blood's £20 000 legal costs.

The only legislative change to be implemented following the McLean report is, at the time of writing, the Human Fertilisation and Embryology (Deceased Fathers) Act 2003 which came into force on 1 December 2003 and specifies the circumstances in which a deceased father can be recorded on the birth certificate.

CODE OF PRACTICE

The HFEA has published and amended a Code of Practice which licensed centres must follow. This covers such topics as the decisions over which persons can obtain IVF treatment. Consultation on the draft of the sixth edition of the Code of Practice took place in 2004.

ACCESS TO FERTILITY SERVICES

There is no legislation which gives a statutory right to access fertility services within the NHS. There are cases outside the NHS where unlikely persons have been given fertility services. For example, a French woman aged 62 was reported as receiving IVF treatment in America with an egg donated by another woman but fertilised by the French woman's brother.[16,17] It was reported[18] in 1991 that doctors in Johannesburg announced the successful delivery by caesarean section of the first baby (a girl – 9 lb 6 oz) born to a human male. A fertilised egg was implanted within the man's abdominal cavity, where it attached to the abdominal wall, developed a placenta and grew to maturity. Sperm and ova were taken from the couple. The wife, who had a 5-year-old child, could not have a second child safely. The man received female hormonal injections throughout the pregnancy and went for regular check-ups.[19] Such events give rise to considerable debate or controversy. It was reported in 2001 that a French woman treated in a London clinic received an embryo created from a donor egg from a younger woman and her brother's sperm. The HFEA is reported to have stated that treating the woman did not contravene British guidelines.[20] There is no enforceable statutory right for an individual to be given IVF treatment and the Code of Practice gives advice to the Licensed Centres on which persons to treat.

There is a statutory duty to

take account of the welfare of any child who may be born as a result of the treatment (including the need of that child for a father), and of any other child who may be affected by the birth (1990 Act s.13(5)) before a woman is provided with treatment services. In one case, this Section was applied to a woman who had a criminal record including offences for prostitution.[21]

In the following case the woman, aged 37 years, brought an action because she had been turned down by the Health Authority when she sought IVF treatment.

Box 27.10 Refusal to provide IVF treatment[22]

The applicant was 37, and was refused IVF treatment by the Health Authority as 35 had been set as the upper limit for such treatment. The judge held that her application for judicial review of this decision must be refused. There was no law to prevent the Health Authority setting limits for its financial expenditure.

Since 2 October 2000 and the coming into force of the Human Rights Act 1998, an application could be made under Article 8 of the European Convention (see Ch. 6 and Appendix 1), which gives a right to respect for private and family life. However, this argument failed when a prisoner sought the right of access to artificial insemination facilities for the purpose of inseminating his wife while he was in prison.[23] The Court of Appeal dismissed the prisoner's appeal saying that the refusal to agree to the request was not breach of the Convention, nor unlawful nor irrational.[24]

In 2000 the Department of Health announced its intention of ending the postcode lottery of infertility treatment[25] following a survey showing considerable variation in access to treatments across England and asked NICE to produce guidelines on access to fertility treatment. In February 2004 the National Institute for Clinical Excellence (NICE) published its guidelines on access to fertility services within the NHS[26] (see Ch. 21 for further discussion of NICE). NICE recommended that couples in which the woman is aged 23–39 years at the time of treatment and who have an identified cause for their infertility problems or who have infertility of at least 3 years duration should be offered up to three stimulated cycles of *in vitro* fertilisation treatment. The guidelines are considered by Ashcroft.[27] In its response to the recommendations,[28] the Department of Health stated it would look for PCTs to offer all women aged 23–39 who meet the NICE clinical criteria a minimum of one full cycle of IVF from April 2005. The Human Fertilisation and Embryology Authority's Guide to Fertility treatment published in 2005 showed that in some areas of the NHS, couples were waiting 5 years for IVF treatment.

SURROGACY

Surrogacy is the use of another person for the production of a child. The surrogate mother might have no genetic link with the child she carries, if an embryo is implanted in her. Or she may herself provide the egg and be inseminated with donor sperm or the sperm of the husband of the couple wishing to have the child. Until the passing of the Surrogacy Arrangements Act 1985, the only law which related to a surrogacy situation was s.50 of the Adoption Act 1958, which prohibits any payment in connection with adoption. The application of this section to a surrogacy situation arose in the case Re A.[29]

Box 27.11 Re A (1987)

In this case, Mr and Mrs A were unable to have children and because of their age had been refused as adoptive parents. They entered into surrogacy arrangements with Mrs B. It was agreed that she would be paid £10 000 to give up her job and have the child. Eventually she accepted £5000 which did not cover her financial losses. The couple applied to adopt the baby. The judge held that a payment to a mother in a surrogacy arrangement did not contravene the Adoption Act if payments made by those others to the natural mother did not include an element of profit or financial reward. Even if they were made for reward, the court had a discretion under the Act to authorise the payments retrospectively. The court granted the adoption order.

The public disquiet over the actions of commercial companies led to the passing of the 1985 Act.

SURROGACY ARRANGEMENTS ACT 1985

This defines 'surrogate mother' as:

a woman who carries a child in pursuance of an arrangement

   a. *made before she began to carry the child, and*

   b. *made with a view to any child carried in pursuance of it being handed over to, and the parental rights being exercised (so far as is practicable) by, another person or other persons*

Section 1(6) as amended by the 1990 Act states:

a woman who carries a child is to be treated for the purposes of subsection (2)(a) above as beginning to carry it at the time of the insemination, or of the placing in her of an embryo, of an egg in the process of fertilisation or of sperm and eggs, as the case may be, that results in her carrying the child.

The legal definition of a surrogacy arrangement in the Act is s.1(3):

An arrangement if, were a woman to whom the arrangement relates to carry a child in pursuance of it, she would be a surrogate mother.

The Act prohibits the making of surrogacy arrangements on a commercial basis. No person on a commercial basis can:

a. initiate or take part in any negotiations with a view to the making of a surrogacy arrangement,

b. offer or agree to negotiate the making of a surrogacy arrangement, or

c. compile any information with a view to its use in making, or negotiating the making of, surrogacy arrangement, and

d. in the UK knowingly cause another to do any of those acts on a commercial basis.

Commercial is defined in s.2(3) in relation to the receipt of payment for oneself or another but payment does not include payment to or for the benefit of a surrogate mother or prospective surrogate mother. Offences are also introduced in relation to advertising of surrogacy arrangements (s.3).

The Warnock Committee recommended that any such surrogacy arrangements, whether on a profit-making basis or not, should not be enforceable. This was enacted by s.36 of the Human Fertilisation and Embryology Act 1990. This adds a new s.1A to the 1985 Act as follows:

No surrogacy arrangement is enforceable by or against any of the persons making it.

The effect of this Section is that if the surrogate mother were to refuse to hand over the baby following the birth, the couple who made the arrangements could not enforce the agreement in court.

If a midwife is told that one of her clients has entered into a surrogacy agreement and is pregnant as a result of this, she should ensure that her duty to the mother and the child comes before the interests of any person on whose account the mother is bearing the child. She should ensure that she is aware of the legal position and that her Supervisor is informed of the situation.

In 1997, the government set up a committee to review surrogacy arrangements in the UK under the chairmanship of Professor Margaret Brazier. Its report[30] recommended that the Surrogacy Arrangements Act 1985 and s.30 of the 1990 Act (see above) should be replaced by new legislation. A Code of Practice on surrogacy should be drawn up by the Department of Health. At the time of writing legislation is awaited.

A recent Court of Appeal case has held that a woman is not entitled to the costs of making a surrogacy arrangement when she had been negligently deprived of the prospect of conceiving and bearing a child naturally.[31] The case is discussed in Chapter 16.

USE OF OVARIAN TISSUE IN EMBRYO RESEARCH AND ASSISTED CONCEPTION

Public concern was raised in 1993 at reports that cells from expelled fetuses were being used in the course of in vitro fertilisation. The Human Fertilisation and Embryology Authority produced a consultation document in January 1994, 'Donated Ovarian Tissue in Embryo Research and Assisted Conception'. The document considered the social and ethical issues which arose from using ovarian tissue obtained from mature women, cadaveric tissue or aborted fetuses. There is a shortage of donated eggs, and the use of tissue from a wider field which could assist in conception would go far in meeting the shortage. The Ethics Committee of the Royal College of Midwives stated that:

– There should be increased public awareness of the need for donated eggs.

– Ovarian tissue could be used in research or for the treatment of infertility subject to a Code of Practice (such as that drawn up by the Polkinghorne Report on the use of fetus and fetal tissue) and subject to the consent of the woman.

– The use of eggs or ovarian tissue from cadavers or fetuses should only be permitted for research into genetic diseases and should not be permitted for research into infertility or for the treatment of infertility.

– The use of ovarian tissue from live donors should continue to be subject to the Code of Practice of the Polkinghorne Report.

– Eggs or ovarian tissue from cadavers or fetuses should not be used in treatment.

– Legislation should be provided to enforce these recommendations.

EMBRYO RESEARCH

The Human Genetics Advisory Commission and the Human Fertilisation and Embryology Authority published a report on Cloning Issues in Reproduction, Science and Medicine in 1998[32] and concluded that the 1990 Act had proved effective in dealing with new developments relating to human cloning. The Report recommended that:

1. The government might wish to consider the possibility of introducing legislation that would effectively ban human reproductive cloning regardless of the technique used, so that the full ban would not depend upon the decision of the Human Fertilisation and Embryology Authority (HFEA) but would be enshrined in statute.

2. The Secretary of State should consider specifying in regulations two further purposes for which HFEA might issue licences for research, so that potential benefits can clearly be explored:

    a. the development of methods of therapy for mitochondrial disease, and

    b. the development of therapeutic treatments for diseased or damaged tissues or organs.

3. Because of the pace of scientific advances in the area of human genetics, the issues are examined again in five years' time in the light of developments and public attitudes towards them.

The government in its response to the report took the view that the 1990 Act was effective in preventing all forms of human cloning[33] and supported the recommendations of HFEA and HGAC and announced the creation of an Advisory Group under the Chief Medical Officer to examine further the potential benefits, risks and alternatives to therapeutic cloning.

The Chief Medical Officer's Expert Advisory Group on Therapeutic Cloning
The Group[34] concluded that:

– stem cells have enormous potential as a source of new tissue for therapeutic use

– the research was warranted across a range of sources of stem cells, including embryos created by *in vitro* fertilisation or cell nuclear replacement

– the existing statutory framework of the 1990 Act would provide the necessary safeguards for this new research.

The Advisory Group also recommended that:

Research Councils fund research into stem cells, including alternative sources of stem cells, and to establish collections of embryonic stem cells to minimise the need for the use of embryos in this research and for the importation of stem cell lines.

The recommendations of this group closely reflected the conclusions of the HFEA/HGAC report. The government responded to the Expert Advisory Group by accepting all its recommendations and undertaking to introduce the necessary regulations. The government emphasised that it would unequivocally ban reproductive cloning by the cell nuclear replacement technique.

NEW REGULATIONS

In December 2000 and January 2001, the House of Commons and the House of Lords passed secondary legislation legalising research on the stem cells of embryos. There was an emotional and heated debate in both Houses.[35] The Statutory Instrument[36] specified the additional purposes for which the Human Fertilisation and Embryology

Authority (HFEA) may grant licences for research involving embryos under the 1990 Act for the purposes of increasing knowledge about the development of embryos or about serious disease, and enabling such knowledge to be applied. This research would be subject to the overriding control and monitoring of the HFEA. The HFEA would have to ensure that there had been explicit consent from individuals whose eggs or sperm were used to create embryos which were subsequently used in research to derive stem cells.

In a report to the House of Lords Scientific Committee which investigated stem cell research, the Royal Society recommended that there should be a world ban on human cloning.[37] The House of Lords Committee reported in February 2002 and stated that stem cell research using embryos should be permitted subject to strict guidelines. Within a few days of the House of Lords report, licences were issued by HFEA for research to be carried out. A decision by the Court of Appeal overruled an earlier High Court decision and held that a cell nuclear replacement organism was an embryo for the purposes of the 1990 Act and therefore subject to the control of HFEA.[38]

Licence for research using cell nuclear transfer

In August 2004, HFEA issued the first licence to create human embryonic stem cells using cell nuclear transfer. Newcastle University was granted permission to create human embryos with three genetic parents to treat women with diseases of the mitochondria. Couples would use IVF treatment to create a fertilised egg. Within hours of fertilisation, the nucleus – containing the DNA from mother and father – would be removed from its original egg and implanted into a donor egg whose own nuclear DNA had been removed. The embryo should then develop normally using the machinery and mitochondria from the donor egg. The scientists will experiment on fertilised eggs from IVF treatment that would otherwise be thrown away. Under the law they would not be allowed to transfer the three-parent embryo to a woman.[39]

Egg freezing

In its Annual Report for 2000, the HFEA stated that carefully controlled use of frozen eggs in fertility treatment can be allowed, but clinics, who must be licensed to offer this treatment, must inform patients of any risks involved and also give clear information about the success rate, which is currently very low. The HFEA has produced a patient leaflet about this procedure.

Egg sharing

This is an arrangement whereby a woman may receive free or subsidised IVF treatment in return for donating her surplus eggs. HFEA has agreed that this practice can take place but only on condition that strict guidelines issued by HFEA were followed to protect all those involved in such arrangements.

Preimplantation Genetic Diagnosis (PGD)

PGD is a technique which is used to detect whether an embryo created *in vitro* is carrying a genetic defect which will give rise to a serious inherited genetic disorder.

HFEA and the Advisory Committee on Genetic Testing (ACGT) (now absorbed into the Human Genetics Commission) issued a consultation paper at the end of 1999. Licences have been issued in 2002 by HFEA for genetic screening and IVF treatment to take place to ensure that an embryo was a compatible donor for a sibling who suffered from a genetic disorder. In one case the sibling suffered from a rare blood disorder which could be treated by a suitable bone marrow transplant.[40]

The HFEA originally took the view that where the embryo does not benefit from the PGD, then a licence will not be granted. However, where there is a benefit to the embryo (as well as to an existing sibling) then PGD will be allowed. The case shown in Box 27.12[41] illustrates one situation where the licence was allowed and the court rejected an application to declare that it was unlawful.

Box 27.12 Tissue-typing for the benefit of a sibling[41]

Raj and Shahana Hashmi wished to bear a child who would be free of the genetic blood disorder, beta thalassaemia major, and whose tissue type would match that of their young son Zain, who suffered from the life-threatening disorder. They hoped that stem cells from blood taken from the umbilical cord of a new born baby with matching tissue would cure their son. They applied to HFEA for a licence for PGD. HFEA decided that tissue-typing would only be permitted where PGD was already necessary to avoid the passing on of a serious genetic disorder and that licences would be granted on a case by case basis and on certain conditions. HFEA granted a licence permitting PGD and tissue-typing as part of the couple's in vitro fertilisation treatment. The granting of the licence was challenged by Josephine Quintavalle on behalf of Comment on Reproductive Ethics who succeeded in an application for judicial review of the lawfulness of HFEA actions. HFEA appealed to the Court of Appeal.

The Court of Appeal held that HFEA had the power to grant a licence to permit simultaneous tests to be carried out on an embryo for the purpose, not only of identifying genetic defects in the embryo, but also of ascertaining whether the tissue type of the embryo would match that of an existing child.

The applicants appealed to the House of Lords[42] who found in favour of the Hashmis. The House of Lords held that the 1990 Act defined in broad terms the HFEA power to grant licences. The authority was specifically created to make ethical distinctions and if Parliament considered it to be failing in that task, it had in reserve its regulatory powers under s.3(3)(c) of the 1990 Act.

In a contrasting case (which must now be read in the light of the HL decision in the Hashmi case), the HFEA turned down the application from the Whitakers to use IVF techniques to select a baby who would be a perfect tissue match for Charlie aged 3 who had a rare blood disorder and required a bone marrow transplant. HFEA refused the application because embryos may be screened only if they might carry a serious genetic risk.[43]

Subsequently the HFEA changed its views and stated that PGD would be permitted to ensure that the implanted embryo was a match for a sibling with a genetic disorder, even though the embryo did not benefit personally.

In January 2005 HFEA announced a new process to speed up applications for PGD.

GENE THERAPY

Concern relating to experimentation with genes which would not be covered by the Human Fertilisation and Embryology Act 1990 (except in so far as it prevented research taking place on embryos after the appearance of the primitive streak or 14th day after mixing) led the government to establish a non-statutory body, the Committee on the Ethics of Gene Therapy, chaired by Sir Cecil Clothier, in November 1989. Its terms of reference were to draw up ethical guidance for the medical profession on treatment of genetic disorders in adults and children by genetic modification of human body cells, to invite and consider proposals from doctors wishing to use such treatment on individual patients, and to provide advice to UK Health Ministers on scientific and medical developments which bear on the safety and efficacy of human gene modification. The Committee reported in January 1992 and its recommendations are shown in Box 27.13.

Box 27.13 Recommendations of the Clothier Committee on the ethics of gene therapy

1. Research should continue but a distinction should be drawn between:

   a. Germ line gene therapy which affects future generations – gene modification of the human gene line should not be done

   b. Somatic cell gene therapy which is concerned only with that person

      i. should be subject to the requirements for other human research

      ii. should initially be for life-threatening diseases or those which cause serious handicap and for which treatment is at present unavailable or unsatisfactory

      iii. should not yet be used for non-disease situations.

▶

2. There should be a new expert/supervisory body to provide scientific and medical advice on matters germane to the safety and efficacy of human gene modification and its use.

3. The approval of local research ethics committees to research projects should be conditional on the approval of the proposed supervisory body. Arrangements for the working of the advisory body and its coordination with LRECs should be made speedily.

4. The attention of the Advisory Committee on Gene Manipulation should be drawn to this report.

5. There should be an effective means of control and discipline from the Local Research Ethics Committees who should bring failures to heed its recommendations to the notice of its appointing body, to the relevant NHS body and to the appropriate professional bodies (GMC etc.). The supervisory body should bring the matter to the attention of the Ministers.

6. The supervisory body should be non-statutory funded by and under the aegis of the Department of Health.

7. Gene therapy work should be confined to a small number of approved centres.

Early proposals to be approved by the Clothier Committee included research into adenosine deaminase deficiency, cystic fibrosis and skin cancer.

The Gene Therapy Advisory Committee was set up to review all proposals for gene therapy in the UK. It is at present chaired by Professor Norman Neven, Professor of Medical Genetics at Belfast City Hospital, and includes lay people such as journalists and church representatives as well as doctors and scientists. Its aims are to consider and advise on:

– acceptability of proposals for gene therapy on human subjects

– working with other agencies with responsibilities in the field

– advising Health Ministers on gene therapy research developments and their implications.

In its eleventh annual report published in 2005[44] it was revealed that most of the approved gene therapy trials focus on cancer. Those trials approved in 2004 included: HIV, brain cancers, cardiovascular disease, colorectal, prostate, and breast cancer, leukaemia and advanced tumours. Funding for gene therapy research into Duchenne

Muscular Dystrophy, cystic fibrosis and childhood blindness is likely to be provided for 2005–2006.

GENDER SELECTION

There has been publicity given to a business which claimed to be able to assist parents in having a child of a specified gender. It used methods which were not covered by the HFEA or the provisions relating to genetic screening. There are at present no laws to prevent the commercialisation of this. Only where the child is born through IVF or where embryos are involved would the activities come under the licensing authorities. The HFEA has licensed four centres to carry out Pre-implantation Genetic Diagnosis (PGD) (see above) which can be used to determine the sex of an embryo where a family is at risk of passing on a serious sex-linked disorder, such as Duchenne Muscular Dystrophy. However, the guidelines of the HFEA do not allow couples to select the sex of their embryos for non-medical reasons. Such selection is available in the USA and there are reports of many couples flying to the States so that they can choose the sex of their babies.[45] Internet sites offer sex selection services which at present do not come under the jurisdiction of HFEA. A report in March 2005 of the House of Commons Science and Technology Select Committee has recommended that parents should be able to choose the sex of their children on social grounds (see below).

GENETIC SCREENING

A project was proposed by Robert Sinsheimer in California in 1984 to identify the protein building blocks which shape human life. Known as the Human Genome Project, it was completed in 2000. The fact of identification of genetic predispositions raises huge ethical and legal dilemmas which are only just being confronted. One of the issues is the right to screen genetically persons for insurance or employment purposes. On the one hand it could be argued that the employer or the insurance company is entitled to receive all relevant information which would affect their decision to take a person on as an employee or for the purposes of insurance cover. On the other hand, it can be seen that without statutory protection against unfair discrimination the person who presents a risk could be subjected to extremely unjust treatment when there is only a probability rather than a certainty that the particular genetic predisposition will materialise.

At present there is no legislation to prohibit an insurance company or employer requiring genetic testing before providing insurance cover or taking a person into employment. There is of course the common law right to refuse to give consent, but this may mean the loss of insurance cover or of employment. The Association of British Insurers has agreed a Code of Practice on insurance and genetic tests (see below).

REPORT BY THE NUFFIELD COUNCIL ON BIOETHICS ON GENETIC SCREENING

The Nuffield Council on Bioethics was established in 1991 to consider the ethical issues presented by advances in biomedical and biological research. The subject of its first report, produced in December 1993, was genetic screening (Nuffield Council on Bioethics 1993). It emphasised the four points shown in Box 27.14.

Box 27.14 Important features of the report on genetic screening

– The difficulty in assessing individual health risks exposed by genetic screening

– The increased complexity of the ethical aspects of confidentiality

– The demands made upon professional and health resources by the required ethical procedures

– The broad framework provided as a safeguard against potential eugenic abuse.

The main conclusions of the report are shown in Box 27.15.

Box 27.15 Conclusions of report on genetic screening

1. Adequately informed consent should be a requirement for all genetic screening programmes.

2. Counselling should be readily available for those being genetically screened, as well as for those being tested on account of a family history of a genetic disorder.

3. Health professionals should seek to persuade individuals, if persuasion should be necessary, to allow the disclosure of relevant genetic information to other family members.

4. Appropriate professional bodies should prepare guidelines to help with the difficult decisions over confidentiality and the passing on of information within the family.

5. The Department of Health should consider with Health Authorities and the appropriate professional bodies, effective arrangements for the preservation

---

559

▶

of confidentiality, particularly in relation to genetic registers, and should issue the necessary guidance.

6. The Department of Employment keeps under review the potential use of genetic screening by employers.

7. Genetic screening of employees for increased occupational risks ought only to be contemplated in specifically defined circumstances such as where there is strong evidence of a clear connection between the working environment and the development of the condition for which genetic screening can be conducted.

8. British insurance companies should adhere to their current policy of not requiring any genetic tests as a prerequisite of obtaining insurance.

9. There should be early discussions between the government and the British insurance industry about the future use of genetic data, and that pending the outcome, the companies should accept a temporary moratorium on requiring the disclosure of genetic data.

10. The need for improving public understanding of human genetics should be borne in mind in any review of the National Curriculum and in the work of all public bodies concerned with the public understanding of science.

11. Its recommendations on adequately informed consent, confidentiality and the central coordination and monitoring of genetic screening programmes are essential to the safeguards about eugenic abuse.

12. The Department of Health in consultation with the appropriate professional bodies should formulate detailed criteria for introducing genetic screening programmes, and establish a central coordinating body to review genetic screening programmes and monitor their implementation and outcome.

INSURERS' CODE OF PRACTICE

The Association of British Insurers published a Code of Practice in 1997. It made further revisions to it in 1999.[46] It is a voluntary code for insurers over genetic tests and gives the following guidance.

1. It should not require a person to take a genetic test in order to obtain insurance cover.

2. If the results of a genetic test are in a person's medical records they can only be taken into account if they apply to one of seven conditions for which the tests

are deemed reliable (these conditions include breast cancer, Alzheimer's and Huntington's disease).

3. If the test is later found to be unreliable then the person is entitled to a refund of overpaid premiums and cheaper future payments.

4. A person is obliged to tell an insurance company if he has had a genetic test and disclose the results.

5. Anyone refused insurance cover or who wishes to complain can contact the ABI.[47]

Some evidence is emerging that contrary to the spokesman of the ABI, some people are being refused insurance cover on the grounds that they have a genetic disorder.[48,49] It may be that either statutory intervention or some form of state insurance cover is necessary to protect those who are vulnerable.

In April 1999, a Genetics and Insurance Committee (GAIC)[50] was established by the Department of Health to develop and publish criteria for the evaluation of specific genetic tests, their application to particular conditions and their reliability and relevance to particular types of insurance. In October 2000, the GAIC recommended new guidelines[51] and suggested that the reliability and relevance of the genetic test for Huntington's Chorea is sufficient for insurance companies to use the result when assessing applications for life insurance. Insurers will not be able to require prospective clients to take the test, but they will be able to ask clients if they have taken tests for Huntington's Chorea, and to ask for the results to be given. The recommendations have been criticised, for example by the National Consumer Council, on the grounds that they will create a genetic underclass and will dissuade people from taking the tests.[52] In addition, scientists are fearful that potential volunteers to genetic tests will refuse to cooperate in this country, thus many scientists would have no option but to work outside this country, where potential research subjects would not have to disclose results to insurance companies.[53]

In its first Annual Report[54] the Genetics and Insurance Committee reported on its work in drawing up criteria and guidelines for insurance providers to submit information on genetic tests that were to be used for insurance purposes. A test must satisfy the three criteria of accuracy, measurement of genetic information, clinical relevance and actuarial relevance, to be approved by the GAIC for consideration by the insurance industry in setting premiums for insurance. The House of Commons Science and Technology Committee Report on Genetics[55] was concerned at the possibility of premiums rising sharply for applicants identified as being of higher risk. The Committee recommended that there should be a 2-year moratorium. In the light of the Committee's report, the Department of Health announced in October 2001 that there was an agreement between the government and the Association of British Insurers that there would be a 5-year moratorium on the use of genetic tests.[56] The Department of Health decided that more time is needed to assess the importance of genetic tests to insurance. For the immediate future, only consumers who want more than £500 000 worth of life insurance, or over £300 000 worth of critical illness, income protection and long-term care insurance will have to disclose genetic test results. There is to be a review of the financial limits after 3 years.

The Human Genetics Commission (HGC) in May 2001 recommended a moratorium on the use of genetic test information by insurance companies and has conducted a review of the legal framework protecting personal genetic information.

The Human Genetics Commission has carried out consultations, now closed, on:

– Genetic testing services supplied direct to the public

– Paternity testing services

– Whose hands on your genes?

It began a national consultation on genetics and reproductive decision making in February 2005. It is also reviewing the issue of genetic testing and employment and relevant papers on this topic are available from its website.[57]

Dangers of reliance on DNA results

An example of the dangers of over-reliance on genetic testing is seen in the report[58] that the Court of Appeal had set aside the conviction of a person on a charge of rape where the main prosecution evidence was of DNA matching. It had been discovered that tests for DNA matching performed by a private laboratory between 1988 and 1990 were flawed and as a result dozens of convictions may be overthrown.

GENETIC DISORDERS AND THE MIDWIFE

The opportunity for genetic screening to take place raises major concerns for the midwife who may be involved in the decision as to whether screening should go ahead. The midwife requires training in this area so that she has the skills to give the appropriate advice to a mother who is contemplating being screened. The midwife should ensure that she is familiar with the ways in which the mother can receive counselling in relation to the disease and the risks in relation to any future pregnancy. She should ensure that:

– the confidentiality of the information received from the mother is protected

– the mother has full information

– the mother knows that she has the right to refuse any genetic testing, and

– the mother should be protected against any zealous researchers anxious to explore the genetics of the mother and child.

In addition, it is foreseeable that a mother might seek advice and comfort from a midwife when told that her child is suffering from a genetic disorder. The midwife should ensure that the mother receives all the appropriate information in relation to that disorder and that the child receives the correct treatment and care. The midwife should protect the rights of the mother and child at a time when the mother is likely to be extremely vulnerable and also protect the mother from any attempt to compel her to allow disclosure of this genetic information to other members of the extended family until such time as the mother is able to make a clear, reasoned decision on her own account.

MISUSE OF GENETIC INFORMATION

Whatever rules are implemented about screening and the use of genetic information, there is always a danger that codes of practice and procedures are not always closely followed, even by the courts, as the following case shows.

The use of DNA, the unique identity marker of each human being, is subject to strict rules in criminal proceedings. Thus the DNA sample taken from an accused on his arrest must be destroyed when he is acquitted.[59] However, in December 2000, the House of Lords held that evidence based on DNA which had been unlawfully retained and not destroyed following the acquittal of an accused, was still admissible in court, subject to the discretion of the trial judge,[60] when the person was charged on a subsequent offence. There is therefore always a danger that if knowledge is available it will be used, despite any regulations to the contrary, on the basis that the ends justify the means.

HOUSE OF COMMONS SCIENCE AND TECHNOLOGY SELECT COMMITTEE REPORT[61] (24 MARCH 2005)

This majority report made significant recommendations to ensure effective regulation of fertility treatment and embryo research in the interests of patients and the public. It recommended that parents should be allowed to choose the sex of their children to achieve a balanced family, that HFEA should be abolished. The minority who opposed the report said that the proposals were too libertarian and fail to uphold the precautionary principle that is at the heart of contemporary legislation and that insufficient regard has been given to public opinion. The pressure group Human Genetics Alert criticised the report[62] and said that social sex selection should not be allowed, because it turns children into consumer items and allows gender stereotypes to determine who gets born. It will throw the door to designer babies wide open.

The chairman of HFEA responded to the report,[63] stated that that the acid test for the report will be how well it deals with the public concerns and meets the need to take these important areas of public interest forward.

EU DIRECTIVE

An EU Directive which introduces new legal requirements in relation to donation, procurement, preservation, testing, processing, storage and distribution of gametes and embryos is due to come into force in the UK in April 2006. (The UK obtained a 1 year delay on its implementation.) Newsletters are being issued by HFEA and are available on its website, which set out the action being taken to implement the new EU rules.

CONCLUSIONS

The area of fertilisation and genetics is one where the law usually lags behind the scientific developments and is always trying to catch up. Criticism of the failure to update laws relating to human fertilisation and embryology were made by the then head of HFEA in August 2003 in a Times interview.[64]

She wished to see the following legislative changes which would:

- Bring under regulation techniques which are not currently controlled. These include Gamete intra-fallopian transfer (GIFT) (in which eggs and sperm are removed and washed, then injected together into the fallopian tubes) and intrauterine insemination (IUI) in which the sperm is injected directly into the womb through a catheter. Any doctor can at present perform GIFT and IUI without a licence.

- Regulate a sex-selection technique where sperm is separated into male and female varieties

- Regulate pre-implantation for genetic diagnosis (PGD), which includes cases where a sibling is conceived who is a genetic match for a child suffering from a genetic disorder.

- Give HFEA more powers and sanctions over clinics which breach regulations.

Baroness Warnock has herself suggested that there should be a new Royal Commission to review the whole field of human fertilisation and embryology. Some small changes have been made as noted above and some are contained in the Human Tissue Act 2004, but substantial legal reforms are still awaited. Under the Human Tissue Act, a Human Tissue Authority has been established, but it is the Government's intention to establish, in 2008, a new authority known as the Regulatory Authority for Fertility and Tissue (RAFT) which will embrace both the current Human Fertilisation and Embryology Authority and the Human Tissue Authority.

Each of the institutions mentioned in this chapter have websites (see Website addresses given earlier in the book) and provide regular updates on their investigations and recommendations which are easily available to the midwife.

QUESTIONS AND EXERCISES

1. A client tells you that she has agreed to bear a child for her sister. How would this affect your work as a midwife?

2. Obtain a copy of the Code issued by the Human Fertilisation and Embryology Authority and discuss the implications for midwifery.

3. A pilot study is being launched for screening for a genetic disposition for coronary heart disease. A client has asked for your advice on whether she should take part with her children. What advice would you give?

4. In what circumstances do you consider that a child should have the right to refuse consent to a genetic screening test?

References

1 Department of Health. Report of the Committee of Inquiry into Fertilisation and Embryology (the Warnock Report) Cmnd 9314. London: HMSO; 1984.

2 Re Attorney General's Reference (No 2 of 2003) [2004] EWCA Crim 785. The Times, 21 April 2004.

3 Criminal Justice and Public Order Act 1994, S. 156.

4 Parental Orders (Human Fertilisation and Embryology) Regulations 1994, SI 1994 No 2767.

5 The Leeds Teaching Hospitals NHS Trust v. Mr A; Mrs A; YA and ZA; The Human Fertility And Embryology Authority, Mr B and Mrs B Lloyds Rep Med [2003] 151.

6 Human Fertilisation and Embryology Authority (Disclosure of Donor Information) Regulations 2004 SI 2004 No 1511.

7 Department of Health. New campaign asks you to 'give life, give hope' to those with fertility problems 2005/0023. London: DoH; January 2005.

8 Frean A. Loss of anonymity deters sperm donors. The Times, 23 March 2005:11.

9 Re R Parental Responsibility: IVF baby. The Times Law Report, 13 May 2005 HL.

10 R. v. Human Fertilisation and Embryology Authority, ex parte Blood [1997] 2 All ER 687 CA.

11 Centre for Reproductive Medicine v. Mrs U. Lloyd's Rep Med [2002] 93.

12 Mrs U v. Centre for Reproductive Medicine. Lloyd's Rep Med [2002] 259.

13 McLean S. Review of Common Law Provisions Relating to the Removal of Gametes and of the Consent Provisions in the Human Fertilisation and Embryology Act 1990. London: HMSO; 1998.

14 Department of Health. Press announcement, 25 August 2000.

15 Rumbelow H. Victory for Mrs Blood changes law of paternity. The Times, 1 March 2003:12.

16 Bremner C. French Woman aged 62 has brother's baby. The Times, 21 June 2001.

17 Pank P. Fertility clinic under attack over 'incest'. The Times, 27 August 2001.

18 News item. Health Alert 1991; 7(123): 331.

19 MIDIRS Midwifery Digest, 1993; March:107.

20 Rogers L. Woman to have brother's IVF child. The Sunday Times, 26 August 2001.

21 R v. Ethical Committee of St Mary's Hospital (Manchester) ex parte H [1988] 1 FLR 512.

22 R v. Sheffield Health Authority ex parte Seale [1994] 25 BMLR 1 QBD.

23 R v. Secretary of State ex parte Mellor. Times Law Report, 5 September 2000.

24 R v. Secretary of State ex parte Mellor. Times Law Report, 1 May 2001.

25 Department of Health. Working towards the ending of postcode lottery of infertility treatment. London: DoH; November 2000.

26 NICE. Fertility: Assessment and treatment for people with fertility problems. NICE; February 2004.

27 Ashcroft RE. In vitro fertilisation for all? BMJ 2003; 327:511–512.

28 Department of Health. Health Secretary welcomes new fertility guidance 2004/0069. London: DoH; February 2004.

29 Re A (an adoption) (surrogacy) [1987] 2 All ER 826.

30 Department of Health. Surrogacy: Review for Health Ministers of Current Arrangements for Payments and Regulation. CM 4068. London: DoH; 1998.

31 Briody v. St Helens and Knowsley AHA (Claim for damages and costs) sub nom Briody v. St Helens and Knowsley AHA [2001] EWCA Civ 1010 [2001] 2 FCR 481 CA.

32 The Human Genetics Advisory Commission and the Human Fertilisation and Embryology Authority. Report on Cloning Issues in Reproduction, Science and Medicine. December 1998.

33 Government Response to the Report by the Human Genetics Advisory Commission and the Human Fertilisation and Embryology Authority on Cloning Issues in Reproduction, Science and Medicine. Cm 4387, June 1999.

34 Department of Health. Chief Medical Officer's Expert Advisory Group on Therapeutic Cloning 'Stem Cells: Medical Progress with Responsibility'. London: HMSO; 2000.

35 Dimond B. The law regarding embryo and stem cell research. Br J Midwifery 2001 9(2):111–114.

36 Human Fertilisation and Embryology (Research Purposes) Regulations 2001 SI 2001 188.

37 Royal Society. Royal Society Report prepared by Professor Richard Gardener. RS; 2001.

38 R (Quintavalle) v. Secretary of State for Health. Times Law Report, 25 January 2002.

39 Derbyshire D. Scientists seeking to create embryos with three parents. Daily Telegraph, 18 October 2004:12.

40 Hawkes N. Couple win right to create life-saving baby. The Times, 23 February 2002.

41 Regina (Quintavalle) v. Human Fertilisation and Embryology Authority. The Times Law Report, 20 May 2003, CA; Lloyd's Rep Med 6[2003] 294.

42 Regina (Quintavalle) v. Human Fertilisation and Embryology Authority. The Times Law Report, 29 April 2005, HL.

43 Peek L. Couple lose fight for designer baby. The Times, 2 August 2002.

44 Department of Health. UK Leads Europe in gene therapy. London: DoH; 2005.

45 Harlow J. Couples fly out for designer babies. The Sunday Times, 7 October 2001.

46 Association of British Insurers. Code of practice for genetic testing. ABI; 1999.

47 Association of British Insurers. Contact: 0207 600 3333.

48 News item. Insurers ignore genetics code. The Sunday Times, 13 December 1998.

49 Winnett R. Medical underclass fears insurance blacklisting. The Sunday Times, 26 March 2000.

50 Department of Health. Online. Available: www.doh.gov.uk/genetics/gaic.htm

51 Department of Health. Committee on Genetics and Insurance Report. London: DoH; 2000.

52 Henderson M. Insurers to check for genetic illness. The Times, 13 October 2000.

53 Henderson M. Scientists attack gene test ruling. The Times, 27 November 2000.

54 Genetics and Insurance Committee. First annual report, April 1999–June 2000. London: DoH; 2000.

55 House of Commons. Science and Technology Committee. Genetics and Insurance. House of Commons; 2001.

56 Department of Health. Health Minister welcomes five year moratorium on genetic tests and insurance. Press release 2001/0494.

57 Human Genetics Commission. Online. Available: www.hgc.gov.uk

58 News item. Sunday Times, 8 May 1994.

59 Police and Criminal Evidence Act 1984, S.64 (3B).

60 R v. B Attorney General's Reference No 3 of 1999. Times Law Report, 14 December 2000.

61 Select Committee on Science and Technology Report on Enquiry into Human Reproductive Technologies and the Law, March 2005.

62 Hawkes N. Let parents choose sex of their children say MPs. The Times, 24 March 2005:8.

63 Human Fertilisation and Embryology Authority. Online. Available: www.hfea.gov.uk

64 Henderson M. Time to review designer baby law, fertility watchdog says. The Times, 30 August 2003:10.

Chapter 28
VACCINE DAMAGE PAYMENTS

Our system of compensation by means of civil action for negligence involves establishing fault, i.e. a breach of the duty of care owed to the person injured. (For further details on the tort of negligence see Ch. 13.) This can be difficult to establish and may mean that many claims are either not brought or are abandoned at an early stage. Critics have demanded a system of no-fault liability such as pertains in New Zealand, Finland and Sweden where compensation is paid for untoward medical accidents without the need to establish that one or more persons is at fault. The present government has indicated that it is prepared to consider the introduction of major changes to our system for compensation including a no-fault system of compensation for certain kinds of harm.[1] A new consultation paper 'Making Amends' was published in 2003[2] (see Ch. 14).

We do have examples of compensation paid on a no-fault liability basis. One such is the payment for vaccine damage. Another statutory scheme for compensation is the criminal injury compensation scheme. The government announced on 26 October 2000 that it was preparing a scheme for compensation and a trust fund for those who have suffered from variant Creutzfeldt–Jakob Disease (CJD) from BSE and their families.

The manufacturers of thalidomide, Distillers, established a fund to pay those who were its victims and this fund was subsequently topped up.

In August 2003 the Secretary of State for Health announced that the Government intended providing compensation to those people who were infected with hepatitis C from contaminated blood products. A fund of £100 million was set up for compensation with the intention that sufferers would obtain between £20 000 and £40 000. The details of the scheme and payments were announced in January 2004.[3]

Under the scheme an *ex gratia* payment of up to £45 000 would be payable to those who were alive on 29 August 2003 and whose Hepatitis C infection is found attributable to NHS treatment with blood or blood products before September 1991. Those people infected will receive an initial lump sum payment of £20 000 and those developing a more advanced stage of the illness such as cirrhosis or liver cancer will get a further £25 000 and people who contracted Hepatitis C through someone infected with the disease will also qualify for payment. The scheme was criticised by some because it excluded widows and those who had already died from the disease.[4]

COMPENSATION FOR VACCINE DAMAGE

It is in the public interest for as many children as possible to be vaccinated against infectious diseases. However, it is recognised that on very rare occasions there can be side-effects of a very crippling kind from vaccines. The Royal Commission on Civil Liability and Compensation for Personal Injuries (The Pearson Report) 1978[5] recommended that where vaccine damage could be proved to have followed from medical procedures recommended by the government, then those who suffered serious damage should be entitled to bring an action in tort against the government on the basis of strict liability. It did not recommend the abandonment of fault liability in other cases of personal injury arising from medical accident. In the light of the Pearson recommendations the government introduced the Vaccine Damage Payments Act 1979 to provide for payments to be made out of public funds in cases where severe disablement occurs as a result of vaccination against certain diseases or of contact with a person who has been vaccinated against any of those diseases. The sum payable was originally £10 000 but this has been increased over the years and since June 2000 stands at £100 000.[6]

The diseases to which the Act applies are shown in Box 28.1.

Box 28.1 Diseases covered by the Vaccine Damage Payments Act 1979

Diphtheria

Tetanus

Whooping cough

Poliomyelitis

Measles

Rubella

Tuberculosis

Smallpox

And any other disease specified by the Secretary of State by statutory instrument.

Haemophilus Type B infection (hib) was added to the list in 1995.[7] Meningococcal Group C was added to the list in 2001.[8]

Severe disability must be established and this is defined in the Act as shown in Box 28.2.

Box 28.2 Definition of severe disability for the purposes of the Vaccine Damage Payments Act

S.1(4) For the purposes of this Act, a person is severely disabled if he suffers disablement to the extent of 80% or more (reduced to 60%) assessed as for the purposes of Social Security legislation.

The Act also covers the situation where a person is severely disabled as the result of a vaccination given to his mother before he was born (s.1(3)).

The conditions of obtaining the payment are set out in Box 28.3.

Box 28.3 Conditions to obtain payment under the Vaccine Damage Payments Act 1979

1. a. Vaccination was carried out in the UK or Isle of Man

   b. on or after 5 July 1948

   c. in the case of smallpox, before 1 August 1971.

2. a. (Except for poliomyelitis and rubella) the vaccination was given whilst the person was under 18 years or during an outbreak of that disease in the UK or Isle of Man.

3. The disabled person was over the age of 2 on the date when the claim was made or, if he died before that date, he died after 9 May 1978 and was over the age of 2 when he died.

Children up to the age of 18 years are now able to bring a claim, but where a claim is made in respect of a vaccination for Meningococcal Group C, the conditions that a person should be under 18 years at the date of the vaccination and that there should be an outbreak of the disease in the UK or Isle of Man do not apply.

Causation

It must be shown that the disablement is the result of the vaccine. Where such causation is in dispute, the Act provides that 'the question whether the severe disablement results from vaccination against any of the diseases shall be determined for the purposes of the Act on the balance of probability'.

Time limits

Provided that the claimant survived both 9 May 1978 and the age of 2, claims can be made in respect of vaccinations carried out since the inception of the NHS in July 1948.

Referral to medical tribunal

The Secretary of State can refer to a tribunal:

- the question of the extent of the disablement suffered by the disabled person

- the question whether he is, or, as the case may be, was immediately before his death disabled as a result of the vaccination to which the claim relates, and

- the question whether, if he is or was so disabled, the extent of his disability is or was such as to amount to severe disablement.

The Act also provides for the payments to or for the benefit of the disabled person and the holding of money by trustees where appropriate.

Offences under the Act

A person, who, for the purpose of obtaining a payment under the Act, whether for himself or for another person, knowingly makes any false statement or representation or produces or furnishes or causes or knowingly allows to be produced or furnished any document or information which he knows to be false in a material particular, is liable to prosecution (s.9(1)).

CIVIL CLAIMS

In comparison with the statutory fixed sum for severe disablement, the awards which are payable by civil action for negligence are much larger. However, as is shown in Chapter 13, all elements necessary to establish liability must be shown or accepted by the defendant. The person seeking compensation must therefore show that:

- a duty of care was owed

- this duty has been broken by a failure to follow the accepted standard of care, and

- as a reasonably foreseeable consequence of this breach

- harm has occurred.

Severe disablement does not have to be shown to recover compensation in the civil courts.

What happens if payment has already been paid out under the Vaccine Damage Payment Act 1979? Does this prevent a civil action taking place? The answer is no. Section 6(4) states that the making of a claim for, or the receipt of, a payment under the Act does not prejudice the right of any person to institute or carry on proceedings in respect of disablement suffered as a result of vaccination against any disease to which the Act applies. However, the fact that a payment has been made under the Act must be taken into account by the court in any civil proceedings where compensation in respect of such disablement is awarded.

Box 28.4 Loveday v. Renton 1988[9]

Mrs Loveday claimed damages on behalf of her daughter Susan, then 17 years, for permanent brain damage after a whooping cough vaccine given in 1970 and 1971. The claim was brought against the Wellcome Foundation, who made the vaccine, and against the doctor who had administered it. The claim was dismissed because she had failed to show on a balance of probabilities that pertussis vaccine could cause permanent brain damage in young children. It thus failed on the issue of causation. The judge stated that if the case had not failed on the issue of causation,

any plaintiff would face insuperable difficulties in establishing negligence on the part of the doctor or nurse who had administered the vaccine.

Such a claim would have to be based on the ground that the vaccination had been given in spite of the presence of certain contraindications, including the possibility that the vaccine was defective.

In contrast to the Loveday case, a claim against the Wellcome Foundation succeeded in an Irish case in 1992 (Best v. Wellcome Foundation).[10]

The High Court had dismissed the plaintiff's claim because of the lack of proof of causation. However the Irish Supreme Court held that the Wellcome Foundation was liable for the negligent manufacture and release of a particular batch of triple vaccine and that the brain damage was caused as a result. It referred the case back to the High Court on the amount of compensation. On 11 May 1993, the High Court approved an award of £2.75 million as compensation for the brain damage sustained in September 1969.

It remains to be seen if there will be any further successful cases brought in the civil courts for vaccine damage. It must be stressed that in the Best case, there was evidence that the particular batch of vaccine was below standard and should not have been released onto the market. However, the contrast between the sums available if fault and causation can be established in the civil courts is clear. The Association of Parents of Vaccine-Damaged Children has been formed to give advice and support to parents.

CONSUMER PROTECTION ACT 1987

If it can be established that a person has been injured as a result of a defect in a product, then there may be a claim under the Consumer Protection Act 1987. In this case it is not necessary to establish fault, merely that there was a defect (see Ch. 9). It has recently been held that a claim can be brought under the Consumer Protection Act 1987 where the claimant was infected with hepatitis through contaminated blood transfusions.[11] This could be used as a precedent for claims in relation to defective vaccines (see Ch. 19).

DISPUTES OVER THE SAFETY OF THE TRIPLE VACCINE

There has been considerable media concern about the triple vaccine (MMR) for mumps, measles and rubella. A report published in the Lancet by Dr Wakefield suggested that the measles vaccine was linked with autism. The result was evidence of a growing number of parents choosing not to allow their babies to have the triple vaccine. The Committee on the Safety of Medicines issued a statement to show that new research showed no link between MMR and autism or bowel disease.[12] Research from Japan in March 2005[13] gave further support to the view that there is no scientific link between autism and MMR.

In spite of the attempted reassurance, figures for cases of mumps are reported to be soaring.[14] Figures provided by the Health Protection Agency in February 2005 showed that 3501 suspected mumps were being seen by doctors across the country, the highest level for 15 years, though many of those infected were teenagers who had missed out when the MMR was introduced in the late 1980s. It is anticipated that the numbers will rise as youngsters whose parents opted not to obtain the MMR are infected.

Another scare relating to the possibility that autism has arisen from mercury being used in vaccines is highlighted in the press.[15]

Midwives are likely to be consulted by mothers over what is best practice for their children and they must ensure that they fulfil their duty of care in providing such information. They should ensure that they have the latest Department of Health and Committee for the Safety of Medicines evidence.

CONCLUSIONS

There is on-going research into the safety of vaccines and since midwives are likely to be consulted by mothers, they need to ensure that they are up-to-date. The Department of Health is considering (see Ch. 14) introducing a new scheme for clinical compensation and this may be comparable to the present Vaccine Damage Payments Act.

QUESTIONS AND EXERCISES

1. A client asks for your advice on whether she should ensure that her children receive the triple vaccine. What advice do you give?

2. What differences are there between a claim for compensation under the Vaccine Damage Payments Act, a claim for compensation under the laws of negligence and a claim under the Consumer Protection Act 1987?

3. Are there any other injuries or disabilities which you consider should be covered by a statutory right to compensation comparable to the Vaccine Damage Payments Act?

References

1 Department of Health. New Clinical Compensation Scheme for the NHS. Press release 2001/0313.

2 Department of Health. Making Amends. A consultation paper setting out proposals for reforming the approach to clinical negligence in the NHS. CMO June 2003.

3 Department of Health. Details of Hepatitis C ex-gratia payment scheme announced. Press release 2004/0025. London: Department of Health; 23 January 2004.

4 Lister S. NHS hepatitis victims to get up to £45,000. The Times, 24 January 2004.

5 The Royal Commission on Civil Liability and Compensation for Personal Injuries (The Pearson Report) Cmnd. 7054 1978.

6 Vaccine Damages Payments, Statutory Instrument 2000 SI 1983.

7 SI 1995 No 1164.

8 Vaccine Damages Payment (Specified Disease) Order 2001 SI 1652.

9 Loveday v. Renton. The Times, 31 March 1988 QBD.

10 Best v. Wellcome Foundation, Dr O'Keefe, the Southern Health Board, the Minister for Health of Ireland and the Attorney General [1994] 5 Med Law Rev; also discussed in Medico Legal J 1994; 61(3):178.

11 A v. National Blood Authority sub nom Hepatitis C Litigation. The Times, 4 April 2001; [2001] 3 All ER 289.

12 Committee on Safety of Medicines. Press release, 13 February 2002.

13 Hawkes N. Study that debunks MMR autism link hailed by doctors. The Times, 4 March 2005:30.

14 Lister S. Mumps soars for teens who missed MMR jab. The Times, 4 February 2005.

15 Waterhouse R. New autism doubt on mercury in vaccines. The Sunday Times, 22 July 2001.

Chapter 29

INFECTIOUS DISEASES AND THE MIDWIFE

The midwife has both a duty to ensure that she does not pass on infections to her clients and also a duty to ensure that she notifies the appropriate authorities in accordance with her duties under the public health legislation. This chapter deals with both these areas and also looks in detail at the midwife and AIDS patients, and fear of contracting AIDS and legal issues arising from cross-infection. Reference should also be made to Chapter 19 on health and safety.

THE MIDWIFE'S HEALTH

There was a requirement under the former Midwives Rules[1] that the midwife be medically examined:

A practising midwife shall, if the Local Supervising Authority deems it necessary for preventing the spread of infection, undergo medical examination by a registered medical practitioner. (former rule 39)

The Local Supervising Authority is the Regional Health Authority in England and the District Health Authority in Wales, in Scotland Health Boards and in Northern Ireland, Health and Social Services Boards (see Ch. 3).

However, this requirement has not been included in the revised Midwives Rules which came into force in August 2004.[2]

This may not be so significant, however, since the requirement to submit to health checks may possibly be implied into a contract of employment of a midwife (or other health professional). There may be an implied duty that she submits herself to an independent medical examination if it is feared that she is not capable, physically or mentally, of being at work (see Ch. 22 on employment law).

Under the statutory duties relating to health and safety, and also under her common law duty of care to her patients, the midwife would have a wider duty in relation to the prevention of cross-infection between patients and she should therefore follow a procedure which would ensure the highest standards of hygiene and infection control.

NOTIFIABLE DISEASES

Certain diseases are defined as notifiable and if the midwife is aware that one of her mothers, or relatives, is infected with such a disease she would have a duty to report it.

Diseases which are notifiable are shown in Box 29.1.

Box 29.1 Notifiable diseases

A. Cholera, plague, relapsing fever, smallpox, typhus

B. Acquired immune deficiency syndrome (AIDS), acute encephalitis, acute polio-myelitis, meningitis, meningococcal septicaemia, anthrax, diphtheria, dysentery, paratyphoid fever, typhoid fever, viral hepatitis, leprosy, leptospirosis, measles, mumps, rubella, whooping cough, malaria, tetanus, yellow fever, ophthalmia neonatorum, scarlet fever, tuberculosis, rabies and viral haemor-rhagic fever.

Those diseases under category A are covered by the duties under the Public Health (Control of Disease) Act 1984.

Those diseases under category B are covered by Regulation 3 of the Public Health (Infectious Diseases) Regulations 1988 and the 1984 Act only applies to the extent set out in column 2 of Schedule 1 of the 1988 Act.

Under s.11 of the 1984 Act, a registered medical practitioner has a duty to notify the proper office of the local authority if he becomes aware, or suspects, that a patient whom he is attending within the district of a local authority is suffering from a notifiable disease or from food poisoning. The duty does not apply if he believes, and has reasonable grounds for believing, that some other registered medical practitioner has complied.

WHAT INFORMATION MUST BE NOTIFIED?

Box 29.2 shows the information which must be notified.

Box 29.2 Information which must be given

– Name, age and sex of the patient and the address of the premises where the patient is

– The disease or, as the case may be, particulars of the poisoning from which the patient is, or is suspected to be, suffering and the date or approximate date of its onset, and

▶

▶

> – If the premises are a hospital, the day on which the patient was admitted, the address of the premises from which he came there and whether or not, in the opinion of the person giving the certificate, the disease or poisoning from which the patient is, or is suspected to be, suffering was contracted in hospital.

POWERS OF THE JUSTICE OF THE PEACE (JP)

Under s.37 of the Public Health (Control of Disease) Act 1984, if the Justice of the Peace is satisfied that a person is suffering from a notifiable disease, and

a. that his circumstances are such that proper precautions to prevent the spread of infection cannot be taken or that such precautions are not being taken, and

b. that serious risk of infection is thereby caused to other persons, and

c. that accommodation is available in a suitable hospital . . .

then the JP can consult with the Health Authority in whose district the area lies and order the person to be removed to it.

Under s.38 the JP can order the detention of a person suffering from a notifiable disease in a hospital for infectious diseases.

OTHER PROVISIONS OF THE PUBLIC HEALTH (CONTROL OF DISEASE) ACT 1984

Section 13 gives the Secretary of State power to make regulations to prevent the spread of notifiable diseases and preventing dangers from the arrival or departure of aircraft or vessels.

Section 43 enables the registered medical practitioner to take precautions in order to prevent the spread of infection where a person suffering from a notifiable disease dies in hospital.

Section 44 requires the person in charge of the premises where a person with a notifiable disease has died to take precautions to prevent anyone coming into contact with the body.

Section 47 of the Act enables the Secretary of State to make regulations relating to the disposal of dead bodies.

Section 48 enables the JP to make an order for the removal of a body and for burial within a specified time to prevent the lives of others being endangered.

Following a report that a person suffering from TB had infected 12 other persons,[3] there have been calls for these public health powers to be strengthened and the Health Protection Agency was asked in 2004 to review the situation and is to report with recommendations on changes to the existing laws. In May 2005 more than 700 patients who had been treated at the Lister Hospital, Stevenage were sent letters urging them to be alert to TB symptoms since an unnamed health worker had been diagnosed with the disease.[4] The BMA called for all children in Britain to be immunised against Hepatitis B since transmission rates were rising and it was 50–100 times more infectious that the AIDS virus.[5]

Role of the midwife
If a midwife knows or suspects that one of her clients may be suffering from an infectious disease or food poisoning she should ensure that the GP of the patient is notified. Alternatively she could herself notify the local authority.

Duty of local authority
The local authority must notify the appropriate Health Authority within 48 hours of the receipt of a certificate of notification.

HIV/AIDS INFECTIONS

The notification provisions described above do not apply to AIDS/HIV infections. These come under the AIDS (Control) Act 1987, which requires periodical reports to be furnished to RHAs and the Secretary of State. The information required includes:

– the number of persons known to be persons with AIDS and the timing of the diagnosis

– the particulars of facilities and services provided by each authority

– the numbers of persons employed by the authority in providing such facilities

– future provision over the next 12 months

– action taken to educate members of the public in relation to AIDS and HIV, to provide training for testing for AIDS, and for the treatment, counselling and care of persons with AIDS or infected with HIV.

The AIDS (Control) (Contents of Reports) Order 1988 has extended the above required information to include that relating to HIV positive persons.

This information is required to enable the appropriate resources to be allocated and plans to be made. Over 3500 new diagnoses of HIV infection have been reported for the UK for 2000, the highest annual total ever. The major routes of infection were: 39% homosexual contact; 49% heterosexual contact; 2.6% IDU; 2.5% mother to baby. Statistics from the Health Protection Agency in 2004 showed that 53 000 adults have the virus which causes AIDS and that up to 14 300 cases are undiagnosed. There were 6000 diagnoses of HIV infection in 2003, a figure expected to exceed 7000 once all the data has been collected, which is more than double the figure for 1998. Each HIV infection is thought to cost between £500 000 and £1 million in treatment and lost productivity.[6]

Under the Public Health (Infectious Diseases) Regulations 1985, local authorities have the power to apply to a Justice of the Peace for the removal of an AIDS sufferer to hospital to be detained there. The JP is also given the power to make an order for a person believed to be suffering from AIDS to be medically examined. There are also powers in relation to the disposal of the body of an AIDS sufferer.

AIDS/HIV AND THE MIDWIFE

The problem of AIDS/HIV gives rise to two different issues:

- First, the midwife as a health professional needs to know her rights and duties in relation to the care of the AIDS/HIV positive pregnant woman and the risk of infection to the midwife during the confinement.

- Second, the midwife herself may contract AIDS or become infected by the HIV virus. What are her rights in employment law? Does she have to disclose this information to her employers? Could she be automatically dismissed?

The UKCC has issued some guidance for practitioners[7] in relation to AIDS/HIV but there appears to have been no guidance specifically for the midwife. The position of the UKCC (now adopted by the NMC) is that the Council is opposed to routine testing of healthcare professionals for HIV infection. Security through safe standards of personal practice supplemented by appropriate re-assignment of infected practitioners whose role involves them in invasive procedures is emphasised. The Royal College of Midwives has published a position paper on AIDS/HIV.[8] The Department of Health has issued guidance on AIDS/HIV infected healthcare workers in 1998[9] which was replaced in 2003.[10] A useful source on HIV in pregnancy and childbirth is a book by J Kennedy.[11]

THE AIDS/HIV PATIENT

The midwife could not refuse to care for a pregnant woman who is suffering from AIDS or is HIV positive. A survey of attitudes of practitioners to HIV/AIDS patients reported that 37% specifically argued that nurses should be allowed to refuse to care for a patient who had developed AIDS.[12] Professional practice, and also legal duty, would however not permit a midwife to refuse. She could be dismissed from a job, removed from the Register and possibly sued by a mother who suffered harm.

Nor could the midwife insist that a person suspected of being an AIDS/HIV carrier should be compulsorily tested. This is not necessarily a disadvantage to the midwife since it is possible to have false negatives and if the person has only recently picked up the infection it may not show up on testing, yet they could still transmit the disease. In addition a recent conference on AIDS highlighted the cases of eight people suffering from full-blown AIDS who did not test positive for HIV. This finding has raised great concerns in relation to testing, blood transfusions, breast milk banks, etc.

How, therefore, can the midwife protect herself against the possibility of being infected? Some deliveries can result in a lot of spilt blood and the midwife is extremely vulnerable.

As an employee, she is entitled to all reasonable care being taken for her safety against reasonably foreseeable risks and dangers (see Ch. 19). The fear of AIDS/HIV infection is one which could be regarded as reasonably foreseeable. This means her employer must take all reasonable care in terms of ensuring that a safe system of work is followed, that staff are trained and competent and that equipment, facilities, buildings and the working environment are safe. The employer's duty derives both from the contract of employment and from the criminal law and the laws relating to health and safety at work.

Any guidance offered by professional groups on what equipment the midwife should use to be reasonably safe should be followed. If the appropriate facilities are not available, the midwife should draw the manager's attention to the deficiencies and ensure that the appropriate steps are taken. If necessary the midwife could use the whistle-blowing procedures (see Ch. 22).

WHAT ARE THE REMEDIES IF NO ACTION IS TAKEN?

The criminal law

A breach of the Health and Safety at Work laws could result in the prosecution of the employer. The Health and Safety Inspectorate has the duty of enforcing the provisions of these laws and making regular inspections of health service premises to ensure that the duties are being observed. If the equipment provided to midwives for home deliveries is inadequate this could also be brought to the attention of the Inspectorate. Obviously, all steps should be taken to ensure that management is made aware of the problems and has the opportunity to remedy them before external assistance is brought in.

There have been recent prosecutions for those, knowing themselves to be HIV positive, who have deliberately inflicted the infection onto others. Stephen Kelly was convicted of knowingly infecting a lover with HIV and was jailed for 5 years (Harris,

2001)[13]. He was prosecuted under the Scottish common law. The Criminal Injury Compensation Scheme recognises that a criminal offence leading to infection with HIV/AIDS should be compensated at level 17 of the tariff (currently £22 000).[14] See Chapter 18 for discussion on the scheme for criminal injury compensation.

In October 2003, Mohammed Dica was found guilty of inflicting biological bodily harm upon two lovers whom he had callously infected with HIV.[15] He was sentenced to 8 years imprisonment, after the judge stated that his behaviour was despicable and he callously conned his victims into having unprotected sex with him. He appealed to the Court of Appeal and won a retrial on the grounds that the trial judge should not have withdrawn from the jury the issue of whether the women consented to intercourse knowing that he was HIV-positive.[16] Following the retrial he was sentenced to $4^1/_2$ years and appeal was refused (R v. Dica (No 2) Times, 9 September 2005). In another case, an African who infected three women with HIV after arriving in Britain as an asylum seeker was given a 10-year prison sentence (Norfolk, Andrew 2004).[17] The judge stated that the grievous bodily harm which he had inflicted on the women fell into the category of the very worst sort.

A woman was jailed for 2 years in July 2005 for infecting her boyfriend, when she knew that she was HIV positive. She had pleaded guilty to unlawfully inflicting grievous bodily harm.[18]

The civil law

Since it is an implied term of the contract of employment that the employer should take all reasonable care for the safety of the employee, failure by the employer to provide reasonable standards of safety would be a breach of the contract of employment. In serious cases, breach of contract gives the innocent party the right to see the contract as at an end. Thus if the midwife was guilty of gross misconduct she could be dismissed instantly without notice. Similarly where the employer is in breach by failing to take reasonable steps to ensure the midwife's safety, the midwife could see the contract as terminated by his conduct and if she has worked for one year or more continuously, she could bring an action for unfair dismissal in the employment tribunal. She would be alleging that there has been a constructive dismissal by virtue of the employer's failures towards her. If she is to take this latter step she must be sure that she has good legal advice and the stages are well documented in writing.

Because it is unknown which mothers are likely to be a danger to the midwife, it is important that every pregnant woman is treated as a potential source of infection and the same high standards are followed for every case. (For further information on health and safety law, see Ch. 19.)

In 2004 the Department of Health issued revised guidance on prevention and testing in children and HIV which also covers advice about hepatitis B and C.[19]

DUTY TO THE AIDS/HIV CLIENT

If the midwife knows that one of her clients is actually suffering from AIDS or is HIV positive, what action should she take? Hopefully her standards of care and safety are such that she would not have to take any additional precautions. However, she should ensure that she has the knowledge to answer the client's questions and advise her on breastfeeding and the problems of infecting the baby with infected milk, if the baby has not already been infected during gestation. The fact that the mother is an HIV carrier or sufferer from AIDS in no way reduces the duty of care that the midwife owes to her. Indeed in some ways it is higher because of the additional information that the midwife should be passing on.

THE HIV POSITIVE CHILD

Where a baby is thought to have contracted the AIDS virus then 'the welfare of the child is the paramount consideration' (see Ch. 32) is the fundamental principle. This was at the heart of a judge's recent decision when he ruled that a baby could be tested for the HIV virus despite the opposition of her parents.[20]

The facts of the case are shown in Box 29.3.[21]

Box 29.3 Facts of case of HIV test on baby[21]

The mother was HIV positive but refused to allow her 4-month-old baby to be tested for the HIV virus. Both parents believed that HIV does not cause AIDS and that the conventional medical treatment of the virus did more harm than good. Judge Wilson noted that both parents were devoted to the baby and that they were knowledgeable and concerned about HIV. However, the judge accepted the current medical view that HIV could lead to AIDS and that drug therapy could be given to minimise the effect of the virus. The mother had refused to accept medical advice to have her baby delivered via a caesarean and not to breastfeed the baby. Instead she arranged for a home delivery and was breastfeeding the baby.

The case in Box 29.3 came to light when a GP carrying out a routine check-up read in the mother's notes that she was HIV positive and raised the issue with Camden Borough Council, which brought the case under the Children Act 1989. The British Medical Association and the Terence Higgins Trust supported the ruling because of the advances made in the treatment of HIV. The National Aids Trust said it was extremely regrettable that court intervention was thought necessary. However, the government policy announced on 13 August 1995[22] by Minister of Health Tessa Jowell, for all pregnant women to be encouraged to have a routine HIV test, is likely to increase the numbers of babies found to be infected and therefore the potential for parental disputes over the babies being tested. A total of 2.5% of the newly reported HIV cases in 2000 were mother-to-baby infections. Midwives need to have the necessary training to advise women on HIV testing, to ensure that they are given the appropriate counselling prior to having the test. The Department of Health has set standards to support the UK antenatal screening programme.[23] The standards cover screening for four infectious diseases: rubella antibody, syphilis, HIV and hepatitis B.

The Department of Health has issued guidance on HIV and infant feeding.[24] This guidance aims to help healthcare professionals provide the necessary information, advice and support to women who are infected with human immunodeficiency virus (HIV) to help them make personal, well-informed decisions about infant feeding.

The case illustrates one of the most difficult dilemmas facing midwives, i.e. when they should seek to intervene against the wishes of the parents, in particular the mother, in order to protect the child. In the case itself, the judge ruled that an HIV test could be carried out, yet he did not rule that the mother should stop breastfeeding the child. Breastfeeding the baby by an HIV positive mother is considered to double the chance of the baby contracting the disease.

If the child's welfare was paramount it could be argued that the risk of contracting the disease through breastfeeding was so great that unless the mother agreed not to feed the baby, then the baby should be taken into care. Yet the judge did not rule on the breastfeeding.

THE MIDWIFE AS THE AIDS/HIV CARRIER

Liability of the midwife
The midwife has a professional duty to notify the Registration body and also her employer that she is suffering from AIDS or is HIV positive. The Court of Appeal ordered a former dentist who was suffering from AIDS to hand over his records so that his patients could be contacted. However, it barred the publication of his name and the name of the Health Authority for whom he worked.[25]

There would probably be civil liability if the midwife gave blood failing to disclose that she was a carrier of AIDS/HIV. If she gave blood deliberately knowing that she could infect others, then as well as being a civil wrong under a principle established in a nineteenth-century case,[26] she could also be guilty of a criminal offence. Stephen Kelly, who was convicted (as described above) of knowingly infecting a lover with HIV, was jailed for 5 years.[13] He was prosecuted under the Scottish common law. In February 2002, a carjacker was imprisoned for 15 years after he threatened victims with an HIV-infected syringe.[27]

Protection of the midwife

She may have protection under the Disability Discrimination Act 1995, but the employer would be entitled to take reasonable measures to ensure that her patients were protected from the risk of cross-infection. We do not have an AIDS/HIV Discrimination Act, so any employee suffering from AIDS or who was HIV positive would have to claim protection from other legislation including the statutory protection from unfair dismissal and the Human Rights Act 1998 and Appendix 1 to this book. A case in 1988 protected the confidentiality of the names of the health professionals who are found to be AIDS/HIV positive against public disclosure.[28]

To remedy the lack of protection for those who are AIDS/HIV sufferers, various organisations have published charters to protect their rights. For example, Marks and Spencer joined with other employers to protect the interests of those who were infected.[29] A charter was drawn up by charities including the Terence Higgins Trust.[30] However, these charters do not in themselves have the force of law.

The guidance issued by the Department of Health on the management of infected healthcare workers and patient notification[31] is based on a new policy (announced in November 2001) on patient notification when a healthcare worker is found to be infected with HIV. It is no longer necessary to notify every patient who has undergone an exposure-prone procedure by an infected healthcare worker because of the low risk of transmission and the anxiety caused to patients and the wider public. The Department of Health recommends that the decision on whether a patient notification exercise should be undertaken should be assessed on a case-by-case basis using a criteria-based framework. Directors of Public Health will be responsible for deciding whether patient notification is necessary, and the United Kingdom Advisory Panel for Health Care Workers infected with Blood-borne Viruses (UKAP) will be available to provide advice.

The Court of Appeal has held that the identify of the healthcare worker who developed HIV and also of his NHS employer should not be published in the newspapers to prevent his being identified. His speciality could however be disclosed.[32]

It has been suggested that one of the main reasons for the increase in HIV positive people is refugee immigrants and in consequence the Department of Health has strengthened its guidelines on the health clearance for serious communicable diseases for new healthcare workers.[33] The House of Lords has held that expulsion of a failed immigrant to a country which could not provide medical treatment equivalent to that which she had received in the UK was not a breach of Article 3 of the European Convention (the right not to be subjected to torture or inhuman and degrading treatment or punishment).[34]

National strategy for sexual health and HIV services

This is considered in Chapter 12.

CROSS-INFECTION AND HOSPITAL-ACQUIRED INFECTIONS

In the care of pregnant and newborn babies, high standards of infection control are vital. In the sixth Annual Report of CESDI[35] it was found that 5% of the deaths analysed were the result of infection: two stillbirths and six neonatal deaths.

A report by the National Audit Office in 2000[36] raised major concerns about the level of hospital-acquired infection (HAI). The report suggested that HAI could be the main or a contributory cause in 20 000 or 4% of deaths a year in the UK and that there are about 100 000 cases of HAI with an estimated cost to the NHS of £1 billion. The NAO drew conclusions on the strategic management of HAI, surveillance and the extent and cost of HAI, and the effectiveness of prevention, detection and control measures. Its recommendations include reviewing the following:

– The value of using an Infection Control Manual

– The 1995 Guidance on Infection Control

– Cost effectiveness of screening patients and staff and isolation of patients, together with standards and guidelines

– The policies on provision of education and training

– The arrangements for monitoring hospital hygiene and hospital practices

– Ensure advice on hand washing is implemented

– Clinical audit arrangements, to ensure infection control is covered

– Isolation facilities

– Guidance on management of HAI outbreaks.

Following this report, the government announced a multi-pronged initiative to tackle hospital-acquired infections. Among the initiatives planned was an antimicrobial strategy including a clampdown on inappropriate antibiotic use and better infection control measures.[37] In addition, there would be independent inspection of hospitals by the Audit Commission and Commission for Health Improvement (now the Healthcare Commission). The government has stated that the Commission for Health Improvement and the Audit Commission would conduct ward inspections and be given the right to seek information on HAI and to publish it.[38,39] The Report on the NHS commissioned by the government from Virgin Group reported that it found grubby wards, litter-strewn entrances and dirty casualty departments throughout the NHS. On 31 July 2000 the Health Minister, Lord Hunt, announced that NHS hospitals were to be given £150 000 each to clean up their wards and disinfect bathrooms as part of a £31 million campaign. The money could be used for extra cleaning staff, materials, equipment and new towels and linen. Patient Environment Action Teams would make unannounced inspections every 6 months and those hospitals that failed to meet standards would be 'named and shamed'. National standards for cleanliness would form part of performance assessment guidelines for hospitals. In

September 2000, eight NHS hospitals were identified by the Department of Health as models for others. They were to assist in drawing up standards for a national action plan for cleanliness. In October 2004, it was agreed that Matrons and nurses at ward level should be able to access cleaning services and in November 2004 the Chief Nursing Officer announced that all staff covered by the Agenda for Change (see Ch. 22) must show that they are able to reduce the risk of healthcare-associated infections including Methicillin-resistant Staphylococcus aureus (MRSA).

METHICILLIN-RESISTANT STAPHYLOCOCCUS AUREUS (MRSA)

One of the greatest challenges in the control of hospital-acquired infection is the eradication of methicillin-resistant Staphylococcus aureus (MRSA). Mandatory Reporting of MRSA began in April 2001 and the first year's results are available on-line.[40] In a press release in February 2002,[41] Lord Hunt, the Health Minister, welcomed the first report for the DoH into rates of hospital infections caused by MRSA,[42] and said that the report had been published because patients have the right to know the rate of infection in their NHS trust.

The Health Protection Agency published a Report in 2004[43] which showed that the number of people dying from the MRSA superbug had risen more than 15-fold in the past decade. It was directly responsible or an underlying cause of 800 deaths in 2002, compared with just 51 cases in 1993. Laboratory reports of MRSA blood poisoning also rose sharply over the same period from 210 cases to more than 5300. MRSA now affects more than 7000 hospital patients a year. A Matron's Charter[44] was published as part of an action plan for cleaner hospitals in October 2004. In November 2004 the Secretary of State set a target for NHS hospitals to reduce the number of MRSA infections by one half by 2008. Figures provided by the Office of National Statistics in February 2005 showed that deaths from MRSA had doubled over the past 5 years, and this was probably an underestimate. Of increasing concern were the findings of a study by the Patients' Association that hundreds of babies just a few days old may have been infected by MRSA.[45] The Health Protection Agency has set up a panel to review equipment, materials and other products which can help improve standards of cleanliness, hygiene and infection control.[46] Linda Bissett has considered how screening and isolating patients could decelerate the MRSA transmission rate.[47]

In July 2005, new legislative proposals were put forward for consultation by the Government to reduce healthcare-associated infections.[48] They include a new code of practice, a new duty on NHS bodies to follow the code with a parallel duty on the Healthcare Commission to assess compliance with it, a new power for the Healthcare Commission to issue an improvement notice and directions for improvement or sanctions which may be taken against those who, in the view of the Secretary of State or Minister, continue significantly to breach the code. The consultation ended on 23 September 2005 and draft legislation is being prepared. Criminal sanctions for breach of the code are at present not being contemplated. It was reported in July 2005 that a South Wales NHS trust had been the first NHS body to award compensation to a patient who had contracted MRSA in hospital. The Bro Morgannwg NHS Trust accepted that it had not followed the correct guidelines on infection control. The infection was discovered the day the patient was due to leave hospital and as a consequence she had to have her new hip removed and was too frail to have a second replacement.[49]

The implications for the midwife of HAI and MRSA in particular are clear: she is personally and professionally responsible for ensuring that her patients are safe and that she works in an environment where high standards of cleanliness and hygiene are maintained.

CONCLUSIONS

Standards of public health and risks of cross-infections both nationally and internationally have come onto the priority agenda of the NHS within recent years. High standards of infection control, implementation of the laws relating to notification of infectious diseases, the guidance on AIDS/HIV infected healthcare professionals and laws relating to the control of infections are all central to the safety of the mother and child. The midwife has a personal and professional role to play in the maintenance of high standards of infection control for which she can be held accountable. She should also be aware of the rules relating to confidentiality which are considered in Chapter 10.

QUESTIONS AND EXERCISES

1. You visit a client and discover that she has been suffering from food poisoning since visiting a restaurant the night before. What action do you take?

2. A client tells you that her husband has just been diagnosed as HIV positive. In what ways, if any, will this affect your practice as a midwife in relation to the client?

3. In the case cited in Question 2, which persons, if any, would you inform of the situation?

4. How can standards of cross-infection control be improved in your own department and in the community?

References

1 UKCC. Midwives Rules and Code of Practice 1998.

2 Nursing and Midwifery Council (Midwives) Rules Order of Council 2004, Statutory Instrument 2004/1764; see also Nursing and Midwifery Council Midwives Rules and Standards, August 2004.

3 Kennedy D. TB Sufferer who refused drugs infects 12 people. The Times, 9 May 2005.

4 News item. The Times, 11 May 2005.

5 News item. Doctors issue hepatitis alert. The Times, 10 May 2005.

6 Fenton K. HIV/AIDS statistics. Health Protection Agency, November 2004.

7 UKCC. Registrar's letter 4/1994 replacing circular Registrar's Letter 12/1993 Updated April 1998; Acquired Immune Deficiency Syndrome and Human Immuno-Deficiency Virus Infection (AIDS and HIV infection); Anonymous testing for the prevalence of the Human Immunodeficiency Virus (HIV); 1994.

8 Royal College of Midwives. HIV and AIDS position paper. London: RCM; 1998.

9 Department of Health. AIDS/HIV Infected Health Care Workers: Guidance on the Management of Infected Health Care Workers and Patient Notification. London: HMSO; 1999.

10 Department of Health. AIDS/HIV Infected Health Care Workers: Guidance on the Management of Infected Health Care Workers and Patient Notification. London: The Stationery Office; 2003.

11 Kennedy J. HIV in pregnancy and childbirth, 2nd edn. Oxford: Books for Midwives; 2003.

12 Akinsanya J, Rouse P. Who will care? A survey of the knowledge and attitudes of hospital nurses to people with HIV/AIDS. J Adv Nurs 1992; 17:400–401.

13 Harris G. Five years for the reckless lover who passed on HIV. The Times, 17 March 2001.

14 Criminal Injuries Compensation Authority (CICA) Glasgow (headquarters) Contact: CICA, Tay House, 300 Bath Street, Glasgow G2 4LN; Tel: 0141 331-2726; Fax: 0141 331-2287; CICA London (headquarters) CICA, Morley House, 26–30 Holborn Viaduct, London EC1A 2JQ; Tel: 020 7842 6800; Fax: 020 7436 0804.

15 Horsnall M. Lover convicted after infecting women with HIV. The Times, 15 October 2003.

16 Ford, R. Man who gave lovers HIV wins a retrial. The Times, 6 May 2004.

17 Norfolk, A. HIV man jailed for infecting women. The Times, 15 May 2004.

18 de Bruxelles S. Woman who knew she had HIV is jailed for infecting boyfriend. The Times, 19 July 2005.

19 Department of Health. Children in need and bloodborne viruses: HIV and Hepatitis. London: DoH; November 2004.

20 Rumbelow H. Judge orders mother to test baby for HIV. The Times, 4 September 1999.

21 Re C (HIV Test) [1999] 2 FLR 1004.

22 Baldwin T, Murray I. All pregnant women must test for Aids. The Times, 13 August 1999.

23 Department of Health. Screening for infectious diseases in pregnancy: Standards to support the UK antenatal screening programme. London: DoH; August 2003.

24 Department of Health. HIV and Infant feeding: Guidance from the UK Chief Medical Officers' Expert Advisory Group on AIDS. London: DoH; 24 September 2004.

25 Horsnall M. Patients to be told of HIV dentist. The Times, 28 February 2002.

26 Wilkinson v. Downton [1987] 2 QB 57.

27 de Bruxelles S. Carjacker held HIV syringe to victims' necks. The Times, 9 February 2002.

28 X v. Y and others [1988] 2 All ER 648.

29 Ashworth J. Charter launched by Sir Evelyn de Rothschild. The Times, 10 July 1992.

30 UK Declaration Working Group August 1991.

31 Department of Health. AIDS/HIV Infected Health Care Workers: Guidance on the management of infected health care workers and patient notification. London: The Stationery Office; 2003.

32 H (a healthcare worker) v. Associated Newspapers Ltd and H (a healthcare worker) v. N (a health authority) [2002] EWCA Civ 195 Lloyd's Rep Med [2002] 210.

33 Department of Health. Health Clearance for serious communicable diseases: new health care workers draft guidance 2003.

34 N v. Secretary of State for the Home Department. The Times, 9 May 2005 HL.

35 Confidential Enquiry into Stillbirths and Deaths in Infancy. 6th Annual Report 1996–1997. London: Maternal and Child Health Research Consortium; 1999.

36 National Audit Office. The Management and Control of Hospital Acquired Infection in Acute NHS Trusts in England. London: HMSO; 2000.

37 Department of Health. Online. Available: www.doh.gov.uk/arbstrat.htm

38 Department of Health. Press release, 12 June 2000.

39 Sherman J. 2000. Infections caught in hospital to be exposed. The Times, 13 June 2000.

40 Public Health Laboratory Service. Online. Available: http//www.phls.org.uk/publications/cdr/PDFfiles/20002/cdr2502.pdf.

41 Department of Health. Lord Hunt welcomes report into rates of MRSA Hospital Infection by NHS Trust. Press release 0066. London: DoH; 2002.

42 Public Health Laboratory Service. Communicable Disease Report 2002. London: Public Health Laboratory Service; 2002.

43 Health Protection Agency Report on MRSA, February 2004.

44 NHS Estates Department of Health. A matron's charter: An action plan for cleaner hospitals, October 2004.

45 Templeton S-K. Hundreds of babies hit by superbug. The Sunday Times, 27 February 2005.

46 Department of Health. Review panel makes progress on helping the NHS to fight MRSA. 2005/0040, February 2005.

47 Bissett L. Controlling the risk of MRSA infection: screening and isolating patients. Br J Nurs 2005; 14(7):386–390.

48 Department of Health. Press release 2005/0247. London: DoH; 15 July 2005.

49 News item. The Times, 22 July 2005.

SECTION F

SPECIFIC SITUATIONS

This final Section looks at specific areas of midwifery practice and client groups including the midwife lecturer, researcher and the law relating to the special needs of children and those suffering from mental illness. Finally, the legal issues arising from the practice of complementary therapies are considered.

Chapter 30

MIDWIFE TEACHERS, CLINICAL INSTRUCTORS, PRECEPTORS AND MENTORS

The NMC Code of Professional Conduct Clause 6.4[1] states:

You have a duty to facilitate students of nursing and midwifery and others to develop their competence

This makes it clear that the instruction and support of other health professionals, at both pre and post registration, is an intrinsic part of a registered practitioner's role.

Most midwives are therefore in some way likely to be involved in the instruction and support of others. Increasingly, this role may be formalised and become part of the contract of employment. Even those who are not employed in a teaching capacity might find that their job description includes responsibilities for the training and mentoring of others. April 2001 marked the end of the transition period for midwives to take on the requirements of post-registration education and practice (PREP) of the UKCC (now replaced by the NMC). An updated PREP handbook was published by the NMC in August 2004.[2] The adoption of the PREP proposals and the requirement for preceptors should result in more midwives being involved in the role of instructor or preceptor (see Ch. 2 on Educational Requirements). For the most part, this is unlikely to give rise to many legal issues. However, in some cases, an awareness of potential dangers and problems could prove to be of considerable advantage. Further information on the legal issues arising in the teaching and assessment process can be seen in the author's chapter in Partners in Learning by Ian Walsh and Caron Swann.[3] Following the UKCC's Education Commission report, 'Fitness for Practice',[4] the UKCC published revised standards for the preparation of teachers of nursing, midwifery and health visiting,[5] which came into force in September 2001. They were reprinted by the NMC in 2002 and August 2004.[6] They cover standards for recording teaching qualifications and standards for mentors and preceptors.

Guidance for those with the responsibility of developing programmes designed to prepare mentors and teachers of nursing, midwifery and health visiting and allied health professionals was published jointly by the English National Board and the Department of Health and is available from the NMC website.[7]

The competencies required for midwifery teachers were considered at an International Confederation of Midwives in 2002[8] and were discussed by JE Thompson[9] who considered that these competencies were important regardless of the level of student taught, type of educational programme or number of years of midwifery experience the learners have.

Reference should also be made to Chapter 31 on Research.

TERMINOLOGY

First, what activities are we considering? Box 30.1 sets out some of the terminology used in the instruction and support of others.

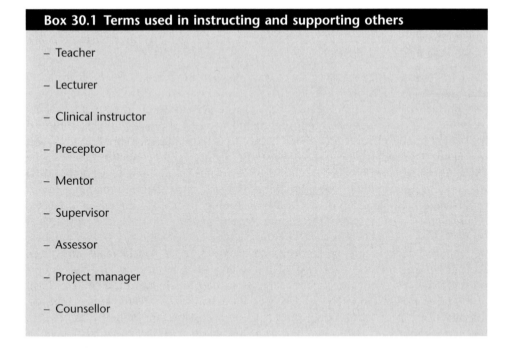

Box 30.1 Terms used in instructing and supporting others

- Teacher

- Lecturer

- Clinical instructor

- Preceptor

- Mentor

- Supervisor

- Assessor

- Project manager

- Counsellor

To make discussion easier in this chapter, the person who is subject to the instruction, mentorship etc. will be referred to as the student, even though the person may well be a registered practitioner.

PRECEPTOR

The definition given by the UKCC within the PREP guidelines is:

a role model and support for about the first four months of practice as a registered practitioner to:

– *provide guidance*

– *be a member of the same team*

– *judge the appropriate level of responsibility*

– *agree objectives and outcomes for the period of support*

– *who may recommend an extension of time.*

MENTOR

Where a (usually) older and more experienced person acts in the nature of a protector for the other for a longer time than would normally be associated with preceptorship, and where the more experienced person provides guidance, support and a concern for the other's advancement and general progress.

TEACHER/INSTRUCTOR/LECTURER

This person would usually be based in a college of education and provide education and training for the student. Normally, she would also have duties to instruct and assess in the workplace and assess the student's progress.

SUPERVISOR

A Supervisor of Midwives has a distinct role set by statute and this role is considered in Chapter 3. The Supervisor of Midwives might, of course, also be a mentor, preceptor or any of the other roles considered in this chapter. Clinical supervision, a form of reflective practice, has been recommended by the UKCC[10] for registered nurses, but, presumably because of the statutory form of supervision, has not been used in midwifery practice. The supervisory needs of midwifery lecturers are considered by Rogers, who reports on the results of an audit of midwife lecturers' experience and needs from supervision and the development of a strategy to meet those needs.[11]

The legal areas which will be discussed in relation to all types of supporters/instructors are shown in Box 30.2.

Box 30.2 Legal areas to be considered

– Statutory requirements

– Duty of care: Liability for negligent advice, delegation and supervision

– Appeals process

– Confidentiality and access to information

– Whistle-blowing

– Contracts of employment

– Health and safety

– NHS agreements

– Giving references

STATUTORY FRAMEWORK

The NMC has the duty of setting the educational requirements for entry onto the Register for its practitioners. This would necessitate keeping in touch with European Directives on changes to the content of professional training. In Chapter 2, Box 2.1, can be found the requirements of the EC for midwifery education and in Box 2.2, the amended requirements of the European Community for the practical and clinical aspects of midwifery programmes added by the European Union Directive 89/594/EEC.

The NMC's standards for pre-registration midwifery programmes[12] are set out in Chapter 2.

It is also a requirement that in order to be placed on the Register, the applicant must satisfy the Council that she is of good health and character (see Ch. 4), as well as having the appropriate professional qualifications. If, therefore, the lecturer becomes aware of evidence about a student which makes it clear that she is not of good character or good health, and therefore should not be placed on the Register, then the lecturer would have a duty to inform the appropriate person. (Where evidence comes to light that a practitioner should not remain on the Register, then this should be reported to the NMC under the fitness to practise procedures which are considered in Chapter 4.) Training schools must be careful that they ensure that the appropriate checks are made before students are taken onto a course, since a student who is told that they cannot be recommended for registration, because of a lack of good health or character which were evident before they started the course, could have an action against the training school for negligence in their being accepted (or failure to advise them during the course of their unsuitability).

In July 2004, the NMC published a consultation paper on the standards for the preparation of mentors and teachers. It closed in October 2004 and reported key themes and issues to Council in March 2005. Its framework to underpin the proposed standard to support training and assessment in practice was to be published in September 2005, following further consultation with employers and other stakeholders.

DUTY OF CARE

It is essential to establish the extent of the duty of care owed to the student/trainee. Rarely is the instructor in a line management relationship with the student but there may be a responsibility when it can be seen that harm may occur to the student or to someone else if no action is taken by the instructor. Reference should be made to Chapter 13 on Negligence and the basic elements to be established before a successful action can be brought.

The following principles emerge:

- There is no concept recognised in law of team liability.

- There is no concept that a superior is vicariously liable for the wrongs of a junior. The superior must be shown to be personally and directly liable. (This is discussed further in Ch. 24 on the Legal Aspects of Management.)

- Standards can differ (see the Bolam Test and Maynards Case).

- Liability can exist for negligent advice.

- Liability can also exist for negligent delegations where the instructor is aware that the student has inadequate experience to undertake a particular activity (see Ch. 24).

- Liability can also exist for negligent supervision if the limited experience of the student indicates that a specific level of supervision is required in order to ensure that the client, the student and others are safe.

The extent of the duty of care

One area in which the teacher would be expected to show competence and have a duty of care would be in ensuring that students were educated in the appropriate areas to obtain registration. The duty is placed upon the lecturer to ensure that the syllabus covered by the student and the standard of teaching, combined with due diligence from the student, is sufficient to enable the student to obtain the necessary qualifications for Registration and practice. The lecturer must therefore ensure that she keeps up-to-date with the statutory requirements for registration.

Incompetent or dangerous students

If it is known that the student is likely to refuse or ignore any advice which is offered and if this refusal is likely to endanger clients, then the teacher would have a responsibility to take the appropriate action to prevent harm. In serious situations this might involve reporting the midwife to the Supervisor of Midwives and/or line manager. In less serious circumstances, and depending upon whether the student is registered or not, it might necessitate warning the student that if the advice is ignored then further action will be taken. Should the instructor take the view that it is not her concern, and harm befalls a client, a defence of 'it was not my business' might not prevail in a hearing before the NMC since the instructor would herself be a registered practitioner and therefore subject to the Code of Professional Conduct: standards for conduct, performance and ethics.[1]

A similar situation would arise if the instructor forms the view that the student is too dangerous to practise. In such circumstances the instructor would have a clear professional responsibility to take any action which is necessary to protect the clients. This would also apply if the instructor fears that the student is mentally disordered. The dangers of such a situation are apparent from the Beverly Allitt case, though there it was not known that the nurse was mentally ill until several children had died.

Where the instructor knows that the student is practising outside her sphere of competence she should ensure that the student's managers are notified and the necessary training is given to the student to enable her to practise safely.

Sometimes, however, the student might confide in the instructor about confidential matters. For example, the student might confess to the instructor that she is disclosing information which has been entrusted to her in confidence. She might tell the instructor that she has passed on to the mother information relating to the unborn child, contrary to the wishes of the Consultant who had wanted to keep that information from the mother for the time being. In such a situation the instructor should ensure that the manager of the midwife is informed and that the mother is receiving all the necessary support. Where the instructor might agree that the student may have been right in her approach, she should be careful not to intervene in a clinical situation for which she is in no way responsible. However, if it appears that the student is in danger of becoming a victim of whistle-blowing, she should ensure that she obtains the required support (see below).

Where the student tells the instructor information about herself in confidence, for example that she is HIV positive, or that she has a drink problem or a criminal record, the instructor should make it clear that she cannot keep silent about such facts and advise the student to notify the Supervisor and her manager and if she fails to do so, then the instructor would be bound to take the necessary action. Where such information is given to the instructor anonymously, the instructor would still have a duty to confront the student and take any necessary action.

Criticisms might also come to the instructor from the ward manager or others about the student's conduct. In such circumstances, the instructor would have a duty to give the student advice and counselling and if necessary advise the head of school.

Students may criticise practice to the instructor. For example, a student might inform the instructor that a doctor is incompetent. In such a case, the instructor would have a responsibility to ensure that the student was supported in taking this further, so that appropriate investigations could be carried out by those with managerial responsibility.

APPEALS PROCESSES

Each education or training institution must ensure that there is a robust, equitable, accessible and just system of appeals. Article 6 of the European Convention on Human Rights (see Appendix 1 of this book) is of particular importance in the assessment process, since it gives a right to a fair trial and is therefore fundamental to any appeals process where results of the assessment or the actual carrying out of an assessment is challenged. Assessors should ensure that, if there is a challenge to their assessment, an independent person reviews the situation and the appropriate appeals machinery is enacted. The principles of natural justice would require that any person involved in hearing an appeal is independent and impartial, hears the evidence from the appellant and ensures that the decision is made in accordance with the evidence received. The decision of an appeals hearing could be challenged in the High Court by way of judicial review if there is an allegation that the principles of natural justice have not been followed or if there is an alleged breach of Article 6. The Appeals process should also cover the timing of assessments and examinations. For example, if an assessor fails to carry out an assessment in time to give the student an opportunity for rectifying any shortcomings, and such an opportunity should have been made available to the student, then the student may well have grounds for appeal.

CONFIDENTIALITY AND ACCESS TO INFORMATION

Since the instructor will not necessarily be professionally concerned with the care of the patient, what right in law does the instructor have to receive information which the student has received in confidence about the patient? It could be argued that the passing on of such information is in the interests of the mother. However, this is very indirect, and it would have to be shown that unless the instructor had this confidential information, harm could arise to the mother or child. An alternative strategy, and one which would be far more open, is for the patient to be told about the situation relating to the instructor/student role and her/his consent obtained to relevant information being passed between them both for the education of the student and for the protection of the patient.

Where the student is concerned about a hazardous situation on the ward which involves confidential information about a patient, notifying the instructor for advice could be seen as an exception to the duty of confidentiality which is in the best interests of the patient or in the public interest. (See Ch. 10 for further discussion on confidentiality.)

WHISTLE-BLOWING

The student should be guided in relation to the procedure for alerting management to any hazardous situations and the instructor should ensure that she is given the appropriate support. Advice should be given on record keeping and letters which are sent to management and copies should be kept (see Ch. 22).

CONTRACTUAL ASPECTS

Midwives employed by NHS Trusts or Primary Care Trusts

Where a midwife is appointed as an instructor, she should ensure that her job description and her terms of service reflect her enlarged duties. Where she is employed by a trust and not by an educational establishment, but is carrying out responsibilities in relation to the latter, she should ensure that her employer is aware of and has agreed to these additional duties and any likely area of conflict is resolved before the agreement is made. If she has any liability towards the educational establishment this should be clarified. She should also have access to the agreement drawn up between the college and the NHS Trust in relation to the practical education of the midwives and their preceptoring or mentoring and any provisions relating to liability.

Midwives employed by education establishments

These midwives should ensure that their duties in relation to the clinical placements are spelt out in writing and they should ensure that they have an input into any agreement drawn up between the college and the trust over the clinical training of midwives and continuing education and preceptoring or mentoring. The agreement should establish clearly responsibility for any harm to the midwife while she is supervising the student on the clinical placement and which organisation is vicariously liable should the midwife cause harm through her negligence.

Consideration for additional duties

It is unlikely that extra payments would be made for midwives to take on the tasks of being mentors or preceptors. However, if certain inducements are offered, the midwife should ensure that these are put in writing.

HEALTH AND SAFETY ASPECTS

Depending on the circumstances of the relationship of instructor to student, the duty of care probably includes duties in relation to health and safety at work. Clearly where the instructor notes that the student is failing to observe instructions in relation to health and safety then she would have a duty in law to inform the student of the dangers and ensure that those who were supervising the student in the workplace were aware of the situation (see Ch. 19 for details of health and safety law).

NHS AGREEMENTS

Agreements for NHS services are increasingly likely to set out the training and educational functions which are expected of the providers. Those who are involved in the instructing/mentoring of others should ensure that the standards both in terms of quantity and quality are detailed in the agreement so that the necessary resources are made available and that this function is specifically itemised for provision by the NHS trust. PREP responsibilities should be clarified so that continuing education and training is provided. While midwives (and all other registered practitioners since the implementation of the PREP provisions) have a statutory duty to undertake refresher courses, the resourcing for this is not always apparent, nor is the provision of paid time off work for study leave. It could be argued that since the employer owes a duty (both under the contract of employment and as part of the duty owed to patients under the law of negligence) to ensure the provision of competent staff, then there is an implied term that the employer will, at its expense, ensure that the competence of professional staff is maintained and that standards of care are improved.

If such duties are built into the agreements for the provision of midwifery services, then this will strengthen midwives' entitlement to receive regular updating and professional development within their paid hours of work. However, ultimately, the duty is on the practitioner to ensure that she keeps up-to-date and receives the necessary study, whatever the policy of the employer in relation to paid study leave.

WRITING REFERENCES

Liability can arise when a midwife is asked to write a reference. If a reference is written negligently then liability can arise both to the recipient of the reference, if in reliance upon that reference she has suffered harm,[13] and also to the person who is the subject of the reference.

Box 30.3 Providing a reference

A midwife is asked to provide a reference for a student who has had a warning at work for coming into work in a dishevelled state. The midwife student asks the midwife not to refer to this incident, assuring her that she now takes considerable care over her appearance and cleanliness. What is the position if the midwife gives the reference without mentioning this warning, and the student obtains the post, and then the employer blames the midwife for an inaccurate reference?

If there is evidence that the student midwife is completely reformed then it would probably not be necessary to mention this in the reference, but much depends upon the questions which are asked. If inaccurate information is given then the person providing the reference could be liable for negligent advice. The recipient of the reference would have to show that harm had occurred as a result of reliance upon the reference. If a person asks for information to be withheld in a reference, the midwife would have to tell the student that she could not give a reference without mentioning specific information. There can also be liability to the person on whose behalf the reference is given, if the reference is written without reasonable care and if harm occurs to the subject of the reference as a result of potential employers relying upon the reference.[14] In one case[15] Sun Alliance Life Ltd appealed against a decision that it had been negligent in its provision of an unfavourable reference in relation to C, a former employee. The Court of Appeal dismissed the appeal, holding that an employer owed a duty of care in providing a reference in respect of a former employee. Sun Alliance had failed to take reasonable care to be fair or accurate with regard to the reference supplied. The reference had inaccurately implied that C had been suspended for serious matters of dishonesty and that the matters had been thoroughly investigated. However, no charges of dishonesty had ever been put to C, let alone investigated.

Every care should be taken to ensure that a reference is written accurately in the light of the facts available.

If a reference is given with due care but is defamatory of the individual, the writer of the reference should be protected from any successful action of defamation whether the comments are correct or they are incorrect, if they were given in a qualified privileged situation without malice by the writer.

CONCLUSION

More and more pressure is placed upon teaching staff, and also those midwives who, although they are not teachers, are expected to fulfil the role of preceptor or mentor or undertake a similar activity. Such activities inevitably carry additional legal responsibilities and midwives must ensure that they have an understanding of the legal implications of any such activity they are asked to undertake. As always, clear and comprehensive documentation of how the activity is carried out is essential.

In October 2001 the Department of Health announced the publication of a prospectus for the NHS University.[16] It was the intention that everyone in the NHS would begin their career with the NHS University through induction courses and direct training. This University would inevitably have a major impact on the current role of nurse lecturers at other institutions and could have paved the way towards a more centralised curriculum and assessments for pre-registration and post-registration courses. Subsequently, in the strategy to reduce the number of NHS quangos it was announced that the NHS Modernisation Agency would be brought together with the NHS Leadership Centre and the NHSU to form an NHS Institute for learning, skills and innovation in July 2005.[17] The NHS Institute would also manage the planned new National Innovation Centre. An advisory board was established to guide the Institute's formation. The NHSU was abolished on 1 August 2005 and the new NHS Institute for Innovation and Improvement came into being on 1 July 2005.[18] It is hoped that the establishment will be accompanied by independent monitoring to analyse its effectiveness in relation to the existing HE institutions.

QUESTIONS AND EXERCISES

1. As a lecturer of midwives, you have been told by a student that a fellow student is acting very oddly and appears to be mentally ill. What action would you take?

2. You are employed by an educational institution but have responsibilities within the field of clinical practice. In the event of your being negligent and causing harm to a client, who would be liable: the educational institution or the trust? How would you find out the answer?

3. In litigation, proof of the instruction which has been given is of increasing importance as a defence. Examine your own record keeping in relation to what you teach or mentor.

References

1 Nursing and Midwifery Council Code of Professional Conduct: standards for conduct, performance and ethics 2002 (renamed) 2004.

2 Nursing and Midwifery Council PREP Handbook (update). Latest revised edition. August 2004.

3 Dimond B. Getting it right: the legal and professional aspects of assessment. In: Walsh I, Swann C, eds. Partners in learning. Abingdon: Radcliffe Medical Press; 2002.

4 UKCC. Fitness for practice. London: UKCC; 1999.

5 UKCC. Standards for the preparation of teachers of nursing, midwifery and health visiting. London: UKCC; 1999.

6 Nursing and Midwifery Council. Standards for the preparation of teachers of nurses, midwives and specialist community public health nurses. NMC; August 2004.

7 English National Board and Department of Health Preparation of Mentors and Teachers, 8 May 2002.

8 International Confederation of Midwives. The Hague: ICM; 2002.

9 Thompson JE. Competencies for midwifery teachers. Midwifery 2002; 18(4):256–259.

10 UKCC. Position statement on clinical supervision. London: UKCC; 1996.

11 Rogers C. The supervisory needs of midwifery lecturers. Br J Midwifery 2002; 10(3):165–168.

12 UKCC. Requirements for pre-registration midwifery programmes. Registrar's Letter 35/2000.

13 Hedley Byrne v. Heller and Partners Ltd House of Lords [1963] 2 All ER 575.

14 Spring v. Guardian Assurance plc and others. Times Law Report, 8 July 1994; [1995] 2 AC 296.

15 Cox v. Sun Alliance Life Ltd [2001] EWCA Civ 649; [2001] IRLR 448 CA.

16 Department of Health. Introducing the NHS University. Press Release 2001/480.

17 Department of Health. New NHS Institute for learning, skills and innovation to be formed in July 2005. London: DoH; 30 November.

18 NHS Institute for Innovation and Improvement. Establishment and Constitution Order, SI 2005 No 1446; Regulations, SI 2005 No 1447.

Chapter 31
MIDWIFERY RESEARCH

The midwife may be involved in research in three ways:
– she may be undertaking it herself as part of her own professional development

– she may be the project manager for someone else's research

– she may be caring for mothers or responsible for staff who are the subjects of a research investigation.

A useful introductory guide to research for midwives has been written by Colin Rees.[1] In addition, since midwifery should be a research-based profession,[2] it is important for the midwife to know when the research results should be incorporated into her standards of practice. Increasingly, the publications of NICE should bring to the attention of practitioners the results of research into midwifery and obstetric practice (see Ch. 21). In its Code of Professional Conduct: standards for conduct, performance and ethics[3] Clause 6.5 the NMC states:

You have a responsibility to deliver care based on current evidence, best practice and, where applicable, validated research when it is available.

The necessity for midwifery to be a research-based profession was emphasised by the Advisory Committee on the Training of Midwives of the Commission of the European Communities in its report and recommendations adopted at its meeting on 14 and 15 January 1992. The Committee's recommendations are shown in Box 31.1.

Box 31.1 Recommendations of the Committee on the Training of Midwives of the EC

1. Research should be included in the curriculum for basic midwifery training. A curriculum should as a minimum include:

   – principles of research

   – elementary research methods including statistics and epidemiology

   – analysis and interpretation of research findings

   – library use

▶
– ethical and moral implications of research

– practical application of research findings.

2.2 The member states should promote the aspects of research in the exercise of the profession of midwifery.

2.3 All research achieved or undertaken by midwives should be entered into a database in the member states.

The issues to be considered in this chapter are shown in Box 31.2.

Box 31.2 Legal issues arising in research

– Consent

– Local Research Ethics Committees

– Confidentiality

– Injuries to the research subject

– Health and safety and the researcher

– Project management

– Research results and the standards of care

– International codes protecting human rights

CONSENT

Consent in relation to treatment and care is considered in Chapters 7 and 8. Chapter 7 looks at the issues relating to trespass to the person and the giving of consent. Chapter 8 looks at the information which must be provided to prevent an action for breach of the duty of care owed in negligence arising. This section builds on these two chapters and considers consent in relation to research.

Box 31.3 illustrates the issues which must be considered in relation to consent to research.

Box 31.3 Issues arising in consent to research

- Nature of the consent

- How consent should be given

- The capacity of the person giving consent

- The information to be given

- Payment and voluntary consent

- Risk of harm to the fetus

- Role of the midwife

- Consent and a records search.

WHAT IS THE NATURE OF CONSENT WHICH IS REQUIRED?

It is essential that the fully informed voluntary consent of the research subject should be obtained before the research progresses. The consent should be given without compulsion and must be given by an adult who has the mental capacity to give consent. The form should explain to the research subject that refusal to participate in the research project will not lead to any prejudice in the care and treatment which is given. Clearly there are advantages in obtaining the mother's consent to participate in a research project about labour, well before labour commences.

SHOULD THE CONSENT BE IN WRITING?

While in practice both written and spoken consent would be defences against an action for trespass to the person, it is easier to prove that consent has been given where it is in writing and the Local Research Ethics Committee (LREC) (see below) would normally require a written consent.

Consent should preferably be obtained both in writing and by word of mouth. The research project should have been before the Local Research Ethics Committee (see below) which would look at the information to be given to the subject and the consent form which is signed.

A research project looking at consent forms for research protocols[4] found that

consent forms for research were more difficult to read than newspaper editorials. Poor read-ability was caused by the use of long paragraphs and long sentences, not by the excessive use of long words.

HOW SHOULD THE COMPETENCE OF THE MOTHER TO GIVE CONSENT BE DETERMINED?

Consent should be given at a time when the mother is capable of giving it. It would not be appropriate to request consent when the mother is part way through labour and does not have the capacity to give consent. The midwife could have an important role in ensuring that consent is not obtained from the mother at a time when she does not have the capacity to make a valid decision. If there are concerns over whether or not the mother has the capacity to give consent, it would be wise to bring in a health professional who is not involved in the research project to make an assessment of the mother's competence and record it in writing.

HOW MUCH INFORMATION SHOULD BE GIVEN TO THE RESEARCH SUBJECT?

While the courts have held that the doctrine of informed consent is not recognised when consent is given for treatment[5] where research is being carried out which has no direct therapeutic benefit for the patient, a higher standard of information giving would probably be required (see Ch. 8 and the Sidaway case). All risks should be explained beforehand. It is doubtful too, if the mother could give consent to a risk of harm to the fetus, unless the risk was so insignificant and the benefits to be obtained by the research outweighed these insignificant risks.

PAYMENT AND VOLUNTARY CONSENT

The general principle is that if the payment is such as materially to affect the patient's attitude, and in a sense buy that consent, there would be concern at the voluntary nature of the consent. Much would of course depend upon the economic circumstances of the mother. Payment of out-of-pocket expenses – travelling if the mother is required to visit the hospital/research centre – would probably not come within the category of a payment which affected the mother's voluntary agreement to participate.

CONSENT AND RISKS TO THE FETUS

What if the mother gives consent to a research project which harms the fetus: could the child when born bring an action against the mother? (This is quite separate from an action against the researcher which might also exist.) Such an action against the mother would not be possible under the Congenital Disabilities (Civil Liability) Act 1976 since under that Act the mother can only be sued if her negligence, which led to the congenital disabilities, occurred when she was driving a car (see Ch. 17). The right of action at common law[6] is no longer available since the implementation of the Congenital Disabilities (Civil Liability) Act 1976.

If the mother gives a valid consent to the research taking place but harm subsequently occurs to the fetus who is born disabled, since the child's right derives from the action in negligence which the mother has, the consent of the mother may well prevent the action from the child succeeding (see s.6 of the Congenital Disabilities Act 1976) unless negligence by the researchers to the mother can be shown.

THE ROLE OF THE MIDWIFE

Where the midwife is aware that researchers are wishing mothers to take part in research projects, she should ensure as protector of the mother that full information is given to the mother, and that the research proceeds only if the mother's consent has been given. If she is not satisfied on these facts, the midwife should be prepared to take up these points with the researchers. She should also make sure that she herself is fully informed about the research. The same principles apply when any medication is being given as part of a research project. If it is an unlicensed medicine which is given on the basis of a personal license to the doctor for a named patient, the midwife should ensure that the mother is fully informed of the situation. If this does not appear to be the case, she should ask the doctor to explain the situation fully to the mother and obtain her full consent.

CONSENT AND RECORDS SEARCH

The giving of consent by the research subject provides a defence against an action for trespass to the person. However, where the nature of the research is the gathering of information from case records, is consent necessary? The answer is yes, since the disclosure of confidential information would be protected by the patient's right to sue for breach of confidentiality by the holder of records in giving access to the researcher. The Data Protection Act 1998 applies to both computerised and manually-held records and there would therefore have to be registration for the additional purpose of research. The consent of the LREC (see below) to undertake the research would also be required. Usually it would be sufficient to assure the mother that there would be no disclosure of personal information relating to her and that in any research publication the research subjects would not be identifiable.

LOCAL RESEARCH ETHICS COMMITTEES

The issues to be discussed here can be seen in Box 31.4.

Box 31.4 Local Research Ethics Committees

– Function and constitution

– Powers and sanctions (if any)

– Role in multi-centre trials

– Financial situation: charging for their services and the legal significance of this.

FUNCTION AND CONSTITUTION

In 1991, the NHS Management Executive issued a booklet entitled 'Local Research Ethics Committees', which gave detailed guidance on the establishment and function of LRECs, and the administrative framework within which they work, the ethical principles to which LRECs should have regard and particular groups of research subjects.[7] It was clearly stated that the responsibility for deciding whether a research project should proceed, within the NHS, lies with the NHS body under whose auspices the research would take place. New guidance on LRECs was issued by the Department of Health in 2001[8] and the new arrangements came into force in April 2002.

The Governance statement defines the purpose of an REC in reviewing the proposed study:

to protect the dignity, rights, safety and well-being of all actual or potential research participants. It shares this role and responsibility with others, as described in the Research Governance Framework for Health and Social Care.[9] (see below)

Research may not be started until ethical approval has been obtained. It is the personal responsibility of the person named as principal investigator to apply for approval by the REC and this person retains responsibility for the scientific and ethical conduct of the research.

Section A of the guidance provided by the Department of Health sets out a Statement of General Standards and Principles and covers the following topics:

– Role of Research Ethics Committees

– The remit of an NHS REC

– Establishment and support of NHS RECs

– Membership requirements and process

– Composition of an REC

– Working procedures

– Multi-centre research

– The Process of ethical review of a research protocol

– Submitting an application

– Glossary.

Section B provides more detailed guidance on operating procedures and the require-ments for general support for RECs. Section C provides a resource for RECs and collates current advice on ethical issues and is to be regularly updated.

In June 2005, the Department of Health announced that improvements were to be carried out to the system by which health researchers gained ethical approval for research in the NHS.[10] The aim is to ensure that applications for good quality research are reviewed consistently, promptly and efficiently by ethics committees. The announcement follows a report by the Ad Hoc Advisory Group on the Operation of NHS Research Ethics Committees whose report has now been passed to the National Patient Safety Agency for consultation on how the improvements are to be effected.

RESEARCH GOVERNANCE FRAMEWORK FOR HEALTH AND SOCIAL CARE[9]

This document from the Department of Health sets standards which should apply to all health and social care research. It emphasises that:

The public has a right to expect high scientific, ethical and financial standards, transparent decision-making processes, clear allocation of responsibilities and robust monitoring arrangements.

With this purpose in mind, it sets standards for ethics, science, information, health and safety, finance and a quality research culture. It identifies responsibilities and accountability generally and also specifically for participants, researchers, the prin-cipal investigator, the research investigator, the research sponsor, universities and other employers of researchers, organisations providing care, the care professionals and the research ethics committees. This framework would be an essential document for any midwife who is either personally involved in a research project or is caring for women and babies who are the subject of research.

Exactly the same principles apply in relation to the duty to recognise and keep con-fidential information obtained during research as apply in the treatment and care of patients. (Reference should therefore be made to Chapter 10. Probably the same exceptions would also exist. However, these have not been tested in court.) Disclosure in the public interest is likely to cause some difficulties and reference should therefore be made to the NMC Code of Professional Conduct: standards for conduct, perfor-mance and ethics.[3]

INJURIES TO THE SUBJECT OF THE RESEARCH

At the present time there has been no implementation of the suggestion made in the Royal Commission on Personal Injuries (The Pearson Report 1978)[11] that those persons who have been injured or harmed as a result of participation in a research project should receive compensation without proof of fault. Any such person must therefore prove that there has been negligence which has caused the harm which he has suffered. However, many research companies and particular drug companies offer compensation without the need to establish that there has been fault. An indemnity is offered both to the researchers and to the subjects when the research is agreed. If the midwife is involved in a research project, whatever her role, she should find out the details of any indemnity provision. The LREC will check the indemnity provisions before agreeing to a research project funded by a pharmaceutical company. The Department of Health at the time of writing is considering a new scheme for compensation for clinical negligence, which may include a partial no-fault liability scheme. If this is implemented, those persons injured during a research project should receive compensation without proving negligence (see Ch. 14).

HEALTH AND SAFETY LAW

The researcher must be aware of all those laws relating to the health and safety of his colleagues and the general public before embarking on any research project. Reference should be made to Chapter 19.

PROJECT MANAGEMENT

Where the midwife is asked to be responsible for a research project she should be aware of the issues shown in Box 31.5.

Box 31.5 Issues arising in research project management

- Negligent advice

- Liability for supervising

- LRECs

- Contracts of employment

- Patients' rights

▶
- Consent

- Data protection

- Confidentiality

- Access to records

- Health and safety

- External funding

Many of these topics are covered in earlier chapters. In this section, emphasis will be placed upon the authorisation of the research project.

It is essential before research is commenced to consider who has the right to control the publication of results and to exercise any censorship over it. Control might vary according to who is funding the research and whether or not it is part of a contract of employment. Box 31.6 illustrates the different forms of projects from the perspective of funding and contracts. Box 31.7 looks at different projects from the perspective of their methods.

Box 31.6 Different forms of funding and control

1. As part of a contract of employment

   - funded externally without the employer's support

   - funded externally with the employer's support

   - for career development, e.g. for higher degree etc. with the financial support of the employer

   - for career development without the financial support of the employer.

2. Outside the contract of employment

   - with external funding

   - with no funding.

Box 31.7 Types of project

- Non-invasive

- Invasive

- Using financial resources

- With no financial resources

- Statistical

- Data collection

- Questionnaires

- Observations, e.g. case study

- Action linked

- Paper/library search

The midwife's role as a supervisor of research is shown in Box 31.8.

Box 31.8 Midwife's role as a supervisor of research

- Coordination

- Commissioning

- Conduct

- Counselling/advising

Areas of potential liability as a supervisor are shown in Box 31.9.

Box 31.9 Areas of potential liability

- Negligent delegation

- Negligent advice

▶

▶

- Failure to support the student

- Failure to obtain funding

- Failure to complete

- Ignorance of earlier research and activities

Before beginning the research project management, the midwife should ensure that she has obtained the relevant permissions to embark on the research. As has been seen, this would include not only the approval of the Local Research Ethical Committee but also the approval of the Health Authority or NHS trust or her educational institute or her employer.

It is advisable to ensure that there is agreement over who has control over publications and editing the research outcomes.

During the project the project manager should ensure that the rules relating to consent are implemented and that the other legal pitfalls mentioned in this chapter are taken into account.

STANDARDS OF CARE AND THE RESULTS OF RESEARCH

One of the most difficult issues is knowing when research results are ready to be incorporated into the standards of care expected of the midwife. Some results are, for example, still of only an exploratory nature and too uncertain to affect current standards of care. An example is the debate over the administration of vitamin K, following research which seemed to suggest that if given intramuscularly it could cause side-effects to babies (see Ch. 14).

This is an area where the midwife should keep alert to any changes in the standards which are required of her and take an immediate note of any instructions from the Committee for the Safety of Medicines and other authorities.

PLAGIARISM

If a midwife researcher were to be found guilty of plagiarism, this could be seen as evidence of lack of fitness to practise by the NMC. In one case[12] two doctors were suspended by the GMC for 3 months for dishonestly plagiarising part of a previously published article in their one medical paper. They admitted the facts but each denied responsibility, leaving the GMC unable to determine who was telling the truth. The Privy Council allowed their appeal on the grounds that there was no justification of making a finding of dishonesty, since it had not been alleged and the GMC conclusion that whoever had not carried out the copying must have known it had been done, did not meet the fundamental principle of fairness. The suspension was substituted for a reprimand.

INTERNATIONAL CODES OF HUMAN RIGHTS

The midwife should be aware of those international codes which attempt to protect the human subject from abuses in research. Any LREC should take into account the principles relating to humane conduct of research.

INTERNATIONAL CONVENTIONS COVERING RESEARCH

NUREMBERG CODE

At the end of the Second World War, military trials were held in Nuremberg where members of the Nazi party, some of the worst perpetrators of crimes against humanity, were prosecuted. In its judgement, the Court set out ten basic principles which should be observed in order to satisfy moral, ethical and legal concepts. These have become known as the Nuremberg Code.[13] The ten principles are summarised in Box 31.10.

Box 31.10 Principles for research from Nuremberg Code

1. The voluntary consent of the human subject is absolutely essential.

2. The experiment should be such as to yield fruitful results for the good of society, unprocurable by other methods.

3. The experiment should be based on results of animal experiments and a knowledge of the natural history of the disease or other problem so that the anticipated results should justify the performance of the experiment.

4. The experiment should be so conducted as to avoid all unnecessary physical and mental suffering and injury.

---

5. No experiment should be conducted where there is an a priori reason to believe that death or disabling injury will occur; except, perhaps, in those circumstances where the experimental physicians also serve as subjects.

6. The degree of risk to be taken should never exceed that determined by the humanitarian importance of the problem to be solved by the experiment.

7. Proper preparations should be made and adequate facilities provided to protect the experimental subject against even remote possibilities of injury, disability or death.

8. The experiment should be conducted only by a scientifically qualified person. The highest degree of skill and care should be required through all stages of the experiment of those who conduct or engage in the experiment.

9. During the course of the experiment the human subject should be at liberty to bring the experiment to an end if he had reached the physical or mental state where continuation of the experiment seems to him to be impossible.

10. During the course of the experiment the scientist in charge must be prepared to terminate the experiment at any stage, if he has probable cause to believe, in the exercise of the good faith, superior skill and careful judgement required of him that a continuation of the experiment is likely to result in injury, disability, or death to the experimental subject.

The above Code and others such as the Declaration of Helsinki have not yet been incorporated into English law. However, they are enforceable through the International Court of Human Rights. The Declaration of Helsinki was amended in Edinburgh in 2000. The European Convention on Human Rights which has been incorporated into the laws of the UK (see Ch. 6 and Appendix 1) will also be relevant in ensuring that research practice respects basic human rights.

EUROPEAN COMMISSION RULES RELATING TO CLINICAL TRIALS

An EC Directive[14] on the implementation of good clinical practice in the conduct of clinical trials on medicinal products for human use stipulates the procedures which must be followed by all member states in carrying out clinical trials. The contents of the Directive are shown in Box 31.11.

Box 31.11 EC Directive on clinical trials

Article 1 Aim of the Directive:

– To establish specific provisions regarding the conduct of clinical trials, including multi-centre trials on human subjects involving medicinal products as defined by Article 1 of Directive 65/66/EEC.

– Good clinical practice to be identified and complied with.

– To adopt and if necessary revise principles of good clinical practice and detailed guidance to be published by the Commission.

– All clinical trials to be designed, conducted and reported in accordance with the principles of good clinical practice.

Article 2 Definitions

Article 3 Protection of clinical trial subjects

Article 4 Clinical trials on minors

Article 5 Clinical trials on incapacitated adults not able to give informed legal consent

Article 6 Ethics Committee

Article 7 Single Opinion

Article 8 Detailed guidance to be published by Commission

Article 9 Commencement of a clinical trial

Article 10 Conduct of a clinical trial

Article 11 Exchange of information

Article 12 Suspension of the trial or infringements

Article 13 Manufacture and import of investigational medicinal products.

Article 14 Labelling

Article 15 Verification of compliance of investigational medicinal products with good clinical and manufacturing practice

▶

▶

Article 16 Notification of adverse events

Article 17 Notification of serious adverse reactions

Article 18 Guidance concerning reports

Article 19 General provisions

Article 20 Adaptation to scientific and technical progress

Article 21 Committee procedure

Article 22 Application

Article 23 Entry into force 4 April 2001

CONCLUSION

The emphasis on practice which is research-based will mean that the midwife will increasingly be required to ensure that her practice is in accordance with clinically effective standards which are based on reputable researched evidence. In addition she will have responsibilities to ensure that the rights of the women she cares for, and who are asked to become research subjects, are respected. Useful databases for midwifery research are MIRIAD[15] and the NHS database known as the National Research Register (NRR).[16]

QUESTIONS AND EXERCISES

1. An obstetrician is researching on pain in childbirth and wants to send a research assistant to accompany you in your work in the community. What questions would you ask about the project and whose responsibility would it be to obtain the consent of the client?

2. You have been told by your manager that a midwifery student has to undertake a research project and you are asked to supervise it. What initial preparations would you make?

3. A client complains that she has just discovered that she has been prescribed a drug which is not generally approved for general use. What action do you take?

References

1 Rees C. Introduction to research for midwives, 2nd edn. Oxford: Books for Midwives Press; 2003.

2 Phillips R. The need for research based midwifery practice. Br J Midwifery 1994; 2(7):335–338.

3 Nursing and Midwifery Council, Code of Professional Conduct: standards for conduct, performance and ethics, 2004.

4 Priestley KA, Campbell C, Valentine CB, et al. Consent forms for research protocols. BMJ 1992; 305:1263–1264. (Reported in MIDIRS Midwifery Digest March 1993; 3:1).

5 Sidaway v. Bethlem Royal Hospital Governors and others 1985 1 All ER 643.

6 Burton v. Islington Health Authority [1992] 3 All ER 833 Court of Appeal.

7 Department of Health. Local Research Ethics Committees. Health Service Circular 1991; (91)5.

8 Department of Health. Governance Arrangements for NHS Research Ethics Committees. London: DoH; 2001; replaces HSG(91)5 (the red book) and HSG(97)23 on multi-centre Research Ethics Committees. Online. Available: www.doh.gov.uk/research/rd1/researchgovernance/corec.htm

9 Department of Health. Research Governance Framework for England, 2nd edn. London: DoH; 2005. Online. Available: www.doh.gov.uk/research/rd3/nhsandd/researchgovernance.htm

10 Department of Health. Improved pathway for health research. Press release 2005/0200. 6 June 2005.

11 Royal Commission on Civil Liability and Compensation for Personal Injury. Chaired by Lord Pearson. Cmnd 7054. London: HMSO; 1978.

12 Salha v. GMC; Abusheika v. GMC [2003] UKPC 80; [2004] ECDR12 PC.

13 Kennedy I, Grubb A. Medical Law, 3rd edn. London: Butterworths; 2000.

14 EC Directive 2001/20/EC. On the implementation of good clinical practice in the conduct of clinical trials on medicinal products for human use.

15 MIRIAD. Online. Available: www.leeds.ac.uk/miru/miriad.htm

16 National Research Register. Online. Available: www.doh.gov.uk/research/nrr.htm

Chapter 32
CHILD PROTECTION

Midwives may become involved in issues relating to child protection. It may be for example that other children of the pregnant woman have to be taken into care, or the midwife might be concerned about the health or safety of the unborn child immediately following delivery. It is essential that the midwife has an understanding of the relevant laws and knows the action which she must take. This has been recently emphasised in a publication by the Chief Nursing Officer.[1] This reviews the nursing, midwifery and health visiting contribution to supporting vulnerable children and young people. In the light of the Green Paper Every Child Matters (see below) it sets a clear strategy for achieving improvements in all services for children and young people. The law relating to consent by a child or young person under 18 years is considered in Chapter 7. Legal issues arising with teenage pregnancies are considered in Chapter 12. More detailed information on child protection and the midwife can be found in a book by Fraser and Nolan[2] and a two-part article by Chapman.[3]

The Children Act 1989 brought into place a new framework for the law relating to children and while not repealing all previous legislation on children, introduced significant new provisions. The main areas covered by the Act are shown in Box 32.1.

Box 32.1 Provisions of the Children Act 1989

1. General principles

2. Orders with respect to children in family proceedings

3. Local authority support for children and families

4. Care and supervision

5. Protection of children

6. Community homes

7. Voluntary homes and voluntary organisations

8. Registered children's homes

▶

9. Private arrangements for fostering children

10. Child minding and day care for young children

11. Secretary of State's supervisory functions and responsibilities

12. Miscellaneous and general.

In this chapter, we shall consider the principles established by the Children Act 1989 and the law relating to child protection. The status of the fetus is considered in Chapter 17. The basic principle is that an unborn child lacks a legal personality and cannot be taken into care, nor made a ward of court.[4]

THE CHILDREN ACT 1989

PART 1: BASIC PRINCIPLES

Part 1 of the Act sets out the basic principles which are to apply in the law relating to children.

They are shown in Box 32.2. Of significance is the fact that the Act places the emphasis upon the duties and responsibilities of the parent rather than the rights of the parent. Even where the child is not living with the parent, this does not remove from the parent his/her responsibilities to the child.

Box 32.2 Principles in the Children Act 1989

1. Welfare of the child:

   i. When a court determines any question in relation to the upbringing of a child or the administration of a child's property and the income from it, the child's welfare shall be the court's paramount consideration.

   ii. In any proceedings relating to the upbringing of the child, the court must have regard to the general principle that any delay in determining the question is likely to prejudice the welfare of the child.

   iii. The court shall have regard in particular to:

      a. the ascertainable wishes and feelings of the child concerned (considered in the light of his age and understanding)

▶

b. his physical, emotional and educational needs

c. the likely effect on him of any change in his circumstances

d. his age, sex, background and any characteristics of his which the court considers relevant

e. any harm which he has suffered or is at risk of suffering

f. how capable each of his parents, and any other person in relation to whom the court considers the question to be relevant, is of meeting his needs

g. the range of powers available to the court under this Act in the proceedings in question.

PARENTAL RESPONSIBILITY FOR CHILDREN

– Where a child's father and mother were married to each other at the time of his birth, they shall each have parental responsibility for the child.

– Where they were not married at the time of his birth, the mother shall have responsibility for the child; the father shall not have parental responsibility for the child unless he acquires it in accordance with the Act.

– Provisions as to how parental responsibility can be acquired are laid down in the Act. (See also Ch. 25 of this book.)

– More than one person may have parental responsibility for the same child at the same time.

– Where more than one person has parental responsibility for a child, each of them may act alone and without the other (or others) in meeting that responsibility.

MEANING OF PARENTAL RESPONSIBILITY

Parental responsibility is defined as:

all rights, duties, powers and responsibilities and authority which by law a parent of a child has in relation to the child and his property.

Parents who fail to take reasonable care for the health and welfare of their children could be guilty of a criminal offence (see below and Ch. 7).

ACQUISITION OF PARENTAL RESPONSIBILITY BY FATHER

The court has the power to provide for the father to have parental responsibility where the couple were not married at the time of the child's birth.

POWERS OF NON-PARENT

The Children Act 1989 gives power to a person who does not have parental responsibility to make decisions on behalf of the child. The Children Act 1989 s.3(5) provides that a person who (a) does not have parental responsibility for a particular child, but (b) has care of the child, may (subject to the provision of this Act) do what is reasonable in all the circumstances of the case for the purpose of safeguarding or promoting the child's welfare. This would probably include giving consent to necessary emergency treatment in the absence of the parents. In addition, professional staff would have a duty of care to take action to save life in such circumstances.

CHILD PROTECTION

Where the midwife has reasonable cause to suspect that a child in the family of a client is being abused she must take the appropriate action. To make a diagnosis of suspected child abuse is a weighty matter. As the 1991 guidelines on inter-agency cooperation (Para. 1.13) stated:[5]

The difficulties of assessing the risk of harm to a child should not be underestimated. It is imperative that everyone who deals with allegations and suspicions of abuse maintains an open and inquiring mind.

Following the Inquiry conducted by Lord Laming into the death of Victoria Climbie[6] the Department of Health published a detailed response, 'Keeping Children Safe'[7] and this was followed by a single source document for safeguarding children.[8] This document aimed to provide a single set of advice for all those involved in the care of children which should replace local guidance. It was followed by a Green Paper, 'Every Child Matters',[9] published in September 2003. The Green Paper focussed on four main areas:

1. Supporting parents and carers

2. Early intervention and effective protection

3. Accountability and integration – locally, regionally and nationally

4. Workforce reform

CHILDREN ACT 2004

Under the Children Act 2004 many of the recommendations of the Green Paper were implemented.

A Children's Commissioner for England (one is already appointed in Wales and another in Scotland) was established with the function of promoting awareness of the views and interests of children. In particular, he is to be concerned with the views and interests of children so far as relating to various aspects of their wellbeing, including:

– Physical and mental health and emotional wellbeing

– Protection from harm and neglect

– Education, training and recreation

– The contribution made by them to society

– Social and economic wellbeing.

The Commissioner can under s.3 conduct an inquiry into a case involving a child if he is satisfied that the case raises issues of public policy, with a view to making recommendations about those issues.

The Children's Commissioners for Scotland and Wales have slightly different functions. Each has a duty to submit an annual report.

Part 2 of the Act is concerned with improving the accountability for children's services within each local authority area. The local authority is required to make arrangements to promote cooperation between the various agencies which are involved in child protection including the police authority, the local probation board, a youth offending team, a strategic health authority and primary care trust and persons providing services under the Learning and Skills Act 2000.

Many specified agencies including primary care trusts, NHS trusts, NHS Foundation Trusts are required to make arrangements together to safeguard and promote the welfare of children. Under s.12 the Secretary of State can by regulations require children's services authorities to establish and operate databases containing information about children at risk.

LOCAL SAFEGUARDING CHILDREN'S BOARD (LSCB)

Each children's services authority must establish a *Local Safeguarding Children's Board (LSCB)* whose membership derives from the agencies specified as partners of the LA in child protection. These LSCBs replace the non-statutory Area Child Protection Committees.

The functions of the LSCB are:

– to coordinate what is done by each person or body represented on the Board for the purpose of safeguarding and promoting the welfare of children in the area of the authority and

– to ensure the effectiveness of what is done by each such person or body for those purposes.

The Secretary of State may prescribe further functions of the LSCB by regulation. In addition regulations can require each children's services authority to prepare and publish a plan setting out the authority's strategy for discharging their functions in relation to children and relevant young persons.

DIRECTOR OF CHILDREN'S SERVICES

Each Children's Services Authority is required to appoint a Director of Children's Services covering both educational and social services functions. In addition a lead member for children's services is to be designated by each children's services authority. This would be a political appointment. Under s.20 joint area reviews of children's services can be carried out by the persons specified in the section. These include the Chief Inspector of Schools, the Commission for Social Care Inspection and the Commission for Healthcare Audit and Inspection (now known as the Healthcare Commission).

Among the many other provisions of the Act, s.58 restricts the grounds on which the battery of a child may be justified as reasonable punishment (see below).

A Minister for Children, Young People and Families has been created in the Department for Education and Skills.

The RCN has published guidance on child protection and the nurse,[10] and emphasises the need of each trust to have a designated or named nurse for child protection, have child protection procedures in place and have a defined policy on raising concerns about colleagues. The establishment of Children's Trusts may assist in improving child protection provisions.

PROCEDURE FOR THE MANAGEMENT OF CHILD ABUSE

There should be in existence an agreed procedure for the management of child abuse cases developed on the lines indicated in the single source document for safeguarding children[8] and the midwife should be acquainted with this. The procedure should specifically refer to the role of the midwifery department if child abuse is suspected. This would require any professional staff working in the department who suspect that there is a possibility of ill-treatment, serious neglect, sexual or emotional abuse of a child, to inform the senior midwife or Consultant in charge of the department who should contact a Consultant paediatrician. If he confirms this possibility, then he should inform the Social Services Department immediately, according to the agreed procedure.

Any midwife must also be alert to the possibility of a colleague causing harm to a patient (see Chs 14 and 19).

What if the doctor disagrees with the midwife?
The midwife should ensure that her concerns are made known to a senior member of the midwifery staff who should decide whether it is appropriate to bring the Consultant in to see the child.

What about the midwife's duty of confidentiality?
Reference to the NMC Code of Professional Conduct: standards for conduct, performance and ethics[11] Clause 5, which covers confidentiality will show that the registration body accepts that there are circumstances when a breach of confidentiality is justified in the public interest. This would include any reasonable suspicion of child abuse. Such information could be passed on to the appropriate agencies without fear of a successful action for breach of confidentiality by the parents (see Ch. 10).

If a suspected case is reported to the police, social services, or NSPCC and it turns out that the suspicions are unfounded, the parents have no right to be given the name of the person reporting them. The House of Lords has held that it is not in the public interest for such information to be disclosed to the parents.[12]

WHAT IF SUSPECTED CHILD ABUSE IS CONFIRMED BY THE CONSULTANT PAEDIATRICIAN?

The agreed arrangements laid down by the LCSB should be followed immediately. The provisions of the Children Act 1989 enable the orders set out in Boxes 32.3, 32.4 and 32.5 to be made.

Box 32.3 Child assessment order (s.43)

This is available where the court is satisfied that the applicant has reasonable cause to suspect that the child is suffering or likely to suffer significant harm. An assessment is required to determine whether or not the child is suffering or is likely to suffer significant harm, and it is unlikely that an assessment can be carried out without an order being made.

Notice must be given of an application for a child assessment order to the child's parents, any person, not the parent, but who has parental responsibility for him, any other person caring for the child and others who have a contact order.

Box 32.4 Emergency protection order (s.44)

If the court is satisfied that there is reasonable cause to believe (in the case of an application by a person) that the child is likely to suffer significant harm if:

a. he is not removed to accommodation provided by or on behalf of the applicant; or

b. he does not remain in the place in which he is then being accommodated;

then the court can order that an emergency protection order be made.

Box 32.5 Removal and accommodation of children by police in cases of emergency

This section enables the child to be taken into police protection. Where a constable believes that a child would be likely to suffer significant harm he may remove the child to suitable accommodation and keep him there. He may also take reasonable steps to ensure that the child's removal from hospital, or other place in which he is being accommodated, is prevented. The section lasts a maximum of 72 hours.

The child assessment order cannot be made if the court is satisfied that there are grounds for making an emergency protection order and that it ought to make that order rather than an assessment order. The order must specify the date by which the assessment is to begin and the period for which it will have effect, such period not exceeding 7 days beginning with the date specified in the order. The effect of the order is that it authorises any person carrying out the assessment, or any part of the assessment, to do so in accordance with the terms of the order (s.43(7)). The child has the right (s.43(8)), if he is of sufficient understanding, to make an informed decision, to refuse to submit to a medical or psychiatric examination or other assessment.

Where the applicant is a local authority it must show that enquiries are being made under s.47(1)(b) (local authority's duty to investigate) and these enquiries are being frustrated by access to the child being unreasonably refused, and the applicant has reasonable cause to believe that access to the child is required as a matter of urgency (s.44(1)(b)). An application may also be made by the NSPCC as an authorised person.

For further details of the sections shown in Boxes 32.3, 32.4 and 32.5 and the other provisions of the Children Act 1989, reference should be made to the Department of Health guides to the Children Act 1989.[13]

UNFOUNDED ALLEGATION OF CHILD ABUSE

In some situations the allegation of child abuse is found to be unjustified and a reason for the child's apparent injuries or disabilities discovered. For example, in one case[14] following a case conference, a baby was taken into care on the basis of medical evidence which suggested that a spiral fracture of her femur was evidence of non-accidental injury. Subsequently, it was discovered that the baby suffered from brittle bone disease and the child was returned to the parents 9 months after the hospital admission. The parents sued and action was also brought in the name of the child arguing a breach of the duty of care owed in the law of negligence, and a breach of Article 8 of the European Convention on Human Rights. The claims failed on the grounds that the child had suffered no injury for which the law recognised a remedy; a duty of care was not owed by the defendants to the parents (the doctor owed a duty of care to the child and his obligations within the multi-disciplinary process militated against the doctor owing any additional duty to the parents in relation to the diagnosis which commenced such a process) and to hold the doctor liable to the parents would cut across the statutory scheme set up for the protection of the child. The Human Rights Act came into force on 2 October 2000, was not retrospective and the cause of action arose in September 1998 and June 1999.

This case, together with other similar cases, was heard by the House of Lords in April 2005 and it was held that healthcare and other child care professionals did not owe a common law duty of care to parents against whom they had made unfounded allegations of child abuse and who, as a result, suffered psychiatric injury.[15]

Lord Nicholls stated that:

the seriousness of child abuse as a social problem demanded that health professionals, acting in good faith in what they believed to be the child's best interests, should not be subject to potentially conflicting duties when deciding whether the child might have been abused, whether their doubts should be communicated to others or what further investigatory or protective steps should be taken.

DUTY OF LOCAL AUTHORITY

Recent cases have held local authorities liable in respect of failures to take action to prevent abuse and in making negligent adoption and fostering arrangements. Thus two people who had been abused as children by their stepfather succeeded in their claim that the local authority had failed to provide an appropriate means of obtaining a determination of their allegations that the local authority had failed to protect them from serious ill-treatment[16] and therefore were in breach of Article 13.

(Article 13 is not included in Schedule 1 of the Human Rights Act 1998 (see appendix) but states that everyone whose rights and freedoms as set forth in this Convention are violated, shall have an effective remedy before a national authority notwithstanding that the violation has been committed by persons acting in an official capacity.)

On the facts of the case there was no breach of Article 3.

In contrast, in another case the European Court of Human Rights recently held that where the local authority failed to protect children from sexual abuse by the stepfather, the local authority was in violation of Article 3 and Article 13 and was held liable to pay damages.[17] In the case of Z. v. UK 1999[18] the Commission found a violation of Articles 3 and 13 arising from the failure of the local authority to take action in respect of serious ill-treatment and neglect caused to four siblings by their parents over a period of more than 4.5 years. In the case of T.P. and K.M. v. the UK,[19] an emergency place of safety, based in large part on video evidence from a child suspected of being abused, was misinterpreted as to the abuser by the local authority and not disclosed to the mother despite her requests. Mother and child complained that the local authority took the child into care on the basis of a careless assumption of fact in violation of Article 8. They also argued violation of Article 6 in that they were denied access by the decision of the domestic courts to sue the local authority and were denied their rights to seek a remedy under Article 13. They succeeded in their claims under Article 3 and 13 but not Article 6.

In another case against a local authority, this time by a couple who adopted a violent child, the couple won their case that they should have been notified by the LA of the boy's serious emotional and behavioural difficulties.[20] The court held that the local authority could be held vicariously liable for negligence by its employees in failing to fulfil their duty of care owed to those who might foreseeably be injured if the duty was carelessly exercised.

PROTECTION OF VULNERABLE ADULTS AND CHILDREN

Various measures have been taken in law to prevent those who are likely to abuse children from having contact with them. The Protection of Children Act 1999, the Sexual Offenders Act 1997 and the Care Standards Act 2000 enable employers to establish if there are grounds for not employing prospective employees.

THE PROTECTION OF CHILDREN ACT 1999

The Protection of Children Act 1999 makes statutory the Department of Health's Consultancy Service Index list and it requires child care organisations to refer the names of individuals considered unsuitable to work with children for inclusion on the list. It also provides rights of appeal against inclusion and requires regulated childcare organisations to check with the list the names of anyone they propose to employ in posts involving regular contact with children and not to employ them if listed. Finally it amends Part V of the Police Act 1997 to allow the Criminal Records Bureau to act as a central access point for criminal records information, List 99[21,22] and the new Department of Health list. In other words, the Criminal Records Bureau will act as a one stop shop in the carrying out of checks.

The effect of the legislation is that organisations such as health trusts who work with children have had a statutory duty from October 2000 to vet prospective employees, paid or unpaid, for work involving contact with children. From October 2000 organisations who have registered with the DoH have been able to check names from their own computers via the internet. In October 2000 there were about 1000 names on the DoH Consultancy Service Index,[23] who had been notified to the DoH because they had been dismissed from childcare posts or who had left such a post in circumstances where the employer considered that a child would be at risk of harm from them.

THE SEXUAL OFFENDERS ACT 1997

The Sexual Offenders Act 1997 was passed in order to ensure that once a sex offender had served his sentence and was about to be released, he would still be subject to some form of supervision to protect persons against the risk of his re-offending. Part 1 of the Act requires the notification of information to the police by persons who have committed certain sexual offences.

SEXUAL OFFENCES (AMENDMENT) ACT 2000

Under this Act, the age at which certain sexual acts (for example homosexual acts in private) are lawful is reduced to 16 years and a new defence is available so that when one party to homosexual activity is below the age of 16 and the other over 16, the younger one does not commit any offence. However, a new offence is introduced for a person 'A' over 18 years to have sexual intercourse with a person or engage in any other sexual activity with another person 'B' if A is in a position of trust in relation to B. 'Position of trust' is defined in s.4 where B is detained in an institution or resident in a home, or cared for in a hospital, residential care home or nursing home, where A is looking after such persons, or A looks after persons under 18 who are receiving full-time education at an educational institution and B is receiving such education.

SEXUAL OFFENCES ACT 2003

This Act follows the White Paper[24] on protecting the public from sex offenders. Part 1 makes new provision about sexual offences, covers non-consensual offences of rape, assault by penetration, sexual assault and causing a person to engage in sexual activity without consent. It is an offence for a person intentionally to penetrate with his penis (s.5) or with any other body part or object (s.6) the vagina, anus or mouth of a child under 13 years. Whether or not the child consented to this penetration is irrelevant. Under s.7 sexual assault of a child under 13 is an offence and under s.8 causing or inciting a child under 13 to engage in sexual activity is an offence. The Act also covers child sex offences and offences involving an abuse of a position of trust towards a child. New offences give protection to persons with a mental disorder. The age of child in the Protection of Children Act 1978 has been amended to 18 and defences are provided for in limited cases where the child is 16 or over and the defendant is the child's partner.

New guidance has been issued by the Department of Health on the Carers and Disabled Children Act 2000 and the Carers (Equal Opportunities) Act 2004 for carers and people with parental responsibility for disabled children.[25]

CARE STANDARDS ACT 2000

Under Part VII of the Care Standards Act statutory provision is made for setting up a list of individuals who are considered unsuitable to work with vulnerable adults. A single list is established for both England and Wales and it will operate in a similar way to the list established under the Protection of Children Act 1999.

TRAINING

It is essential that all midwives should be given the opportunity to be trained in the local child protection procedure and the role and function of the ACPC and its procedures. It is essential that in this emotive area the midwife should feel confident in her knowledge of the policy and procedures which should be followed. The training should also include an understanding of the provisions of the Children Act 1989 and the recommendations of the reports of inquiries into the handling of child abuse cases, such as the Cleveland Report and the Laming Report.

RECORD KEEPING

Whether or not child abuse is confirmed at the time of the visit, the records of the midwife relating to that visit could be extremely significant evidence in the future. If there is a case conference and a court case, the midwife might well be required to give evidence of her meeting with the parent and child and the examination which she carried out. Since this might take place at an uncertain date in the future, she will be extremely reliant upon the comprehensiveness and clarity of her records.

DISPUTES WITH PARENTS

Parents may not always take the best course for their children and the question arises at what stage a midwife would be justified in intervening. For example, in Chapter 29 a case is discussed when the judge ordered an HIV test on a baby, contrary to the wishes of the mother. The situation in relation to triple vaccine gives rise to similar issues (see Ch. 28). Midwives must act in the best interests of the child.

CRIMINAL OFFENCE

In some circumstances the failure of a parent to take approved medical advice for their child can result in criminal proceedings. A Rastafarian couple who had refused on religious grounds to allow their diabetic daughter who was 9 years old to be given insulin were convicted of manslaughter on 28 October 1993 in Nottingham. The father was given a sentence of imprisonment and the mother a suspended sentence.[26] They believed in using homeopathic medicine.[27] This is, of course, an extreme circumstance. In 2001 parents[28] who had fed their baby daughter a fruit-only diet pleaded guilty of cruelty to a child, when she died of a chest infection brought on by malnutrition. A manslaughter charge was left on the file. In 2005 a mother was convicted of feeding her child excessive salt.

APPROVED MEDICAL OPINION

As in the HIV case, in almost all cases where parents have disputed medical recommendations about treatment for their patients, the courts have supported the doctors' views. One significant case where this did not happen was where parents refused to permit a liver transplant to take place on their toddler. The Court of Appeal held that in the very specific circumstances of the case (the parents lived abroad and as health professionals they believed the transplant not to be in the best interests of the child) the transplant would not be ordered against their wishes.[29] In contrast, there are several cases where the courts have ordered blood transfusions to be given to children of Jehovah's Witnesses[30] (see Ch. 7). For recent cases relating to disputes over whether severely disabled children should be allowed to die see Chapter 9.

PARENTAL RIGHTS AND RESPONSIBILITIES

The Children Act 1989 placed the emphasis on parental responsibilities rather than parental rights. Such responsibilities remain after divorce and care orders and will only cease with the death of the parent or the death or adoption of the child or order of the court.

Unmarried fathers and parental responsibility
Where the parents are unmarried, only the mother has parental responsibilities unless the father has taken steps to ensure that he is legally recognised as having

parental responsibilities. From December 2003, it has been possible for the unmarried couple to register the birth of the child together and thereby the unmarried father acquires parental responsibilities.

Corporal punishment

Gradually the room for manoeuvre of decision making of the parents is reducing. A decision of the European Court of Human Rights ruled that it was unlawful for a parent to use corporal punishment on a child[31] (see Ch. 6). A father was given an admonishment after he was found guilty of smacking his child in a dentist's waiting room.[32] It is illegal for corporal punishment to be used by teachers in schools in this country. The extension of s.548 of the Education Act 1996 banning corporal punishment in all schools was challenged by head teachers, teachers and parents at four independent schools on the grounds that it was incompatible with their rights under Schedule 1 Part 1 Article 9 and Schedule 1 Part 2 Article 2 of the European Convention on Human Rights. The House of Lords held that while the beliefs of the appellants in the use of corporal punishment could be respected, Parliament was entitled to decide that the manifestation of these beliefs in practice was not in the best interests of children and the extension of the corporal punishment ban was not therefore incompatible with the ECHR.[33]

In the Children Act 2004 s.58 states:

(1) In relation to any offence specified in subsection (2) below, battery of a child cannot be justified on the ground that it constituted reasonable punishment.

(2) The offences referred to in sub-section (1) are:

   a. an offence under s.18 or 20 of the Offences against the Person Act 1861 (wounding and causing grievous bodily harm)

   b. An offence under s.47 of that Act (assault occasioning actual bodily harm)

   c. An offence under s.1 of the Children and Young Persons Act 1933 (cruelty to persons under 16)

(3) Battery of a child causing actual bodily harm to a child cannot be justified in any civil proceedings on the ground that it constituted reasonable punishment

(4) For the purposes of sub-section (3) 'actual bodily harm' has the same meaning as it has for the purposes of s.47 of the Offences against the Person Act 1861

(5) In s.1 of the Children and Young Persons Act 1933, omit sub-section (7). (Section 1(7) made the right any parent or person having lawful control or charge of a child to administer punishment an exception of the offence of assaulting or wilfully ill treating a child.)

The result of these changes is that a parent who causes actual bodily harm on his or her child cannot defend the action by claiming that it was reasonable chastisement of an unruly child. What is meant by actual bodily harm? The authoritative textbook of Archbold on criminal procedure and evidence[34] states that actual bodily harm has its ordinary meaning and includes any hurt or injury calculated to interfere with the health or comfort of the victim: such hurt or injury need not be permanent, but must be more than merely transient or trifling. It may include a momentary loss of consciousness, where there is injurious impairment to the victim's sensory functions. It is also capable of including psychiatric injury, but it does not include mere emotions, such as fear, distress or panic.

Could the parents have access to the midwife's and other professionals' records?

The provisions of the Data Protection Act 1998 apply to both computerised and manually-held records. Where the patient is a child, an application for access can be made by a person having parental responsibility for the patient. However, access can be permitted if the holder of the record is satisfied either:

a. that the patient has consented (this would not be possible in the case of a very young child), or

b. that the patient is incapable of understanding the nature of the application and the giving of access would be in his best interests.

In addition, partial access must be refused by the holder to any part of the record which in the opinion of the holder of the record, would disclose:

a. information provided by the patient in the expectation that it would not be disclosed to the applicant, or

b. information obtained as a result of any examination or investigation to which the patient consented in the expectation that the information would not be so disclosed (s.5(3)) (see Ch. 10).

CHILDREN, YOUNG PEOPLE AND MATERNITY SERVICES NATIONAL SERVICE FRAMEWORK

In September 2004 the NSF for Children, Young People and Maternity Services was published.[35] It marks the achievement of many working groups considering different aspects of child healthcare. It provides minimum standards for child healthcare across a range of specialities which can be used by health professionals and parents/young people alike but clearly the allocation of resources for its implementation will have a considerable influence on its effectiveness.

CONCLUSIONS

Midwives have a significant role to play in child protection and may become involved in giving evidence. They should take advice from senior management or from lawyers to the trust. Their documentation is likely to come under close scrutiny in any conflict (see Ch. 15). This is a greatly changing field with the implementation of the Children Act 2004, and changing statutory responsibilities. It is hoped that the new strategy of the Chief Nursing Officer will ensure the NMC registered practitioners play a major role in protecting these vulnerable persons. A children's health and maternity services E-bulletin has been set up by the Department of Health to enable healthcare practitioners to have regular updates on activities supporting the Every Child Matters: Change for Children agenda.[36]

QUESTIONS AND EXERCISES

1. A 15-year-old is expecting a child and an internal examination is necessary. The client is considered too young to give a valid consent. Could consent be given by an aunt who is accompanying her?

2. There is concern about the possibility of a client abusing her 2-year-old child, and about the future safety of the unborn child. What action should the midwife take?

3. A 13-year-old girl who is expecting a baby is considered to be in need of care; what should the midwife do?

References

1 Chief Nursing Officer. Department of Health Review of the nursing, midwifery and health visiting contribution to vulnerable children and young people. London: DoH; 2004.

2 Fraser J, Nolan M. Child protection: a guide for midwives. Oxford: Elsevier; 2004.

3 Chapman T. Safeguarding the welfare of children, Parts 1 and 2. Br J Midwifery 2002; 10(9):569–572; 2003; 11(2):116–119.

4 Re F (in utero) [1988] 2 All ER 193.

5 Home Office, Department of Health, Department of Education and Science, Welsh Office. Working Together Under the Children Act 1989: a guide to arrangements for inter-agency co-operation for the protection of children from abuse. London: HMSO; 1991.

6 Inquiry. Online. Available: http://www.victoria-climbie-inquiry.org.uk

7 Department of Health. Keeping children safe. London: Stationery Office; 2003.

8 Department of Health. What to do if you're worried a child is being abused. DoH; 2003. Online. Available: www.doh.gov.uk/safeguardingchildren/index.htm

9 Department of Health. Every child matters. Green Paper, September 2003.

10 Royal College of Nursing Child Protection: every nurse's responsibility 002 045 June 2003. Online. Available: www.rcn.org.uk

11 Nursing and Midwifery Council. Code of Professional Conduct: standards for conduct, performance and ethics. NMC; 2004.

12 D v. NSPCC [1977] 1 All ER 589.

13 Department of Health. An introductory guide to the Children Act for the NHS. London: HMSO; 1990.

14 RK and MK v. Oldham NHS Trust Lloyd's Rep Med 1[2003] 1.

15 D. v. East Berkshire Community Health NHS Trust and Another; MAK and Another v. Dewsbury Healthcare NHS Trust and Another; RK and Another v. Oldham NHS Trust and Another. The Times Law Report, 22 April 2005 HL.

16 D.P. and J.C. v United Kingdom (Application No 38719/97). The Times Law Report, 23 October 2002, European Court of Human Rights.

17 E and others v. United Kingdom (Application No 33218/96). The Times Law Report, 4 December 2002, ECHR.

18 Z. v. UK (1999) 28 EHRR CD 65.

19 T.P and K.M. v. the UK No 28945/95 10.9.99.

20 A and Another v. Essex County Council. Times Law Report, 24 January 2003.

21 List 99. A list held by the Department for Education and Employment of those considered unsuitable to work with children. It has always been a statutory list.

22 Department of Health. An introductory guide to the Children Act for the NHS. London: HMSO; 1990.

23 Department of Health. Press Notice, 2 October 2000.

24 White Paper. Protecting the Public: strengthening protection against sex offenders and reforming the law on sexual offences CM 5668. Home Office; November 2002.

25 Department of Health Carers and Disabled Children Act 2000 and the Carers (Equal Opportunities) Act 2004 for carers and people with parental responsibility for disabled children. Combined Draft Policy Guidance, January 2005.

26 News item. The Times, 29 October 1993.

27 News item. The Times, 6 November 1993.

28 Gregoriadis L, Peek L. Baby starved to death on fruit diet. The Times, 14 July 2001.

29 Re C (a minor) (medical treatment – refusal of parental consent) [1997] 8 Med LR 166 CA.

30 For example Re E (a minor) (wardship: medical treatment) Family Division [1993] 1 FLR 386.

31 A v. The United Kingdom (100/1997/884/1096) judgement on 23 September 1998.

32 Cramb A. Father who smacked his daughter goes free. The Daily Telegraph, 10 June 1999.

33 R (On the application of Williamson) v. Secretary of State for Education and Employment: sub nom Williamson v Secretary of State for Education and Employment [2005] UKHL 15; [2005] 2 WLR 590.

34 Archbold (this issue edited by Richardson PJ). Criminal pleading, evidence and sentencing. London: Sweet and Maxwell; 2005.

35 Department of Health. Online. Available: www.doh.gov.uk/nsf/children

36 Department of Health. E-bulletin; MB-Childrens-NSF@dh.gsi.gov.uk

Chapter 33

MENTAL DISORDER AND MENTAL INCAPACITY

Suicide is the leading cause of maternal death[1] in the UK and there are clear implications for the role of the midwife and her records and information sharing.[2] The midwife may encounter women who suffer from mental disorder and/or those who lack mental capacity to make specific decisions. Because of the dangers of postnatal depression and puerperal fever to the mother and child it is essential that the midwife has a good understanding of the help which is to hand, the legal powers which exist if intervention is necessary and what action she should take. It is not the intention here to provide the midwife with a comprehensive account of the law relating to mental disorder and to those who lack mental capacity, but rather to raise her awareness of the issue and to enable her to know how to seek further information.

MENTALLY INCAPACITATED ADULTS

Since 1990 proposals for providing statutory provision for decisions on behalf of mentally incapacitated adults have been discussed. The Law Commission published a series of consultation documents on various aspects of the protection of those adults who are unable to make decisions themselves. This culminated in a report in 1995 containing draft legislation for Mental Incapacity.[3] No action was taken after its publication but in 1997, the Lord Chancellor issued another consultation document.[4] This was followed by a White Paper in 1999.[5] Subsequently draft legislation[6] was published which was examined by a joint committee of Parliament which published its recommendations.[7] The Mental Capacity Act 2005 is due to be brought into force in 2007 and as a consequence some of the principles of law which were recognised at common law will have statutory force. These principles are set out in Chapter 7. At the same time the Department of Health is consulting on how the gap (known as the 'Bournewood gap') in statutory protection, for those admitted to psychiatric hospital and who lack mental capacity, can be filled[8] (see Ch 7).

Where a midwife is aware that one of her clients suffers from learning disabilities, she would need to determine the capacity of the woman to make decisions, bringing if necessary expert assistance to determine capacity. The principles set out by the Court of Appeal in the case of Re MB[9] and discussed in Chapter 7 (Box 7.9) should be followed. The vast majority of those with learning disabilities are unlikely to come within the definition of mental disorder for the purposes of the Mental Health Act

639

1983 and are therefore unlikely to be compulsorily admitted to hospital for treatment. When the Mental Capacity Act 2005 comes into force, the Court of Protection will have an expanded role to take on decisions in relation to care and treatment, and can appoint deputies with specified powers to act on behalf of a person who lacks the requisite capacity. In addition individuals can appoint persons to have lasting powers of attorney under which they can make decisions on his or her behalf. A new office of Public Guardian will be created to establish and maintain a register of lasting powers of attorney and of orders appointing deputies and supervising deputies as set out in s.58 of the 2005 Act.

In addition under the Sexual Offences Act 2003 (see Chs 32 and 12) new offences are created in relation to sexual activity with persons with a mental disorder impeding choice, causing a person with a mental disorder to engage in sexual activity and with care workers inciting persons with a mental disorder to have sexual activity. These provisions are designed to provide more protection for vulnerable persons.

MENTALLY DISORDERED: AN INTRODUCTION

At present the law relating to compulsory admission of mentally disordered patients is laid down in the Mental Health Act 1983. There have however been an expert report (in 1998), White Papers, draft bills considering the reform of the Mental Health legislation. The main point of controversy is whether it is lawful to lock up those who present a severe risk to public safety, even though they have committed no crimes. At the time of writing a revised Bill has been drafted and is being subjected to pre-legislative scrutiny by a Committee of the Houses of Parliament. Legislation is at present awaited and is unlikely to be in force before April 2007.

The philosophy behind the Mental Health Act 1983 is that where possible, patients suffering from mental disorder should be treated without admission to psychiatric hospitals. If admission is required then it should be on the basis of informal admission. Only where there is no alternative to detention should the powers of compulsory admission in the Act be used.

Most patients would therefore be cared for in the community with assistance from the community psychiatric nurse, with overall responsibility taken by the General Practitioner assisted by out-patient referrals to a Consultant psychiatrist. Mothers may require specialist help and advice if they are taking anti-psychotic or anti-depressant medication when they become pregnant. The midwife should ensure that she is aware of any possible contraindications for medication at all times during and after the pregnancy. If admission to hospital becomes necessary, most patients would agree to informal (i.e. voluntary) admission. The midwife should discuss with the patient and the hospital staff the antenatal care required by the mother and the arrangements to be made when labour commences, trying to ensure that the mother's wishes are obtained and respected.

Unfortunately, one of the characteristics of some forms of mental disorder is an absence of insight and therefore it is necessary in certain exceptional circumstances to arrange for the admission of a person compulsorily to hospital for in-patient treatment. This may be necessary following confinement if it is suspected that the mother is suffering from puerperal disorder or severe postnatal depression. Most districts now have a mother and baby unit and the midwife should ensure that she is aware of the location of these, since it may be that, with assurance, the mother might be prepared to accept informal admission to such a unit if she knows that she can take the baby with her. If the midwife is aware that no such provision has been made, she could take up the issue with her supervisor and the NHS trust or strategic health authority. It may be possible for admission to such a unit to be provided on the basis of an out of the catchment area referral. A national audit has been carried out of joint mother and baby admissions to UK psychiatric hospitals since 1996.[10] The value of the midwife contributing to a multi-disciplinary service for the mental health needs of women is clear.

DEFINITION OF MENTAL DISORDER

No person can be compulsorily detained under the Mental Health Act 1983 unless she is suffering from mental disorder as defined in the Act. The definition is set out in Box 33.1.

Box 33.1 Definition of mental disorder

Mental illness, arrested or incomplete development of mind, psychopathic disorder and any other disorder or disability of mind.

All the terms except 'mental illness' are further defined in the Act.

Mental impairment means:

A state of arrested or incomplete development of mind (not amounting to severe mental impairment) which includes significant impairment of intelligence and social functioning and is associated with abnormally aggressive or seriously irresponsible conduct on the part of the person concerned.

The Act makes if clear that a person cannot be dealt with under the Act as suffering from mental disorder 'by reason only of promiscuity or other immoral conduct, sexual deviancy or dependence on alcohol or drugs'. This means that if a woman is pregnant and abusing drugs she cannot be detained under the Mental Health Act 1983 unless she is shown to be suffering from mental disorder apart from the drug abuse.

COMPULSORY ADMISSION

There are three main sections for the compulsory admission of the mentally dis-ordered person (other than through the courts). These are shown in Box 33.2.

Box 33.2 Compulsory admission for mental disorder

Section 4 emergency admission for assessment for up to 72 hours

Section 2 admission for assessment for up to 28 days

Section 3 admission for treatment for up to 6 months.

Section 4

This is an emergency admission section and enables a person to be detained for up to 72 hours on the basis of one medical recommendation. It must be established that it is of urgent necessity for the admission for assessment and that compliance with the provisions for two medical recommendations would involve undesirable delay. The patient can be detained under s.4 for up to 72 hours. The requirements for ss.2 and 4 are shown in Box 33.3.

Box 33.3 Medical requirements for ss.2 and 4

a. The patient is suffering from mental disorder of a nature or degree which war-rants the detention of the patient in a hospital for assessment (or for assessment followed by medical treatment) for at least a limited period; and

b. he ought to be so detained in the interests of his own health or safety or with a view to the protection of other persons.

The applicant is usually an approved social worker, though, as with the other two Sections, it could be the 'nearest relative'. The approved social worker is 'approved' because she/he has undergone a special training in mental health. In applying for a s.4 admission the approved social worker has to explain why a second medical recommendation for admission could not be obtained. The application is made to the managers of the appropriate hospital and the application gives authority to ambulance men or police to transfer the patient to the hospital.

Section 2

This is an application for assessment and under this the person can be detained for up to 28 days. There must be two medical recommendations, one of them from a doctor who is recognised as having the required expertise in psychiatric medicine, i.e. he is approved under s.12 of the Act and is colloquially called a 'Section 12 doctor'. One of the two doctors should have had previous acquaintance with the patient and if this is not possible the approved social worker must explain the reasons why on the application form. The medical requirements shown in Box 33.3 must be present.

Section 3

This is an admission for treatment and can last up to six months. Two medical recommendations are required but unlike s.2, a specific form of mental disorder must be specified (see Box 33.4). The other requirements shown in Box 33.4 must be present. Again one of the medical recommendations must be by a s.12 approved doctor and preferably at least one of the doctors should have had previous acquaintance with the patient. The nearest relative should be consulted over the application by the approved social worker and has the right to object to the application being made.

Box 33.4 Medical requirements for s.3 admission

a. He is suffering from mental illness, severe mental impairment, psychopathic disorder or mental impairment and his mental disorder is of a nature or degree which makes it appropriate for him to receive medical treatment in a hospital; and

b. in the case of psychopathic disorder or mental impairment, such treatment is likely to alleviate or prevent a deterioration of his condition; and

c. it is necessary for the health or safety of the patient or for the protection of other persons that he should receive such treatment and it cannot be provided unless he is detained under this section.

Definition of nearest relative

The relative who is 'nearest' is defined by statute (s.26 of the Mental Health Act 1983). Where the patient is married it would be the spouse. A co-habitee would count as the nearest relative where the couple had been living together for a period of not less than 6 months. A person other than a relative could be classified as a relative if he/she had been ordinarily living with the patient for at least 5 years.

TREATMENT FOR MENTAL DISORDER

Compulsory treatment for mental disorder can be given under the Act to the patient detained under either s.2 or s.3, but not to the patient who is detained under s.4. This is so even though s.2 is described as admission for assessment.

Box 33.5 shows the treatments which can be given and the conditions required.

Box 33.5 Treatment for mental disorder

Section 57 Surgery destroying brain tissue, hormonal implants to control sexual urge. The patient must consent and the understanding of the patient to consent should be certified by three persons appointed by the Mental Health Act Commission, one of whom must be a registered medical practitioner. The latter must certify that the treatment should be given.

Section 58 Medication after 3 months and electroconvulsive therapy. The patient must either consent or a second opinion must be obtained from an independent doctor appointed by the Mental Health Act Commission.

Section 63 Any treatment not covered by ss.57 and 58 which is given for mental disorder under the direction of the responsible medical officer.

Section 62 Enables the provisions of the above Sections to be dispensed with in an emergency situation.

It should be noted that if medication is required after 3 months and the mother is either unable or unwilling to give consent, a second opinion doctor must be called in to decide if the treatment should be given. He has a duty to examine the patient, determine whether the patient is incapable of giving consent or is refusing consent, talk to the responsible medical officer about the proposed treatment, and decide whether the treatment should be given against the patient's will. Before he decides he must consult with two persons: one a nurse who is professionally concerned with the treatment of the patient, the other who is neither doctor nor nurse who is also professionally concerned with the patient. This latter person could be a midwife if she is sufficiently involved with the patient. The second opinion advisory doctor (SOAD) merely has to record on the statutory form (Form 39) the names of the nurse and the other professional whom he has consulted. He does not have to record what their advice was. If the midwife were to be the second professional to be consulted it would be advisable for her to ensure that she records in her patient records the content of her advice to the SOAD.

The midwife must of course take particular precautions to ensure that any treatment being given for mental disorder will not be harmful to the pregnancy or breastfeeding.

In one case[11] (which is discussed in Ch. 7) the judge decided that the woman, who was suffering from paranoid schizophrenia, was detained in a psychiatric hospital under s.3 and was refusing to have a caesarean operation, could be given a caesarean operation under s.63 of the Mental Health Act 1983 as being treatment for mental disorder. This decision is highly disputed and since the decision in Re MB[12] and in the case of St George's Hospital,[13] is unlikely to be followed (see Ch. 7).

AFTERCARE SERVICES S.117 MENTAL HEALTH ACT 1983

It is a statutory duty for the health service and local authorities, in conjunction with the voluntary sector, to provide aftercare services for patients who have been detained under specific sections including s.3 and s.37, and are discharged from hospital. Charges cannot be made for these services.

THE MENTAL HEALTH (PATIENTS IN THE COMMUNITY) ACT 1995

The Mental Health (Patients in the Community) Act 1995 saw the introduction of aftercare under supervision, or supervised discharge as it has become known.[14] The power to place patients under aftercare under supervision applies only to patients who are detained under ss.3, 37 or 47 and 48. It must be applied for while the patient is still under section.

The grounds for aftercare under supervision are that:

1. the patient is suffering from a specified form of mental disorder, i.e. mental illness, severe mental impairment, psychopathic disorder, or mental impairment;
2. there would be a substantial risk of serious harm to:
    (a) the health of the patient; or
    (b) the safety of the patient; or
    (c) the safety of other persons; or
    (d) of the patient being seriously exploited if he were not to receive the aftercare services to be provided for him under s.117 after he leaves hospital; and
3. his being so subject to aftercare under supervision is likely to help secure that he receives the aftercare services to be so provided.

The application is made by the responsible medical officer who must consult with the following:

1. the patient;
2. one or more persons who have been professionally concerned with the patient's medical treatment in hospital;
3. one or more persons who will be professionally concerned with the aftercare services to be provided for the patient under s.117;

4. any person who, the RMO believes, will play a substantial part in the care of the patient after he leaves hospital, but will not be professionally concerned with any of the aftercare services to be so provided;

5. the person appearing to be the nearest relative.

Aftercare under supervision lasts for 6 months, but can be renewed if the specified conditions are present. The patient has the right of appeal to a Mental Health Review Tribunal against the imposition of aftercare under supervision. The purpose of the supervision is to ensure that the patient obtains the aftercare services specified under s.117. Specific requirements can be laid down with which the patient must comply. However, failure to comply does not lead to automatic readmission to psychiatric hospital, but would lead to a review by the multi-disciplinary team over the appropriate action to be taken. A person is nominated as the supervisor of the patient, who together with the named community psychiatrist would be responsible for monitoring the care and compliance of the patient.

COMMON LAW POWERS

If life-saving treatment is required for the patient who is admitted under s.4 then it could be given under the powers which exist at common law under the Re F ruling, until the provisions of the Mental Capacity Act 2005 come into force. (For further discussion on this, see Ch. 7.)

Again, any treatment must take into account the pregnancy or if the mother is feeding the baby.

THE INFORMAL IN-PATIENT

If the mother is already in hospital as an informal patient and wishes to take her own discharge and it would be dangerous to her health or safety or to other people for her to do so, she could be detained under the provisions of the Mental Health Act 1983. (See Boxes 33.6 and 33.7.)

Box 33.6 Holding power of the nurse (s.5(4))

This enables a nurse qualified in mental disorder to prevent an informal patient who is being treated for mental disorder from leaving the hospital. The detention can exist for up to 6 hours but it will end as soon as the patient's own doctor (or his nominee) arrives to see the patient. He may then, following an examination of the patient, decide to detain the patient further.

Box 33.7 Power of doctor to detain an in-patient (s.5(2))

This enables the patient's doctor or his nominee to detain the patient for up to 72 hours to enable an application to be considered for admission under the Mental Health Act 1983. It may be that after the doctor has examined the patient it is decided that compulsory admission is not necessary and the section will then end and the patient will become informal. Alternatively, following examination by the patient's own doctor and by another doctor and the approved social worker an application is made under s.2 or s.3. For s.5(2) to be used the in-patient need not have been admitted for the treatment of mental disorder. Section 5(2) could therefore be used on non-psychiatric wards.

RENEWAL

Sections 4, 2, 5(4) and 5(2) are not renewable. A patient on s.2 who needs to be detained for longer can be further detained on s.3. Section 3 can be renewed for a further 6 months and then for 1 year at a time. The procedure for the renewal is that the responsible medical officer in charge of the patient's care examines the patient, within the period of 2 months ending with the date the section is due to end and, if it appears to him that the specific condition of mental disorder is present and the other conditions required by s.20 are present, he must furnish to the managers a report to that effect and the patient's detention is then renewed. The managers in their review can decide that the patient should be discharged.

APPEALS AGAINST DETENTION

The patient can appeal to a Mental Health Review Tribunal (MHRT) for discharge or to the managers of the hospital. There are set times for applying to the MHRT but not to the managers. The nearest relative also has the right to apply to an MHRT if his/her attempt to discharge the patient under s.23 has been barred by the responsible medical officer under s.25. Either patient or nearest relative can apply to the MHRT if the specific form of mental disorder is reclassified under s.16.

Where a patient has not himself applied for a Mental Health Review Tribunal hearing during the first 6 months and after that at least once every 3 years, the managers of the hospital have a duty to refer the patient to the MHRT. (In the case of those under 16 years, the time limit is every year.)

It may be that, if the midwife has remained in close contact with the patient during a period of detention, a report and/or oral evidence might be required from the midwife at the hearing giving her views upon the discharge. Article 5 of the European Convention on Human Rights recognises that:

Everyone has the right to liberty and security of person. No one shall be deprived of his liberty save in the following cases and in accordance with a procedure prescribed by law. One of the cases listed is:

(e) the lawful detention of persons for the prevention of the spreading of infectious diseases, of persons of unsound mind, alcoholics or drug addicts or vagrants

This exception covers those suffering from mental disorder providing they are detained in accordance with a procedure established by law. There have been several successful appeals to the European Court of Human Rights by patients detained under the Mental Health Act 1983 because their human rights have not been respected. In the case of Osman v. United Kingdom[15] the European Court of Human Rights held that Article 2 placed upon authorities a positive duty to prevent suicide attempts through risk assessments and appropriate polices and staffing levels. Placing a detained patient under seclusion was challenged by judicial review as being contrary to Article 3 of the European Convention on Human Rights, i.e. 'inhuman and degrading treatment or punishment'.[16] The High Court held that seclusion is capable of infringing a patient's rights under Article 3; it did not *per se* amount to a breach of those rights. There are many cases where patients have alleged that waiting too long for a hearing before a Mental Health Review Tribunal is a breach of their human rights.[17]

INFORMATION TO THE PATIENT

One of the duties on the managers introduced by the 1983 Act is to ensure that the patient receives both in writing and orally information relating to her Section, the right to apply to the managers and the Mental Health Review Tribunal, and the rules relating to consent to treatment. This duty is usually delegated by the managers to the nursing staff or the medical records staff. Leaflets are available giving the information for each of the different Sections and these are available in a wide variety of languages. A midwife who has a client detained in hospital should ask to see the leaflet so that she herself understands the implications of the Section the patient is under.

Information to the nearest relative

The information which is given to the patient must also be given in writing to the nearest relative. However, the patient has a statutory right to object to this information being given to the nearest relative.

The managers

In respect of an NHS trust these are the non-executive board members and only they, with their co-opted members, can carry out the function of hearing appeals to the managers by the patient against detention or renewing the patient's detention following a report from the responsible medical officer. Other functions in respect of the Mental Health Act can be delegated to officers.

THE MENTAL HEALTH ACT COMMISSION

In 1983 a watchdog for detained patients was established, known as the Mental Health Act Commission. It consists of about 90 different professionals and lay people whose jurisdiction is to visit the detained patients and to take up any complaints from them where they are not satisfied by the response from the managers, or any other complaint relating to the exercise of powers and duties under the Mental Health Act. It also has statutory duties in relation to the withholding of mail in the special hospitals (i.e. Broadmoor, Rampton and Ashworth). It also has a duty every other year to provide a report to the Secretary of State which he must place before each House of Parliament. Plans are being considered at present to abolish the Mental Health Act Commission and transfer its functions to the Healthcare Commission (Commission for Healthcare Audit and Inspection).

CODE OF PRACTICE

The Secretary of State has a duty to prepare and revise as appropriate a Code of Practice. Midwives who are involved in the care of mothers with a mental disorder would find this a useful tool of reference.

Caesareans and mental disorder

There have been examples where pregnant women being treated for mental disorder under the Mental Health Act 1983 have been compelled to undergo a caesarean section. These are considered in Chapter 7, where the guidance from the Court of Appeal is discussed.

Protection of vulnerable adults

Legislation establishing lists of those who are a potential danger to children and vulnerable adults, and statutory requirements to consult these lists, are considered in Chapter 32. Midwives caring for women with learning disabilities have a responsibility as part of their duty of care to take into account their level of capacity to make decisions and should ensure that their standards of information giving and communication with the women take into account the disabilities. In November 2001 an Oxford midwife who shouted at a mother and her partner (both of whom had a learning disability), and told them that their newborn twins would be taken away from them by social services, was removed from the Register following a hearing before the UKCC Professional Conduct Committee.[18]

FUTURE CHANGES

Major changes to our present mental health law are currently being proposed. An expert committee was set up by the government in 1998 under the chairmanship of Professor Richardson to review the Mental Health Act 1983. Its terms of reference included the degree to which the current legislation needs updating, and to ensure that there is a proper balance between safety (both of individuals and the wider community) and the rights of individual patients. It was required to advise the government on how mental health legislation should be shaped to reflect contemporary patterns of care and treatment and to support its policy as set out in Modernising Health Services.[19] The Expert Committee presented its preliminary proposals, which set out the principles on which any future legislation should be based, in April 1999, and its full report was published in November 1999.[20] The government presented its proposals for reform in 1999, with a final date for response by 31 March 2000.[21] The proposals include the reasons for proposed changes and cover the following topics:

– Guiding principles for a new mental health act

– Processes of applying compulsory powers

– Criteria for compulsory care and treatment

– The new tribunal's remit

– Discharge and aftercare

– Interface with the criminal justice system

– Treatment

– Safeguards.

At the time of writing, a new draft bill has been published and is being subjected to pre-legislative scrutiny.

NATIONAL SERVICE FRAMEWORKS

The government has published National Service Frameworks for different specialties to ensure that there is a minimum standard of provision across the country. The National Service Frameworks for Mental Health were published in 1999 and set standards in five areas:

– Standard one: Mental health promotion

– Standards two and three: Primary care and access to services

– Standards four and five: Effective services for people with severe mental illness

– Standard six: Caring about carers

– Standard seven: Preventing suicide.

The implementation of these standards is overseen by the Healthcare Commission (Commission for Healthcare Audit and Inspection which replaced the Commission for Health Improvement).

CONCLUSION

Major changes are to take place in the care of the mentally disordered. It is essential that the rights of the mentally disordered pregnant woman are safeguarded and appropriate provision made for the care of the mother and baby. Midwives have an important role to play in ensuring that high standards are set and implemented and in order to secure this a good understanding of the mental health laws is essential. They also need to ensure that the rights of the mentally ill pregnant woman are protected, particularly in relation to the law of consent and compulsory caesareans. This is considered in Chapter 7, which also looks at the law relating to mental capacity). There is evidence that at present midwives often neglect the needs of women with mental illness[22] and developments in Northern Ireland[23] to provide an awareness of maternal mental illness and service provision may be relevant to the work of many midwives in the UK.

QUESTIONS AND EXERCISES

1. You are concerned that a patient of yours who is extremely depressed and is 36 weeks pregnant might be in need of assistance. You have discussed this with her but she refuses to see her General Practitioner or seek other help. What action do you take?

2. You visit a mother who gave birth two days ago, and she seems very disturbed and irrational. You are worried about her mental health. She has made it clear that she would refuse to see her General Practitioner and would not be prepared to consider informal admission for treatment. What action do you take and what is your legal liability?

References

1 Cantwell R, Cox JL. Psychiatric disorders in pregnancy and the puerperium. Curr Obstet Gynaecol 2003; 13(1):7–13.
2 Robinson J. The perils of psychiatric records. Br J Midwifery 2002; 10(3):173.
3 Law Commission. Mental Incapacity Report No 231. London: HMSO; 1995.
4 Lord Chancellor. Who Decides? Decision making on behalf of mentally incapacitated adults. London: HMSO; 1997.
5 Lord Chancellor. Making decisions on behalf of mentally incapacitated adults. London: HMSO; 1999.
6 Department of Health. Draft Mental Incapacity Bill CM 5859, June 2003. Online. Available: http://www.parliament.uk/parliamentary_committees/jcmib.cfmw
7 House of Lords and House of Commons Joint Committee on the Draft Mental Incapacity Bill Session 2002–2003 HL paper 189-1; HC 1083-1.
8 Department of Health. Bournewood Consultation: The approach to be taken in response to the judgement of the European Court of Human Rights in the "Bournewood" case. DoH, March 2005.
9 Re MB (an adult: medical treatment) [1997] 2 FLR 426.
10 Salmon MP, Abel K, Webb R. et al. A national audit of joint mother and baby admissions to UK psychiatric hospitals: an overview of findings. Arch Women's Mental Health 2004; 7(1):65–70.

11 Tameside and Glossop Acute Services Trust v. CH [1996] 31 BMLR 93.

12 Re MB (an adult: medical treatment) [1997] 2 FLR 426.

13 St George's Healthcare NHS Trust v. S; R. v. Collins *ex parte* S [1998]; 44 BMLR 160 CA.

14 Dimond B. The Mental Health (Patients in the Community) Act 1995. Dinton, Wilts: Quay Books Mark Allan Press; 1996.

15 Osman v. United Kingdom [2000] 29 EHRR 245.

16 S v. Airedale National Health Service Trust. The Times Law Report, 25 July 2003; Lloyd's Rep Med [2003] 21.

17 Jones R. Mental Health Act Manual, 8th edn. London: Sweet and Maxwell; 2003.

18 NMC news item. UKCC news 2001.

19 Department of Health. Modernising Mental Health Services. London: HMSO; 1998.

20 Department of Health. Expert Committee Review of the Mental Health Act 1983. London: HMSO; 1999.

21 Department of Health. Reform of the Mental Health Act 1983. London: HMSO; 1999.

22 Hamilton S. Mind . . . the gap! Maternal mental illness. In: Wickham S, ed. Midwifery: best practice 2. Edinburgh: Books for Midwives; 2004:92–94.

23 Murray K, Hamilton S. Perinatal mental health: A Northern Ireland experience. MIDIRS Midwifery Digest 2005; 15(1):121–124.

Chapter 34
COMPLEMENTARY THERAPIES

The popularity of complementary and alternative therapies has increased dramatically over recent years both within and outside the NHS. Midwives are increasingly likely to be caring for women who are interested in using in place of, or in addition to, orthodox treatments a wide variety of complementary and alternative therapies. This chapter briefly sets out the law relating to complementary therapy practice in relation to midwifery practice and considers the following topics:

– Definition of complementary therapies

– Clients who are involved in a complementary therapy:

   - disclosure to the midwife

   - ignorance on the part of the midwife

– The midwife as complementary therapist

   - agreement of employer

   - consent of the woman

   - defining standards

– Use of complementary therapies in midwifery

– National developments.

More detailed analysis of the law for the practitioner in a complementary therapy and the legal implications of many different therapies are to be found in Dimond (1998).[1] The RCM has also issued a position paper on complementary therapies and the midwife.[2]

Midwives are affected by the increase in the popularity of complementary therapies in two ways:

– Some are undertaking training in a therapy regarded as complementary to conventional medicine.

– Others are aware that the mothers they care for are consulting practitioners in complementary medicine therapies and may be taking homeopathic or herbal remedies or other treatment at the same time as receiving orthodox treatments.

DEFINITION OF COMPLEMENTARY THERAPIES

'Complementary' is defined as: completing: together making up a whole ... of medical treatment, therapies, etc ... (Pamphlet of the British Complementary Medicine Association, BCMA).[3] It is thus seen to work in parallel with orthodox medicine. The BCMA therefore states that therapy groups which are represented by the BCMA advise and encourage patients to see their doctor wherever appropriate. The House of Lords Select Committee on Science and Technology held an inquiry into complementary medicine. It reported[4] in November 2000 and recommended that there should be regulation of complementary and alternative medicines and there should be further research to evaluate their effectiveness. It divided such therapies into three groups:

a. Professionally organised therapies, where there is some scientific evidence of their success, though seldom of the highest quality, and there are recognised systems for treatment and training of practitioners. This group includes acupuncture, chiropractic, herbal medicine, homeopathy and osteopathy.

b. Complementary medicines where evidence that they work is generally lacking but which are used as an adjunct rather than a replacement for conventional therapies, so that lack of evidence may not matter so much. Included in this group are Alexander Technique, aromatherapy, nutritional medicine, hypnotherapy and Bach and other flower remedies.

c. Techniques that offer diagnosis as well as treatment, but for which scientific evidence is almost completely lacking. This group cannot be supported and includes naturopathy, crystal therapy, kinesiology, radionics, dowsing and iridology.

The Select Committee of the House of Lords considered that some remedies such as acupuncture and aromatherapy should be available on the NHS, and NHS patients should have wider access to osteopathy and chiropractics. The implementation of these recommendations will lead to fundamental changes in how complementary and alternative therapies are viewed in relation to orthodox medicine and within the NHS.

THE CLIENT IN COMPLEMENTARY THERAPY

DISCLOSURE TO THE MIDWIFE

When a woman is referred to a midwife in the NHS, then information relating to that person's care within the NHS would also be given. Thus the midwife should have basic information about the client in order to determine the care which is required by the woman. In addition, the midwife would usually have access to health records kept on the woman, to ensure that her care is compatible with other treatment that she is receiving.

In contrast, where the woman is receiving treatment from a complementary thera-pist, there is usually no official way in which this information can be made known to the midwife other than through the woman. The midwife therefore relies upon the openness of the woman in disclosing information which may be relevant to the care and treatment provided during the pregnancy.

Clearly, the importance of this communication between woman and midwife will depend upon the relevance of the complementary therapy to the pregnancy. Some therapies may have little effect; others, such as acupuncture and homeopathy, may have a significant effect on the recommendations the midwife may make. If there is a conflict between the two treatments, then the midwife and therapists need to discuss this with the woman, who should be given the choice over which course to pursue.

IGNORANCE ON THE PART OF THE MIDWIFE

Does it matter if the midwife has no knowledge of the complementary therapy which the patient is undergoing? The answer is that it may have an important effect, and had the midwife been aware of certain information about the therapy she might have advised the woman differently. Where harm has occurred, expert evidence on causation would be required to show whether anything the midwife had done could have caused that harm. It is hoped that in reviewing the practice of the midwife, it would be revealed that the woman had been receiving treatment from other persons. In the light of this, any liability on the part of each of these persons could be analysed. Reasonable practice would require that once a midwife ascertains that the woman is receiving alternative or complementary therapies, then the midwife should make all reasonable inquiries (e.g. from the complementary therapist or from others who could reasonably be expected to point out any contraindications) so that the woman and baby are reasonably safe.

THE MIDWIFE AS COMPLEMENTARY MEDICINE THERAPIST

AGREEMENT OF EMPLOYER

It is recognised that many midwives are considering the use of complementary therapies in the care of mothers and babies. If a midwife obtains a training in a complementary therapy, she should ensure that she obtains the agreement of the employer before she uses this skill as part of her practice as a midwife. If she fails to do this and causes harm to the patient while using her complementary therapy skills, then her employer could argue that she was not acting in course of employment when she caused the harm. It is therefore not vicariously liable for the harm, but the midwife must accept personal liability for the harm which has been caused. (In the light of a recent case such an argument by the employer may not succeed: see the discussion on vicarious liability in Chapter 13.)

If the NHS trust or PCT gives expressed or implied consent to complementary thera-pies being used by a midwife then her work in this field could be seen as being in the course of employment, in which case the NHS trust or PCT would be vicariously liable for the harm which has been caused. On the other hand, if the NHS trust or PCT were unaware of the complementary therapy work, then it may refuse to accept vicarious liability for any harm caused by her complementary therapy, arguing that the work was not performed in the course of her employment as a practitioner (see Ch. 13 on Vicarious liability). In this case the midwife would be personally liable.

It is also essential for the midwife to obtain the consent of the employer if she intends to use her complementary therapy skills privately during working hours. In the case of Watling v. Gloucester County Council Employment[5] an occupational therapist was dismissed when he saw private patients for alternative therapy during working hours. His application for unfair dismissal failed. He had been warned by his employ-ers not to conduct his private business during his working hours and lunch times were for a break, not for private work.

CONSENT OF THE WOMAN

It is also essential that the woman should explicitly give consent before the midwife is allowed to use any complementary therapies on her. The basic principles of obtain-ing consent apply (see Ch. 7) but since a woman would not normally expect a midwife to be providing complementary therapies, it is imperative that the midwife gives full details of all that is involved and makes it absolutely clear that the mother is fully entitled to receive the treatment usually provided by the midwife even though she refuses the complementary medicine treatment and care. It is preferable to obtain the consent in writing and to put in a leaflet the information which the woman should be told about the treatment.

DEFINING STANDARDS

One of the difficulties of some complementary therapies is that there may not be a clear definition of the expected standard of care. If harm were to occur to a woman and the woman wished to claim compensation, she would have to establish that the midwife, in using her complementary therapy skills, failed to use the reasonable standard of care which she was entitled to expect from her. This may not be easy to prove. Reference must be made to the various bodies providing accreditation for individual therapies on what would be regarded as the reasonable standards of their specific therapy in those particular circumstances.

The issue of the standards within Chinese medicine arose in a recent case.

Box 34.1 Standard of care of a complementary therapist[6]

S, who was suffering from a skin condition, consulted a practitioner of traditional Chinese herbal medicine. After taking nine doses of the herbal remedy, S became ill and later died of acute liver failure, which was attributable to a rare and unpredictable reaction to the remedy. His widow brought proceedings against the practitioner but failed. The High Court held that on the evidence before it the actions of the herbalist had been consistent with the standard of care appropriate to traditional Chinese herbal medicine in accordance with established requirements.

In May 2001[7] a woman was awarded £6500 in her case against a hypnotist. She alleged that she had become a suicidal zombie as a result of being hypnotised on stage, which reawakened the trauma of childhood sex abuse. The judge held that a suggestion by the hypnotist that she should imagine going back to being a child was negligent. This could be seen as age regression, which is expressly forbidden in a Home Office Circular in 1989 which states that no stage performance should include age regression.

ADVICE OF THE NMC

In its Midwives Rules and Standards which were revised in August 2004[8] the NMC provided guidance on Rule 7 in relation to the administration of medicines which states that a practising midwife shall only supply and administer those medicines, including analgesics, in respect of which she has received the appropriate training as to use, dosage and methods of administration. Included in the guidance are provisions relating to homeopathic and herbal medicines:

Homeopathic and herbal medicines are subject to the licensing provisions of the Medicines Act 1968. A number of these, however, have product licences, but have not been evaluated for their efficacy, safety or quality and you should look to the best available evidence to inform women.

A woman has the right to use homeopathic and herbal medicines. However, if you believe that using the medicines might be counterproductive you should discuss this with the woman.

The emphasis in the guidance that the midwife should look to the best available evidence echoes the NMC Code of Professional Conduct: standards for conduct, performance and ethics[9] which states in Clause 6.5:

You have a responsibility to deliver care based on current evidence, best practice and, where applicable, validated research when it is available.

The implications are that the midwife must keep up to date with the standards in complementary medicine, whether she is practising them or not when she knows the woman is making use of them.

USE OF COMPLEMENTARY THERAPIES IN MIDWIFERY

There are several general works describing the role which complementary therapies can play in nursing and midwifery.[10,11] Denise Tiran has described the use of aromatherapy for pregnancy and childbirth[12] and has also reviewed the use of alternative therapies alongside conventional treatments in breech presentation.[13] She has set up Expectancy Ltd, an expectant parents' complementary therapies consultancy, which will provide evidence-based website information to women on the safe and effective use of complementary therapies and natural remedies during pregnancy and childbirth.[14] Mandy Curry describes the introduction of complementary therapies into the Peterborough Maternity Unit,[15] and the importance of ensuring that standards and practices of staff within a maternity service are maintained at a high and safe level. The March 2002 issue of The Practising Midwife (5(3)) focuses on the use of complementary therapies and their use antenatally and during labour. Articles include the use of chiropractic, self-hypnosis, cranio-sacral therapy and massage in midwifery, and the development of a database on the use of complementary therapies in midwifery by Maggie Evans. In the January 2005 issue of the Practising Midwife articles by Denise Tiran, Anne Haines with Linda Kimber, Nerissa Fields, Sue Spencer and Irene Carter consider topics such as the role of complementary medicine in pregnancy and birth, yoga, hypnosis and ginger. Yates and Anderson have considered the role of shiatsu for midwives,[16] Finlay and Gough have provided a practical guide to reflexivity for health researchers[17] and Nerissa Fields has provided a video on yoga for pregnancy and childbirth.[18]

ACUPUNCTURE IN PREGNANCY

One of the obvious therapies which complement orthodox practice is that of acupuncture. Michele Denny described the setting up of an acupuncture clinic within the NHS to provide acupuncture in pregnancy.[19] The clinic offered treatment for backache, sciatica, muscle and ligament pain, nausea and vomiting, carpal tunnel syndrome, constipation, headaches and heartburn. She concluded, following an audit of the service, that women were enthusiastic about the service and wanted the acupuncture service to be offered for labour and the puerperium. She suggested that if funding could be secured, a specialist clinical midwife could be employed to promote the benefits of complementary therapies to pregnant and childbearing women. A pilot study conducted in an Australian antenatal clinic evaluated the use of acupuncture in maternity care and found that the women concerned stated that the acupuncture had improved their wellbeing.[20]

AROMATHERAPY IN CHILDBIRTH

Ethel Burns and others[21] undertook a study to assess a cohort of mothers who all used aromatherapy during childbirth. The authors concluded that aromatherapy oils had the potential to reduce anxiety, fear or pain and suggested that the integration of aromatherapy into mainstream practice is worth exploring as a means of enabling midwives to gain greater confidence in their holistic skills and improve the quality of midwifery care. However, the authors realised that further research including randomised controlled trials were required.

Spiritual midwifery care[22] is recommended by Jennifer Hall, not in the sense of organised religion, but as part of the holistic care of the woman required by the Midwives Rules. Rosemary Ann Garratt also explores holistic woman-centred care through the use of complementary therapies in the healing role of the midwife.[23] Pat Hung explores traditional Chinese customs and practices for the postnatal care of Chinese mothers.[24] Psychotherapy is considered by Diane Gosden and Ann Saul[25] to have a valuable part to play in midwifery, but they warn against the midwife becoming too interventionist and disempowering of the woman.

However, the findings of many of these studies are not supported by the rigorous research which is now required for orthodox medicine.

NATIONAL DEVELOPMENTS

There is no doubt about the interest which now exists in complementary or alternative therapies. It is estimated that one-third of the population have tried its remedies or visited its practitioners. The Health Education Authority has published an A to Z guide which covers 60 therapies.[26] Much research needs to be done on the efficacy of these therapies and the Health Authority Council has approved a research project to be undertaken by the National Association of Health Authorities and Trusts into the prevalence of complementary therapies and their services for patients, purchasers and providers. The Health Authority Council has appointed a steering and working group to coordinate the project, which will be undertaken by Blueprint Consultancy.

The Prince of Wales suggested the setting up of a group to consider the current positions of orthodox, complementary and alternative medicine in the UK and how far it would be appropriate and possible for them to work more closely together. Four working groups looking at

- research and development
- education and training

– regulation, and

– delivery mechanisms

were established under a steering group chaired by Dr Manon Williams, Assistant Private Secretary to HRH The Prince of Wales. It reported in 1997 and made extensive recommendations.[27] These include encouraging more research and the dissemination of its results; emphasising the common elements in the core curriculum of all health-care workers, both orthodox and complementary, and alternative medicine; establishing statutory self-regulatory bodies for those professions which could endanger patient safety; and identifying areas of conventional medicine and nursing which are not meeting patients' needs at present. It also recommended the establishment of an Independent Standards Commission for Complementary and Alternative Medicine. Subsequently the Prince of Wales has established a Foundation for Integrated Health,[28] from which further information on complementary therapies can be obtained. An information pack for primary care on complementary medicine has been sponsored by the Department of Health.[29] The pack was initiated after a survey found that 1 in 4 adults would use alternative therapies at some point in their lives. The Select Committee on Science and Technology of the House of Lords[30] (see above) considered that some remedies such as acupuncture and aromatherapy should be available on the NHS, and NHS patients should have wider access to osteopathy and chiropractics. The implementation of these recommendations will lead to fundamental changes in how complementary and alternative therapies are viewed in relation to orthodox medicine and within the NHS.

In September 2001 the Medicines Control Agency (MCA) called upon the UK traditional Chinese medicines sector to improve the quality and safety standards of its medicines.[31] The MCA has started consultations with the ethnic medicine sector with the intention of extending the list of potent or toxic ingredients which are not permitted in unlicensed herbal medicines in order that the public should be protected. The MCA has issued guidance on traditional ethnic medicines and its compliance with the law.[32]

HERBAL MEDICINES AND ACUPUNCTURE

Working groups were set up by the Department of Health to consider the regulation of herbal medicine practitioners and acupuncturists.[33] As a result of their recommendations in March 2004 the Department of Health put forward a consultation paper proposing the establishment of a Complementary and Alternative Medicine Council.[34] This would have similar powers to the GMC or NMC and would assess qualifications in herbal medicine and acupuncture and would require possession of a registration certificate to practise in these fields. Following the consultation, the Department of Health announced considerable support for a new council and a draft order for the new council was to be published.[35] Julie Stone has reviewed the significance of this new council in the light of the past 10 years of regulation of complementary and alternative therapies.[36]

In December 2004 the Department of Health announced almost a £1 million grant to improve the regulation of complementary and alternative healthcare.[37] The funding was to be made available to the Prince of Wales's Foundation for Integrated Health over the next 3 years to support the Foundation's work in developing robust systems of regulation for the main complementary healthcare professions. The aim was that effective voluntary self-regulation schemes would be set up for homeopathy, aromatherapy and reflexology.

A strategy to develop research capacity in complementary and alternative medicine[38] was put forward by the Department of Health, which invited Higher Education Institutions (HEIs) to register their interest in hosting research into this field.[39]

TRADITIONAL CHINESE MEDICINES AND HERBAL MEDICINES

In September 2004 the Medicines and Healthcare Products Regulatory Agency (MHRA) issued advice to consumers and the herbal sector about the poor quality of some traditional chinese medicines (TCMs) on the UK market.[40] Under current regulations unlicensed herbal medicines do not have to meet set standards of quality and safety (see s.12 of the Medicines Act 1968). However, if products are found containing illegal or potent ingredients, such as prescription only medicines, the MHRA can remove them from sale. The MHRA was investigating a dietary supplement which contained a banned substance and also a product which contained high levels of mercury. The Chairman of MHRA stated that the advice to consumers is not to take TCMs if they are not labelled in English. Good labelling is in itself not a guarantee of a good quality product. It also recommends that a patient if consulting a doctor or pharmacist should tell him if the patient was taking TCMs or other herbal remedies. The same advice also applies to anyone consulting a midwife.

REGULATION OF HERBAL MEDICINE PRACTITIONERS

The MHRA also consulted on proposals to improve the regulation of herbal remedies made-up by herbalists for individual patients, and are currently considering the responses to this. As a result of this consultation, a new Herbal Medicines Advisory Committee is to be set up under the Medicines and Healthcare products Regulatory Agency (MHRA), under the provisions of the Medicines Act 1968. This Advisory Committee would look at both unlicensed medicines and those registered from October 2005 onwards under the new EU Directive on Traditional Herbal Medicines.

The European Directive on Traditional Herbal Medicines, setting out clear standards for the safety and quality of over the counter traditional herbal medicines, is due to be implemented in 2005.

The Herbal Medicines Advisory Committee would work alongside the existing Advisory Board for the Registration of Homeopathic Products.

CONCLUSIONS

The current interest in and use of complementary and alternative medicines shows no sign of abating. The Department of Health's initiative in setting up a Council for the state regulation of herbal medicine and acupuncture is likely to be followed by state regulation of other complementary and alternative therapies to the benefit of both practitioners and patients. Such therapies are increasingly likely to be available via the NHS as primary care trusts explore cheaper, but effective, alternatives to conventional medicine. The British Medical Association at its Conference in 2000 recommended that acupuncture should be available on the NHS. The big stumbling block at present is that research-based evidence is not available for many of the claims made by practitioners. Following the recommendations of the House of Lords Select Committee on Science and Technology there will be more requirements for research-based evidence of the clinical effectiveness of many complementary therapists so midwives are likely to become involved in this area. In October 2005, a report commissioned by the Prince of Wales[41] was published, which recommended that complementary therapies such as acupuncture and osteopathy should play a greater role in the NHS. The debate which followed showed that unless there were clear research findings on the efficacy of such treatments, orthodox medicine would not embrace them.[42] Perhaps the time has come for the National Institute for Health and Clinical Excellence to investigate the research evidence for many complementary and alternative therapies and practices.

QUESTIONS AND EXERCISES

1. You have decided that you would like to undertake a training in aromatherapy and eventually use it as part of your practice as a midwife. What actions would you take to ensure that your plans are compatible with your professional role as a registered midwife?

2. Identify the ways in which the knowledge that a woman was receiving complementary therapy treatment could affect the tests, care or treatment which you give that person.

3. Do you consider that those complementary therapists who so wished should be permitted to have registered status under the Health Professions Council? If not, what criteria would you lay down for a profession to receive registered status?

4. Which complementary therapies do you consider could be seen as most effective in supporting a woman during and after her pregnancy?

References

1 Dimond B. The legal aspects of complementary therapy practice. Edinburgh: Churchill Livingstone; 1998.

2 Royal College of Midwives. Complementary therapies and midwifery. London: RCM; 1999.

3 British Complementary Medicine Association. Further information can be obtained from: BCMA at Exmoor Street, London W10 6DZ.

4 House of Lords Select Committee on Science and Technology. 6th Report: Complementary and alternative medicine. Session 1999–2000; 21 November 2000.

5 Watling v. Gloucester County Council Employment Tribunal EAT/868/94 17 March 1995, 23 November 1994, Lexis transcript.

6 Shakoor (Administratrix of the Estate of Shakoor (Deceased)) v. Situ (T/A Eternal Health Co). The Independent, 25 May 2000.

7 Horsnell M. Abused woman wins case against hypnotist. The Times, 26 May 2001.

8 Nursing and Midwifery Council. Midwives Rules and Standards. NMC; August 2004.

9 Nursing and Midwifery Council. NMC Code of Professional Conduct: standards for conduct, performance and ethics. NMC; November 2004.

10 Rankin-Box A. Complementary therapies: A guide for nursing and the caring profession. London: Croom-Helm; 1998.

11 Tiran D, Mack S, eds. Complementary therapies for pregnancy and childbirth. London: Baillière Tindall; 1995.

12 Tiran D. Clinical aromatherapy for pregnancy and childbirth, 2nd edn. Edinburgh: Churchill Livingstone; 2000.

13 Tiran D. Breech presentation: increasing maternal choice. Complementary Therapies in Nursing and Midwifery 2004; 10:233–238.

14 Tiran D. Breech complementary therapies in maternity care: personal reflexions on the last decade. Compl Ther Clin Pract 2005; 11:48–50.

15 Curry M. Complementing practice. Practising Midwife 1998; 1(5):32–34.

16 Yates S, Anderson T. Shiatsu for midwives. Oxford: Books for Midwives; 2003.

17 Finlay L, Gough B, eds. Reflexivity: A practical guide for researchers in health and social sciences. Oxford: Blackwell Publishing; 2003.

18 Fields N. Yoga for pregnancy and childbirth with Nerissa (video). Online. Available: www.yogawithnerissa.co.uk

19 Denny M. Acupuncture in pregnancy. Practising Midwife 1999; 2(4): 29–31.

20 Hope-Allan N, Adams J, Sibritt D, Tracy S. The use of acupuncture in maternity care. Compl Ther Nursing and Midwifery 2004; 10:229–232.

21 Burns E, Blamey C, Lloyd AJ. Aromatherapy in childbirth: an effective approach to care. Br J Midwifery 2000; 8(10):639–643.

22 Hall J. Spiritual midwifery care: old practice for a new millennium. Br J Midwifery 2000; 8(2):82.

23 Hung P. Traditional Chinese customs and practices for the postnatal care of Chinese mothers. Compl Ther Nurs Midwifery 2001; 7(4):202–206.

24 Gosden D, Saul A. Reflections on the use of psychotherapy in midwifery. Br J Nurs 1999; 7(9):543–546.

25 Laurance J. Alternative health: An honest alternative or just magic? The Times, 5 February 1996.

26 Health Education Authority. A–Z guide on complementary therapies. HEA; 1995.

27 Foundation for Integrated Medicine. Integrated healthcare: A Way forward for the next five years. Foundation for Integrated Medicine; 1997.

28 Foundation for Integrated Health. Online. Available: www.fihealth.org.uk

29 Department of Health. Complementary medicine information pack for primary care. Online. Available: www.doh.gov.uk

30 House of Lords Select Committee on Science and Technology. 6th Report: Complementary and Alternative Medicine. Session 1999–2000; 21 November 2000.

31 Department of Health. Concern over quality and safety standards of traditional Chinese medicines. Press Release 2001/0448.

32 Medicines Control Agency. Traditional ethnic medicines, public health and compliance with medicines law. Online. Available: www.mca.gov.uk

33 Department of Health. Online. Available: www.doh.gov.uk/herbalmedicinewg/index.htm; www.doh.gov.uk/acupuncturewg/index.htm

34 Department of Health. Regulation of herbal medicine and acupuncture. DoH; March, 2004.

35 Department of Health. Backing for crackdown on bogus alternative medical practitioners. DoH; 14 February 2005.

36 Stone J. Regulation of CAM practitioners: reflecting on the last 10 years. Compl Ther Clin Pract 2005; 11.

37 Department of Health. Better Regulation of Complementary healthcare. Press notice 2004/0464.

38 Pighills A, Bailey C. Developing research capacity in complementary and alternative medicine. A strategy for action. DoH; April 2002.

39 Department of Health. Online. Available: www.doh.gov.uk/research/rd1/cam.htm

40 Department of Health. MHRA issues advice about quality of traditional Chinese medicines. Press release, 3 September 2004.

41 Smallwood C. Complementary Therapies and the NHS. Report commissioned by the Prince of Wales.

42 Rose D. Prince backs alternative treatments on the NHS. The Times, 7 October 2005.

HUMAN RIGHTS ACT 1998

SCHEDULE 1: The Articles of the European Convention on Human Rights

PART I

**THE CONVENTION
RIGHTS AND FREEDOMS**

ARTICLE 2

RIGHT TO LIFE

1. Everyone's right to life shall be protected by law. No one shall be deprived of his life intentionally save in the execution of a sentence of a court following his conviction of a crime for which this penalty is provided by law.

2. Deprivation of life shall not be regarded as inflicted in contravention of this Article when it results from the use of force which is no more than absolutely necessary:

   (a) in defence of any person from unlawful violence;

   (b) in order to effect a lawful arrest or to prevent the escape of a person lawfully detained;

   (c) in action lawfully taken for the purpose of quelling a riot or insurrection.

ARTICLE 3

PROHIBITION OF TORTURE

No one shall be subjected to torture or to inhuman or degrading treatment or punishment.

ARTICLE 4

PROHIBITION OF SLAVERY AND FORCED LABOUR

1. No one shall be held in slavery or servitude.

2. No one shall be required to perform forced or compulsory labour.

3. For the purpose of this Article the term "forced or compulsory labour" shall not include:

   (a) any work required to be done in the ordinary course of detention imposed according to the provisions of Article 5 of this Convention or during conditional release from such detention;

   (b) any service of a military character or, in case of conscientious objectors in countries where they are recognised, service exacted instead of compulsory military service;

   (c) any service exacted in case of an emergency or calamity threatening the life or wellbeing of the community;

   (d) any work or service which forms part of normal civic obligations.

ARTICLE 5

RIGHT TO LIBERTY AND SECURITY

1. Everyone has the right to liberty and security of person. No one shall be deprived of his liberty save in the following cases and in accordance with a procedure prescribed by law:

   (a) the lawful detention of a person after conviction by a competent court;

   (b) the lawful arrest or detention of a person for non-compliance with the lawful order of a court or in order to secure the fulfilment of any obligation prescribed by law;

   (c) the lawful arrest or detention of a person effected for the purpose of bringing him before the competent legal authority on reasonable suspicion of having committed an offence or when it is reasonably considered necessary to prevent his committing an offence or fleeing after having done so;

   (d) the detention of a minor by lawful order for the purpose of educational supervision or his lawful detention for the purpose of bringing him before the competent legal authority;

   (e) the lawful detention of persons for the prevention of the spreading of infectious diseases, of persons of unsound mind, alcoholics or drug addicts or vagrants;

   (f) the lawful arrest or detention of a person to prevent his effecting an unauthorised entry into the country or of a person against whom action is being taken with a view to deportation or extradition.

2. Everyone who is arrested shall be informed promptly, in a language which he understands, of the reasons for his arrest and of any charge against him.

3. Everyone arrested or detained in accordance with the provisions of paragraph1(c) of this Article shall be brought promptly before a judge or other officer authorised

by law to exercise judicial power and shall be entitled to trial within a reasonable time or to release pending trial. Release may be conditioned by guarantees to appear for trial.

4. Everyone who is deprived of his liberty by arrest or detention shall be entitled to take proceedings by which the lawfulness of his detention shall be decided speedily by a court and his release ordered if the detention is not lawful.

5. Everyone who has been the victim of arrest or detention in contravention of the provisions of this Article shall have an enforceable right to compensation.

ARTICLE 6

RIGHT TO A FAIR TRIAL

1. In the determination of his civil rights and obligations or of any criminal charge against him, everyone is entitled to a fair and public hearing within a reasonable time by an independent and impartial tribunal established by law. Judgment shall be pronounced publicly but the press and public may be excluded from all or part of the trial in the interest of morals, public order or national security in a democratic society, where the interests of juveniles or the protection of the private life of the parties so require, or to the extent strictly necessary in the opinion of the court in special circumstances where publicity would prejudice the interests of justice.

2. Everyone charged with a criminal offence shall be presumed innocent until proved guilty according to law.

3. Everyone charged with a criminal offence has the following minimum rights:

   (a) to be informed promptly, in a language which he understands and in detail, of the nature and cause of the accusation against him;

   (b) to have adequate time and facilities for the preparation of his defence;

   (c) to defend himself in person or through legal assistance of his own choosing or, if he has not sufficient means to pay for legal assistance, to be given it free when the interests of justice so require;

   (d) to examine or have examined witnesses against him and to obtain the attendance and examination of witnesses on his behalf under the same conditions as witnesses against him;

   (e) to have the free assistance of an interpreter if he cannot understand or speak the language used in court.

ARTICLE 7

NO PUNISHMENT WITHOUT LAW

1. No one shall be held guilty of any criminal offence on account of any act or omission which did not constitute a criminal offence under national or

international law at the time when it was committed. Nor shall a heavier penalty be imposed than the one that was applicable at the time the criminal offence was committed.

2. This Article shall not prejudice the trial and punishment of any person for any act or omission which, at the time when it was committed, was criminal according to the general principles of law recognised by civilised nations.

ARTICLE 8

RIGHT TO RESPECT FOR PRIVATE AND FAMILY LIFE

1. Everyone has the right to respect for his private and family life, his home and his correspondence.

2. There shall be no interference by a public authority with the exercise of this right except such as is in accordance with the law and is necessary in a democratic society in the interests of national security, public safety or the economic well-being of the country, for the prevention of disorder or crime, for the protection of health or morals, or for the protection of the rights and freedoms of others.

ARTICLE 9

FREEDOM OF THOUGHT, CONSCIENCE AND RELIGION

1. Everyone has the right to freedom of thought, conscience and religion; this right includes freedom to change his religion or belief and freedom, either alone or in community with others and in public or private, to manifest his religion or belief, in worship, teaching, practice and observance.

2. Freedom to manifest one's religion or beliefs shall be subject only to such limitations as are prescribed by law and are necessary in a democratic society in the interests of public safety, for the protection of public order, health or morals, or for the protection of the rights and freedoms of others.

ARTICLE 10

FREEDOM OF EXPRESSION

1. Everyone has the right to freedom of expression. This right shall include freedom to hold opinions and to receive and impart information and ideas without interference by public authority and regardless of frontiers. This Article shall not prevent States from requiring the licensing of broadcasting, television or cinema enterprises.

2. The exercise of these freedoms, since it carries with it duties and responsibilities, may be subject to such formalities, conditions, restrictions or penalties as are

prescribed by law and are necessary in a democratic society, in the interests of national security, territorial integrity or public safety, for the prevention of disorder or crime, for the protection of health or morals, for the protection of the reputation or rights of others, for preventing the disclosure of information received in confidence, or for maintaining the authority and impartiality of the judiciary.

ARTICLE 11

FREEDOM OF ASSEMBLY AND ASSOCIATION

1. Everyone has the right to freedom of peaceful assembly and to freedom of association with others, including the right to form and to join trade unions for the protection of his interests.

2. No restrictions shall be placed on the exercise of these rights other than such as are prescribed by law and are necessary in a democratic society in the interests of national security or public safety, for the prevention of disorder or crime, for the protection of health or morals or for the protection of the rights and freedoms of others. This Article shall not prevent the imposition of lawful restrictions on the exercise of these rights by members of the armed forces, of the police or of the administration of the State.

ARTICLE 12

RIGHT TO MARRY

Men and women of marriageable age have the right to marry and to found a family, according to the national laws governing the exercise of this right.

ARTICLE 14

PROHIBITION OF DISCRIMINATION

The enjoyment of the rights and freedoms set forth in this Convention shall be secured without discrimination on any ground such as sex, race, colour, language, religion, political or other opinion, national or social origin, association with a national minority, property, birth or other status.

ARTICLE 16

RESTRICTIONS ON POLITICAL ACTIVITY OF ALIENS

Nothing in Articles 10, 11 and 14 shall be regarded as preventing the High Contracting Parties from imposing restrictions on the political activity of aliens.

ARTICLE 17

PROHIBITION OF ABUSE OF RIGHTS

Nothing in this Convention may be interpreted as implying for any State, group or person any right to engage in any activity or perform any act aimed at the destruction of any of the rights and freedoms set forth herein or at their limitation to a greater extent than is provided for in the Convention.

ARTICLE 18

LIMITATION ON USE OF RESTRICTIONS ON RIGHTS

The restrictions permitted under this Convention to the said rights and freedoms shall not be applied for any purpose other than those for which they have been prescribed.

PART II

THE FIRST PROTOCOL

ARTICLE 1

PROTECTION OF PROPERTY

Every natural or legal person is entitled to the peaceful enjoyment of his possessions. No one shall be deprived of his possessions except in the public interest and subject to the conditions provided for by law and by the general principles of international law. The preceding provisions shall not, however, in any way impair the right of a State to enforce such laws as it deems necessary to control the use of property in accordance with the general interest or to secure the payment of taxes or other contributions or penalties.

ARTICLE 2

RIGHT TO EDUCATION

No person shall be denied the right to education. In the exercise of any functions which it assumes in relation to education and to teaching, the State shall respect the right of parents to ensure such education and teaching in conformity with their own religious and philosophical convictions.

ARTICLE 3

RIGHT TO FREE ELECTIONS

The High Contracting Parties undertake to hold free elections at reasonable intervals by secret ballot, under conditions which will ensure the free expression of the opinion of the people in the choice of the legislature.

PART III

THE SIXTH PROTOCOL

ARTICLE 1

ABOLITION OF THE DEATH PENALTY

The death penalty shall be abolished. No one shall be condemned to such penalty or executed.

ARTICLE 2

DEATH PENALTY IN TIME OF WAR

A State may make provision in its law for the death penalty in respect of acts committed in time of war or of imminent threat of war; such penalty shall be applied only in the instances laid down in the law and in accordance with its provisions. The State shall communicate to the Secretary General of the Council of Europe the relevant provisions of that law.

CONGENITAL DISABILITIES (CIVIL LIABILITY) ACT 1976

(1976 c.28; 46 Halsbury's Statutes (3rd edn.) 1837)
Amended by 1977 Unfair Contract Terms Act and
by Human Fertilisation and Embryology Act 1990

1. CIVIL LIABILITY TO A CHILD BORN DISABLED

(1) If a child is born disabled as the result of such an occurrence before its birth as is mentioned in subsection (2) below, and a person (other than the child's own mother) is under this section answerable to the child in respect of the occurrence, the child's disabilities are to be regarded as damage resulting from the wrongful act of that person and actionable accordingly at the suit of the child.

(2) An occurrence to which this section applies is one which –

(a) affected either parent of the child in his or her ability to have a normal, healthy child; or

(b) affected the mother during her pregnancy, or affected her or the child in the course of its birth, so that the child is born with disabilities which would not otherwise have been present.

(3) Subject to the following subsections, a person (here referred to as 'the defendant') is answerable to the child if he was liable in tort to the parent or would, if sued in due time, have been so; and it is no answer that there could not have been such liability because the parent suffered no actionable injury, if there was a breach of legal duty which, accompanied by injury, would have given rise to the liability.

(4) In the case of an occurrence preceding the time of conception, the defendant is not answerable to the child if at that time either or both of the parents knew the risk of their child being born disabled (that is to say, the particular risk created by the occurrence); but should it be the child's father who is the defendant, this subsection does not apply if he knew of the risk and the mother did not.

(5) The defendant is not answerable to the child, for anything he did or omitted to do when responsible in a professional capacity for treating or advising the parent,

if he took reasonable care having due regard to then received professional opinion applicable to the particular class of case; but this does not mean that he is answerable only because he departed from received opinion.

(6) Liability to the child under this section may be treated as having been excluded or limited by contract made with the parent affected, to the same extent and subject to the same restrictions as liability in the parent's own case; and a contract term which could have been set up by the defendant in an operation by the parent, so as to exclude or limit his liability to him or her, operates in the defendant's favour to the same, but no greater, extent in an action under this section by the child.

(7) If in the child's action under this section it is shown that the parent affected shared the responsibility for the child being born disabled, the damages are to be reduced to such extent as the court thinks just and equitable having regard to the extent of the parent's responsibility.

1A(1) In any case where:

   (a) a child carried by a woman as the result of the placing in her of an embryo or of sperm and eggs or her artificial insemination is born disabled;

   (b) the disability results from an act or omission in the course of the selection, or the keeping or use outside the body, of the embryo carried by her or the gametes used to bring about the creation of the embryo, and

   (c) a person is under this section answerable to the child in respect of the act or omission the child's disabilities are to be regarded as damage resulting from the wrongful act of the person and actionable accordingly at the suit of the child.

(2) Subject to subsection (3) below and the applied provisions of section 1 of this Act, a person (here referred to as 'the defendant') is answerable to the child if he was liable in tort to one or both of the parents, (here referred to as 'the parent or parents concerned') or would, if sued in due time, have been so; and it is no answer that there could not have been such liability because the parent or parents concerned suffered no actionable injury, if there was a breach of the legal duty which, accompanied by injury, would have given rise to the liability.

(3) The defendant is not under this section answerable to the child if at the time the embryo, or the sperm and eggs, are placed in the woman or the time or her insemination (as the case may be) either or both of the parents knew of the risk of their child being born disabled (that is to say, the particular risk created by the act or omission).

(4) Subsection (5) to (7) of section 1 of this Act apply for the purposes of this section as they apply for the purposes of that section but as if reference to the parent or the parent affected were references to the parent or parents concerned.

2. LIABILITY OF A WOMAN DRIVING WHEN PREGNANT

A woman driving a motor vehicle when she knows (or ought reasonably to know) herself to be pregnant is to be regarded as being under the same duty to take care for the safety of her unborn child as the law imposes on her with respect to the safety of other people; and if in consequence of her breach of that duty her child is born with disabilities which would not otherwise have been present, those disabilities are to be regarded as damage resulting from her wrongful act and actionable accordingly at the suit of the child.

3. DISABLED BIRTH DUE TO RADIATION

(1) Section 1 of this Act does not affect the operation of the Nuclear Installations Act 1965 as to liability for, and compensation in respect of, injury or damage caused by occurrences involving nuclear matter or the emission of ionising radiations.

(2) For the avoidance of doubt anything which –

    (a) affects a man in his ability to have a normal, healthy child; or

    (b) affects a woman in that ability, or so affects her when she is pregnant that her child is born with disabilities which would not otherwise have been present, is an injury for the purposes of that Act.

(3) If a child is born disabled as the result of an injury to either of its parents caused in breach of a duty imposed by any of sections 7 to 11 of that Act (nuclear persons, etc.) the child's disabilities are to be regarded under the subsequent provisions of that Act (compensation and other matters) as injuries caused on the same occasion, and by the same breach of duty, as was the injury to the parent.

(4) As respects compensation to the child, section 13(6) of that Act (contributory fault of person injured by radiation) is to be applied as if the reference there to fault were to the fault of the parent.

(5) Compensation is not payable in the child's case if the injury to the parent pre-ceded the time of the child's conception and at that time either or both of the parents knew the risk of their child being born disabled (that is to say, the par-ticular risk created by the injury).

4. INTERPRETATION AND OTHER SUPPLEMENTARY PROVISIONS

(1) References in this Act to a child being born disabled or with disabilities are to its being born with any deformity, disease or abnormality, including predisposi-

tion (whether or not susceptible of immediate prognosis) to physical or mental defect in the future.

(2) In this Act –

(a) 'born' means born alive (the moment of a child's birth being when it first has a life separate from its mother), and 'birth' has a corresponding meaning; and

(b) 'motor vehicle' means a mechanically propelled vehicle intended or adapted for use on roads.

(3) Liability to a child under section 1 or 2 of this Act is to be regarded –

(a) as respects all its incidents and any matters arising or to arise out of it; and

(b) subject to any contrary context or intention, for the purpose of construing references in enactments and documents to personal or bodily injuries and cognate matters, as liability for personal injuries sustained by the child immediately after its birth.

(4) No damages shall be recoverable under either of those sections in respect of any loss of expectation of life, nor shall any such loss be taken into account in the compensation payable in respect of a child under the Nuclear Installations Act 1965 as extended by section 3, unless (in either case) the child lives for at least 48 hours.

(5) This Act applies in respect of births after (but not before) its passing, and in respect of any such birth it replaces any law in force before its passing, whereby a person could be liable to a child in respect of disabilities with which it might be born; but in section 1 (3) of this Act the expression 'liable in tort' does not include any reference to liability by virtue of this Act, or to liability by virtue of any such law.

(6) References to the Nuclear Installations Act 1965 are to that Act as amended; and for the purposes of section 28 of that Act (power by Order in Council to extend the Act to territories outside the United Kingdom) section 3 of this Act is to be treated as if it were a provision of that Act.

5. CROWN APPLICATION

This Act binds the Crown. (N.B. The Act was passed on 22nd July, 1976.)

GLOSSARY

Acceptance - An agreement to the terms of an offer which leads to a binding legal obligation, i.e. a *contract*

Accusatorial - A system of court proceedings where the two sides contest the issue (contrast with *inquisitorial*)

Act - Of Parliament, *statute*

Action - Legal proceedings

Actionable per se - A court action where the claimant does not have to show loss, *damage* or harm to obtain compensation, e.g. an action for *trespass to the person*

Actus reus - The essential element of a crime which must be proved to secure a conviction, as opposed to the mental state of the accused (*mens rea*)

Adversarial - The approach adopted in an accusatorial system

Advocate - A person who pleads for another: it could be paid and professional, such as a *barrister or solicitor*, or it could be a lay advocate either paid or unpaid; a witness is not an advocate

Affidavit - A statement given under oath

Alternative dispute - Methods to resolve a dispute without going to court such as: resolution; mediation

Appellate court - A court which hears appeals from lower courts, e.g. Court of Appeal and House of Lords

Approved social worker - A social worker qualified for the purposes of the Mental Health Act

Arrestable offence - An offence defined in s.24 of the Police and Criminal Evidence Act 1984, which gives to the citizen the power of arrest in certain circumstances without a warrant

Assault - A threat of unlawful contact (*trespass to the person*)

Bailee - A person who undertakes to care for the property of another

Bailment - The transfer of property from a bailor to a bailee

Bailor - One who leaves property in the care of another

Balance of probabilities - The standard of proof in *civil* proceedings

Barrister - A lawyer qualified to take a case in court

Battery - An unlawful touching (see *Trespass to the person*)

Bench - The *magistrates*, Justices of the Peace

Bolam test - The test laid down by Judge McNair in the case of Bolam v. Friern HMC on the standard of care expected of a professional in cases of alleged *negligence*

Bona fide - In good faith

Breach - Breaking, usually of a legal duty

Burden of proof - The duty of a party to litigation to establish the facts, or in criminal proceedings the duty of the prosecution to establish both the *actus reus* and the *mens rea*

Case citation - The reference to an earlier reported case made possible because of the reference system, e.g. 1981 1 All ER 267 means the first volume of the All England Reports for 1981 at p.267 which is the reference for the case of Whitehouse v. Jordan, where Whitehouse is the plaintiff, Jordan the defendant and 'v.' stands for versus, i.e. against. Other law reports include: AC Appeals Court; QB Queens Bench Division; WLR Weekly Law Reports

Cause of action - The facts that entitle a person to sue

Certiorari - An action taken to challenge an administrative or judicial decision (literally: to make more certain)

Civil action - Proceedings brought in the civil courts

Civil wrong - An act or omission which can be pursued in the civil courts by the person who has suffered the wrong (see *torts*)

Claimant - The person bringing a civil action (originally *plaintiff*)

Committal proceedings - Hearings before the magistrates to decide if a person should be sent for *trial* in the Crown Court

Common law - Law derived from the decisions of judges, case law, judge-made law

Conditional fees - A system whereby client and lawyer can agree that payment of fees is dependent upon the outcome of the court action; also known as 'no win, no fee'

Conditions - Terms of a *contract* (see *warranties*)

Criminal courts - Courts such as magistrates and crown courts hearing criminal prosecutions

Constructive knowledge - Knowledge which can be obtained from the circumstances

Continuous service - The length of service which an employee must have served to be entitled to receive certain statutory or contractual rights

Contract - An agreement enforceable in law

Contract for services - An agreement, enforceable in law, whereby one party provides services, not being employment, in return for payment or other consideration from the other

Contract of service - A contract for employment

Coroner - A person appointed to hold an inquiry (inquest) into a death in unexpected or unusual circumstances

Counter-offer - A response to an offer which suggests different terms and is therefore counted as an offer not an acceptance

Cross examination - Questions asked of a witness by the lawyer for the opposing side: leading questions can be asked

Criminal wrong - An act or omission which can be pursued in the criminal courts

Damage - Harm which has occurred

Damages - A sum of money awarded by a court as compensation for a tort or breach of contract

Declaration - A ruling by the court, setting out the legal situation

Defamation - The publication of a statement which tends to lower a person in the estimation of right thinking members of society generally. If spoken it is known as slanderous; if in permanent form, a libel

Disclosure - Documents made available to the other party

Dissenting judgement - A judge who disagrees with the decision of the majority of judges

Distinguished (of cases) - The rules of precedent require judges to follow decisions of judges in previous cases, where these are binding upon them. However, in some circumstances it is possible to come to a different decision because the facts of the earlier case are not comparable with the case now being heard, and therefore the earlier decision can be 'distinguished'

Domiciliary - At the home

Ethics - The science of morals, moral principles and rules of conduct

Eugenics - The science of the production of fine offspring

Euthanasia - Bringing about gentle and easy death, mercy killing

Examination in chief - The witness is asked questions in court by the lawyer of the party who has asked the witness to attend. Leading questions cannot be asked

Ex gratia - As a matter of favour, e.g. without admission of *liability*, of payment offered to a claimant

Ex parte - On one side only, where the other side is not a party to the action

Expert witness - Evidence given by a person whose general opinion based on training or experience is relevant to some of the issues in dispute (contrast with *witness of fact*)

Frustration (of contracts) - The ending of a contract by operation of law, because of the existence of an event not contemplated by the parties when they made the contract, e.g. imprisonment, death, blindness

Re F ruling - A professional who acts in the best interests of an incompetent person who is incapable of giving consent, does not act unlawfully if he follows the accepted standard of care according to the *Bolam Test*

Guardian ad litem - A person with a social work and child care background who is appointed to ensure that the court is fully informed of the relevant facts which relate to a child and that the wishes and feelings of the child are clearly established. The appointment is made from a panel set up by the local authority

Guilty - A finding in a criminal court of responsibility for a criminal offence

Gynaecology - The branch of medicine which devotes itself to the care and prevention of genital tract disorders in women and which for the most part is not concerned with pregnancy

Hearsay - Evidence which has been learnt from another person

Hierarchy - The recognised status of courts which results in lower courts following the decisions of higher courts (see *precedent*). Thus decisions of the House of Lords must be followed by all lower courts, unless they can be *distinguished* (see above)

HSC - Health Service Circular issued by Department of Health

Honorary - Without payment

In camera - Court proceedings heard in private

Indemnity - Security against loss or damage, compensation for loss occurred

Indictable - Can be tried on an indictment (i.e. before the crown court; some crimes are triable either way, i.e. before the crown court and summarily before magistrates)

Indictment - Written accusation against a person, charging him with a serious crime, triable by jury

Informal - Of a patient who has entered hospital without any statutory requirements

Injunction - An order of the court restraining a person

Inquisitorial - a system of justice whereby the truth is revealed by an inquiry into the facts conducted by the judge, e.g. coroner's court

Invitation to treat - The early stages in negotiating a contract, e.g. an advertisement, or letter expressing interest. An invitation to treat will often precede an offer which when accepted leads to the formation of an agreement which, if there is consideration and an intention to create legal relations, will be binding

Judicial review - An application to the High Court for a judicial or administrative decision to be reviewed and an appropriate order made, e.g. declaration

Judiciary - Judges

Justice of the peace (JP) - A lay *magistrate,* i.e. not legally qualified, who hears summary (minor) offences and sometimes indictable (serious) offences in the magistrates court in a group of three (*bench*)

Liable/liability - Responsible for the wrongdoing or harm in civil proceedings

Litigation - Civil proceedings

Live birth - The birth of a child born alive (s.41 of 1953 Act)

Magistrate - A person (see *JP* and *stipendiary*) who hears summary (minor) offences or indictable offences which can be heard in the magistrates court

Mens rea - The mental element in a crime (contrasted with *actus reus*)

Misconduct - Conduct unworthy of a registered nurse, midwife or health visitor, as the case may be, and includes obtaining registration by fraud (Rule 1(2)(k) Professional Conduct Rules SI 1993 No 893)

Negligence (1) - A breach by the defendant of a legal duty to take reasonable care not to injure the plaintiff or cause him loss

Negligence (2) - The attitude of mind of a person committing a civil wrong as opposed to intentionally

Next friend - A person who brings a court action on behalf of a minor

Non-executive - A person who does not hold office, used in relation to NHS board members who are directors but who do not hold office within the authority

Notifiable - A disease which must be notified to the authorities by law

Nuisance - A wrong which interferes with the use and enjoyment of a person's land

Obstetrics - The field of medicine dealing with the care of women during childbirth

Offer - A proposal made by a party which if accepted can lead to a contract. It often follows an *invitation to treat.*

Ombudsman - A Commissioner (e.g. Health, Local Government) appointed by the Government to hear complaints

Payment into court - An offer to settle a dispute at a particular sum, which is paid into court. The claimant's failure to accept the offer means that the claimant is liable to pay costs, if the final award is the same or less than the payment made.

Pedagogic - Of the science of teaching

Plaintiff - Term formerly used to describe one who brings an action in the civil courts. Now the term *claimant* is used.

Plea in mitigation - A formal statement to the court aimed at reducing the sentence to be pronounced by the judge

Postpartum - Occurring after childbirth or pertaining to the period following delivery or childbirth

Practice direction - Guidance issued by the head of the court to which they relate on the procedure to be followed

Pre-action protocol - Rules of the Supreme Court provide guidance on action to be taken before legal proceedings commence

Precedent - A decision which may have to be followed in a subsequent court hearing (see *heirarchy*)

Prima facie - At first sight, or sufficient evidence brought by one party to require the other party to provide a defence.

Privilege - In relation to evidence, being able to refuse to disclose it to the court

Privity - The relationship which exists between parties as the result of a legal agreement

Professional misconduct - Conduct of a registered health practitioner which could lead to conduct and competence proceedings by the Registration Body

Proof - Evidence which secures the establishment of a claimant's or prosecution's or defendant's case

Prosecution - The pursuing of criminal offences in court

Quantum - The amount of compensation, or the monetary value of a claim

Queen's counsel (QC) - A senior barrister, also known as a 'silk'

Ratio - The reasoning behind the decision in a court case

Reasonable doubt - To secure a conviction in criminal proceedings the prosecution must establish 'beyond reasonable doubt' the guilt of the accused

Rescission - Where a contract is ended by the order of a court, or by the cancellation of the contract by one party entitled in law to do so

Res ipsa loquitur - The thing speaks for itself

Sanctions - Penalties, remedies following civil or criminal wrong

Solicitor - A lawyer who is qualified on the register held by the Law Society

Stillborn child - A child which has issued forth from its mother after the 24th week of pregnancy and which did not at any time after being completely expelled from its mother breathe or show any other signs of life, and the expression 'stillbirth' shall be construed accordingly (s.41 Births and Deaths Registration Act 1953 (as amended))

Standard of proof - The level that the party who has the burden of proof must satisfy, e.g. on a balance of probabilities (civil courts); beyond all reasonable doubt (criminal courts)

Statute Law (Statutory) - Law made by Acts of Parliament

Statutory Instrument - Orders and regulations having binding force. They must usually be laid before Parliament and will usually become law if they are confirmed by a simple resolution of both Houses (affirmative resolution). Some become law after they have been laid for a prescribed period unless they are annulled by resolution of either House (negative resolution)

Stipendiary magistrate - A legally qualified magistrate who is paid (i.e. has a stipend)

Strict liability - liability for a criminal act where the mental element does not have to be proved; in civil proceedings liability without establishing *negligence*

Subpoena - An order of the court requiring a person to appear as a witness (subpoena *ad testificandum*) or to bring records/documents (subpoena *duces tecum*)

Summary offence - A lesser offence which can only be heard by *magistrates*

Summary judgement - A procedure whereby the claimant can obtain judgement without the defendant being permitted to defend the action

Surrogacy - An arrangement whereby a person carries a child for another mother or couple

Tort - A civil wrong excluding breach of contract. It includes: *negligence, trespass (to the person*, goods or land), nuisance, breach of statutory duty and defamation

Trespass to the person - A wrongful direct interference with another person. Harm does not have to be proved

Trial - A court hearing before a judge

Trustee - One who holds property in trust for another (e.g. has duties to care for it)

Ultra vires - Outside the powers given by law (e.g. of a statutory body or company)

Vicarious liability - The liability of an employer for the wrongful acts of an employee committed while in the course of employment

Void - Invalid or not legally binding

Voidable - Can be made void

Volenti non fit injuria - To the willing there is no wrong; the voluntary assumption of risk

Ward of court - A minor placed under the protection of the High Court, which assumes responsibility for him or her and all decisions relating to his or her care must be made in accordance with the directions of the court

Warranties - Terms of a contract which are considered to be less important than the terms described as conditions: breach of a condition entitles the innocent party to see the contract as ended, i.e. repudiated by the other party (breach of warranties entitles the innocent party to claim damages)

Wednesbury principle - The court will intervene to prevent or remedy abuses of power by public authorities if there is evidence of unreasonableness or perversity. Principle laid down by the Court of Appeal in the case of Associated Provincial Picture House Ltd v. Wednesbury Corporation [1948] 1 KB 233

Without prejudice - Without detracting from or without disadvantage to. The use of the phrase prevents the other party using the information to the prejudice of the one providing it

Witness of fact - A person who gives evidence of what they saw, heard, did or failed to do (contrast with *expert witness*)

Writ - A form of written command, e.g. the document which used to commence civil proceedings. Now a claim form is served

Midwifery terms taken from definitions contained in the Midwives Rules (August 2004)

In these rules - Interpretation

Attendance upon - Providing care or advice to a woman or care to a baby whether or not the midwife is physically present

Approved educational institution - An institution or part of an institution or a combination of institutions approved by the Council under Article 15(6) of the Order for conducting the whole or part of a midwifery programme of education

Childbirth - Includes the antenatal, intranatal and postnatal periods

Education - Includes training

Emergency - A sudden, unexpected event relating to the health or condition of a woman or baby which requires immediate attention

Local supervising authority midwifery officer - The midwifery officer appointed by a local supervising authority in accordance with Rule 13(1)

Main area of practice - The geographical location where the midwife has been, or will be, practising most often in the 12-month period related to the most recent notification of intention to practise

Midwifery programme of education - An integrated theoretical and clinical practice programme that meets the standards established by the Council under Article 15(1)(a) of the Order

The Order - The Nursing and Midwifery Order 2001

Postnatal period - The period after the end of labour during which the attendance of a midwife upon a woman and baby is required, being not less than 10 days and for such longer period as the midwife considers necessary

Practising midwife - A registered midwife who notifies her intention to practise to a local supervising authority and who has updated her practice in accordance with the standards published by the Council, and who—

(a) is in attendance upon a woman and baby during the antenatal, intranatal or postnatal period; or

(b) holds a post for which a midwifery qualification is required

Supervisor of Midwives - A person appointed by a local supervising authority to exercise supervision over midwives practising in its area in accordance with Rule 11(1)

Woman and baby - Any woman, regardless of her age, and where reference is made to 'baby' in conjunction with 'woman', it shall be taken as including reference to the woman's unborn baby during the antenatal and intranatal periods

Appelbe GE, Wingfield J, eds. Dale and Appelbe's Pharmacy: Law and Ethics, 8th edn. London: The Pharmaceutical Press; 2005.

Beddard R. Human Rights and Europe, 3rd edn. Cambridge: Grotius Publications; 1992.

Brazier M. Medicine, Patients and the Law. Harmondsworth: Penguin; 1992.

Brazier M, ed. Street on Torts, 8th edn. London: Butterworths; 1998.

British Medical Association. Consent, Rights and Choices in Health Care for Children and Young People. London: BMJ Books; 2001.

Clarkson CMV, Keating HM. Criminal Law Text and Materials, 2nd edn. London: Sweet & Maxwell; 1990.

Clerk and Lindsell. Clerk and Lindsell on Torts, 18th edn. London: Sweet & Maxwell; 2000.

Dimond B. Legal Aspects of Child Health Care. London: Mosby; 1996.

Dimond B. Legal Aspects of Care in the Community. London: Macmillan; 1997.

Dimond B. Legal Aspects of Complementary Therapy Practice. Edinburgh: Churchill Livingstone; 1998.

Dimond B. Legal Aspects of Physiotherapy. Oxford: Blackwell Science; 1999.

Dimond B. Patients' Rights, Responsibilities and the Nurse: Central Health Studies, 2nd edn. Lancaster: Quay Publishing; 1999.

Dimond B. Legal Aspects of Pain Management. Dinton, Salisbury: Quay Publications, Mark Allen Press; 2002.

Dimond B. Legal Aspects of Patient Confidentiality, Dinton, Salisbury: Quay Publications, Mark Allen Press; 2002.

Dimond B. Legal Aspects of Consent. Dinton, Salisbury: Quay Publications, Mark Allen Press; 2003.

Dimond B. Legal Aspects of Nursing, 4th edn. Hemel Hempstead: Pearson Education; 2004.

Dimond B. Legal Aspects of Occupational Therapy, 2nd edn. Oxford: Blackwell Scientific; 2004.

Dimond B. Legal Aspects of Health and Safety. Dinton, Salisbury: Quay Publications, Mark Allen Press; 2005.

Dimond B. Legal Aspects of Medicines. Dinton, Salisbury: Quay Publications, Mark Allen Press; 2005.

English National Board. Preparation for Supervisors of Midwives Open Learning Programme. London: ENB; 1992.

Finch J. Speller's Law Relating to Hospitals, 7th edn. London: Chapman and Hall Medical; 1994.

Gann R. The NHS A to Z, 2nd edn. Winchester: The Help for Health Trust; 1993.

Henderson C, Macdonald S, eds. Mayes' Midwifery, 13th edn. London: Baillière Tindall; 2004.

Hendrick J. Law and Ethics in Nursing and Healthcare. London: Stanley Thomas; 2000.

Heywood JI, ed. The UKCC Code of Conduct: a critical guide. London: Nursing Times Books; 1999.

Hoggett B. Mental Health Law, 4th edn. London: Sweet & Maxwell; 1996.

Howarth DR, O'Sullivan JA. Hepple, Howarth and Matthews Tort: Cases and Materials, 5th edn. London: Butterworths; 2000.

Hunt G, Wainwright P, eds. Expanding the Role of the Nurse. Oxford: Blackwell Scientific; 1994.

Hurwitz B. Clinical Guidelines and the Law. Abingdon: Radcliffe Medical Press; 1998.

James PS. Introduction to English Law, 9th edn. London: Butterworths; 1976.

Jay R, Hamilton A. Data Protection Law and Practice. London: Sweet & Maxwell; 1999.

Jones, M. Medical Negligence. London: Sweet and Maxwell; 1996.

Jones MA. Textbook on Torts, 8th edn. Oxford: Oxford University Press; 2002.

Jones MA, Morris AE. Blackstone's Statutes on Medical Law, 3rd edn. Oxford: Oxford University Press; 2003.

Jones R. Mental Health Act Manual, 8th edn. London: Sweet & Maxwell; 2003.

Keenan D. Smith and Keenan's English Law, 14th edn. London: Pearson Longman; 2004.

Kennedy I, Grubb A. Medical Law and Ethics, 3rd edn. London: Butterworths; 2000.

Kidner R. Blackstone's Statutes on Employment Law, 3rd edn. London: Blackstones; 1993.

Kloss D. Occupational Health Law, 3rd edn. Oxford: Blackwell Scientific; 2000.

Korgaonkar G, Tribe D. Law for Nurses. London: Cavendish; 1995.

Leach P. Taking a Case to the European Court of Human Rights. London: Blackstone; 2001.

Maclean A. Briefcase of Medical Law. London: Cavendish; 2001.

Mandelstam M. An A–Z of Community Care Law. London: Jessica Kingsley; 1998.

Deakin S, Johnston A, Markensinis B. Markensinis and Deakin's Tort Law, 5th edn. Oxford: Clarendon; 2003.

Mason D, Edwards P. Litigation: A Risk Management Guide for Midwives. London: Royal College of Midwives; 1993.

Mason JK, McCall-Smith A. Law and Medical Ethics, 6th edn. London: Butterworths; 2002.

McHale J, Fox M, with Murphy J. Health Care Law. London: Sweet and Maxwell; 1997.

McHale J, Tingle J. Law and Nursing, 2nd edn. Oxford: Butterworth-Heinemann; 2001.

Miers D, Page A. Legislation, 2nd edn. London: Sweet & Maxwell; 1990.

Montgomery J. Health Care Law, 2nd edn. Oxford: Oxford University Press; 2003.

Morgan D, Lee RG. Human Fertilisation and Embryology Act 1990. London: Blackstone; 1991.

Mowbray A. Cases and Materials on the European Convention on Human Rights. London: Butterworths; 2001.

Painter RW, Holmes A. Cases and Materials on Employment Law. Oxford: Oxford University Press; 2004.

Pyne RH. Professional Discipline in Nursing, Midwifery and Health Visiting, 2nd edn. Oxford: Blackwell Scientific; 1991.

Rowson R. An Introduction to Ethics for Nurses. Harrow: Scutari Press; 1990.

Royal College of Midwives. Examples of Effective Midwifery Management. London: RCM; 1993.

Royal College of Midwives. The Midwife: Her Legal Status and Accountability. London: RCM; 1993.

Rumbold G. Ethics in Nursing Practice, 2nd edn. London: Baillière Tindall; 1993.

Selwyn N. Selwyn's Law of Employment, 12th edn. London: Butterworth; 2002.

Silverton L. The Art and Science of Midwifery. London: Pearson Education; 1998.

Sims S. Practical Approach to Civil Procedure, 4th edn. London: Blackstone; 2000.

Slapper G, Kelly D. The English Legal System, 6th edn. London: Cavendish; 2001.

Stauch M, Wheat K, Tingle J. Source Book on Medical Law, 2nd edn. London: Cavendish; 2002.

Steiner J. Textbook on EC Law, 3rd edn. London: Blackstone; 1992.

Stone J, Matthews J. Complementary Medicine and the Law, 2nd edn. Oxford: Oxford University Press; 1996.

Storch J. Towards a Moral Horizon. Nursing Ethics for Leadership and Practice. Toronto: Pearson Education; 2004.

Symon A. Obstetric Litigation from A to Z. Wiltshire: Mark Allen Publishing; 2001.

Tingle J, Foster C. Clinical Guidelines: law, policy and practice. London: Cavendish; 2002.

Tolley's Health and Safety at Work Handbook, 15th edn. Croydon: Tolley; 2003.

Tschudin V, Marks MD. Ethics: A Primer for Nurses. London: Baillière Tindall; 1993.

Vincent C, ed. Clinical Risk Management. London: BMJ Books; 1995.

Wheeler J. The English Legal System. Harlow: Pearson Education; 2002.

White R, Carr P, Lowe N. A Guide to the Children Act 1989, 3rd edn. Oxford: Butterworths; 2002.

Wilkinson R, Caulfield H. The Human Rights Act: a Practical Guide for Nurses. London: Whurr; 2000.

Wyndham-Kay J (Chairman). Report of Royal College of Midwives' Commission on Legislation Relating to Midwives. London: RCM; 1991.

Young AP. Legal Problems in Nursing Practice, 2nd edn. London: Harper and Rowe; 1989.

Young AP. Law and Professional Conduct in Nursing, 2nd edn. Harrow: Scutari Press; 1994.

Reference should also be made to the many articles on different legal aspects of midwifery practice which can be found in *The Practising Midwife*, *The British Journal of Midwifery*, *The Midwives Chronicle*, *Midwifery Matters*, *Midwife* and similar journals for registered practitioners in general. The Midwives Information and Resource Service (MIDIRS) provides an extremely useful guide to articles relevant to midwifery published in other journals. A bibliography of general and specialist books on midwifery, nursing and medical books is available from Meditec, Nursing Book Service, York House, 26 Bourne Road, Coldersworth, Lincolnshire NG33 5JE.

WEBSITE ADDRESSES

Audit Commission	www.audit-commission.gov.uk
Bristol Inquiry (Kennedy Report)	www.bristol-inquiry.org.uk
Civil Procedure Rules	www.open.gov.uk/lcd/civil/procrules_fin/ crules.htm
Commission for Racial Equality	www.cre.gov.uk/
Department of Constitutional Affairs	www.dca.gov.uk
Department of Health	www.dh.gov.uk
Department of Trade and Industry	www.dti.gov.uk/
Domestic Violence	www.domesticviolence.gov.uk
Health and Safety Commission	www.hsc.gov.uk
Health and Safety Executive	www.hse.gov.uk
Health Professions Council	www.hc-uk.org
Human Fertilisation and Embryology Authority	www.hfea.gov.uk/
Human Rights	www.humanrights.gov.uk
Medicines and Healthcare Products Regulatory Agency	www.mhra.gov.uk
MIDIRS	www.midirs.gov.uk
National Audit Office	www.nao.gov.uk
National Patient Safety Agency	www.npsa.gov.uk
National Treatment Agency	www.nta.nhs.uk/
NHS Direct	www.nhsdirect.nhs.uk
NHS Professionals	www.nhsprofessionals.nhs.uk

NHS website	www.nhs.uk
NICE	www.nice.org.uk
Nursing and Midwifery Council	www.nmc-uk.org/
Open Government	www.open.gov.uk
Pain website	www.pain-talk.co.uk
Royal College of Midwives	www.rcm.org.uk
Royal College of Nursing	www.rcn.org.uk
Shipman Inquiry	www.the-shipman-inquiry.org.uk/reports.asp
UK Parliament	www.parliament.uk
Victoria Climbie Inquiry	www.victoria-climbie.org.uk

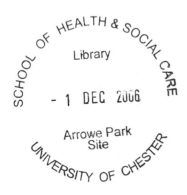